Current Diagnosis and Treatment in Dermatology

Current Diagnosis and Treatment in Dermatology

Editor: Heidi Mueller

AMERICAN
MEDICAL PUBLISHERS
www.americanmedicalpublishers.com

AMERICAN
MEDICAL PUBLISHERS
www.americanmedicalpublishers.com

Cataloging-in-Publication Data

Current diagnosis and treatment in dermatology / edited by Heidi Mueller.
p. cm.
Includes bibliographical references and index.
ISBN 979-8-88740-029-7
1. Skin--Diseases. 2. Skin--Diseases--Diagnosis. 3. Skin--Diseases--Treatment.
4. Dermatology. I. Mueller, Heidi.
RL71 .C87 2023
616.5--dc23

American Medical Publishers,
41 Flatbush Avenue,
1st Floor, New York,
NY 11217, USA

ISBN 979-8-88740-029-7 (Hardback)

Contents

Preface

The purpose of the book is to provide a glimpse into the dynamics and to present opinions and studies of some of the scientists engaged in the development of new ideas in the field from very different standpoints. This book will prove useful to students and researchers owing to its high content quality.

Dermatology is the branch of medicine concerned with the study, research, diagnosis, and management of diseases that affect the skin including membranes, nails and hair. There are several types of dermatologic conditions, including warts, cold sore, fungal infections, acne, psoriasis, eczema, dermatitis, etc. Various tests such as biopsy, culture, skin patch test, diascopy, dermoscopy, and Tzanck test are utilized for the diagnosis of skin diseases. A number of dermatological therapies can be used for the treatment of skin conditions. The most common type of treatment is topical medication, which is directly applied to the affected area in order to achieve the desired result. Some of the other treatment therapies include laser therapy, phototherapy, systemic medications, surgery, radiotherapy, dermahistopathology, surgery, photodynamic therapy, and immunotherapy. This book contains some path-breaking studies in the field of dermatology. It strives to provide a fair idea about this discipline and to help develop a better understanding of the latest advances in the diagnosis and treatment of skin diseases. This book is an essential guide for both academicians and those who wish to pursue this discipline further.

At the end, I would like to appreciate all the efforts made by the authors in completing their chapters professionally. I express my deepest gratitude to all of them for contributing to this book by sharing their valuable works. A special thanks to my family and friends for their constant support in this journey.

Editor

1

Autoreactive T-Lymphocytes in Inflammatory Skin Diseases

Wolf-Henning Boehncke[1,2]* *and Nicolo Costantino Brembilla*[1]

[1] *Department of Pathology and Immunology, Faculty of Medicine, University of Geneva, Geneva, Switzerland,* [2] *Divison of Dermatology and Venereology, Geneva University Hospitals, Geneva, Switzerland*

Correspondence:
Wolf-Henning Boehncke
wolf-henning.boehncke@hcuge.ch

The presence of one or several autoantigen(s) and a response by the adaptive immune system are the key criteria to classify a pathology as an autoimmune disease. The list of entities fulfilling this criterion is currently growing in the light of recent advancements in the pathogenetic understanding of a number of important dermatoses. The role of autoreactive T-lymphocytes differs amongst these pathologies. While they are directly involved as effector cells attacking and sometimes killing their respective target in some diseases (e.g., vitiligo), they provide help to B-lymphocytes, which in turn produce the pathogenic autoreactive antibodies in others (pemphigus and pemphigoid). Atopic dermatits is a chimera in this regard, as there is evidence for both functions. Psoriasis is an example for an entity where autoantigens were finally identified, suggesting that at least a subgroup of patients should be classified as suffering from a true autoimmune rather than autoinflammatory condition. Identification of resident memory T-lymphocytes (T_{RM}) helped to understand why certain diseases relapse at the same site after seemingly effective therapy. Therefore, the in-depth characterization of autoreactive T-lyphocytes goes way beyond an academic exercise and opens the door toward improved therapies yielding durable responses. T_{RM} are particularly suitable targets in this regard, and the clinical efficacy of some established and emerging therapeutic strategies such as the inhibition of Janus Kinase 3 or interleukin 15 may rely on their capacity to prevent T_{RM} differentiation and maintenance. Research in this field brings us closer to the ultimate goal in the management of autoimmunity at large, namely resetting the immune system in order to restore the state of tolerance.

Keywords: resident memory T-lymphocytes, psoriasis, atopic dermatitis, bullous pemphigoid, pemphigus, alopecia areata, vitiligo, scleroderma

INTRODUCTION

During T-cell development, T-cell receptors (TCR) are generated randomly and subsequently undergo a selection process in the thymus (**Figure 1**). This includes a positive round of selection to guarantee selfMHC-restriction and a negative round to eliminate T-cells that recognize self-antigens too strongly. The fate of a developing T-cell depends on the strength and duration of the interaction between its TCR on the one hand and the self-peptide-MHC complexes presented by thymic cells on the other hand. While TCRs with theoretically infinitive affinity may be generated, developing T-cells have to match a binary destiny: life or death. The intrinsic mechanism of selection is thus prone to the development of auto-reactive cells, especially those harboring TCRs with affinity close to the threshold for negative selection (1). Another issue comprises the

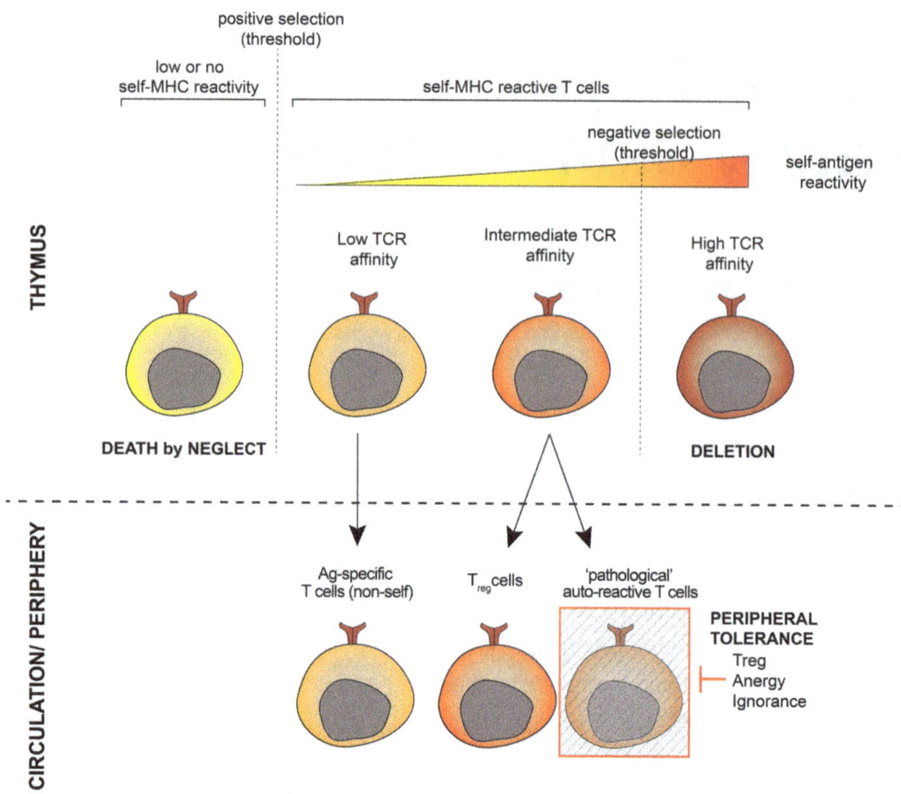

FIGURE 1 | Shaping the T-cell repertoire. T-lymphocytes undergo positive selection to ensure restriction to the host's antigen presenting molecules as well as negative selection to eliminate strongly autoreactive cells in the thymus prior to populating the periphery. T-cells whose TCR affinity is close to the threshold for negative selection have a high potential for autoreactivity and escape thymic negative selection. A subset of these cells is programmed to become T_{reg} cells, others (the potentially pathogeneic autoreactive cells) are kept under the control of the peripheral tolerance.

presence of tissue-specific genes that are not expressed in the thymus and poorly regulated by the autoimmune regulator [AIRE, (2)], toward which T-cells are not depleted during thymic selection. As a result of these mechanisms, autoreactive T-cells are released into the circulation and inevitably exist in all individuals (3). Autoreactive T-lymphocytes behave just like "normal" ones, namely, they recognize antigenic peptides presented to them in the context of a host's antigen presenting HLA molecule and become activated if the appropriate signals are provided. The difference lies in the antigenic peptide, which for "normal" T-lymphocytes is a foreign structure, e.g., part of a pathogen, while autoreactive T-lymphocytes are specific for peptides representing "self," e.g., part of an anchoring protein of keratinocytes.

The autoreactive compartment comprises at least two types of cells: self-reactive cells programmed during development to control the immune response as a part of a peripheral tolerance mechanism (this is the case for regulatory T-cells, T_{regs}), and autoreactive cells that may turn to be harmful and cause autoimmunity. The latter are, however, found at low frequencies in the peripheral T-cell pool, and their functions are hidden by peripheral tolerance mechanisms. Harmful autoreactive T-cells that escape central tolerance are indeed rendered inoffensive via anergy, ignorance, and active suppression by T_{regs} [reviewed in (4)].

T_{regs} can be classified into thymic T_{regs}, peripheral T_{regs}, and *in vitro* induced T_{regs} (5). These subsets show functional and phenotypic similarities, but differ epigenetically. T_{regs} interact directly with different cell types of the innate and adaptive immune systems, but also exhibit their anti-inflamamtory effects via cytokines such as IL-10, IL-35, TGF-β, and galectin-1.

The frequency of autoreactive T-cells specific for a given self-antigen has been evaluated by peptide-MHC tetramer technology to be similar to those specific for foreign antigens, in the order of 1 to 10 per million T-cells (6). The study of the total autoreactive T-cell repertoire in healthy individuals is, however, hampered by the fact that peripheral tolerance mechanisms make autoreactive T-cells functionally indistinguishable. Richards and colleagues addressed this issue by analyzing the "exposed" self-reactive T-cells upon removal of T_{reg} cells in Foxp3^{DTR} mice. Self-reactivity was observed in about 4% of peripheral CD4+ and CD8+ T-cells, a frequency similar to the responses to allo-MHC complexes or superantigens (7).

Thus, autoreactive T-cells are readily detectable in healthy individuals, but they are efficiently controlled by peripheral tolerance. When the tolerance is broken, autoreactive T-cells

TABLE 1 | The role of autoreactive T-lymphocytes in inflammatory skin diseases.

Entity	HLA association	autoantigen	T-cell involvement
Vitiligo	Yes	Melanocyte-dervied antigens	• CD8+, destroying melanocytes • T RM
Alopecia areata	Yes	• Trichohyalin? • Tyrosinase-related protein-2	• CD8 • (CD4+ needed in animal models for maximal induction)
Psoriasis	Yes	• ADAMTS-like protein 5 • (LL-37) • (neolipid antigens)	• CD8+ • T RM
Scleroderma	Yes	Unknown (Nuclear antigens (Topo1, RNApolIII, centromere) recognized by autoantibodies)	• CD4+, CD8+
Bullous pemphigoid	Yes	NC16A domain of BP180	CD4+
Pemphigus vulgaris	Yes	Desmoglein 3	CD4+
Atopic dermatitis	No	Hom s 2 (α-NAC)	CD8+, producing IL-4 and IFN-γ

may become activated and generate overt autoimmunity. In that regard, interesting insights are being generated by the therapeutical use of checkpoint inhibitors, e.g., CTLA-4 and programmed cell death protein 1 (PD-1) blocking antibodies. These compounds represent a promising approach to treat various cancers since they boost specific anti-tumor T-cell immunity by restraining tolerogenic mechanisms exploited by the tumor. The drawback is that peripheral tolerance is weakened and patients may develop so called immune-related adverse events (irAEs). These irAEs differ from "classic" organ-specific autoimmune disease in as much as they affect a broader range of organs and cells (8). These data clearly show how autoreactive T-cells may be reactivated in particular situations.

How tolerance is broken or evaded during "classical" autoimmunity is a complex and incompletely understood matter. Autoimmune responses are currently thought to arise from a combination of genetic and environmental factors. For example, HLA polymorphisms could result in altered regulation or reduced threshold for autoreactive T-cells, with environmental factors constituting the initial triggering for inappropriate activation (9). Regarding peripheral tolerance, T_{regs} may become dysfunctional through at least 4 distinct mechanisms, namely plasticity (capacity to produce IL-17 after loss of the transcription factor FOXP3), reduced CD18 expression, epigenetic changes, and inhibitory mRNA targeting FOXP3. This allows proinflammatory cells such as Th1 and TH17 lymphocytes to escape regulation and to perform their effector functions in an uncontrolled manner (10).

Activation of autoreactive T-lymphocytes is a key event in almost any kind of autoimmune response: while T-cells are important effectors in some entities (e.g., psoriasis), their principal mode of action in other diseases is to provide help for B-lymphocytes produce the disease-mediating auto-antibodies (e.g., bullous pemphigoid). A clinical consequence is that drugs targeting T-cell function are highly effective to treat the former, while B-cell directed drugs currently represent the gold standard for the latter.

We will now discuss the current pathophysiological concepts of the clinically most relevant inflammatory skin diseases for which a role of autoreactive T-lymphocytes is either well-established or suggested based on the evidence.

VITILIGO

Vitiligo (11) (**Table 1**) occurs in about 1% of the population worldwide and is thus the most common cause of acquired skin, hair, and oral depigmentation. It is characterized by the occurence of well-demarked whitish macules. The histology of lesional skin is characterized by a dermal inflammatory infiltrate along with hypopigmentation in the basal layer of the epidermis, the latter being caused by destruction of melanocytes. The hypothesis of it representing a T-cell mediated autoimmune disease is backed up by its HLA association, the identification of melanocyte-derived potential autoantigens (12, 13), and demonstration of CD8+ T-lymphocytes targeting and destroying melanocytes (14). Consequently, most of the strategies used to treat vitiligo have an impact on T-cell function. This holds true for topical glucocorticosteroids and calcineurin inhibitors as well as phototherapies, while the use of other systemic immunosuppressants is not recommended based on current guidelines (15).

Frequently, rapid recurrences at identical locations are observed after stopping therapy (16), arguing in favor of a persisting cutaneous autoimmune memory, which reactivates the disease once the treatment has been stopped. Resident memory T-lymphocytes (T_{RM}) are candidates representing this memory (17), and several groups have described their presence in vitiligo (18–20). Efforts to provide evidence in favor of their direct pathogenetic involvement are hampered, as there are currently no tools at disposition that allow for their specific removal or blockade without affecting other T-cell populations. Recently, Richmond et al. confirmed the T_{RM} phenotype of autoreactive T-lymphocytes within lesions of vitiligo patients (21). Using a mouse model, they went on to demonstrate that blocking the receptor for interleukin-15 (IL-15)—a crucial cytokine for T_{RM} generation and function—with a specific antibody reverses the disease and depletes T_{RM} after long-term therapy. Interestingly, even short-term local intradermal treatment provided durable repigmentation without depletion of autoreactive T-lymphocytes. Taken together, the authors suggest that autoreactive T-lymphcytes are recruited to the skin, encounter IL-15 presented to them by keratinocytes, up-regulate interferon gamma (IFN-γ), and depend on IL-15 for survival once they become resident in the epidermis.

ALOPECIA AREATA

Alopecia areata (AA) (22) (**Table 1**) has a cumulative lifetime incidence of about 2%. It manifests in the form of non-scarring, patchy hair loss, with a narrowing of the hair shaft near the scalp as a hallmark. Histology reveals a peribulbar lymphocytic infiltrate, comprising CD8+ T-lymphocytes within the follicular epithelium, and CD4+ T-lymphocytes around the hair follicules. Evidence in favor of an autoimmune pathogenesis comes from its HLA association (23), association with other autoimmune diseases such as vitiligo (24), and response to immunosupressive therapies (25).

Similar to the central nervous system or the placenta, the hair follicule is considered an immune privileged site. Evidence in favor of this hypothesis comes from experiments showing survival of melanocytes in hair follicules grafted from black guinea pig skin onto albino guinea pigs, and viability of human dermal sheath tissues within sex-mismatched transplants (26, 27). It is the loss of this immune privilege that is considered a cornerstone in the pathogenesis of AA. The mechanisms of immune privilege preservation in hair follicles as well as potential causes of its collapse have recently been reviewed elsewhere (28).

Several lines of evidence, including elegant experiments using human scalp explants grafted onto severely immunocompromised mice, point toward CD8+ T-lymphocytes as important effector cells. However, maximal induction of the AA phenotype requires the help of CD4+ T-lymphocytes (29, 30) Using a well-established C3H/HeJ mouse model (31), characterized by spontaneous development of alopecia and recapitulating many pathologic features of human AA, Xing et al. identified a subset of cytotoxic memory T-lymphocytes (CD8+NKG2D+) as the relevant effector cells for the autoimmune response toward the hair follicle, and postulated that IFN-γ secreted from CD8+ T-lymphocytes erases the immune priviledge in the hair follicle, inducing the production of IL-15 and promoting further cellular autoimmunity (32). This hypothesis is strikingly similar to the current pathogenic concept in vitiligo (see above).

Progress toward identifying putative autoantigens in AA was made using a two-step screening approach: first, candidate peptides derived from proteins expressed by keratinocytes or melanocytes (as the suspected targets of autoreactive T-lymphjocytes) were designed *in silico* based on their affinity to the AA-associated allele HLA-A*0201. These were then screened for their capacity to activate CD8+ T-lymphocytes from AA patients. Using this approach, the hair follicle antigens trichohyalin and tyrosinase-related protein-2 were identified as putative autoantigens, with trichohyalin being capable of inducing mononuclear cells to secrete proapoptotic factors harmful to hair follicle keratinocytes (33).

PSORIASIS

Psoriasis (34) (**Table 1**) affects around 2% of the population. The characteristic red scaly plaques, which often occur on elbows, knees, and scalp, but can affect any site of the body, already highlight the two major pathogenetic processes active in parallel in psoriasis, namely inflammation (explaining the redness) and epidermal hyperproliferation (hence the scaly plaque). This is histologically reflected by epidermal acanthosis (thickening of viable layers), hyperkeratosis (thickened cornified layer), and parakeratosis (cell nuclei present in the cornified layer). Rete ridges reach deep into the papillary dermis, resulting in profound indentation of both layers. Within the dermis, blood vessels are dilated, contorted, and reach into the tips of the dermal papillae. Finally, there is a mixed epidermo-dermal mononuclear inflammatory infiltrate rich in T-lymphocytes, along with increased numbers of macrophages, mast cells and neutrophils. The epidermal accumulation of the latter results in the so-called pustules of Kogoj and subcorneal microabscesses (Munro's microabscesses).

Ever since the introduction of ciclosporine A into the therapeutic armentarium, psoriasis has been regarded as a T-cell driven disease, and the important role of T-lymphocytes triggering psoriasis has been shown using T-cell transfer experiments in a xenogeneic transplantation model (35). The observation by Boyman et al. that skin grafts from non-lesional skin of psoriasis patients transferred onto immunodeficient mice spontaneously developed the phenotype of lesional skin was taken as evidence for the presence of T_{RM} (36). A clinical study evaluating E-selectin blockade as a means to prevent the extravazation of T-lymphocytes into the skin showed little therapeutic efficacy in treating psoriasis (37). This was taken as evidence that psoriasis depends primarily on skin resident T-lymphocytes rather than recirculating T-lymphocytes. On the other hand, inhibiting CD8+ T-cell migration into the epidermis blocked the psoriatic transformation of the grafts in the model used by Boyman et al. (38), and the blockade of LFA-1, another adhesion molecule involved in T-cell trafficking into the skin, does show clinical efficacy (39). The discrepancy between the two clinical studies cited here may be explained by the complexity of the interplay of adhesion molecules as well as mediators in the recruitment of lymphocytes into the skin (40). Whether or not interference with lymphocyte recruitment to the skin has a therapeutic efficacy, it may thus depend on the exact molecular target(s) as well as the degree to which functional inhibition of a given adhesion molecule is achieved *in vivo*. The above-mentioned observations support the idea of ongoing psoriasis exhausting the pool of skin-resident pathogenic T-lymphocytes and requiring substitution from lymphoid organs, where these clones might reside as central memory T-lymphocytes (41).

HLA association, namely with HLA class I (42, 43), and the oligoclonality of the T-cell infiltrate (44) have been interpreted as evidence for an antigen-driven, possibly autoimmune pathogenesis. To date, HLA-C*06:02 is considered the most important psoriasis risk allele (45). In a series of elegant experiments, Arakawa et al. set out to identify potential autoantigens (46). First, they identified HLA-C*06:02 expressing melanocytes as targets for T-cell hybridomas expressing a receptor, which was previously identified as being functionally relevant in patients. They went on to identify the melanocyte ADAMTS-like protein 5 as putative autoantigen and observed T-lymphocytes attacking melanocytes in psoriasis lesions of patients.

Another potential autoantigen LL-37 is generated by extracellular cleavage of a 170 amino acid cathelicidin antimicrobial peptide (47). However, to the knowledge of the authors, it has yet to be shown that the antigen processing and presentation machinery of the target cell is capable of generating an HLA class-I restriced peptide from the original protein. Without such confirmation, a role as autoantigen for CD8+ T-lymphocytes needs to be interpreted with care (48).

Finally, neolipid antigens generated by mast cell phospholipase have been described as targets for psoriatic CD1a restricted T-cells (49).

Besides autoreactive T-lymphocytes, T_{regs} are also thought to contribute to psoriasis through ineffective control of proinflammatory cells: while $CD4^{+}CD25^{+}FOXP3^{+}$ cells are readily detectable in the blood of psoriasis patients, they are unable to suppress Th1 effects. In contrast, T_{regs} isolated from healthy individuals and co-cultured with Th1 cells from psoriasis patients were able to suppress biological effects of the latter (50). In line with this finding, a positive correlation between T_{regs} and Th17 cells (key effector cells in the context of the psoriatic inflammation) in psoriasis has been shown (51, 52) suggesting that the immune system attempts to downregulate the ongoing inflammation through increased presence of T_{regs}, but these are unable to effectively inhibit the disease. As outlined in the introduction, there are at least four mechanisms of rendering T_{regs} dysfunctional.

SCLERODERMA

Scleroderma (Systemic Sclerosis, SSc) (53) (**Table 1**) occurs in around one in 10,000 people worldwide and has a remarkable female predominance. Although rare, scleroderma is associated with high mortality, greater than any other rheumatic disease. Clinical manifestations are heterogeneous, and progression may vary from somewhat stable situations to sometimes rapidly progressive disease. Cases of scleroderma are generally classified into one of two major subsets according to the extent of skin fibrosis: the limited form is defined by skin involvement distal from elbows and knees, whereas patients affected by the diffuse form present extensive cutaneous and internal organ involvement.

The pathophysiology of scleroderma includes three main peculiarities: progressive fibrosis, diffuse fibroproliferative microangiopathy, and inflammation. While the exact etiology remains unknown as of now, environmental as well as genetic factors are considered to be important in the initial phase of the disease. Several lines of evidence suggest that autoreactive T-cells and chronic inflammatory events participate in the initiation or maintenance of the fibrotic process (54).

The first hint comes from genetic and epigenetic studies. Loci in the HLA class II region show the strongest genetic association with the disease, followed by genes involved in B- and T-cell activation and innate immunity. Similarly, epigenetic alterations generally include genes with a role in autoimmunity and T-cell function or regulation (55).

Next, assessment of scleroderma skin revealed that a mononuclear cell infiltrate precedes the fibrotic change and that synthesis of collagen is maximal above it (56, 57). Interestingly, T-cells infiltrating the affected skin show a limited TCR usage, suggesting that they have undergone clonal expansion in response to a specific autoantigen (58).

Another aspect underlying the autoimmune nature of scleroderma is the characteristic presence of anti-nuclear antibodies, including anti-centromere, anti-topoisomerase 1 (anti-topo1) and anti-RNA polymerase III (RNApolIII) antibodies. Anti-topo1 antibodies have high specificity for scleroderma (20–40% of patients) and predict more severe disease and mortality (59). Confirming the involvement of autoreactive T cell-dependent B-cell help, anti-topo1 antibodies are known to exhibit class switching and show strong associations with specific HLA alleles (60). Seminal works from Boin and Wright's groups proved that tolerance to topo1 antigens is effectively broken and topo1-autoreactive T-cells are found in patients presenting these antibodies (61, 62). The possible pathogenic role of nucelar antibodies remains, however, debated, while the frequency of circulating autoreactive CD4+ T-cells was shown to predict interstitial-lung disease development (62).

Regarding the presence of autoantibodies, a striking feature is that patients having anti-RNApolIII antibodies but not the other types show a temporal clustering between the onset of cancer and scleroderma. Rosen et al. provided some evidence in favor of a causative link and proposed that somatic mutation of the RNApolIII in the tumor may actually trigger the activation of autoreactive T-cells that cross-react with the tumor mutated antigen, leading to the initiation of the autoimmune scleroderma response (63).

Finally, three randomized controlled trials tested the efficacy of autologous stem cell transplantation for treating scleroderma. A durable improvement in skin fibrosis, pulmonary functions and quality-of-life measures were achieved, suggesting that immune "replacement" and thus deletion of possible autoreactive lymphocytes might be beneficial (64).

While autoreactive T-cells likely represent an integral or causative part of the pathogenesis of scleroderma, the autoantigens and the mechanisms involved remain largely unknown.

Besides autoreactive T-cells, the quantification of T_{regs} in patient tissues generated contradictory results: most studies reported a reduced frequency while some found an increase in T_{reg} numbers, particularly in early and active disease. Nonetheless, T_{regs} appear to consistenly harbor a defective suppressing capacity in scleroderma, leading to a weaker peripheral tolerance (65, 66).

BULLOUS PEMPHIGOID

Bullous pemphigoid (BP) (67) (**Table 1**) develops in 12 to 66 individuals per million people per year. It is characterized by tense blisters and erosions, often preceded by urticarial lesions. Blisters often arise on the flexor sites of the extremities as well as the trunk; they may persist for several days before transforming into secondary lesions, namely erosions and crusts.

Histopathology of lesional skin specimen shows subepidermal splitting, leaving the dermo-epidermal junction intact, and a dense infiltrate rich in granulocytes, primarily eosinophils and neutrophils.

Contrary to the entities discussed so far, BP is considered an antibody-mediated autoimmune disease. It is characterized by immunoglobulin (Ig) G and E autoantibodies recognizing BP230 and BP180, both antigens localizing to the hemidesmosomes. While BP230 represents an intracellular component, BP180 is a transmembrane glycoprotein of keratinocytes constituting the basal layer. The collagen type XVII extracellular NC16A domain of BP180 comprises immunodominant B-cell epitopes. Numerous *in-vitro* experiments as well as animal models have established a pivotal role for Fc receptor-mediated effects in the process of blister formation (68).

Repetitively, reports on a possible involvement of CD4+ helper T-lymphocytes were published (69, 70). However, while the key role of autoantibody responses to BP180 is well-established in BP, the evidence and clinical relevance of disease-specific T-lymphocyte responses remained unclear. More recent work by Pickford et al. shed more light on the T-lymphocyte participation in BP autoreactivity (71). They tested proliferative and cytokine responses of peripheral blood mononuclear cells from patients and controls to recombinant NC16A and a panel of overlapping peptides spanning this region of BP180. They identified numerous disease-associated factors which influence the composition of the cytokine responses. The strongest association with BP was observed for specific IL-4 and IgE responses, suggesting a potential role for autoreactive Th2 lymphocytes. These results align well with older observations using a humanized mouse model, where the importance of NC16A specific Th-lymphocytes was demonstrated (72, 73). Interestingly, this NC16A response by T-lymphocytes was restricted to HLA-DQB1*0301, a known BP susceptibility allele (74).

A role of T_{regs} in BP was recently documented by Haeberle et al. in a mouse model for BP: they showed that autoantibodies against different known autoantigens, including BP230, develop spontaneously in T_{reg} deficient scurfy mice, leading to blister formation. This study suggests that autoreactive T-lymphocytes initiate the disease in the absence of proper immune control (75).

PEMPHIGUS VULGARIS

Pemphigus vulgaris (PV) (76) is another blistering autoimmune disease with an immunopathogenesis comparable to pemphigoid. Its incidence is in the order of 1–5 new cases per million people per year. Clinically, PV often starts progressively with mucosal lesions and subsequently extensive flacid skin blisters. Blister formation occurs intraepidermally. Autoreactive IgG antibodies recognize desmoglein (Dsg) 3 and 1 within desmosomes, adhesion complexes between keratinocytes. HLA-DRB1*04:02 and HLA-DQB1*05:03 have been identified as disease-associated HLA class II alleles.

Similar to BP, a role for autoreactive helper T-lymphocytes has long been postulated in PV, but was difficult to demonstrate. Several years ago, Emig et al. showed in a humanized HLA-DRB1*04:02 transgenic mouse model that T-lymphocytes recognize human desmoglein 3 epitopes in the context of HLA-DRB1*04:02 leading to the induction of pathogenic IgG autoantibodies, which in turn trigger intra-epidermal blister formation (77). Activation of Dsg3-reactive CD4+ T-lymphocytes is restricted to the HLA-DRB1*04:02 allele. IgG autoantibodies are produced following CD40-CD40L-dependent T-cell—B-cell interactions and exhibit specificities to both N- and C-terminal epitopes of the human Dsg3 ectodomain. Since then, additional evidence has been generated for an active role of CD4+ helper T-lymphocytes (78), but functional studies in patients are still lacking, and most groups working in the field do not assign a high priority to this aspect of translational research in PV (79).

ATOPIC DERMATITIS

Atopic dermatitis (AD) (80) (**Table 1**) has a lifetime prevalence in the order of 10–20% in developed countries with pruritus being the leading symptom. Eczematous lesions can be acute, subacute or chronic, and predilection sites change with age. Co-occurrence of altered epidermal structure and function on the one hand and cutaneous inflammation triggered by pathologic immune responses to antigens encountered in the skin on the other hand are characteristic for AD.

Numerous cell types contribute to antigen presentation in AD, including dermal dendritic cells, epidermal Langerhans cells, and inflamamtory dendritic epidermal cells expressing a high-affinity receptor for IgE (81). The latter explains how these cells can present allergens typically triggering type-I (immediate-type) allergic reactions, subsequently inducing T-lymphocyte mediated type-IV (delayed-type) reactions.

Autoreactivity is a known phenomenon in atopic dermatitis. A systematic review provided evidence that up to a third of patients exhibit autoreactive IgE antibodies (82). This may be based on molecular mimicry, as several IgE-binding keratinocyte-derived antigens show homology with environmental allergens (83). Besides, reports on autoreactive T-lymphocytes date back to the beginning of this decade (84, 85). Based on these observations, which suggested a role for the autoallergen Hom s 2, the α-chain of the nascent polypeptide-associated complex (α-NAC), Roesner et al. performed an in-depth analysis of α-NAC specific CD8+ T-cell responses (86). They found higher numbers of α-NAC specific, terminally differentiated peripheral T-lymphocytes in sensitized atopic patients compared with non-atopic controls. These cells secrete IL-4 and IFN-γ, suggesting a pathogenic role in AD.

As in psoriasis, there is also evidence for substantial dysregulation of T_{regs} in atopic dermatitis. The positive correlation of these cells with disease severity both in mouse models as well as in patients (87, 88) documents the immune

TABLE 2 | Innovative therapeutic strategies exploring the role of T-lymphocytes.

Target	approach	Evidence	References
T_{RM} differentiation and maintenance	JAK3 inhibition	Clinically effective in vitiligo, alopecia areata	(23, 94, 95)
T_{RM} differentiation and maintenance	Anti IL-15 antibodies	Effective in a mouse model of vitiligo	(21)
Preventing T_{reg} transformation	Anti IL-23	Clinically effective in psoriasis	(91)
Autoreactive B-lymphocytes	Chimeric antigen receptor T-lymphocytes	Effective in a mouse model of pemphigus vulgaris	(96)
Immune reconstitution	Multiple • Chemotherapies • Depleting antibodies • AHSCT	Clinically effective in multiple sclerosis, scleroderma	(64, 97, 98)
T_{reg} expansion	mTOR inhibition	Clinically effective in lupus erythematosus, psoriasis	(99–101)

AHSCT, autologous hematopoietic stem cell transplantation.

system's attempt to downregulate the ongoing inflammation through increased presence of T_{regs}, which, however, are unable to inhibit the disease.

THERAPEUTIC PERSPECTIVES

So far, we have reviewed the established or potential role of autoreactive T-lymphocytes in a number of different inflammatory skin diseases. These T-lymphocytes fall principally into two major categories: (1) they function either as effector cells or represent the immunological memory in the skin that may be responsible for relapsing disease or (2) they provide help to B-lymphocytes to produce the pathogenic autoantibodies, as is the case of BP and PV. In atopic dermatitis, there is evidence for both roles.

To date, targeted therapies such as biologics or small molecules allow to directly and specifically interfere with the central pathomechanisms. These therapies are often more effective when compared with conventional anti-inflammatory therapies, making these agents the key compounds of current treatment algorithms (89, 90). However, despite therapeutic effects, which sometimes go way beyond the respective molecules' half-lifes (91), all of these currently available therapies cannot prevent relapse, once they are stopped. Discussions to which extent such currently available therapies are disease-modifying, as we increasingly witness in the context of company-sponsored projects, e.g., in the field of psoriasis (92), seem therefore premature. Instead, remission might be a more appropriate term in this context.

As pointed out in the different chapters above, T_{RM} are a particularly important subpopulation in the pathophysiology of several autoimmune skin diseases. Their presence elegantly explains recurrance of such diseases after seemingly successful therapy. This makes T_{RM} attractive targets to achieve durable responses. Boniface and Senechal recently pointed out potential strategies in this regard, looking at vitiligo as a model for a skin memory disease (93) (**Table 2**):

- Strategies to prevent T_{RM} differentiation and maintenance in the skin could target relevant mediators of this process, including IL-15, as discussed above. While effective depletion of skin-resident T_{RM} through direct blockade of the IL-15 receptor has been shown in a mouse model (21), data from patients are not yet available. Another way to inhibit the IL-15 signaling pathway is through inhibition of Janus Kinase 3 (JAK3). Noteworthy, a clinical trial demonstrated the efficacy of the non-specific JAK inhibitor tofacitinib in combination with phototherapy to treat vitiligo (95).
- Next, strategies to prevent accumulation of T_{RM} in the skin might be warranted. As T_{RM} are likely to accumulate after repetitive flares of the disease, maintenance therapies after successful initial disease control could be an adequate approach. In line with this hypothesis, maintenance therapy using a topical calcineurin inhibitor twice weekly in patients with repigmented lesions reduces the recurrance of old vitiligo lesions (16).
- Finally, while T_{RM} depletion remains to be demonstrated in patients, it seems feasible to aim at dampening T_{RM} activation through the long-term use of immunomodulating agents. In fact, both clinical studies cited above provide evidence for the efficacy of such an approach (16, 95). The study by Liu et al. assessed the effects of JAK inhibition and phototherapy separately, allowing for the conclusion that phototherapy seems necessary for melanocyte regeneration, while JAK inhibition suppresses T-cell mediators of vitiligo (95).

Noteworthy, the current pathogenetic concept of AA also suggests a role for memory T-lymphocytes, IFN-γ, and IL-15 (32). In that very publication, the authors went on to demonstrate therapeutic efficacy of the non-specific JAK inhibitor tofacitinib as well as the JAK1/2 inhibitor ruxolitinib not only in their mouse model, but also in all three AA patients treated with ruxolitinib (32). As in vitiligo, therapeutic application of JAK inhibitors is currently being explored further in AA (94).

Turning to bullous autoimmune diseases, engineering chimeric antigen receptor (CAR) T-lymphocytes may bear a potential (**Table 2**). This approach proved effective in leukemia, where a CD19-specific CAR, composed of an extracellular single-chain variable fragment antibody fused to cytoplasmic signaling domains, triggers cytotoxic T-cell reactions upon contact with CD19+ B-lymphocytes, which results in specific and permanent elimination of the respective B-lymphocytes, yielding durable remission (102). Ellebrecht et al. applied this concept to PV, suggesting that expression of Dsg3 as the extracellular domain of a CAR should specifically target cytotoxic responses to those B-lymphocytes bearing anti-Dsg3 B-cell receptors; this should result in a targeted therapy avoiding general immunosuppression (96). Using a mouse model, they succeeded to show that such cells expand, persist, and specifically eliminate Dsg3 autoreactive B-lymphocytes.

While the strategies discussed so far document the substantial efforts to attack pro-inflammatory elements, much less studies assess the potential to strengthen regulatory elements. In this regard, recent observations in the field of psoriasis are of interest. A much cited hypothesis regards the IL-23/IL-17 axis as central in its pathogenesis, with IL-23 triggering the production of IL-17A in numerous cell types, mainly T-lymphocytes; IL-17A is itself a valid target for highly effective therapies (34, 103). As IL-23 inhibition exhibits long-lasting therapeutic efficacy way beyond the half-life of the biologics used (91), one might speculate that additional effects beyond the postulated "upstream" inhibition of IL-17A production might be clinically relevant. T_{regs} are potential targets in this regard. These lymphocytes exhibit substantial plasticity. They can lose their immunosuppressive function under the influence of pro-inflammatory cytokines such as IL-23, IL-1β, and IL-2 through the loss of FOXP3, ultimately switching toward a pro-inflammatory function (104). IL-23 blockade may hamper this transformation. In line with this concept is the observation by Maxwell et al. who used a mouse model of colitis to show that a regulatory, anti-inflammatory environment in the gut can be promoted through blockade of IL-23 (105). Investigating the role of regulatory elements as potential therapeutic targets may deserve more attention in the future (10).

The "holy grail" of treating autoimmune diseases is the re-establishment of peripheral tolerance, may be best reflected by the concept of immune reconstitution therapy (**Table 2**). Multiple sclerosis has become a model disease in this regard. Numerous approaches have been explored in this disease to "reset" the immune system, including pulsed lympho- or myeloablative treatments through chemotherapies, monoclonal antibodies such as alemtuzumab, and autologous hematopoietic stem cell transplantation (AHSCT). The pivotal trial documenting feasibility of AHSCT in multiple sclerosis was published in 1997 (97). The current status of this field of research has recently been reviewed in this journal (98), supporting the concept of re-establishing a state of peripheral tolerance through deletion of pathogenic clones, achievable via direct ablation in combination with inducing lymphopenia, the latter favoring replicative senescence and clonal attrition. Normalization of genetic signatures along with altered regulatory T-cell populations provide evidence that a restoration of the regulatory network of the immune system really takes place. Moreover, AHSCT is likely to initiate a "rebooting" of the intrathymic selection program that potentially results in the regeneration of a diversified repertoire of naïve T-cells that will again be capable of appropriately modulating immune responses to future antigenic encounters. Similar observations have been made in the field of sceroderma (64).

An alternative approach is emerging in rheumatology, but could also be explored in the inflammatory skin diseases discussed above. This strategy is based on the role of the mechanistic target of rapamycin (mTOR) as a central regulator of T-cell lineage specification (106). Both mTOR complexes 1 (mTORC1) and 2 (mTORC2) need to be blocked simultaneously to allow T_{reg} differentiation. Studying systemic lupus erythematosus (SLE), Kato and Perl showed that IL-21, identified as a key proinflamamtory cytokine in this disease, stimulated both TORC-1 and−2, and abrogated differentiation as well as function of T_{regs} along with autophagy, a phenomenon underlying T_{reg} dysfunction in SLE (99). In turn, dual blockade of TORC-1 and -2 by 4 weeks of rapamycin treatment induced autophagy and corrected T_{reg} function. Progressive improvement in disease activity, associated with a correction of pro-inflamamtory T-cell lineage specification was also observed in in patients with active SLE during 12 months of sirolimus treatment (100). This approach might have the potential to restore tolerance in other autoimmune diseases as well, including psoriasis (101).

In summary, it is evident that there are multiple pathways through which autoreactive T-lymphocytes contribute to the pathogenesis of inflammatory skin diseases, some of which have only recently been identified as classical autoimmune disorders. In all of these diseases, targeting the autoreactive T-cell subpopualtion is a promising and in some cases already well-estabilshed therapeutic strategy. T_{RM} are particularly suitable targets to ensure long-lasting therapeutic effects; the same holds true for the strategies that strengthen the immunosuppressive functions of T_{regs}. Observations in multiple sclerosis and scleroderma suggest that resetting the immune system in order to restore the state of tolerance as the ultimate goal in the management of autoimmunity at large may be feasible.

AUTHOR CONTRIBUTIONS

W-HB and NB jointly selected the topic for the review, performed the literature review, wrote the manuscript, and designed the figure along with tables.

REFERENCES

1. Koehli S, Naeher D, Galati-Fournier V, Zehn D, Palmer E. Optimal T-cell receptor affinity for inducing autoimmunity. *Proc Natl Acad Sci USA.* (2014) 111:17248–53. doi: 10.1073/pnas.1402724111
2. Eldershaw SA, Sansom DM, Narendran P. Expression and function of the autoimmune regulator (Aire) gene in non-thymic tissue. *Clin Exp Immunol.* (2011) 163:296–308. doi: 10.1111/j.1365-2249.2010.04316.x
3. Richards DM, Kyewski B, Feuerer M. Re-examining the nature and function of self-reactive T cells. *Trends Immunol.* (2016) 37:114–25. doi: 10.1016/j.it.2015.12.005
4. Mueller DL. Mechanisms maintaining peripheral tolerance. *Nat Immunol.* (2010) 11:21–7. doi: 10.1038/ni.1817
5. Shevach EM, Thornton AM. tTregs, pTregs, and iTregs: similarities and differences. *Immunol Rev.* (2014) 259:88–102. doi: 10.1111/imr.12160
6. Yu W, Jiang N, Ebert PJ, Kidd BA, Muller S, Lund PJ, et al. Clonal deletion prunes but does not eliminate self-specific alphabeta CD8(+) T lymphocytes.

Immunity. (2015) 42:929–41. doi: 10.1016/j.immuni.2015.05.001

7. Richards DM, Ruggiero E, Hofer AC, Sefrin JP, Schmidt M, von Kalle C, et al. The contained self-reactive peripheral T cell repertoire: size, diversity, and cellular composition. *J Immunol.* (2015) 195:2067–79. doi: 10.4049/jimmunol.1500880
8. Kong YC, Flynn JC. Opportunistic autoimmune disorders potentiated by immune-checkpoint inhibitors anti-CTLA-4 and anti-PD-1. *Front Immunol.* (2014) 5:206. doi: 10.3389/fimmu.2014.00206
9. Rosenblum MD, Remedios KA, Abbas AK. Mechanisms of human autoimmunity. *J Clin Invest.* (2015) 125:2228–33. doi: 10.1172/JCI78088
10. Uttarkar S, Brembilla NC, Boehncke WH. Regulatory cells in the skin: pathophysiological role and potential targets for anti-inflammatory therapies. *J Allergy Clin Immunol.* (2019) 143:1302–10. doi: 10.1016/j.jaci.2018.12.1011
11. Boniface K, Seneschal J, Picardo M, Taieb A. Vitiligo: focus on clinical aspects, immunopathogenesis, and therapy. *Clin Rev Allergy Immunol.* (2018) 54:52–67. doi: 10.1007/s12016-017-8622-7
12. Yang C, Wu J, Zhang X, Wen L, Sun J, Cheng Y, et al. Fine-mapping analysis of the MHC region for vitiligo based on a new Han-MHC reference panel. *Gene.* (2018) 648:76–81. doi: 10.1016/j.gene.2018.01.053
13. Yi X, Cui T, Li S, Yang Y, Chen J, Guo S, et al. Identification of the risk HLA-A alleles and autoantigen in han chinese vitiligo patients and the association of CD8+T cell reactivity with disease characteristics. *Med Sci Monit.* (2018) 24:6489–97. doi: 10.12659/MSM.910515
14. van den Boorn JG, Konijnenberg D, Dellemijn TA, van der Veen JP, Bos JD, Melief CJ, et al. Autoimmune destruction of skin melanocytes by perilesional T cells from vitiligo patients. *J Invest Dermatol.* (2009) 129:2220–32. doi: 10.1038/jid.2009.32
15. Taieb A, Alomar A, Bohm M, Dell'anna ML, De Pase A, Eleftheriadou V, et al. Guidelines for the management of vitiligo: the European dermatology forum consensus. *Br J Dermatol.* (2013) 168:5–19. doi: 10.1111/j.1365-2133.2012.11197.x
16. Cavalie M, Ezzedine K, Fontas E, Montaudie H, Castela E, Bahadoran P, et al. Maintenance therapy of adult vitiligo with 0.1% tacrolimus ointment: a randomized, double blind, placebo-controlled study. *J Invest Dermatol.* (2015) 135:970–4. doi: 10.1038/jid.2014.527
17. Clark RA. Resident memory T cells in human health and disease. *Sci Transl Med.* (2015) 7:269rv261. doi: 10.1126/scitranslmed.3010641
18. Cheuk S, Schlums H, Gallais Serezal I, Martini E, Chiang SC, Marquardt N, et al. CD49a Expression defines tissue-resident CD8(+) T cells poised for cytotoxic function in human skin. *Immunity.* (2017) 46:287–300. doi: 10.1016/j.immuni.2017.01.009
19. Malik BT, Byrne KT, Vella JL, Zhang P, Shabaneh TB, Steinberg SM, et al. Resident memory T cells in the skin mediate durable immunity to melanoma. *Sci Immunol.* (2017) 2:eaam6346. doi: 10.1126/sciimmunol.aam6346
20. Boniface K, Jacquemin C, Darrigade AS, Dessarthe B, Martins C, Boukhedouni N, et al. Vitiligo skin is imprinted with resident memory CD8 T cells expressing CXCR3. *J Invest Dermatol.* (2018) 138:355–64. doi: 10.1016/j.jid.2017.08.038
21. Richmond JM, Strassner JP, Zapata L Jr., Garg M, Riding RL, Refat MA, et al. Antibody blockade of IL-15 signaling has the potential to durably reverse vitiligo. *Sci Transl Med.* (2018) 10:eaam7710. doi: 10.1126/scitranslmed.aam7710
22. Trueb RM, Dias M. Alopecia areata: a comprehensive review of pathogenesis and management. *Clin Rev Allergy Immunol.* (2018) 54:68–87. doi: 10.1007/s12016-017-8620-9
23. Betz RC, Petukhova L, Ripke S, Huang H, Menelaou A, Redler S, et al. Genome-wide meta-analysis in alopecia areata resolves HLA associations and reveals two new susceptibility loci. *Nat Commun.* (2015) 6:5966. doi: 10.1038/ncomms6966
24. Goh C, Finkel M, Christos PJ, Sinha AA. Profile of 513 patients with alopecia areata: associations of disease subtypes with atopy, autoimmune disease and positive family history. *J Eur Acad Dermatol Venereol.* (2006) 20:1055–60. doi: 10.1111/j.1468-3083.2006.01676.x
25. Gordon KA, Tosti A. Alopecia: evaluation and treatment. *Clin Cosmet Investig Dermatol.* (2011) 4:101–6. doi: 10.2147/CCID.S10182
26. Barker CF, Billingham RE. Analysis of local anatomic factors that influence the survival times of pure epidermal and full-thickness skin homografts in guinea pigs. *Ann Surg.* (1972) 176:597–604. doi: 10.1097/00000658-197211000-00004
27. Reynolds AJ, Lawrence C, Cserhalmi-Friedman PB, Christiano AM, Jahoda CA. Trans-gender induction of hair follicles. *Nature.* (1999) 402:33–4. doi: 10.1038/46938
28. Rajabi F, Drake LA, Senna MM, Rezaei N. Alopecia areata: a review of disease pathogenesis. *Br J Dermatol.* (2018) 179:1033–48. doi: 10.1111/bjd.16808
29. Gilhar A, Ullmann Y, Berkutzki T, Assy B, Kalish RS. Autoimmune hair loss (alopecia areata) transferred by T lymphocytes to human scalp explants on SCID mice. *J Clin Invest.* (1998) 101:62–7. doi: 10.1172/JCI551
30. Gilhar A, Landau M, Assy B, Shalaginov R, Serafimovich S, Kalish RS. Mediation of alopecia areata by cooperation between CD4+ and CD8+ T lymphocytes: transfer to human scalp explants on Prkdc(scid) mice. *Arch Dermatol.* (2002) 138:916–22. doi: 10.1001/archderm.138.7.916
31. Sundberg JP, Cordy WR, King LE Jr. Alopecia areata in aging C3H/HeJ mice. *J Invest Dermatol.* (1994) 102:847–56. doi: 10.1111/1523-1747.ep12382416
32. Xing L, Dai Z, Jabbari A, Cerise JE, Higgins CA, Gong W, et al. Alopecia areata is driven by cytotoxic T lymphocytes and is reversed by JAK inhibition. *Nat Med.* (2014) 20:1043–9. doi: 10.1038/nm.3645
33. Wang EHC, Yu M, Breitkopf T, Akhoundsadegh N, Wang X, Shi FT, et al. Identification of autoantigen epitopes in alopecia areata. *J Invest Dermatol.* (2016) 136:1617–26. doi: 10.1016/j.jid.2016.04.004
34. Boehncke WH, Schon MP. Psoriasis. *Lancet.* (2015) 386:983–94. doi: 10.1016/S0140-6736(14)61909-7
35. Boehncke WH, Dressel D, Zollner TM, Kaufmann R. Pulling the trigger on psoriasis. *Nature.* (1996) 379:777. doi: 10.1038/379777a0
36. Boyman O, Hefti HP, Conrad C, Nickoloff BJ, Suter M, Nestle FO. Spontaneous development of psoriasis in a new animal model shows an essential role for resident T cells and tumor necrosis factor-alpha. *J Exp Med.* (2004) 199:731–6. doi: 10.1084/jem.20031482
37. Bhushan M, Bleiker TO, Ballsdon AE, Allen MH, Sopwith M, Robinson MK, et al. Anti-E-selectin is ineffective in the treatment of psoriasis: a randomized trial. *Br J Dermatol.* (2002) 146:824–31. doi: 10.1046/j.1365-2133.2002.04743.x
38. Conrad C, Boyman O, Tonel G, Tun-Kyi A, Laggner U, de Fougerolles A, et al. Alpha1beta1 integrin is crucial for accumulation of epidermal T cells and the development of psoriasis. *Nat Med.* (2007) 13:836–42. doi: 10.1038/nm1605
39. Frampton JE, Plosker GL. Efalizumab: a review of its use in the management of chronic moderate-to-severe plaque psoriasis. *Am J Clin Dermatol.* (2009) 10:51–72. doi: 10.2165/0128071-200910010-00009
40. Schon MP, Zollner TM, Boehncke WH. The molecular basis of lymphocyte recruitment to the skin: clues for pathogenesis and selective therapies of inflammatory disorders. *J Invest Dermatol.* (2003) 121:951–62. doi: 10.1046/j.1523-1747.2003.12563.x
41. Gaide O, Emerson RO, Jiang X, Gulati N, Nizza S, Desmarais C, et al. Common clonal origin of central and resident memory T cells following skin immunization. *Nat Med.* (2015) 21:647–53. doi: 10.1038/nm.3860
42. Tiilikainen A, Lassus A, Karvonen J, Vartiainen P, Julin M. Psoriasis and HLA-Cw6. *Br J Dermatol.* (1980) 102:179–84. doi: 10.1111/j.1365-2133.1980.tb05690.x
43. Schmitt-Egenolf M, Eiermann TH, Boehncke WH, Stander M, Sterry W. Familial juvenile onset psoriasis is associated with the human leukocyte antigen (HLA) class I side of the extended haplotype Cw6-B57-DRB1*0701-DQA1*0201-DQB1*0303: a population- and family-based study. *J Invest Dermatol.* (1996) 106:711–4. doi: 10.1111/1523-1747.ep12345600
44. Menssen A, Trommler P, Vollmer S, Schendel D, Albert E, Gurtler L, et al. Evidence for an antigen-specific cellular immune response in skin lesions of patients with psoriasis vulgaris. *J Immunol.* (1995) 155:4078–83.
45. Lenz TL, Deutsch AJ, Han B, Hu X, Okada Y, Eyre S, et al. Widespread non-additive and interaction effects within HLA loci modulate the risk of autoimmune diseases. *Nat Genet.* (2015) 47:1085–90. doi: 10.1038/ng.3379
46. Arakawa A, Siewert K, Stohr J, Besgen P, Kim SM, Ruhl G, et al. Melanocyte antigen triggers autoimmunity in human psoriasis. *J Exp Med.* (2015) 212:2203–12. doi: 10.1084/jem.20151093

47. Lande R, Botti E, Jandus C, Dojcinovic D, Fanelli G, Conrad C, et al. The antimicrobial peptide LL37 is a T-cell autoantigen in psoriasis. *Nat Commun.* (2014) 5:5621. doi: 10.1038/ncomms6621
48. Prinz JC. Human leukocyte antigen-class I alleles and the autoreactive T cell response in psoriasis pathogenesis. *Front Immunol.* (2018) 9:954. doi: 10.3389/fimmu.2018.00954
49. Cheung KL, Jarrett R, Subramaniam S, Salimi M, Gutowska-Owsiak D, Chen YL, et al. Psoriatic T cells recognize neolipid antigens generated by mast cell phospholipase delivered by exosomes and presented by CD1a. *J Exp Med.* (2016) 213:2399–412. doi: 10.1084/jem.20160258
50. Bovenschen HJ, van de Kerkhof PC, van Erp PE, Woestenenk R, Joosten I, Koenen HJ. Foxp3+ regulatory T cells of psoriasis patients easily differentiate into IL-17A-producing cells and are found in lesional skin. *J. Invest. Dermatol.* (2011) 131:1853–60. doi: 10.1038/jid.2011.139
51. Ma L, Xue HB, Guan XH, Shu CM, Wang F, Zhang JH, et al. The imbalance of Th17 cells and CD4+CD25highFoxp3+ Treg cells in patients with atopic dermatitis. *J Euro Acad Dermatol Venereol.* (2013) 28:1079–86. doi: 10.1111/jdv.12288
52. Zhang L, Li Y, Yang X, Wei J, Zhou S, Zhao Z, et al. Characterization of Th17 and FoxP3(+) treg cells in paediatric psoriasis patients. *Scand J Immunol.* (2016) 83:174–80. doi: 10.1111/sji.12404
53. Denton CP, Khanna D. Systemic sclerosis. *Lancet.* (2017) 390:1685–99. doi: 10.1016/S0140-6736(17)30933-9
54. Chizzolini C, Brembilla NC, Montanari E, Truchetet ME. Fibrosis and immune dysregulation in systemic sclerosis. *Autoimmun Rev.* (2011) 10:276–81. doi: 10.1016/j.autrev.2010.09.016
55. Tsou PS, Sawalha AH. Unfolding the pathogenesis of scleroderma through genomics and epigenomics. *J Autoimmun.* (2017) 83:73–94. doi: 10.1016/j.jaut.2017.05.004
56. Kahari VM, Sandberg M, Kalimo H, Vuorio T, Vuorio E. Identification of fibroblasts responsible for increased collagen production in localized scleroderma by in situ hybridization. *J Invest Dermatol.* (1988) 90:664–70. doi: 10.1111/1523-1747.ep12560826
57. Prescott RJ, Freemont AJ, Jones CJ, Hoyland J, Fielding P. Sequential dermal microvascular and perivascular changes in the development of scleroderma. *J Pathol.* (1992) 166:255–63. doi: 10.1002/path.1711660307
58. Sakkas LI, Platsoucas CD. Is systemic sclerosis an antigen-driven T cell disease? *Arthritis Rheum.* (2004) 50:1721–33. doi: 10.1002/art.20315
59. Nihtyanova SI, Denton CP. Autoantibodies as predictive tools in systemic sclerosis. *Nat Rev Rheumatol.* (2010) 6:112–6. doi: 10.1038/nrrheum.2009.238
60. Kuwana M, Medsger TA Jr., Wright TM. T cell proliferative response induced by DNA topoisomerase I in patients with systemic sclerosis and healthy donors. *J Clin Invest.* (1995) 96:586–96. doi: 10.1172/JCI118071
61. Kuwana M, Medsger TA Jr., Wright TM. Analysis of soluble and cell surface factors regulating anti-DNA topoisomerase I autoantibody production demonstrates synergy between Th1 and Th2 autoreactive T cells. *J Immunol.* (2000) 164:6138–46. doi: 10.4049/jimmunol.164.12.6138
62. Fava A, Cimbro R, Wigley FM, Liu QR, Rosen A, Boin F. Frequency of circulating topoisomerase-I-specific CD4 T cells predicts presence and progression of interstitial lung disease in scleroderma. *Arthritis Res Ther.* (2016) 18:99. doi: 10.1186/s13075-016-0993-2
63. Joseph CG, Darrah E, Shah AA, Skora AD, Casciola-Rosen LA, Wigley FM, et al. Association of the autoimmune disease scleroderma with an immunologic response to cancer. *Science.* (2014) 343:152–7. doi: 10.1126/science.1246886
64. Del Papa N, Pignataro F, Zaccara E, Maglione W, Minniti A. Autologous hematopoietic stem cell transplantation for treatment of systemic sclerosis. *Front Immunol.* (2018) 9:2390. doi: 10.3389/fimmu.2018.02390
65. Brembilla NC, Chizzolini C. T cell abnormalities in systemic sclerosis with a focus on Th17 cells. *Eur Cytokine Netw.* (2012) 23:128–39. doi: 10.1684/ecn.2013.0325
66. Frantz C, Auffray C, Avouac J, Allanore Y. Regulatory T cells in systemic sclerosis. *Front Immunol.* (2018) 9:2356. doi: 10.3389/fimmu.2018.02356
67. Schmidt E, Zillikens D. Pemphigoid diseases. *Lancet.* (2013) 381:320–32. doi: 10.1016/S0140-6736(12)61140-4
68. Liu Z, Diaz LA, Troy JL, Taylor AF, Emery DJ, Fairley JA, et al. A passive transfer model of the organ-specific autoimmune disease, bullous pemphigoid, using antibodies generated against the hemidesmosomal antigen, BP180. *J Clin Invest.* (1993) 92:2480–8. doi: 10.1172/JCI116856
69. Eming R, Budinger L, Riechers R, Christensen O, Bohlen H, Kalish R, et al. Frequency analysis of autoreactive T-helper 1 and 2 cells in bullous pemphigoid and pemphigus vulgaris by enzyme-linked immunospot assay. *Br J Dermatol.* (2000) 143:1279–82. doi: 10.1046/j.1365-2133.2000.03901.x
70. Lin MS, Fu CL, Giudice GJ, Olague-Marchan M, Lazaro AM, Stastny P, et al. Epitopes targeted by bullous pemphigoid T lymphocytes and autoantibodies map to the same sites on the bullous pemphigoid 180 ectodomain. *J Invest Dermatol.* (2000) 115:955–61. doi: 10.1046/j.1523-1747.2000.00153.x
71. Pickford WJ, Gudi V, Haggart AM, Lewis BJ, Herriot R, Barker RN, et al. T cell participation in autoreactivity to NC16a epitopes in bullous pemphigoid. *Clin Exp Immunol.* (2015) 180:189–200. doi: 10.1111/cei.12566
72. Budinger L, Borradori L, Yee C, Eming R, Ferencik S, Grosse-Wilde H, et al. Identification and characterization of autoreactive T cell responses to bullous pemphigoid antigen 2 in patients and healthy controls. *J Clin Invest.* (1998) 102:2082–9. doi: 10.1172/JCI3335
73. Thoma-Uszynski S, Uter W, Schwietzke S, Schuler G, Borradori L, Hertl M. Autoreactive T and B cells from bullous pemphigoid (BP) patients recognize epitopes clustered in distinct regions of BP180 and BP230. *J Immunol.* (2006) 176:2015–23. doi: 10.4049/jimmunol.176.3.2015
74. Delgado JC, Turbay D, Yunis EJ, Yunis JJ, Morton ED, Bhol K, et al. A common major histocompatibility complex class II allele HLA-DQB1* 0301 is present in clinical variants of pemphigoid. *Proc Natl Acad Sci USA.* (1996) 93:8569–71. doi: 10.1073/pnas.93.16.8569
75. Haeberle S, Wei X, Bieber K, Goletz S, Ludwig RJ, Schmidt E, et al. Regulatory T-cell deficiency leads to pathogenic bullous pemphigoid antigen 230 autoantibody and autoimmune bullous disease. *J. Allergy Clin. Immunol.* (2018) 142:1831–1842.e1837. doi: 10.1016/j.jaci.2018.04.006
76. Bystryn JC, Rudolph JL. Pemphigus. *Lancet.* (2005) 366:61–73. doi: 10.1016/S0140-6736(05)66829-8
77. Eming R, Hennerici T, Backlund J, Feliciani C, Visconti KC, Willenborg S, et al. Pathogenic IgG antibodies against desmoglein 3 in pemphigus vulgaris are regulated by HLA-DRB1*04:02-restricted T cells. *J Immunol.* (2014) 193:4391–9. doi: 10.4049/jimmunol.1401081
78. Sezin T, Vorobyev A, Sadik CD, Zillikens D, Gupta Y, Ludwig RJ. Gene expression analysis reveals novel shared gene signatures and candidate molecular mechanisms between pemphigus and systemic lupus erythematosus in CD4(+) T Cells. *Front Immunol.* (2017) 8:1992. doi: 10.3389/fimmu.2017.01992
79. Spindler V, Eming R, Schmidt E, Amagai M, Grando S, Jonkman MF, et al. Mechanisms causing loss of keratinocyte cohesion in pemphigus. *J Invest Dermatol.* (2018) 138:32–7. doi: 10.1016/j.jid.2017.06.022
80. Weidinger S, Novak N. Atopic dermatitis. *Lancet.* (2016) 387:1109–22. doi: 10.1016/S0140-6736(15)00149-X
81. Novak N. An update on the role of human dendritic cells in patients with atopic dermatitis. *J Allergy Clin Immunol.* (2012) 129:879–86. doi: 10.1016/j.jaci.2012.01.062
82. Tang TS, Bieber T, Williams HC. Does "autoreactivity" play a role in atopic dermatitis? *J. Allergy Clin. Immunol.* (2012) 129:1209–15.e1202. doi: 10.1016/j.jaci.2012.02.002
83. Zeller S, Rhyner C, Meyer N, Schmid-Grendelmeier P, Akdis CA, Crameri R. Exploring the repertoire of IgE-binding self-antigens associated with atopic eczema. *J Allergy Clin Immunol.* (2009) 124:278–85, 285.e271–7. doi: 10.1016/j.jaci.2009.05.015
84. Balaji H, Heratizadeh A, Wichmann K, Niebuhr M, Crameri R, Scheynius A, et al. Malassezia sympodialis thioredoxin-specific T cells are highly cross-reactive to human thioredoxin in atopic dermatitis. *J. Allergy Clin. Immunol.* (2011) 128:92–9 e94. doi: 10.1016/j.jaci.2011.02.043
85. Heratizadeh A, Mittermann I, Balaji H, Wichmann K, Niebuhr M, Valenta R, et al. The role of T-cell reactivity towards the autoantigen alpha-NAC in atopic dermatitis. *Br J Dermatol.* (2011) 164:316–24. doi: 10.1111/j.1365-2133.2010.10090.x
86. Roesner LM, Heratizadeh A, Wieschowski S, Mittermann I, Valenta R, Eiz-Vesper B, et al. alpha-NAC-specific autoreactive CD8+ T cells in atopic dermatitis are of an effector memory type and secrete IL-4 and IFN-gamma. *J Immunol.* (2016) 196:3245–52. doi: 10.4049/jimmunol.1500351

87. Gaspar K, Barath S, Nagy G, Mocsai G, Gyimesi E, Szodoray P, et al. Regulatory T-cell subsets with acquired functional impairment: important indicators of disease severity in atopic dermatitis. *Acta Derm Venereol.* (2015) 95:151–5. doi: 10.2340/00015555-1882
88. Roesner LM, Floess S, Witte T, Olek S, Huehn J, Werfel T. Foxp3(+) regulatory T cells are expanded in severe atopic dermatitis patients. *Allergy.* (2015) 70:1656–60. doi: 10.1111/all.12712
89. Feliciani C, Joly P, Jonkman MF, Zambruno G, Zillikens D, Ioannides D, et al. Management of bullous pemphigoid: the European dermatology forum consensus in collaboration with the European academy of dermatology and venereology. *Br J Dermatol.* (2015) 172:867–77. doi: 10.1111/bjd.13717
90. Nast A, Amelunxen L, Augustin M, Boehncke WH, Dressler C, Gaskins M, et al. S3 Guideline for the treatment of psoriasis vulgaris, update - short version part 2 - special patient populations and treatment situations. *J Dtsch Dermatol Ges.* (2018) 16:806–13. doi: 10.1111/ddg.13538
91. Krueger JG, Ferris LK, Menter A, Wagner F, White A, Visvanathan S, et al. Anti-IL-23A mAb BI 655066 for treatment of moderate-to-severe psoriasis: Safety, efficacy, pharmacokinetics, and biomarker results of a single-rising-dose, randomized, double-blind, placebo-controlled trial. *J. Allergy Clin. Immunol.* (2015) 136:116–24.e117. doi: 10.1016/j.jaci.2015.01.018
92. Iversen L, Eidsmo L, Austad J, de Rie M, Osmancevic A, Skov L, et al. Secukinumab treatment in new-onset psoriasis: aiming to understand the potential for disease modification - rationale and design of the randomized, multicenter STEPIn study. *J Eur Acad Dermatol Venereol.* (2018) 32:1930–9. doi: 10.1111/jdv.14979
93. Boniface K, Seneschal J. Vitiligo as a skin memory disease: The need for early intervention with immunomodulating agents and a maintenance therapy to target resident memory T cells. *Exp Dermatol.* (2019). doi: 10.1111/exd.13879. [Epub ahead of print].
94. Damsky W, King BA. JAK inhibitors in dermatology: the promise of a new drug class. *J Am Acad Dermatol.* (2017) 76:736–44. doi: 10.1016/j.jaad.2016.12.005
95. Liu LY, Strassner JP, Refat MA, Harris JE, King BA. Repigmentation in vitiligo using the Janus kinase inhibitor tofacitinib may require concomitant light exposure. *J. Am. Acad. Dermatol.* (2017) 77:675–82.e671. doi: 10.1016/j.jaad.2017.05.043
96. Ellebrecht CT, Bhoj VG, Nace A, Choi EJ, Mao X, Cho MJ, et al. Reengineering chimeric antigen receptor T cells for targeted therapy of autoimmune disease. *Science.* (2016) 353:179–84. doi: 10.1126/science.aaf6756
97. Fassas A, Anagnostopoulos A, Kazis A, Kapinas K, Sakellari I, Kimiskidis V, et al. Peripheral blood stem cell transplantation in the treatment of progressive multiple sclerosis: first results of a pilot study. *Bone Marrow Transplant.* (1997) 20:631–8. doi: 10.1038/sj.bmt.1700944
98. Massey JC, Sutton IJ, Ma DDF, Moore JJ. Regenerating immunotolerance in multiple sclerosis with autologous hematopoietic stem cell transplant. *Front Immunol.* (2018) 9:410. doi: 10.3389/fimmu.2018.00410
99. Kato H, Perl A. Blockade of treg cell differentiation and function by the interleukin-21-mechanistic target of rapamycin axis via suppression of autophagy in patients with systemic lupus erythematosus. *Arthritis Rheumatol.* (2018) 70:427–38. doi: 10.1002/art.40380
100. Lai ZW, Kelly R, Winans T, Marchena I, Shadakshari A, Yu J, et al. Sirolimus in patients with clinically active systemic lupus erythematosus resistant to, or intolerant of, conventional medications: a single-arm, open-label, phase 1/2 trial. *Lancet.* (2018) 391:1186–96. doi: 10.1016/S0140-6736(18)30485-9
101. Leducq S, Giraudeau B, Tavernier E, Maruani A. Topical use of mammalian target of rapamycin inhibitors in dermatology: a systematic review with meta-analysis. *J Am Acad Dermatol.* (2019) 80:735–42. doi: 10.1016/j.jaad.2018.10.070
102. Schuster SJ, Svoboda J, Chong EA, Nasta SD, Mato AR, Anak O, et al. Chimeric antigen receptor T cells in refractory B-cell lymphomas. *N Engl J Med.* (2017) 377:2545–54. doi: 10.1056/NEJMoa1708566
103. Hawkes JE, Chan TC, Krueger JG. Psoriasis pathogenesis and the development of novel targeted immune therapies. *J Allergy Clin Immunol.* (2017) 140:645–53. doi: 10.1016/j.jaci.2017.07.004
104. Kannan AK, Su Z, Gauvin DM, Lippert SE, Marie HP, McGaraughty SP, et al. IL-23 induces regulatory T cell plasticity with implications for inflammatory skin diseases. *J. Immunol.* (2017) 198(1 Suppl):220.213–20.213.
105. Maxwell JR, Zhang Y, Brown WA, Smith CL, Byrne FR, Fiorino M, et al. Differential roles for Interleukin-23 and Interleukin-17 in Intestinal Immunoregulation. *Immunity.* (2015) 43:739–50. doi: 10.1016/j.immuni.2015.08.019
106. Delgoffe GM, Pollizzi KN, Waickman AT, Heikamp E, Meyers DJ, Horton MR, et al. The kinase mTOR regulates the differentiation of helper T cells through the selective activation of signaling by mTORC1 and mTORC2. *Nat Immunol.* (2011) 12:295–303. doi: 10.1038/ni.2005

2

Lichen Planus Pemphigoides: From Lichenoid Inflammation to Autoantibody-Mediated Blistering

Franziska Hübner[1†], *Ewan A. Langan*[1,2†] *and Andreas Recke*[1,3*]

[1] Department of Dermatology, University of Lübeck, Lübeck, Germany, [2] Dermatological Sciences, University of Manchester, Manchester, United Kingdom, [3] Lübeck Institute of Dermatological Research, University of Lübeck, Lübeck, Germany

***Correspondence:**
Andreas Recke
Andreas.Recke@uksh.de

[†] *These authors have contributed equally to this work*

Lichen planus pemphigoides (LPP) is a very rare autoimmune sub-epidermal blistering disease associated with lichenoid skin changes. Initially thought to be a mere variant of more common inflammatory dermatoses, particularly Bullous Pemphigoid (BP) or Lichen Planus (LP), a growing body of evidence suggests that it is a disease entity in its own right. In common with a range of autoimmune blistering diseases, including BP, pemphigoid gestationis (PG), mucous membrane pemphigoid (MMP) and linear IgA dermatosis (LAD), a key feature of the disease is the development of autoantibodies against type XVII collagen (COL17). However, accurately establishing the diagnosis is dependent on a careful correlation between the clinical, histological and immunological features of the disease. Therefore, we present an up to date summary of the epidemiology and etiopathogenesis of LPP, before illustrating the predisposing and precipitating factors implicated in the development of the disease. In addition to a selective literature search, we compare reports of potential drug-induced cases of LPP with pharmacovigilance data available via OpenVigil. We subsequently outline the cardinal clinical features, important differential diagnoses and current treatment options. We conclude by demonstrating that an improved understanding of LPP may not only lead to the development of novel treatment strategies for the disease itself, but may also shed new light on the pathophysiology of more common and treatment-refractory autoimmune blistering diseases.

Keywords: Lichen planus pemphigoides, autoantibodies, Bullous Pemphigoid, Lichen Planus, BP180, BP230

INTRODUCTION

First described by Kaposi over a century ago (1), Lichen planus pemphigoides (LPP, syn. Lichen ruber pemphigoides) is commonly considered to be a variant of Lichen Planus (LP), characterized and complicated by the formation of tense blisters and bullae.

In addition to the clinical findings, including lichenoid plaques and tense blisters, the gold standard for the diagnosis of LPP is the demonstration of autoantibody deposition along the dermal-epidermal junctional zone in perilesional skin biopsies; first reported by Stingl and Holubar in 1975 (2). Almost two decades later, Tamada et al. established that the autoantigen in LPP is a 180 kDa protein expressed in the hemidesmosomes of the dermal-epidermal junction (3). Interestingly, the same autoantigen is responsible for the development of Bullous Pemphigoid (BP), namely type XVII collagen (COL17) (4).

DEFINITION

Lichen planus pemphigoides can be best defined as an autoimmune dermatosis, the hallmarks of which are lichenoid and bullous skin lesions, which develop in the context of autoantibodies targeting type XVII collagen COL17.

Clinically, the diagnosis relies on carefully distinguishing the disease phenotype from that seen in bullous LP. Given the potential clinical, histological and immunological overlap between LPP, bullous LP and BP, the clinician must also determine which disease is present, although they may occasionally occur simultaneous, which may further complicate reaching the correct diagnosis(ses). Several clinical features can support reaching the correct diagnosis. For example, bullous LP classically describes the formation of blisters on pre-existing lichenoid plaques. In contrast to bullous LP, the blisters of LPP are typically located outside of LP lesions. However, several cases of LPP with blistering restricted to the lichenoid plaques have been reported, casting doubt on the utility of blister localization to clinically differentiate between LPP and Bullous LP with any degree of certainty (5, 6). The blisters in Bullous Pemphigoid tend to occur on urticated plaques and may evolve into erosions and crusts.

Moreover, there are other subtle differences in the clinical presentation of BP and LPP. For example, the typical age of onset of LPP is significantly younger than that in BP (7, 8). Furthermore, LPP lesions are predominantly found on the extremities, whereas in BP they are more often generalized (8) and associated with pruritus. The clinical course of LPP is usually less protracted and generally milder than that in BP.

Ultimately, the detection of autoantibodies to the dermal-epidermal junction is central to supporting and securing the diagnosis. In contrast to LPP, the skin changes seen in bullous LP develop in the absence of autoantibodies against structural proteins of the skin, especially COL17 (9). In terms of pathogenesis, given that in the majority of cases of LPP the development of lichenoid skin lesions precedes the formation of blisters, it has been hypothesized that lichenoid inflammation itself may actually promote the development of an autoimmune response, targeting proteins of the epidermal basement membrane (10–14).

In fact, Kromminga et al. identified subtle differences in the epitope specificity of autoantibodies in the sera of patients with LPP, BP, and mucous membrane pemphigoid (MMP) (15), using recombinant fragments of the NC16A subdomain of COL17. The sera of 12 patients with BP, 6 with gestational pemphigoid (PG), 10 with MMP and 4 with LPP were examined using nine overlapping dihydrofolate reductase-fused subfragments with a size of 13–18 amino acids of the NC16A (amino acids E_{490}-L_{565} of COL17, Uniprot entry Q9UMD9) to evaluate the epitope binding pattern by immunoblotting (15). Here, most BP and PG patient sera bound to fragments representing amino acids E_{490}-G_{532}; MMP patient sera preferentially bound to fragments E_{490}-R_{507} and D_{514}-L_{565}; while LPP sera generally lacked binding to E_{490}-R_{507} but showed reactivity with fragments comprising D_{514}-L_{565}. Kromminga et al. did not perform any statistical evaluation as to whether these differences are significant. However, on the basis of the published data it was possible to carry out a statistical analysis[1]. We found that the differences between BP and LPP ($p = 0.0032$), MMP and LPP ($p = 1.07 \times 10^{-13}$) and LPP and PG ($p = 3.08 \times 10^{-43}$) were actually highly significant. In addition, BP and PG ($p = 3.82 \times 10^{-13}$) and MMP and PG ($p = 1.95 \times 10^{-24}$) had significantly different binding patterns, while MMP and BP did not.

EPIDEMIOLOGY

The exact prevalence of LPP is unknown. Only 4 cases of LPP were identified in a cohort of 68 patients with blistering diseases from Kuwait; equivalent to an incidence of 0.3/1,000,000 inhabitants (16). A study from India reported 3 patients with LPP in a series of 268 cases with autoimmune blistering dermatoses (17). In contrast, epidemiological studies in patients with blistering dermatoses, based in France, Germany, Greece, Serbia, and Singapore, with patient numbers ranging from 41 to 1,161, did not identify any cases of LPP (18–23). Based on ICD10 classification data from health insurance providers in Germany, the reported prevalence of L12.8 (other pemphigoid diseases) was 4.7 per million patients and 259 per million patients for BP (L12.0) (7). Unfortunately, the LPP ICD10 code L43.1, was not specifically evaluated. However, the epidemiological data analysis based upon ICD10 codes is complicated by the fact that the ICD10 code L43.1 is shared between LPP and bullous LP. Nevertheless, based on the available data the prevalence may be estimated at about 1 per 1,000,000 patients.

The sex ratio (male/female) is described to be roughly 0.8/1 in adults and 3.3/1 in children and adolescents (8), failing to support a specific predilection according to sex. The mean age of onset is approximately 46 years (range between 4 and 85), which is well below the typical age of onset of BP (7). Interestingly, it is not exceptionally rare for LPP to affect children and adolescents. Indeed, in a case report collection with 78 patients, 13 (~16%) were children or adolescents (8).

ETIOPATHOGENESIS

LPP is characterized by autoantibodies against type XVII collagen (COL17, BPAG2), a structural protein that resides in hemidesmosomes at the dermal-epidermal junction (4, 24, 25). Similarly to BP, autoantibodies in LPP may also bind to the 230 kDa BPAG1 (3). In most cases, the COL17-specific autoantibodies in LPP react with the membrane-proximal NC16A subdomain (amino acid residues 490–565 of UniProt entry Q9UMD9) (4, 24). In addition, the C-terminal portion of COL17 and desmoglein 1 have been identified as epitopes and antigens, respectively, in LPP (26). Other autoantibodies against unidentified antigens with a molecular weight of 130 kDa (27) and 200 kDa (28) have also been described. The reported variability in autoantigen specificity may result in clinical variants of LPP which appear similar to BP, with

[1]Using multinomial regression (R open source statistical software, packages *nnet* for the function *multinom* and *car* for the function *Anova*) and the Benjamini-Hochberg correction for multiple testing.

autoantibodies against NC16A (24, 29), and MMP with mucosal lesions and autoantibodies against the C-terminal portion of COL17 (26, 30).

In fact, COL17 is a common autoantigen in a variety of autoimmune blistering dermatoses (31, 32), including LPP, BP, linear IgA dermatosis (33, 34), PG, MMP and paraneoplastic pemphigus (35). Autoantibodies against COL17 have been demonstrated to induce inflammation and blistering due to the effector functions of the Fc portion (36–38). Moreover, a deposition of complement factor C3 at the dermal-epidermal junction found in skin biopsies of LPP indicates an involvement of complement in the pathogenesis. In case of BP and epidermolysis bullosa acquisita, a similar subepidermal blistering disease, the activation of the complement system has been described as a crucial event in the pathogenesis (39, 40).

However, a growing evidence suggests that both complement-dependent and complement-independent mechanisms may both be relevant and effective in subepidermal blistering dermatoses (41–44). The amount of complement-activating IgG1 and non-activating IgG4 autoantibodies (45) is variable between patients. Cases with only IgG4 autoantibodies and without any complement deposition at the derma-epidermal junction exist, suggesting complement-independent mechanisms in blister formation (43). Binding of leporine autoantibodies to type XVII collagen was demonstrated to induce skin fragility, both in a complement-dependent and independent manner, in a murine model for bullous pemphigoid (44). This was confirmed in a similar mouse model, additionally indicating a disease mitigating effect of complement receptor C5aR2 (42).

Although not specifically demonstrated for all diseases, the pathogenic mechanisms ultimately resulting in subepidermal cleavage and macroscopic may be similar and/or shared between distinct autoimmune blistering dermatoses.

The development of autoantibodies against COL17 in LP appears to be a primary event in the development of LPP. This is supported by the fact that blistering almost exclusively follows the appearance of the typical lichenoid skin lesions (8).

In more than 40% of cases with vulvar LP, the NC16A domain of COL17 has been demonstrated to be a target for circulating T cells with rapid effector function (10). The authors used an ELISpot assay that detected IFNγ-producing autoreactive T cells, i.e., the only determined Th1 responses. The T-cell responses in bullous pemphigoid have been investigated with more detail: it appears that most patients have a Th2 or mixed Th1/Th2 response to the complete extracellular portion of BP180 (46). The situation of T cell responses in LPP is unknown. One may speculate that the Th1 response in LP could protect from conversion to a blistering disease, and that a dysregulated Th2 response to NC16A might be necessary for the development of LPP.

In addition to T cell responses, several authors have reported the presence of circulating autoantibodies against COL17 in patients with LP, especially oral or genital LP (10–14). A clinical course similar to LPP was observed in LP-type chronic graft-vs.-host disease, where the patient developed autoantibodies against COL17 and mucous membrane pemphigoid (47). In summary, the development of autoantibodies against COL17 in LPP appears to be linked to the T cell-mediated lichenoid inflammation.

CLINICAL FEATURES AND ESTABLISHMENT OF DIAGNOSIS

Diagnosis is based on careful correlation of the clinical, histopathological and immunopathological features.

In LPP, two discrete primary skin lesions occur: lichenoid papules/plaques and tense blisters. Cases of LPP exclusively restricted to mucous membranes have also been reported (48, 49). The nail apparatus may also be affected by LPP, resulting in nail atrophy or even loss of the nail plate (50). This suggests that LPP is in fact a very heterogeneous disease, whose clinical symptoms and immunologic markers can mimic both BP and mucous membrane pemphigoid (49).

The lichenoid eruption consists of pruritic violaceous polygonal papules and plaques with a shiny surface (**Figures 1A,B**). On the mucosa, patterned white streaks may be found, most prominently on the buccal and the outer genital mucosa (48, 51). Blisters and erosions typically appear after the development of the lichenoid skin changes and classically on previously unaffected skin. Histopathology of a bullous lesion shows the typical feature of BP (2, 31): subepidermal separation with multiple eosinophils in the blister fluid and an eosinophilic infiltrate, whereas histopathology of a lichenoid lesion shows the typical features of lichen planus with focal hyperkeratosis, hypergranulosis, subepidermal band-like lymphocytic infiltrate, and Interface dermatitis with vacuolar change at the dermal-epidermal junction and apoptotic keratinocytes (so called Civatte bodies) (2, 51, 52).

IgG and complement factor C3 deposition at the dermal-epidermal junction zone can be detected using direct immunofluorescence of perilesional biopsies (2) (**Figures 1C,D**). In contrast, direct immunofluorescence studies of lichenoid lesions may show typical features of LP: irregular band of fibrinogen at the dermal-epidermal junction and colloid bodies in the papillary dermis (53). Circulating autoantibodies in patient sera that bind to the NC16A or C-terminal domains of COL17 or desmogleins may be detected using routine methods including indirect immunofluorescence on monkey esophagus or human neonatal foreskin (54), ELISA and immunoblotting of human keratinocyte extracts (32, 55). In addition to this, circulating autoantibodies will bind to the roof of the artificial blister in indirect immunofluorescence on 1M NaCl-salt split skin (56).

The gold standard for the diagnosis of LPP is the combination of the typical clinical features and the demonstration of autoantibodies binding to the dermal-epidermal junction.

DIFFERENTIAL DIAGNOSIS

In addition to BP and bullous LP, several other dermatoses form the differential diagnosis. For example, erythema multiforme has morpho- and histo-logical features that resemble LPP, most notably a lichenoid or interface dermatitis and blistering (57).

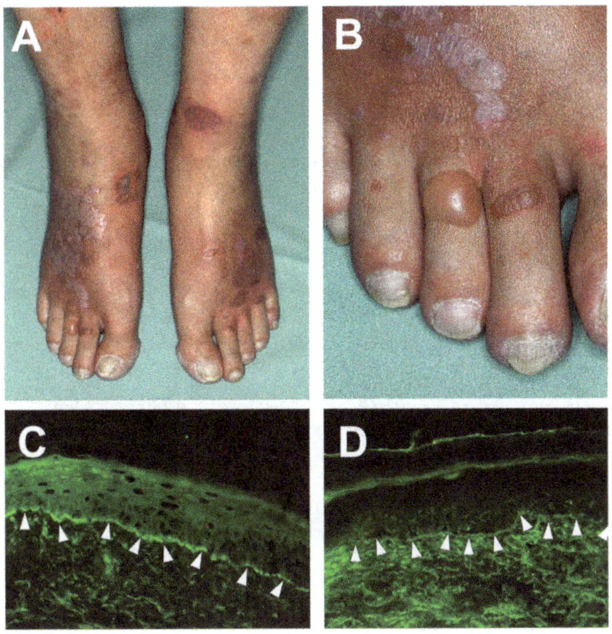

FIGURE 1 | Clinical features of Lichen planus pemphigoides. **(A)** Violaceous plaques with polygonal configuration affecting the dorsal aspects of the feet, with tense blisters and erosions on non-lesional skin. **(B)** Close-up view of the right foot. **(C)** detection of complement factor C3 deposition and, **(D)** IgG deposition at the dermal-epidermal junction in a punch biopsy from perilesional skin, using direct immunofluorescence microscopy (magnification 200×).

Atypical subacute cutaneous lupus erythematosus may present with similar clinical features as LPP (57, 58), underscoring the importance of a complete immunologic work-up to demonstrate autoantibodies against structural proteins of the skin, and especially the NC16A domain of BP180. Furthermore, in case of atypical clinical presentation, antinuclear antibody and dsDNA antibody testing is recommended.

Paraneoplastic pemphigus may present with similar skin changes and immunological features are those in LPP (59, 60), including autoantibodies against BP180. However, paraneoplastic pemphigus serum autoantibodies typically cause an intercellular binding pattern in the epidermis and can bind to rat bladder epithelia and to envoplakin and periplakin (61).

During the course of disease, LPP may even evolve into other types of autoimmune blistering skin diseases, such as pemphigoid nodularis (62), also known as non-bullous pemphigoid.

DRUGS AND CONDITIONS ASSOCIATED WITH LPP

Several reports describe an association between the development of LPP and medication and/or and pre-existing medical conditions.

LPP and Drugs

Relying solely on observational evidence, several drugs have been associated with the development of LPP (**Table 1**). A causal association is at least conceivable when the LPP developed shortly after the intake of new medication and fully resolved after cessation of the suspected drug-trigger. Perhaps the strongest evidence for drug-induced LPP is in the context angiotensin-converting enzyme (ACE) inhibitor use. There are four reports of an association of LPP with different angiotensin-converting enzyme (ACE) inhibitors (64, 67, 68, 74). Nevertheless, it should be acknowledged that in the majority of published reports of medication-induced LPP, drug re-challenge was either not performed or not associated with disease recurrence.

LPP and Infections

LPP has also been reported to be a complication of infection, particularly viral infections (**Table 1**), for example varicella (72, 73) and hepatitis B (77, 78). In fact, all of the published cases of LPP and viral hepatitis to date have been in association with hepatitis B (77, 78) and not hepatitis C infection. This is in contrast to LP, in which only hepatitis C has been reported as a trigger factor. The odds ratio to develop LP, especially oral LP, is described to be 2.5–4.5 for individual who are seropositive for HCV (80). Vice versa, a meta-analysis showed that the odds ratio to have a positive serology of HCV was 2.73–13.48 in patients with oral LP (81).

LPP and Cancer

An association of LPP with colon adenocarcinoma points raises the possibility of a paraneoplastic variant of the disease (82).

Medication as a Trigger of Both LP and BP

If one considers the possibility that LPP occurs as a complication of LP, it is conceivable that drugs that trigger the more prevalent disease LP also increase the risk of developing LPP. In fact, a large number of drugs have been described as possibly related to the development of LP, including ACE inhibitors. Several drugs are reportedly associated with the development of LP, including antimalarials, thiazide diuretics, NSAIDs, quinidine, beta-blockers, gold compounds, and tumor necrosis factor alpha inhibitors (51). The list of drugs that have been reported to induce BP is more extensive than the equivalent list for LP. It includes antibiotics, Calcium channel antagonists, ACE inhibitors, beta-blockers, angiotensin 1 antagonists, vaccines, NSAIDs, diuretics, Gliptins, TNF-alpha inhibitors, D-penicillamine, and tiobutarid (52). An induction of BP by PUVA has been reported only anecdotally (83, 84).

Comparison of Case Report Data With Pharmacovigilance Information

Pharmacovigilance databases provide another valuable resource to identify drugs that may trigger the development of LPP. However, one major drawback is that LPP is not specified as a disease in the WHO list of adverse events. Instead, the terms "lichen planus" and "pemphigoid" were used to analyze pharmacovigilance data using the OpenVigil database tool (URL: http://openvigil.pharmacology.uni-kiel.de/openvigilfda.php). Pharmacovigilance report analyses are compared with case reports in **Table 1**, supported the observation of LPP cases that were caused by ACE inhibitors (enalapril, capropril, and ramipril), but also simvastatin and pembrolizumab. With the

TABLE 1 | Drugs and conditions that were reported to be associated with LPP.

Drug	Reference[c]	Pharmacovigilance data disproportionality analysis[a,b]			
		Lichen planus		Pemphigoid	
		Chi squared (Yates)	Reporting odds ratio (95%-CI)	Chi squared (yates)	Reporting odds ratio (95%-CI)
Cinnarizine	(63)	n.r.	n.r.	n.r.	n.r.
Enalapril	(64)	**7.93***	**3.1 (1.48–6.53)**	**35.93***	**3.79 (2.41–5.95)**
Narrowband UVB	(27)	*n.a.*	*n.a.*	*n.a.*	*n.a.*
Chinese herbs	(65)	*n.a.*	*n.a.*	*n.a.*	*n.a.*
"weight reduction drug"	(66)	*n.a.*	*n.a.*	*n.a.*	*n.a.*
Captopril	(67, 68)	**17.93***	**6.48 (2.69–15.62)**	0.03	0.58 (0.08–4.11)
Simvastatin	(69)	**11.09***	**1.79 (1.28–2.51)**	**51.79***	**2.13 (1.73–2.62)**
Pembrolizumab	(70)	**88.22***	**10.1 (5.71–17.83)**	**427.24***	**14.06 (10.15–19.46)**
PUVA	(71)	*n.a.*	*n.a.*	*n.a.*	*n.a.*
Varicella Chickenpox	(72, 73)	*n.a.*	*n.a.*	*n.a.*	*n.a.*
Ramipril	(74)	**43.95***	**3.63 (2.44–5.4)**	**279.96***	**5.41 (4.34–6.75)**
Renal tuberculosis[d]	(75)	*n.a.*	*n.a.*	*n.a.*	*n.a.*
Isoniazide[d]	(75)	n.r.	n.r.	n.r.	n.r.
Rifampin[d]	(75)	n.r.	n.r.	n.r.	n.r.
Ethambutol[d]	(75)	0.56	5.51 (0.78–39.21)	0.02	2.47 (0.35–17.58)
Pyrazinamide[d]	(75)	0.00016	2.04 (0.29–14.48)	1.81	2.75 (0.88–8.52)
Gestodene + Ethinylestradiol	(76)	n.r.	n.r.	n.r.	n.r.
Hepatitis B Virus	(77, 78)	*n.a.*	*n.a.*	*n.a.*	*n.a.*

[a]*Disproportionality analyses were performed using OpenVigil. A possible association requires a minimum report count of N > 3, a reporting odds ratio > 2 and a Chi-Squared value > 4 (79). An asterisk (*) indicates a possible relationship between drug and disease. Drugs associated with both lichen planus and pemphigoid are indicated by bold font face.*
[b]*n.r., respective condition not reported; n.a., no data available.*
[c]*Each of the references describes a single case of drug-induced LPP.*
[d]*The case report by Demirçay et al. (75) describes one patient with renal tuberculosis who developed LPP after treatment with isoniaziade, rifampin, ethambutol and pyrazinamide.*

exception of captopril, both LP and pemphigoid disease were found to be putative side effects of these drugs. The reported association of anti-tuberculosis drugs with LPP could not be confirmed by pharmacovigilance data. For all other drugs and conditions that were suspected to be associated with LPP, no data could be found.

Identification of Putative Triggers for LPP, LP, and BP From Pharmacovigilance Information

In addition, pharmacovigilance data also allows the identification of drugs that are not yet reported as possible triggers for LPP but are putative triggers for LP and/or pemphigoid (**Table 2**). Drugs that were reported as possible triggers for both LP and pemphigoid were hydrochlorothiazide, candesartan, sitagliptine, amlodipine, losartan, fluoxetine, and terbinafine. In addition, vildagliptine has been identified as a potent trigger for the development of BP (90), though OpenVigil did not contain any entries with this drug.

For some drugs, pharmacovigilance report analyses do not overlap or even contradict the published literature (**Table 2**). In case of Ibuprofen, the association with pemphigoid could be confirmed, but not in case of LP. The same holds true for sulfasalazine and risperidone. In case of gabapentin, a negative association with pemphigoid was found. For TNFα inhibitors, pharmacovigilance data indicates a negative association of etanercept and adalimumab with pemphigoid and no association with LP. A negative association (odds ratio below 1) may indicate here a protective effect of the respective drug regarding pemphigoid, although gabapentin, etanercept and adalimumab are no established treatment options for this disease. Alternatively, this negative association may be the result of a statistical phenomenon where patients who tend to develop pemphigoid are less likely to be treated with the aforementioned drugs. In the other hand, infliximab seems to be positively associated with LP, but not with pemphigoid.

It has to be noted that pharmacovigilance data is based on physician-initiated reports about possible adverse events and not on a prospective data collection. Common belief about possible relationships between drugs and adverse events may lead to further skewing of data. Moreover, it is difficult to control for confounders or interactions. If a certain drug is used to treat a disease that predisposes for LP, BP or LPP, the disproportionality analysis cannot distinguish this from a drug-related predisposition. Furthermore, it is not possible to distinguish whether a certain drug truly causes LPP or whether it just increases the probability for a clinical manifestation in patients that are otherwise predisposed to LPP.

TABLE 2 | Drugs and conditions not yet reported to be associated with LPP, but with LP or pemphigoid.

Drug	**Reference[c]**		**Pharmacovigilance data disproportionality analysis[a,b]**			
	LP	**Pemphigoid**	**Lichen planus**		**Pemphigoid**	
			Chi squared (Yates)	**Reporting odds ratio (95%-CI)**	**Chi squared (yates)**	**Reporting odds ratio (95%-CI)**
Ibuprofen	(51)	(52)	0.22	1.16 (0.72–1,87)	**8.3***	**2.2 (1.3–3.8)**
Hydrochlorothiazide	(51)	(52)	**190.2***	**4.9 (3.8–6.3)**	100*	**2.84 (2.3–3.5)**
Infliximab	(51)	(52)	**36.9***	**2.9 (2.0–4.0)**	2.6	1.34 (0.9–1.9)
Etanercept	(51)	(52)	0.8	1.14 (0.9–1.5)	**53.3****	**0.29 (0.2–0.4)**
Adalimumab	(51)	(52)	11.7	1.57 (1.2–2.0)	**14.4****	**0.59 (0.5–0.8)**
Hydroxychloroquine	(51)		**89.23***	**6.22 (4.1–9.5)**	2.6	0.37 (0.1–1.2)
Candesartan[d]	*no ref.[e]*		**16.43***	**3.64 (2–6.8)**	**149***	**6.09 (4.4–8.4)**
Sitagliptine	(85)	(52)	**7.48***	**2.22 (1.29–3.9)**	**1689***	**13.25 (11.3–15.6)**
Furosemide		(52)	0.56	1.2 (0.8–1.7)	**382***	**3.96 (3.4–4.6)**
Verapamil		(52)	n.r.	n.r.	**9.8***	**4.38 (1.82–10.5)**
Ciprofloxacine		(52)	0.04	1.2 (0.5–2.7)	**13.4***	**2.14 (1.43–3.2)**
Amoxicillin	*no ref.[e]*	(52)	**9.6***	**2.5 (1.4–4.5)**	0.07	1.13 (0.64–2)
Cephalexin		(52)	2.6	2.7 (1–7.1)	**51.5***	**5.1 (3.2–8.2)**
Spironolactone		(52)	1.7	1.7 (0.9–3.4)	**13.9**	**2.2 (1.5–3.3)**
Amlodipin	(86)	(52)	**33.3***	**2.3 (1.7–3.0)**	**194***	**3.1 (2.6–3.7)**
Losartan	*no ref.[e]*	(52)	**37.7***	**3.0 (2.1–4.4)**	**13**	**1.8 (1.3–2.5)**
Sulfasalazine	(87)	(52)	**8.8***	**3.0 (1.5–6.0)**	0.03	0.8 (0.4–2)
Fluoxetine	*no ref.[e]*	(52)	**19.4***	**2.6 (1.7–4.1)**	**15.4**	**2 (1.4–2.8)**
Gabapentine		(52)	0.1	0.9 (0.6–1.5)	**17.8****	**0.3 (0.2–0.6)**
Galantamine hydrobromide		(52)	n.r.	n.r.	**21.9***	**9.3 (3.5–24.9)**
Levetiracetam		(52)	0.07	1.2 (0.6–2.5)	**23.3***	**2.4 (1.7–3.4)**
Terbinafine	(88)	(52)	**8.4***	**4.8 (1.8–12.8)**	**11.5***	**3.8(1.8–7.9)**
Omeprazole		(52)	11.9	1.7 (1.3–2.3)	9.7	1.4 (1.1–1.8)
Risperidone	(89)	(52)	0.8	0.5 (0.1–1.8)	**19.6***	**2.5 (1.7–3.7)**
Hepatitis C virus	(51)		n.a.	n.a.	n.a.	n.a.

[a]*Disproportionality analyses were performed using OpenVigil. A possible association requires a minimum report count of N > 3, a reporting odds ratio > 2 and a Chi-Squared value > 4 (79). An asterisk (*) and bold face indicates a possible relationship between drug and disease. Drugs associated with both lichen planus and pemphigoid are indicated by bold font face. A double asterisk (**) indicates a negative relationship between drug and disease. The corresponding drug names and relationship parameter values are highlighted in red.*

[b]*n.r., respective condition not reported; n.a., no data available.*

[c]*Drug associations for pemphigoid as summarized by Stavropoulos et al. (52), for lichen planus as summarized by Arnold et al. (51) and reported by Swale and McGregor (86).*

[d]*Candesartan was not reported by name previously, only by drug class.*

[e]*No ref. indicates that pharmacovigilance data analysis suggests an association of drug and disease, but the search term "lichen planus" plus drug name did not retrieve any pubmed records.*

TREATMENT

In a selective PubMed literature review of case reports published from the year 2000 onward, we were able to find treatment information from $N = 53$ patients in $N = 43$ articles (**Table 3**). Most reports ($N = 42$) describe the use of corticosteroids (mainly oral prednisolone) in various doses, from very low dose in some Japanese cases up to 2 mg/kg body weight. High doses of prednisolone are used for treatment of LPP in children. Topical corticosteroids were used in $N = 20$ cases, followed by dapsone in $N = 15$ cases.

In a case of oral lichen planus pemphigoides, topical gel ointment containing fluocinonid or dexamethasone was reportedly effective (48).

Although in most of the reported cases, patients were successfully treated with systemic corticosteroids, this might not be the best option given the side-effect profile. Other treatment options include topical corticosteroids, dapsone, and acitretin, whose use may be associated with fewer side-effects. This situation may be compared with that in BP. Here, systemic oral corticosteroids had been considered as standard treatment for decades (110) until Joly et al. effected a paradigmatic shift in treatment by demonstrating the equivalent efficacy of highly potent topical steroids, with fewer side-effects (111). On the other hand, given that patients with LPP tend to be younger, with fewer co-morbidities, one could argue that systemic treatment would be less hazardous and may result in speedier disease resolution.

TABLE 3 | Reported treatment options for LPP since 2000.

Treatment[a]	Success *N* cases	Failure *N* cases	References
Acitretin	2	1	(70, 91, 92)
Azathioprin	3	1	(2, 17, 93, 94)
Ciclosporin (systemic)	2		(95, 96)
Corticosteroids (systemic)	**38**	**4**	(2, 5, 8, 12, 17, 26–28, 48, 62, 65, 67, 70–73, 75–77, 82, 91, 93–104)
Corticosteroids (topically)	**15**	**5**	(2, 8, 48, 49, 64, 72, 92, 93, 95, 97–99, 104–107)
Ciclosporine (topically)	Ø	1	(49)
Dapsone	**13**	**2**	(12, 26, 65, 66, 70, 75, 77, 91, 94, 98–100, 103, 108)
Doxycycline	1	Ø	(107)
Hydroxychloroquine	Ø	1	(94)
IVIG	3	Ø	(49, 62)
MTX	1	1	(95, 102)
Mycophenolatmofetile	2	1	(48, 62, 94)
PUVA	Ø	2	(70, 91)
Rituximab	Ø	1	(70)
Sirolimus	Ø	1	(70)
Tacrolimus (topically)	1	Ø	(48)
Tetracycline/Nicotinamide	2	1	(70, 94, 105)
Ustekinumab	1	Ø	(94)
Termination of the triggering medication or tumor resection	**8**	**2**	(49, 64–67, 69, 70, 76, 82, 93, 109)
Non-termination of potentially triggering medication	1	Ø	(70)

[a] *The listed treatment may be part of a combination therapy. Individual cases may be counted multiple times with different drugs. Treatment options with at least 10 reports are highlighted in bold font. Some publications report more than one case.*

Another interesting observation made during the review of the case reports is the very low doses of corticosteroids that were used for treatment in some Japanese cases (71, 97). Here, a dose of 15 mg, irrespective of body weight, was reportedly effective. In contrast, corticosteroid doses in cases from other countries are often between 0.5 and 1 mg/kg body weight, i.e., 2 to 4-fold higher.

From our experience (112), a combination of topical dexamethasone, prednisolone pulse therapy (100 mg/day for 3 days, initially every 3rd week) and acitretin (20 mg/day p.o.) is often sufficient to induce remission of blistering within 3 months and disappearance of LP lesions within 1 year. Similar observations have been reported in the literature (91).

Alternatives or additives to corticosteroid treatment could include dapsone (100 mg/daily), tetracycline (2 × 500 mg/daily) in combination with nicotinamide (2 × 500 mg/daily), mycophenolate mofetil (1000–1500 mg/daily in two doses), cyclosporine A (2 mg/kg body weight in 2 doses/day), methotrexate (7.5–20 mg/week or 0.5 mg/kg body weight/week in children).

Our PubMed literature search also retrieved the use of hypnotic suggestion for the treatment of LPP (113), though this article was published in 1959.

In 10 cases, a triggering medication or condition such as a underlying malignancy was identified and treated, resulting in resolution of skin lesions in 8 cases. One report describes the management of LPP associated with pembrolizumab therapy in a patient with malignant melanoma (70). In this patient, dapsone led to resolution of LPP, allowing the treatment with pembrolizumab to be continued. In this context, pembrolizumab was not necessarily the direct trigger of LPP *per se*, but may have been an important co-factor for the clinical manifestation of a subclinical disease, potentially related to its mode of action.

CONCLUSION

LPP is a very rare disease entity that belongs to a larger family of diseases characterized by autoantibodies against COL17. It is a heterogenic disease, but shared common clinical features with other autoimmune blistering diseases, including BP and MMP. Its pathognomonic feature is the association with LP, supported by the demonstration of IgG and complement factor C3 deposition at the dermal-epidermal junction. Several case reports indicate an association with ACE inhibitors, simvastatin and checkpoint inhibitors, but also with HBV infection. There is no current consensus on the optimal treatment regime for LPP. However, combinations of systemic with topical corticosteroids, potentially in combination with dapsone or acitretin are worth considering. An improved understanding of the pathophysiology of LPP may help to shed new light on the mechanisms that lead to the development of autoantibodies against COL17 and subsequent blister formation.

AUTHOR CONTRIBUTIONS

FH, EL and AR discussed data and wrote the manuscript. AR identified the patient, performed literature search, and pharmacovigilance data analyses.

ACKNOWLEDGMENTS

We thank all people not mentioned here who were involved in patient care and routine laboratory diagnostics.

REFERENCES

1. Kaposi M. Lichen ruber pemphigoides. *Arch Derm Syph.* (1882) 24:345–6.
2. Stingl G, Holubar K. Coexistence of lichen planus and bullous pemphigoid. A immunopathological study. *Br J Dermatol.* (1975) 93:313–20. doi: 10.1111/j.1365-2133.1975.tb06497.x
3. Tamada Y, Yokochi K, Nitta Y, Ikeya T, Hara K, Owaribe K. Lichen planus pemphigoides: identification of 180 kd hemidesmosome antigen. *J Am Acad Dermatol.* (1995) 32:883–7. doi: 10.1016/0190-9622(95)91554-0
4. Zillikens D, Caux F, Mascaro JM, Wesselmann U, Schmidt E, Prost C, et al. Autoantibodies in lichen planus pemphigoides react with a novel epitope within the C-terminal NC16A domain of BP180. *J Invest Dermatol.* (1999) 113:117–21. doi: 10.1046/j.1523-1747.1999.00618.x
5. Matos-Pires E, Campos S, Lencastre A, João A, Mendes-Bastos P. Lichen planus pemphigoides. *J Dtsch Dermatol Ges J Ger Soc Dermatol.* (2018) 16:335–7. doi: 10.1111/ddg.13434_g
6. Archer CB, Cronin E, Smith NP. Diagnosis of lichen planus pemphigoides in the absence of bullae on normal-appearing skin. *Clin Exp Dermatol.* (1992) 17:433–6. doi: 10.1111/j.1365-2230.1992.tb00253.x
7. Hübner F, Recke A, Zillikens D, Linder R, Schmidt E. Prevalence and age distribution of pemphigus and pemphigoid diseases in Germany. *J Invest Dermatol.* (2016) 136:2495–8. doi: 10.1016/j.jid.2016.07.013
8. Zaraa I, Mahfoudh A, Sellami MK, Chelly I, El Euch D, Zitouna M, et al. Lichen planus pemphigoides: four new cases and a review of the literature. *Int J Dermatol.* (2013) 52:406–12. doi: 10.1111/j.1365-4632.2012.05693.x
9. Liakopoulou A, Rallis E. Bullous lichen planus - a review. *J Dermatol Case Rep.* (2017) 11:1–4. doi: 10.3315/jdcr.2017.1239
10. Baldo M, Bailey A, Bhogal B, Groves RW, Ogg G, Wojnarowska F. T cells reactive with the NC16A domain of BP180 are present in vulval lichen sclerosus and lichen planus. *J Eur Acad Dermatol Venereol.* (2010) 24:186–90. doi: 10.1111/j.1468-3083.2009.03375.x
11. Buijsrogge JJA, Hagel C, Duske U, Kromminga A, Vissink A, Kloosterhuis AJ, et al. IgG antibodies to BP180 in a subset of oral lichen planus patients. *J Dermatol Sci.* (2007) 47:256–8. doi: 10.1016/j.jdermsci.2007.05.011
12. Barnadas MA, Roé E, Dalmau J, Alomar A, Martínez L, Gelpí C. Lichen planus pemphigoides: detection of anti-BP 180 antibodies by ELISA and immunoblotting tests. *J Eur Acad Dermatol Venereol.* (2010) 24:1360–1. doi: 10.1111/j.1468-3083.2010.03632.x
13. Herrero-González JE, Parera Amer E, Segura S, Mas Bosch V, Pujol RM, Martínez Escala ME. Epithelial antigenic specificities of circulating autoantibodies in mucosal lichen planus. *Int J Dermatol.* (2016) 55:634–9. doi: 10.1111/ijd.12990
14. Shipman AR, Cooper S, Wojnarowska F. Autoreactivity to bullous pemphigoid 180: is this the link between subepidermal blistering diseases and oral lichen planus? *Clin Exp Dermatol.* (2011) 36:267–9. doi: 10.1111/j.1365-2230.2010.03878.x
15. Kromminga A, Sitaru C, Meyer J, Arndt R, Schmidt E, Christophers E, et al. Cicatricial pemphigoid differs from bullous pemphigoid and pemphigoid gestationis regarding the fine specificity of autoantibodies to the BP180 NC16A domain. *J Dermatol Sci.* (2002) 28:68–75. doi: 10.1016/S0923-1811(01)00144-X
16. Nanda A, Dvorak R, Al-Saeed K, Al-Sabah H, Alsaleh QA. Spectrum of autoimmune bullous diseases in Kuwait. *Int J Dermatol.* (2004) 43:876–81. doi: 10.1111/j.1365-4632.2004.02292.x
17. De D, Khullar G, Handa S, Saikia UN, Radotra BD, Saikia B, et al. Clinical, demographic and immunopathological spectrum of subepidermal autoimmune bullous diseases at a tertiary center: A 1-year audit. *Indian J Dermatol Venereol Leprol.* (2016) 82:358. doi: 10.4103/0378-6323.175928
18. Wong SN, Chua SH. Spectrum of subepidermal immunobullous disorders seen at the National Skin Centre, Singapore: a 2-year review. *Br J Dermatol.* (2002) 147:476–80. doi: 10.1046/j.1365-2133.2002.04919.x
19. Bertram F, Bröcker E-B, Zillikens D, Schmidt E. Prospective analysis of the incidence of autoimmune bullous disorders in Lower Franconia, Germany. *J Dtsch Dermatol Ges J Ger Soc Dermatol.* (2009) 7:434–40. doi: 10.1111/j.1610-0387.2008.06976.x
20. Zillikens D, Wever S, Roth A, Weidenthaler-Barth B, Hashimoto T, Bröcker EB. Incidence of autoimmune subepidermal blistering dermatoses in a region of central Germany. *Arch Dermatol.* (1995) 131:957–8. doi: 10.1001/archderm.131.8.957
21. Bernard P, Vaillant L, Labeille B, Bedane C, Arbeille B, Denoeux JP, et al. Incidence and distribution of subepidermal autoimmune bullous skin diseases in three French regions. bullous diseases French study group. *Arch Dermatol.* (1995) 131:48–52. doi: 10.1001/archderm.1995.01690130050009
22. Patsatsi A, Lamprou F, Kokolios M, Stylianidou D, Trigoni A, Kalampalikis D, et al. Spectrum of autoimmune bullous diseases in Northern Greece. A 4-year retrospective study and review of the literature. *Acta Dermatovenerol Croat.* (2017) 25:195–201.
23. Milinković MV, Janković S, Medenica L, Nikolić M, Reljić V, Popadić S, et al. Incidence of autoimmune bullous diseases in Serbia: a 20-year retrospective study: Incidence of autoimmune bullous diseases. *J Dtsch Dermatol Ges.* (2016) 14:995–1005. doi: 10.1111/ddg.13081
24. Skaria M, Salomon D, Jaunin F, Friedli A, Saurat JH, Borradori L. IgG autoantibodies from a lichen planus pemphigoides patient recognize the NC16A domain of the bullous pemphigoid antigen 180. *Dermatol Basel Switz.* (1999) 199:253–5. doi: 10.1159/000018257
25. Hsu S, Ghohestani RF, Uitto J. Lichen planus pemphigoides with IgG autoantibodies to the 180 kd bullous pemphigoid antigen (type XVII collagen). *J Am Acad Dermatol.* (2000) 42:136–41. doi: 10.1016/S0190-9622(00)90024-0
26. Sekiya A, Kodera M, Yamaoka T, Iwata Y, Usuda T, Ohzono A, et al. A case of lichen planus pemphigoides with autoantibodies to the NC16a and C-terminal domains of BP180 and to desmoglein-1. *Br J Dermatol.* (2014) 171:1230–5. doi: 10.1111/bjd.13097
27. Mandy Chan WM, Lee JSS, Thiam Theng CS, Chua SH, Boon Oon HH. Narrowband UVB-induced lichen planus pemphigoide. *Dermatol Rep.* (2011) 3:e43. doi: 10.4081/dr.2011.e43
28. Yoon KH, Kim SC, Kang DS, Lee IJ. Lichen planus pemphigoides with circulating autoantibodies against 200 and 180 kDa epidermal antigens. *Eur J Dermatol.* (2000) 10:212–4.
29. Giudice GJ, Emery DJ, Zelickson BD, Anhalt GJ, Liu Z, Diaz LA. Bullous pemphigoid and herpes gestationis autoantibodies recognize a common non-collagenous site on the BP180 ectodomain. *J Immunol.* (1993) 151:5742–50. doi: 10.1016/0923-1811(93)90940-Q
30. Lee JB, Liu Y, Hashimoto T. Cicatricial pemphigoid sera specifically react with the most C-terminal portion of BP180. *J Dermatol Sci.* (2003) 32:59–64. doi: 10.1016/S0923-1811(03)00035-5
31. Witte M, Zillikens D, Schmidt E. Diagnosis of autoimmune blistering diseases. *Front Med.* (2018) 5:296. doi: 10.3389/fmed.2018.00296
32. van Beek N, Zillikens D, Schmidt E. Diagnosis of autoimmune bullous diseases. *J Dtsch Dermatol Ges.* (2018) 16:1077–91. doi: 10.1111/ddg.13637
33. Pas HH, Kloosterhuis GJ, Heeres K, van der Meer JB, Jonkman MF. Bullous pemphigoid and linear IgA dermatosis sera recognize a similar 120-kDa keratinocyte collagenous glycoprotein with antigenic cross-reactivity to BP180. *J Invest Dermatol.* (1997) 108:423–9. doi: 10.1111/1523-1747.ep12289703
34. Hashimoto T, Ishii N, Tsuruta D. Production of neoepitopes by dynamic structural changes on BP180/type XVII collagen. *J Invest Dermatol.* (2017) 137:2462–4. doi: 10.1016/j.jid.2017.09.001
35. Yashiro M, Nakano T, Taniguchi T, Katsuoka K, Tadera N, Miyazaki K, et al. IgA paraneoplastic pemphigus in angioimmunoblastic T-cell lymphoma with antibodies to desmocollin 1, type VII collagen and laminin 332. *Acta Derm Venereol.* (2014) 94:235–6. doi: 10.2340/00015555-1660
36. Sitaru C, Schmidt E, Petermann S, Munteanu LS, Bröcker E-B, Zillikens D. Autoantibodies to bullous pemphigoid antigen 180 induce dermal-epidermal separation in cryosections of human skin. *J Invest Dermatol.* (2002) 118:664–71. doi: 10.1046/j.1523-1747.2002.01720.x
37. Shimanovich I, Mihai S, Oostingh GJ, Ilenchuk TT, Bröcker E-B, Opdenakker G, et al. Granulocyte-derived elastase and gelatinase B are required for dermal-epidermal separation induced by autoantibodies from patients with epidermolysis bullosa acquisita and bullous pemphigoid. *J Pathol.* (2004) 204:519–27. doi: 10.1002/path.1674
38. Hirose M, Recke A, Beckmann T, Shimizu A, Ishiko A, Bieber K, et al. Repetitive immunization breaks tolerance to type XVII collagen and leads to bullous pemphigoid in mice. *J Immunol.* (2011) 187:1176–83. doi: 10.4049/jimmunol.1100596

39. Liu Z, Giudice GJ, Swartz SJ, Fairley JA, Till GO, Troy JL, et al. The role of complement in experimental bullous pemphigoid. *J Clin Invest.* (1995) 95:1539–44. doi: 10.1172/JCI117826
40. Mihai S, Chiriac MT, Takahashi K, Thurman JM, Holers VM, Zillikens D, et al. The alternative pathway of complement activation is critical for blister induction in experimental epidermolysis bullosa acquisita. *J Immunol.* (2007) 178:6514–21. doi: 10.4049/jimmunol.178.10.6514
41. Iwata H, Ujiie H. Complement-independent blistering mechanisms in bullous pemphigoid. *Exp Dermatol.* (2017) 26:1235–9. doi: 10.1111/exd.13367
42. Karsten CM, Beckmann T, Holtsche MM, Tillmann J, Tofern S, Schulze FS, et al. Tissue destruction in bullous pemphigoid can be complement independent and may be mitigated by C5aR2. *Front Immunol.* (2018) 9:488. doi: 10.3389/fimmu.2018.00488
43. Dainichi T, Nishie W, Yamagami Y, Sonobe H, Ujiie H, Kaku Y, et al. Bullous pemphigoid suggestive of complement-independent blister formation with anti-BP180 IgG4 autoantibodies. *Br J Dermatol.* (2016) 175:187–90. doi: 10.1111/bjd.14411
44. Natsuga K, Nishie W, Shinkuma S, Ujiie H, Nishimura M, Sawamura D, et al. Antibodies to pathogenic epitopes on type XVII collagen cause skin fragility in a complement-dependent and -independent manner. *J Immunol.* (2012) 188:5792–9. doi: 10.4049/jimmunol.1003402
45. Recke A, Sitaru C, Vidarsson G, Evensen M, Chiriac MT, Ludwig RJ, et al. Pathogenicity of IgG subclass autoantibodies to type VII collagen: induction of dermal-epidermal separation. *J Autoimmun.* (2010) 34:435–44. doi: 10.1016/j.jaut.2009.11.003
46. Büdinger L, Borradori L, Yee C, Eming R, Ferencik S, Grosse-Wilde H, et al. Identification and characterization of autoreactive T cell responses to bullous pemphigoid antigen 2 in patients and healthy controls. *J Clin Invest.* (1998) 102:2082–9. doi: 10.1172/JCI3335
47. Hanafusa T, Azukizawa H, Nishioka M, Tanemura A, Murota H, Yoshida H, et al. Lichen planus-type chronic graft-versus-host disease complicated by mucous membrane pemphigoid with positive anti-BP180/230 and scleroderma-related autoantibodies followed by reduced regulatory T cell frequency. *Eur J Dermatol.* (2012) 22:140–2. doi: 10.1684/ejd.2011.1587
48. Sultan A, Stojanov IJ, Lerman MA, Kabani S, Haber J, Freedman J, et al. Oral lichen planus pemphigoides: a series of four cases. *Oral Surg Oral Med Oral Pathol Oral Radiol.* (2015) 120:58–68. doi: 10.1016/j.oooo.2015.03.012
49. Mignogna MD, Fortuna G, Leuci S, Stasio L, Mezza E, Ruoppo E. Lichen planus pemphigoides, a possible example of epitope spreading. *Oral Surg Oral Med Oral Pathol Oral Radiol Endod.* (2010) 109:837–43. doi: 10.1016/j.tripleo.2009.12.044
50. Khullar G, Handa S, De D, Saikia UN. Bullous lichen planus of the nails. *JAMA Dermatol.* (2015) 151:674–5. doi: 10.1001/jamadermatol.2014.5701
51. Arnold DL, Krishnamurthy K. Lichen, Planus. In: *StatPearls.* Treasure Island, FL: StatPearls Publishing. (2019). Available online at: http://www.ncbi.nlm.nih.gov/books/NBK526126/
52. Stavropoulos PG, Soura E, Antoniou C. Drug-induced pemphigoid: a review of the literature. *J Eur Acad Dermatol Venereol.* (2014) 28:1133–40. doi: 10.1111/jdv.12366
53. Yamanaka Y, Yamashita M, Innocentini LMA, Macedo LD, Chahud F, Ribeiro-Silva A, et al. Direct immunofluorescence as a helpful tool for the differential diagnosis of oral lichen planus and oral lichenoid lesions. *Am J Dermatopathol.* (2018) 40:491–7. doi: 10.1097/DAD.0000000000001071
54. Emtenani S, Yuan H, Lin C, Pan M, Hundt JE, Schmidt E, et al. Normal human skin is superior to monkey oesophagus substrate for detection of circulating BP180-NC16A-specific IgG antibodies in bullous pemphigoid. *Br J Dermatol.* (2018) 180:1099–1106. doi: 10.1111/bjd.17313
55. van Beek N, Dähnrich C, Johannsen N, Lemcke S, Goletz S, Hübner F, et al. Prospective studies on the routine use of a novel multivariant enzyme-linked immunosorbent assay for the diagnosis of autoimmune bullous diseases. *J Am Acad Dermatol.* (2017) 76:889–94.e5. doi: 10.1016/j.jaad.2016.11.002
56. Zillikens D, Kawahara Y, Ishiko A, Shimizu H, Mayer J, Rank CV, et al. A novel subepidermal blistering disease with autoantibodies to a 200-kDa antigen of the basement membrane zone. *J Invest Dermatol.* (1996) 106:1333–8. doi: 10.1111/1523-1747.ep12349283
57. Gru AA, Salavaggione AL. Lichenoid and interface dermatoses. *Semin Diagn Pathol.* (2017) 34:237–49. doi: 10.1053/j.semdp.2017.03.001
58. Inoue Y, Adachi A, Ueno M, Fukumoto T, Nishitani N, Fujiwara N, et al. Atypical subacute cutaneous lupus erythematosus presenting as lichen planus pemphigoides with autoantibodies to C-terminus of BP180, desmoglein 1 and SS-A/Ro antigen. *J Dermatol.* (2012) 39:960–2. doi: 10.1111/j.1346-8138.2012.01536.x
59. Stevens SR, Griffiths CE, Anhalt GJ, Cooper KD. Paraneoplastic pemphigus presenting as a lichen planus pemphigoides-like eruption. *Arch Dermatol.* (1993) 129:866–9. doi: 10.1001/archderm.1993.01680280054010
60. Hsiao CJ, Hsu MM, Lee JY, Chen WC, Hsieh WC. Paraneoplastic pemphigus in association with a retroperitoneal Castleman's disease presenting with a lichen planus pemphigoides-like eruption. A case report and review of literature. *Br J Dermatol.* (2001) 144:372–6. doi: 10.1046/j.1365-2133.2001.04030.x
61. Probst C, Schlumberger W, Stöcker W, Recke A, Schmidt E, Hashimoto T, et al. Development of ELISA for the specific determination of autoantibodies against envoplakin and periplakin in paraneoplastic pemphigus. *Clin Chim Acta.* (2009) 410:13–8. doi: 10.1016/j.cca.2009.08.022
62. Sakuma-Oyama Y, Powell AM, Albert S, Oyama N, Bhogal BS, Black MM. Lichen planus pemphigoides evolving into pemphigoid nodularis. *Clin Exp Dermatol.* (2003) 28:613–6. doi: 10.1046/j.1365-2230.2003.01401.x
63. Miyagawa S, Ohi H, Muramatsu T, Okuchi T, Shirai T, Sakamoto K. Lichen planus pemphigoides-like lesions induced by cinnarizine. *Br J Dermatol.* (1985) 112:607–13. doi: 10.1111/j.1365-2133.1985.tb15272.x
64. Onprasert W, Chanprapaph K. Lichen planus pemphigoides induced by enalapril: a case report and a review of literature. *Case Rep Dermatol.* (2017) 9:217–24. doi: 10.1159/000481449
65. Xu H-H, Xiao T, He C-D, Jin G-Y, Wang Y-K, Gao X-H, et al. Lichen planus pemphigoides associated with Chinese herbs. *Clin Exp Dermatol.* (2009) 34:329–32. doi: 10.1111/j.1365-2230.2008.02900.x
66. Rosmaninho A, Sanches M, Oliveira A, Alves R, Selores M. Lichen planus pemphigoides induced by a weight reduction drug. *Cutan Ocul Toxicol.* (2011) 30:306–8. doi: 10.3109/15569527.2011.566234
67. Ben Salem C, Chenguel L, Ghariani N, Denguezli M, Hmouda H, Bouraoui K. Captopril-induced lichen planus pemphigoides. *Pharmacoepidemiol Drug Saf.* (2008) 17:722–4. doi: 10.1002/pds.1618
68. Flageul B, Foldes C, Wallach D, Vignon-Pennamen MD, Cottenot F. Captopril-induced lichen planus pemphigoides with pemphigus-like features. A case report. *Dermatologica.* (1986) 173:248–55. doi: 10.1159/000249262
69. Stoebner P-E, Michot C, Ligeron C, Durand L, Meynadier J, Meunier L. [Simvastatin-induced lichen planus pemphigoides]. *Ann Dermatol Venereol.* (2003) 130:187–90.
70. Schmidgen MI, Butsch F, Schadmand-Fischer S, Steinbrink K, Grabbe S, Weidenthaler-Barth B, et al. Pembrolizumab-induced lichen planus pemphigoides in a patient with metastatic melanoma. *J Dtsch Dermatol Ges J Ger Soc Dermatol.* (2017) 15:742–5. doi: 10.1111/ddg.13272
71. Kuramoto N, Kishimoto S, Shibagaki R, Yasuno H. PUVA-induced lichen planus pemphigoides. *Br J Dermatol.* (2000) 142:509–12. doi: 10.1046/j.1365-2133.2000.03366.x
72. Ilknur T, Akarsu S, Uzun S, Özer E, Fetil E. Heterogeneous disease: a child case of lichen planus pemphigoides triggered by varicella. *J Dermatol.* (2011) 38:707–10. doi: 10.1111/j.1346-8138.2011.01220.x
73. Mohanarao TS, Kumar GA, Chennamsetty K, Priyadarshini T. Childhood lichen planus pemphigoides triggered by chickenpox. *Indian Dermatol Online J.* (2014) 5:S98–100. doi: 10.4103/2229-5178.146169
74. Ogg GS, Bhogal BS, Hashimoto T, Coleman R, Barker JN. Ramipril-associated lichen planus pemphigoides. *Br J Dermatol.* (1997) 136:412–4. doi: 10.1111/j.1365-2133.1997.tb14956.x
75. Demirçay Z, Baykal C, Demirkesen C. Lichen planus pemphigoides: report of two cases. *Int J Dermatol.* (2001) 40:757–9. doi: 10.1046/j.1365-4362.2001.01334.x
76. Laureano A, Rafael M, Marques Pinto G, Cardoso J. Lichen planus pemphigoides possibly induced by hormone therapy. *Eur J Dermatol.* (2013) 23:903–4. doi: 10.1684/ejd.2013.2180
77. Jang SH, Yun SJ, Lee SC, Lee JB. Lichen planus pemphigoides associated with chronic hepatitis B virus infection. *Clin Exp Dermatol.* (2015) 40:868–71. doi: 10.1111/ced.12530

78. Flageul B, Hassan F, Pinquier L, Blanchet-Bardon C, Dubertret L. [Lichen pemphigoid associated with developing hepatitis B in a child]. *Ann Dermatol Venereol.* (1999) 126:604–7.
79. Evans SJ, Waller PC, Davis S. Use of proportional reporting ratios (PRRs) for signal generation from spontaneous adverse drug reaction reports. *Pharmacoepidemiol Drug Saf.* (2001) 10:483–6. doi: 10.1002/pds.677
80. Le Cleach L, Chosidow O. Clinical practice. Lichen planus. *N Engl J Med.* (2012) 366:723–32. doi: 10.1056/NEJMcp1103641
81. Alaizari NA, Al-Maweri SA, Al-Shamiri HM, Tarakji B, Shugaa-Addin B. Hepatitis C virus infections in oral lichen planus: a systematic review and meta-analysis. *Aust Dent J.* (2016) 61:282–7. doi: 10.1111/adj.12382
82. Hamada T, Fujimoto W, Okazaki F, Asagoe K, Arata J, Iwatsuki K. Lichen planus pemphigoides and multiple keratoacanthomas associated with colon adenocarcinoma. *Br J Dermatol.* (2004) 151:252–4. doi: 10.1111/j.1365-2133.2004.06074.x
83. George PM. Bullous pemphigoid possibly induced by psoralen plus ultraviolet A therapy. *Photodermatol Photoimmunol Photomed.* (1996) 11:185–7. doi: 10.1111/j.1600-0781.1995.tb00166.x
84. Lutowiecka-Wranicz A, Sysa-Jedrzejowska A, Skwarczynska-Banyś E. [Effect of drugs and ultraviolet rays on the development of pemphigoid]. *Przegl Dermatol.* (1980) 67:641–6.
85. Ohtani A, Takenaka Y, Ishiguro N, Kawashima M. Case of lichen planus induced by sitagliptin phosphate hydrate. *J Dermatol.* (2017) 44:1081–2. doi: 10.1111/1346-8138.13624
86. Swale VJ, McGregor JM. Amlodipine-associated lichen planus. *Br J Dermatol.* (2001) 144:920–1. doi: 10.1046/j.1365-2133.2001.04172.x
87. Ghosh S, Jain VK, Chaudhuri S, Mathur SK. Sulfasalazine induced lichen planus in a patient of rheumatoid arthritis. *Indian J Dermatol Venereol Leprol.* (2013) 79:541–4. doi: 10.4103/0378-6323.113103
88. Zheng Y, Zhang J, Chen H, Lai W, Maibach HI. Terbinafine-induced lichenoid drug eruption. *Cutan Ocul Toxicol.* (2017) 36:101–3. doi: 10.3109/15569527.2016.1160101
89. Woo V, Bonks J, Borukhova L, Zegarelli D. Oral lichenoid drug eruption: a report of a pediatric case and review of the literature. *Pediatr Dermatol.* (2009) 26:458–64. doi: 10.1111/j.1525-1470.2009.00953.x
90. Varpuluoma O, Försti A-K, Jokelainen J, Turpeinen M, Timonen M, Huilaja L, et al. Vildagliptin significantly increases the risk of bullous pemphigoid: a finnish nationwide registry study. *J Invest Dermatol.* (2018) 138:1659–61. doi: 10.1016/j.jid.2018.01.027
91. Kolb-Mäurer A, Sitaru C, Rose C, Bröcker E-B, Goebeler M, Zillikens D. [Treatment of lichen planus pemphigoides with acitretin and pulsed corticosteroids]. *Hautarzt.* (2003) 54:268–73. doi: 10.1007/s00105-002-0459-0
92. Hackländer K, Lehmann P, Hofmann SC. Successful treatment of lichen planus pemphigoides using acitretin as monotherapy: Clinical Letter. *J Dtsch Dermatol Ges.* (2014) 12:818–9. doi: 10.1111/ddg.12380
93. Davis AL, Bhocal BS, Whitehead P, Frith P, Murdoch ME, Leigh IM, et al. Lichen planus pemphigoides: its relationship to bullous pemphigoid. *Br J Dermatol.* (1991) 125:263–71. doi: 10.1111/j.1365-2133.1991.tb14753.x
94. Knisley RR, Petropolis AA, Mackey VT. Lichen Planus Pemphigoides Treated With Ustekinumab. *Cutis.* (2017) 100:415–418.
95. Malakar S, Saha A. Successful treatment of resistant lichen planus pemphigoides with cyclosporine: a new hope. *Indian J Dermatol.* (2016) 61:112–4. doi: 10.4103/0019-5154.174067
96. Washio K, Nakamura A, Fukuda S, Hashimoto T, Horikawa T. A case of lichen planus pemphigoides successfully treated with a combination of cyclosporine A and prednisolone. *Case Rep Dermatol.* (2013) 5:84–87. doi: 10.1159/000350285
97. Kabuto M, Fujimoto N, Yamaguchi A, Tanaka T. Evaluation of mononuclear cells in lichen planus pemphigoides. *Acta Derm Venereol.* (2016) 96:276–8. doi: 10.2340/00015555-2191
98. Cohen DM, Ben-Amitai D, Feinmesser M, Zvulunov A. Childhood lichen planus pemphigoides: a case report and review of the literature. *Pediatr Dermatol.* (2009) 26:569–74. doi: 10.1111/j.1525-1470.2009.00988.x
99. Goldscheider I, Herzinger T, Varga R, Eming R, Ruzicka T, Flaig MJ, et al. Childhood lichen planus pemphigoides: report of two cases treated successfully with systemic glucocorticoids and dapsone. *Pediatr Dermatol.* (2014) 31:751–3. doi: 10.1111/pde.12214
100. Conde Fernandes I, Pinto Almeida T, Mendes I, Cunha Velho G, Alves R, Selores M. Lichen planus pemphigoides in a child. *Eur J Dermatol.* (2012) 22:570–1. doi: 10.1684/ejd.2012.1764
101. von Stebut E, Steinbrink K, Bräuninger W. Lichen ruber pemphigoides. *Aktuelle Dermatol.* (2004) 30:73–6. doi: 10.1055/s-2004-814476
102. Duong B, Marks S, Sami N, Theos A. Lichen planus pemphigoides in a 2-year-old girl: response to treatment with methotrexate. *J Am Acad Dermatol.* (2012) 67:e154–6. doi: 10.1016/j.jaad.2011.12.024
103. Skvara H, Stingl G. Lichenoid eruption with single plantar blisters: a very rare case of lichen planus pemphigoides. *J Eur Acad Dermatol Venereol.* (2009) 23:596–7. doi: 10.1111/j.1468-3083.2008.02982.x
104. Loyal J, Rashtak S. Vulvar lichen planus pemphigoides. *Int J Womens Dermatol.* (2017) 3:225–7. doi: 10.1016/j.ijwd.2017.07.002
105. Shimada H, Shono T, Sakai T, Ishikawa K, Takeo N, Hatano Y, et al. Lichen planus pemphigoides concomitant with rectal adenocarcinoma: fortuitous or a true association? *Eur J Dermatol.* (2015) 25:501–3. doi: 10.1684/ejd.2015.2619
106. Jensen AØ, Steiniche T, Veien NK, Deleuran MS. Lichen planus pemphigoides in a 6-year-old child. *Acta Paediatr.* (2009) 98:2–3. doi: 10.1111/j.1651-2227.2008.01069.x
107. Solomon LW, Helm TN, Stevens C, Neiders ME, Kumar V. Clinical and immunopathologic findings in oral lichen planus pemphigoides. *Oral Surg Oral Med Oral Pathol Oral Radiol Endodontol.* (2007) 103:808–13. doi: 10.1016/j.tripleo.2006.03.020
108. Harjai B, Mendiratta V, Kakkar S, Koranne R. Childhood lichen planus pemphigoides - a rare entity. *J Eur Acad Dermatol Venereol.* (2006) 20:117–8. doi: 10.1111/j.1468-3083.2005.01346.x
109. Zhu YI, Fitzpatrick JE, Kornfeld BW, Fitzpatrick JE. Lichen planus pemphigoides associated with ramipril. *Int J Dermatol.* (2006) 45:1453–5. doi: 10.1111/j.1365-4632.2006.02711.x
110. Fine JD. Management of acquired bullous skin diseases. *N Engl J Med.* (1995) 333:1475–84. doi: 10.1056/NEJM199511303332207
111. Joly P, Roujeau J-C, Benichou J, Picard C, Dreno B, Delaporte E, et al. A comparison of oral and topical corticosteroids in patients with bullous pemphigoid. *N Engl J Med.* (2002) 346:321–7. doi: 10.1056/NEJMoa011592
112. Recke A, Schmidt E, Zillikens D, Shimanovich I. Lichen planus pemphigoides. *J. Deusch. Dermatol. Gesellschaft* 9(Suppl. 1):251–5. doi: 10.1111/j.1610-0387.2011.07633.x
113. Suvorov VA. [Lichen ruber planus pemphigoides in a patient treated by hypnotic suggestion]. *Sov Med.* (1959) 23:112–3.

3

Serological Diagnosis of Autoimmune Bullous Skin Diseases

Sandra Saschenbrecker, Ingolf Karl, Lars Komorowski, Christian Probst, Cornelia Dähnrich, Kai Fechner, Winfried Stöcker and Wolfgang Schlumberger*

Institute for Experimental Immunology, Euroimmun AG, Lübeck, Germany

***Correspondence:**
Sandra Saschenbrecker
s.saschenbrecker@euroimmun.de

Autoimmune bullous dermatoses (AIBD) encompass a variety of organ-specific autoimmune diseases that manifest with cutaneous and/or mucosal blisters and erosions. They are characterized by autoantibodies targeting structural proteins of the skin, which are responsible for the intercellular contact between epidermal keratinocytes and for adhesion of the basal keratinocytes to the dermis. The autoantibodies disrupt the adhesive functions, leading to splitting and blister formation. In pemphigus diseases, blisters form intraepidermally, whereas in all other disease types they occur subepidermally. Early identification of autoimmune bullous dermatoses is crucial for both treatment and prognosis, particularly as regards tumor-associated disease entities. The diagnosis is based on clinical symptoms, histopathology, direct immunofluorescence to detect antibody/complement deposits, and the determination of circulating autoantibodies. The identification of various target antigens has paved the way for the recent development of numerous specific autoantibody tests. In particular, optimized designer antigens and multiplex test formats for indirect immunofluorescence and ELISA have enhanced and refined the laboratory analysis, enabling highly efficient serodiagnosis and follow-up. This review elaborates on the current standards in the serological diagnostics for autoimmune bullous dermatoses.

Keywords: autoantibody, autoimmune bullous dermatosis, biochip, ELISA, indirect immunofluorescence, pemphigoid, pemphigus, serology

INTRODUCTION

Autoimmune bullous dermatoses (AIBD) are associated with autoantibodies that bind to structural proteins in the skin and mucous membranes, which are components of desmosomes (e.g., desmogleins, desmocollins, plakins) and hemidesmosomes (e.g., BP180, BP230, plectin, $\alpha6\beta4$ integrin, laminin 332, laminin $\gamma1$, type VII collagen) [**Figure 1**, (1)]. These autoimmune reactions interfere with intercellular connections and anchoring mechanisms within the epidermis and dermal-epidermal junction, leading to the separation of skin layers and the formation of blisters and/or erosions (2, 3). The most important AIBD types and corresponding target antigens are summarized in **Table 1**.

Intraepidermal Blistering Diseases

In pemphigus diseases, the autoimmune system targets primarily the cadherin-type transmembrane adhesion molecules desmoglein (Dsg) 1 and 3. Desmogleins, together with desmocollins, provide cohesion between epidermal keratinocytes, and are linked intracellularly to the intermediate filament network via different types of plakins (**Figure 1**). In response to

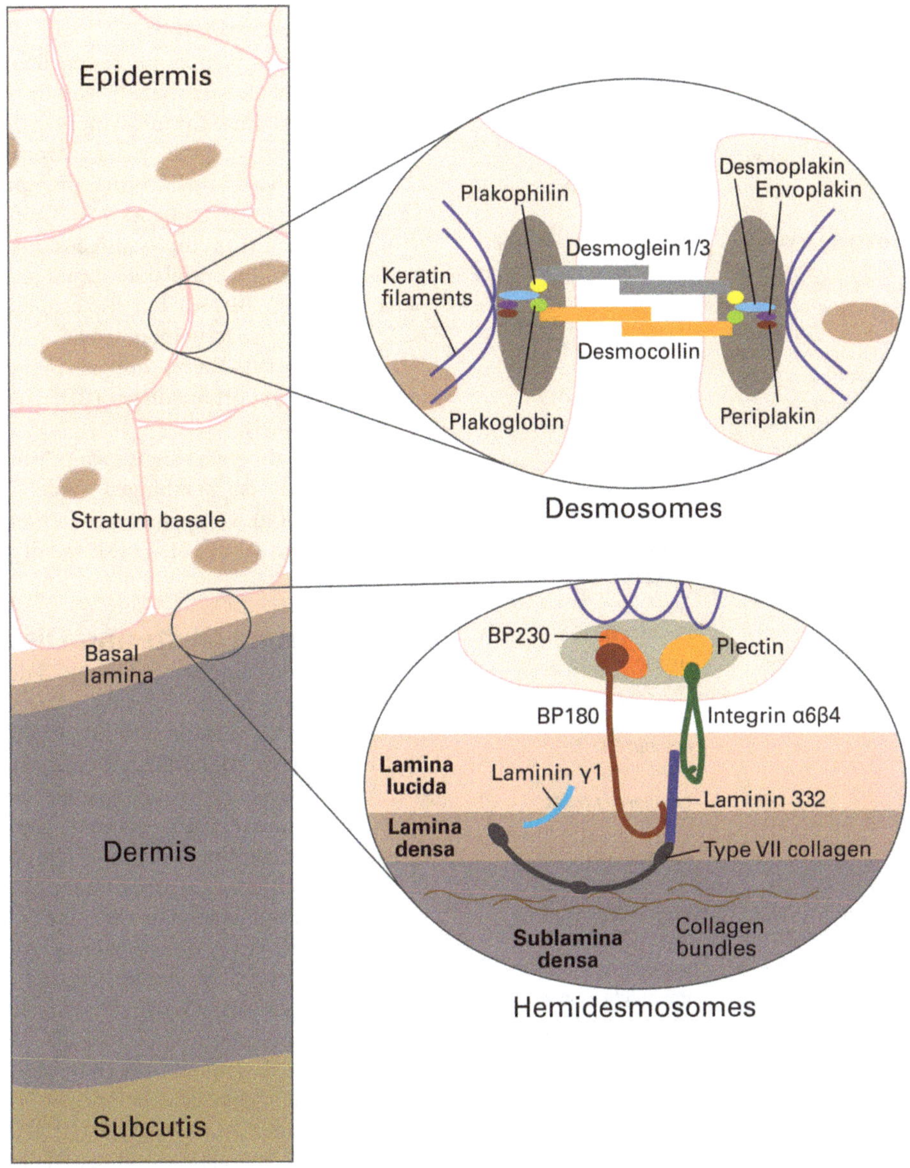

FIGURE 1 | Schematic presentation of human skin, depicting the targets of autoantibodies in autoimmune bullous dermatoses, reproduced from Gosink and Schlumberger, MEDLAB Magazine 2016 (1) with permission of MEDLAB Magazine. Top circle: antigenic structural components of desmosomes, which interconnect the cytoskeletons of neighboring keratinocytes in the epidermis. Bottom circle: antigenic structural components of hemidesmosomes, which anchor the cells of the epidermal stratum basale in the underlying basal lamina at the dermal-epidermal junction.

autoantibody binding, cell metabolism, intracellular signaling and desmosome structure are subject to alterations that cause the loss of cell-to-cell adhesion (acantholysis) and intra-epidermal split formation, resulting in flaccid blisters and erosions in the skin and/or mucous membranes (4, 5).

The clinical phenotype of pemphigus (i.e., the site of blister formation) is determined by the underlying antibody profile and the normal tissue distribution of Dsg1 and Dsg3. Dsg1 is predominantly expressed on the surface of the epidermis, whereas Dsg3 accumulates mainly in deeper epidermal layers and in the mucous membranes. As pemphigus foliaceus (PF) is associated only with IgG autoantibodies against Dsg1, blistering is confined to the upper skin, while there is no apparent mucosal involvement. In pemphigus vulgaris (PV), Dsg3 is the major autoantigen, but 50–60% of patients have additional autoantibodies to Dsg1. PV manifests as three different subtypes (2): [i] in mucosal-dominant PV, antibodies are restricted to Dsg3 and induce blisters in deep layers of the oral mucosa; [ii] patients with mucocutaneous PV exhibit reactivity against both Dsg1 and Dsg3 and show involvement of the epidermis in addition to the mucous membranes; [iii] the cutaneous PV type is less frequent and associated with blistering in deep epidermal layers owing to anti-Dsg1 and pathogenically weak anti-Dsg3. In contrast to PF, acantholysis takes place in the lower skin layers (2, 6–11). PV is

TABLE 1 | Autoantibody specificities in autoimmune bullous dermatoses.

Blistering	Disease	Ig type	Target antigen[a,b,c]
Intra-epidermal	Pemphigus foliaceus	IgG	**Dsg1**
	Pemphigus vulgaris	IgG	**Dsg3**, Dsg1
	IgA pemphigus	IgA	**Dsg1, Dsg3, *Dsc1***, *Dsc2, Dsc3*
	Paraneoplastic pemphigus	IgG	**Dsg3**, Dsg1, **envoplakin**, ***periplakin***, *desmoplakin I, desmoplakin II, epiplakin, plectin*, BP230, *Dsc1, Dsc2, Dsc3, α2-macroglobulin-like protein 1*
	Pemphigus vegetans	IgG	Dsg3, Dsg1, *Dsc3*
	Pemphigus erythematosus	IgG	Dsg1
	Pemphigus herpetiformis	IgG	**Dsg1**, Dsg3, *Dsc1*, *Dsc3*
	Drug-induced pemphigus	IgG	**Dsg1**, Dsg3
Sub-epidermal	Bullous pemphigoid	IgG	**BP180***, BP230
	Pemphigoid gestationis	IgG	**BP180***, BP230
	Linear IgA dermatosis	IgA	***BP180***$^{**/***}$, BP180*, BP230
	Mucous membrane pemphigoid	IgG/IgA	*BP180*****, BP180*, ***laminin 332***, BP230, *α6β4 integrin*
	Anti-laminin γ1/p200 pemphigoid	IgG	***Laminin γ1 (p200)***
	Lichen planus pemphigoides	IgG	**BP180***, BP230
	Epidermolysis bullosa acquisita	IgG	**Type VII collagen**
	Dermatitis herpetiformis	IgA (IgG)	**Epidermal transglutaminase**, tissue transglutaminase, endomysium, deamidated gliadin

[a] *Main target antigens are indicated in bold.*

[b] *Parameters for which commercial monospecific detection assays are not available are indicated in italics.*

[c] *Immunodominant regions: Dsg1: N-terminal ectodomain, Dsg3: N-terminal ectodomain, BP180: *NC16A/**LABD97/***LAD-1/****C-terminal epitopes; BP230: globular C-terminal domain; type VII collagen: N-terminal NC1 domain.*

the most frequent intraepidermal AIBD, accounting for 80% of all pemphigus cases and, for the most part, affecting middle-aged and elderly persons.

In patients with PV, numerous autoantibodies have been identified that target other structural and metabolic proteins, such as desmocollins (Dsc) 1 and 3, muscarinic and nicotinic acetylcholine receptors, mitochondrial antigens, thyroid peroxidase, hSPCA1, plakophilin 3, plakoglobin, and E-cadherin. Studies on the pathogenic role of some of these non-Dsg autoantibodies suggest that they synergistically complement the classic effects of anti-Dsg autoantibodies in the complex process of pemphigus pathogenesis (12–15).

IgA pemphigus (also referred to as "intercellular IgA dermatosis") (16, 17) has been found in association with serum IgA reactivity against desmosomal cadherins, i.e., Dsc1, Dsc2, Dsc3, Dsg1, and Dsg3 (18–21).

Paraneoplastic pemphigus is a life-threatening form of pemphigus that is associated with a neoplasm (e.g., non-Hodgkin's lymphoma, chronic lymphocytic leukemia, Castleman tumor, thymoma, sarcoma, Waldenstrom's macroglobulinemia) (22). Pathogenesis is based on a combination of humoral and cellular autoimmune responses (23). Circulating autoantibodies are directed against multiple antigens, including predominantly plakins (envoplakin, periplakin, desmoplakin I, desmoplakin II, epiplakin, plectin, BP230), but also cadherins (Dsg3, Dsg1, Dsc1, Dsc2, Dsc3), α2-macroblobulin-like 1 (24–34). Due to their high specificity (91–100%), anti-envoplakin autoantibodies are considered an important diagnostic marker for paraneoplastic pemphigus (35–38).

In addition, the pemphigus group includes several (atypical) variants, such as pemphigus vegetans (39), pemphigus erythematosus (40, 41), pemphigus herpetiformis (42), endemic pemphigus (fogo selvage etc.) (43), and drug-induced pemphigus (44, 45).

Subepidermal Blistering Diseases

The heterogenous group of pemphigoid diseases is characterized by subepidermal blister formation, which can occur in the skin and mucous membranes (3). Circulating autoantibodies target components of the dermal-epidermal junction (**Figure 1**) (46). As the targeted hemidesmosomal proteins and structural filaments provide contact between the epidermal cells and the basement membrane, the autoimmune reactions cause the epidermis to peel away from the underlying dermis.

Bullous pemphigoid (BP) is the most common AIBD and occurs primarily in the elderly (onset in the late 70s) (47). It manifests with tense, bulging blisters on inflamed or non-inflamed skin, while mucous membranes are rarely affected. Patient serum contains IgG targeting mainly the hemidesmosomal proteins BP180 and BP230. BP180 is a transmembrane glycoprotein whose major immunogenic epitopes are located in the extracellular 16th non-collagenous domain (BP180-NC16A) (48). Due to their high prevalence, anti-BP180 autoantibodies represent the most important serological marker for BP. BP230 is a cytoplasmic protein which interacts with BP180. Its globular C-terminal domain mediates the attachment of keratin filaments to the hemidesmosomal plaque and contains the majority of immunoreactive sequences (49). Anti-BP230 positivity occurs in a subset of anti-BP180 negative BP patients, making it an important additional marker (50–54). Many BP sera also exhibit reactivity against antigenic sites outside the immunodominant domains of BP180 and BP230, which should be addressed in those BP patients unreactive with the immunodominant domains (<10%) (52, 55).

Pemphigoid gestationis is a manifestation of BP occurring in pregnant women and in puerperium, presenting with urticarial plaques and/or tense blisters. BP180-NC16A is the main target (90%) of autoantibodies in patients with pemphigoid gestationis, while anti-BP230 reactivity is less prevalent (56, 57).

The serological hallmark in linear IgA dermatosis is anti-basement membrane reactivity of class IgA autoantibodies recognizing the 120 kDa ectodomain fragment of BP180, referred to as linear IgA disease antigen 1 (LAD-1) and a derivative thereof (linear IgA bullous disease antigen of 97 kDa, LABD97) (58–61). A small proportion of sera recognizes BP180-NC16A or BP230 (62–64).

Mucous membrane pemphigoid affects one or more mucous membranes (e.g., oral, ocular, genital, anal) and may also involve the skin. Patients exhibit low-titer IgG/IgA autoantibodies directed against components of the basement membrane zone, with BP180 and laminin 332 presenting the two major targets (65). Anti-BP180 reactivity is not only directed against the NC16A domain, but also against C-terminal extracellular epitopes (66–69). The identification of anti-laminin 332 positive patients is vitally important as they have an increased relative risk for cancer, with malignancies occurring in about 25–30% of cases (70–73). Furthermore, patients with mucous membrane pemphigoid may exhibit increased IgG/IgA against BP230 (74, 75) or α6β4 integrin, the latter indicating the presence of ocular lesions (76, 77).

In anti-laminin γ1/p200 pemphigoid, tense blisters can be found on erythematosus or normal skin, with a high tendency to affect acral surfaces (78, 79). The associated autoantibodies target a 200-kDa basement membrane protein, referred to as laminin γ1 (80, 81).

Lichen planus pemphigoides emerges with bullous skin lesions in conjunction with lichen planus. Compared to BP, this disease has a much lower incidence, affects younger patients (onset 40–50 years), is usually less severe and arises mainly on the limbs (82). Serum reactivity is preferentially directed against C-terminal epitopes in the immunodominant NC16A domain of BP180 (83, 84).

Epidermolysis bullosa acquisita (EBA) is a rare, subepidermal blistering disease that can occur at any age. Patients suffer from chronic inflammation, blistering and scarring of the skin and mucous membranes. (85, 86). A characteristic feature is the presence of autoantibodies directed against type VII collagen, the main constituent of anchoring fibrils at the dermal-epidermal junction, with the major antigenic epitopes located within the amino-terminal non-collagenous domain (NC1) (87–90).

Dermatitis herpetiformis (Duhring's disease) is the cutaneous manifestation of coeliac disease (sprue, gluten-sensitive enteropathy), affecting about 10% of coeliac patients. It is characterized by blisters forming in deeper (subepidermal) layers of the skin, while the mucous membranes do not show any blistering. The targets of circulating IgA antibodies are epidermal/tissue transglutaminase, endomysium, and deamidated gliadin (91–95). Since the underlying gluten-sensitive enteropathy is frequently associated with selective IgA deficiency, the additional determination of class IgG antibodies can be diagnostically indicated (96).

DIAGNOSTIC APPROACH

The diagnosis of AIBD is detailed in recent publications (97–104). Commonly recommended approaches are based on several pillars that cover symptomatic evaluation and laboratory tests.

Firstly, the clinical characteristics have to be determined, including patient history, physical examination, and assessment of the disease activity (105).

Secondly, histopathology is performed on lesional skin or mucosal biopsy. Although of limited diagnostic value, the observation of intra-/subepidermal cleavage and inflammatory infiltrates can give a first information for differentiation between pemphigus and pemphigoid diseases.

Thirdly, direct immunofluorescence (DIF) microscopy using cryosections of perilesional biopsy specimens is performed to detect tissue-bound autoantibodies. This method is still the diagnostic gold standard, with a sensitivity in the range of 82–91% and a specificity of 98% (106–110), but it provides only limited information on the target antigens. DIF microscopy narrows down the diagnosis according to the deposited Ig subclass and binding pattern (103). For example, intercellular deposition of IgG and/or C3 in the epidermis is characteristic of PV, PF, and paraneoplastic pemphigus. By contrast, linear binding of IgG and/or C3 at the dermal-epidermal junction can be found in pemphigoid diseases, with further differentiation options based on the serration pattern (u-serration vs. n-serration) (103, 111). Granular IgA deposits along the basement membrane zone and at the dermal papillae tips are observed in dermatitis herpetiformis.

The fourth pillar addresses the serological detection and differentiation of circulating autoantibodies. Serology has the advantage of being minimally invasive, which is particularly helpful in cases where biopsy specimens cannot be obtained (children, uncooperative adults). In many cases, serological testing may even suffice to establish the diagnosis in conjunction with a compatible clinical picture (112). Serum analysis relies on indirect immunofluorescence (IIF) microscopy using native tissue sections and recombinant proteins as substrates. Recombinant antigens are also applied in immunoblot or immunoprecipitation analyses and in enzyme-linked immunosorbent assays (ELISA), the latter having additional relevance to the monitoring of disease activity. Conventionally, the serological diagnosis of AIBD follows a multi-step approach that is based on initial IIF screening using one or two tissue substrates, followed by individual antigen-specific assays (ELISA, immunoblot) that correspond to the clinical suspicion and the IIF screening results. Meanwhile, alternative approaches for highly efficient and expeditious testing are available utilizing multiparametric analysis tools (113, 114). In clinical practice, routine serological results should be interpreted with care, taking into consideration the possibility of discrepancies between IIF and ELISA or negative serology in biopsy-proven patients. Assay results may even be positive in cases without other laboratory or clinical evidence of pemphigus (109, 115). Such inconsistent findings complicate decision-making, bearing the risk of misdiagnosis. Where available, alternative serological methods (e.g., keratinocyte binding assay) may provide additional information to ascertain or rule out a diagnosis, especially when no biopsy is available (115).

Early diagnosis and differentiation of AIBD is crucial for the initiation of an appropriate treatment. In most AIBD entities (e.g., BP, linear IgA disease, anti-laminin γ1/p200 pemphigoid), systemic corticosteroids in combination with further immunosuppressants/-modulants are sufficient to induce clinical remission, whereas treatment of pemphigus remains challenging as reflected by a mortality of 8–42% in mucocutaneous PV (116). However, prognosis has improved due to the development of new therapy options, including immunoadsorption, intravenous immunoglobulins, and anti-CD20 monoclonal antibodies (2, 112, 116–124). In paraneoplastic pemphigus and anti-laminin 332 mucous membrane pemphigoid, the disease prognosis may be unfavorable due to associated neoplasia in 100% and in up to 30% of cases, respectively (73, 125).

SEROLOGICAL SCREENING USING TISSUE SUBSTRATES IN IIF

IIF microscopy using tissue substrates has traditionally been performed as a standard method for the detection of autoantibodies in AIBD. Due to their high sensitivity, these substrates have priority for screening purposes. However, they do not allow definite determination of the autoantibodies' specificity (e.g., differentiation between anti-Dsg1 and anti-Dsg3).

Esophagus

Esophagus from monkey or guinea pig is a highly sensitive substrate. Two characteristic immunofluorescence patterns can be differentiated on this tissue. [i] Pemphigus-specific autoantibodies result in a honeycomb-like fluorescence of the intercellular substance in the stratum spinosum. These autoantibodies are directed against prickle cell desmosomes, reacting with surface antigens of keratinocytes (**Figure 2A**). [ii] A fine linear staining between the stratum basale and the connective tissue is caused by anti-basement membrane zone autoantibodies, which are associated with pemphigoid diseases or EBA (**Figure 2B**).

When pemphigus serum is applied, monkey esophagus yields a sensitivity of 81–100% and a specificity of 89–100%, making it the optimal substrate in the screening for intercellular antibodies in suspected cases of PV and PF (113, 126–132). This substrate has often been reported to be more sensitive for PV than for PF as monkey esophagus is a mucosal tissue with high expression of Dsg3, the major target in PV, in contrast to lower Dsg1 expression (132). The predictive value of a negative test result is highly reliable to exclude the diagnosis of pemphigus, and false-positive results (intercellular staining of non-pemphigus sera) is not associated with an increased risk of developing pemphigus subsequently (132). In BP, 68–73% of cases were reported positive for anti-basement zone antibodies, at a specificity of 97% (51, 106, 133). It should be taken into account that antibodies against blood group antigens A and B may lead to unspecific desmosome fluorescence on monkey esophagus, potentially leading to false positive results. As this interference may account for up to 10% of healthy blood donors, adsorption reagents should be applied in suspected cases (e.g., blocking with soluble A/B antigens or with red blood cells from an AB-positive donor) (134).

Salt-Split Skin

Skin, in which partial dermal-epidermal splitting is induced by incubation with a 1 M NaCl solution, presents the IIF substrate of choice when screening for autoantibodies in subepidermal AIBD (135, 136). It is optimally suited for the detection of anti-basement membrane zone autoantibodies, as reflected by a reported sensitivity of 73–96% and a specificity of 97% (106, 108, 133, 137). In addition, it allows the differentiation between autoantibodies with different antigenic binding properties. Anti-BP180, anti-BP230, and anti-α6β4 integrin stain the epidermal side of the artificial split (blister roof), as detectable in BP, pemphigoid gestationis, linear IgA dermatosis, and anti-BP180-type mucous membrane pemphigoid (**Figure 2C**). In contrast, anti-type VII collagen, anti-laminin 332, and anti-laminin γ1 bind along the dermal side of the split (blister floor), pointing toward EBA, anti-laminin-332-type mucous membrane pemphigoid, and anti-laminin γ1/p200 pemphigoid, respectively (**Figure 2D**) (100, 138).

Urinary Bladder

In suspected cases of paraneoplastic pemphigus, IIF on rat (or monkey) urinary bladder is performed to detect autoantibodies against plakins and to distinguish paraneoplastic pemphigus from other pemphigus diseases. As envoplakin, periplakin, and desmoplakins (but not Dsg1 and Dsg3) are highly expressed in bladder tissue, and owing to the high specificity of this substrate (74% sensitivity, 99–100% specificity), positive IgG reactivity with the urothelium is considered a diagnostic indication of paraneoplastic pemphigus (38, 139) (**Figure 2E**). However, negative IIF on bladder does not exclude the diagnosis of paraneoplastic pemphigus and should entail other serological techniques (36, 38).

Liver

Tissue sections of primate liver are best suited to visualize autoantibodies (IgA) against endomysium in dermatitis herpetiformis. Positive reactivity is indicated by a fluorescent filamentous lining of the intralobular sinusoids (140) (**Figure 2F**).

ANTIGEN-SPECIFIC SEROLOGICAL ASSAYS

The identification of the autoantibodies' target antigens can be accomplished using monospecific IIF, ELISA and/or immunoblot tests. For this purpose, many antigenic substrates have been made available by means of recombinant expression systems. By selecting only immunoreactive epitopes and deleting domains that cause unspecific reactions, the sensitivity and specificity of the resulting assay can often be improved (141). For example, a recombinant tetramer of the immunodominant NC16A domain of BP180, termed BP180-NC16A-4X, was designed to multiply the number of antibody binding sites per molecule, thereby optimizing the immunoreactivity and diagnostic efficiency in BP serology. A second example concerns a gliadin-analogous fusion peptide (GAF-3X), which contains three repetitive modified copies of formerly described peptides recognized

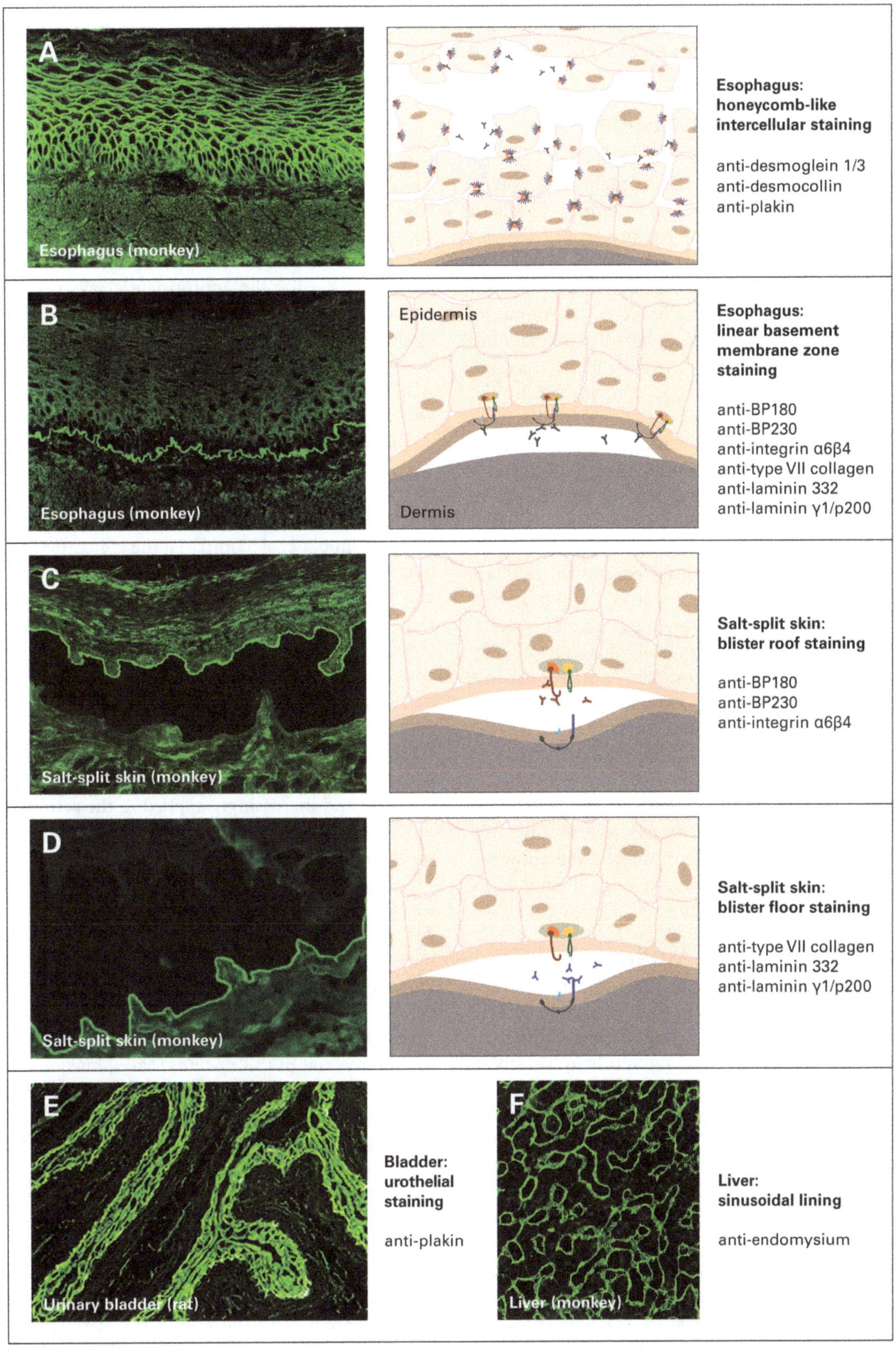

FIGURE 2 | Indirect immunofluorescence staining of different tissue substrates in autoimmune bullous dermatoses. **(A,B)** Monkey esophagus, **(C,D)** monkey salt-split skin, **(E)** rat urinary bladder and **(F)** monkey liver. Graphics and annotations on the right indicate the staining patterns and possible underlying reactivities, reproduced and modified from Euroimmun customer leaflet, with permission of Euroimmun, Germany.

by autoantibodies in most patients with coeliac disease and dermatitis herpetiformis (142). After expression and purification from *Escherichia coli*, those two antigens were applied in IIF and ELISA (142–145).

Recombinant Monospecific Substrates in IIF

Compared to classic tissue sections that contain a multitude of different antigens and sometimes require specialist knowledge for reliable interpretation, recombinant substrates considerably simplify IIF evaluation and may allow a *prima vista* differentiation between AIBD-associated diseases. Recombinant IIF assays are based on BIOCHIP technology (Euroimmun, Lübeck, Germany), in which the substrates are coated onto millimeter-sized BIOCHIPs and arranged on the reaction fields of microscope slides. The slides are incubated using the Titerplane technique, which provides parallel incubation of multiple samples under standardized, identical conditions (146). Two types of recombinant IIF substrates can be distinguished:

In the first case, the target antigen is expressed in the human cell line HEK293, which provides authentic conformational folding and post-translational modification (141, 147). Since transfected and mock-transfected control cells are coated onto the BIOCHIPs side by side, it is straightforward to distinguish true-positive sera containing antigen-specific antibodies (smooth to fine granular cytosolic fluorescence only in the subset of transfected cells) from sera reacting against other cell components (nuclear or cytoplasmic staining of all cells). Available recombinant cell-based substrates for AIBD serology include Dsg1, Dsg3, BP230, and type VII collagen (**Figures 3A–D**) (144, 149).

In the second case, purified recombinant antigens (e.g., BP180-NC16A-4X and GAF-3X) are coated directly onto the BIOCHIPs. If a positive serum sample is applied, the antigenic areas will fluoresce in a particular pattern (e.g., diamonds or circles) against a dark background (**Figures 3E,F**).

Multiparametric BIOCHIP Mosaics in IIF

The recombinant monospecific IIF substrates can be analyzed side by side with classic tissue sections in standardized BIOCHIP mosaics (Euroimmun; **Figure 4**). The combination of different substrates in the same test field allows autoantibody screening and confirmatory discrimination to be carried out in a single incubation, thus facilitating differential diagnosis among the various types of AIBD. Particularly in diagnostically difficult cases, this multiparametric technique is cost- and time-effective compared to the conventional multi-step approach (113, 150).

Several studies have been performed on the diagnostic performance of the mosaic-based IIF technique. Cumulative findings indicate that this method is highly sensitive and specific for pemphigus and BP (150–152). For example, monkey esophagus yielded sensitivities of 83–100% (PV), 98% (PF), and 69% (mixed pemphigus panel), with specificities in the range of 89–100%. Anti-Dsg1 was detectable with a sensitivity of 19–52% (PV), 90% (PF), and 38% (mixed pemphigus panel) and a specificity of ≥99%. The sensitivity of anti-Dsg3 detection amounted to 98–100% (PV) and 87% (mixed pemphigus panel), with specificities ranging from 97 to 100% (113, 152–154). In BP, basement membrane zone staining on esophagus and/or salt-split skin provided a sensitivity and specificity of 50–99 and 77–100%, respectively. The sensitivity and specificity for anti-BP180 detection were reported to be 83–100 and 97–100%, respectively, and for anti-BP230 detection 30–67 and 97–100%, respectively (113, 144, 152, 154, 155). van Beek et al. (113) compared the performance of the "Dermatology Mosaic 7" (**Figure 4A**) with the conventional multi-step procedure (156). Between both approaches, high diagnostic agreement (94%, kappa 0.88–0.97) was observed. In <5% of the cases, final diagnosis could only be made by using the appropriate assays within the multi-step approach, because additional substrates would have to be added to the standard IIF mosaic for these rare disorders. Meanwhile, however, further mosaics adjusted to the diagnosis of particular AIBD types have been evaluated, including the detection of [i] anti-BP180 in pemphigus gestationis (100% sensitivity, 100% specificity) (157), [ii] anti-type VII collagen NC1 in EBA (92% sensitivity, 100% specificity) (149), [iii] anti-laminin 332 in mucous membrane pemphigoid (77–84% sensitivity, 100% specificity) (72), and [iv] anti-Dsc in atypical pemphigus variants (158). Tampoia et al. compared the concordance between results obtained by mosaic-based IIF vs. ELISA (MBL/Euroimmun) and found excellent agreements for the determination of anti-Dsg3 (kappa 0.97–1.00) and anti-BP180 (kappa 0.94–0.90) (154). Özkesici et al. reported correlations between mosaic-based IIF and ELISA (Euroimmun) of 85% (anti-Dsg1), 94% (anti-Dsg3), and 98% (anti-BP180) (152).

Enzyme-Linked Immunosorbent Assays

ELISA systems based on recombinant target antigens are widely available and increasingly applied in the serological diagnosis of AIBD. They are used to confirm and differentiate autoantibody specificities, supporting the diagnostic attribution of AIBD subtypes. Moreover, ELISA allow quantitative measurement of antibody levels, enabling disease and therapy monitoring, as described below. In most cases, ELISA are sufficient to support the diagnosis and cheaper than other complex techniques. Further advantages include standardization, objective data, easy handling, automated processing, high throughput, and (for most parameters) commercial availability.

Commercial ELISA systems (MBL, Euroimmun) are available for the detection of autoantibodies against Dsg1 and Dsg3 in pemphigus (147, 159) and against envoplakin in paraneoplastic pemphigus (36). In pemphigoid diseases, commercial ELISA (MBL, Euroimmun) include BP180 (143, 160), BP230 (50, 54), and type VII collagen (149, 161). Importantly, the highest detection rate among BP patients is achieved by combining the ELISA results for anti-BP180 and anti-BP230 (87–100%), reflecting a diagnostic added value compared to mere anti-BP180 testing (50–54). Therefore, in cases with clinically suspected cases of BP, where anti-BP180 testing is negative, it is recommended to analyze serum reactivity against BP230 (97). Moreover, ELISA for the detection of autoantibodies against deamidated gliadin and transglutaminase (92) are available, supporting the diagnosis of dermatitis herpetiformis. Besides, less standardized in-house ELISA systems are applied in specialized laboratories, including

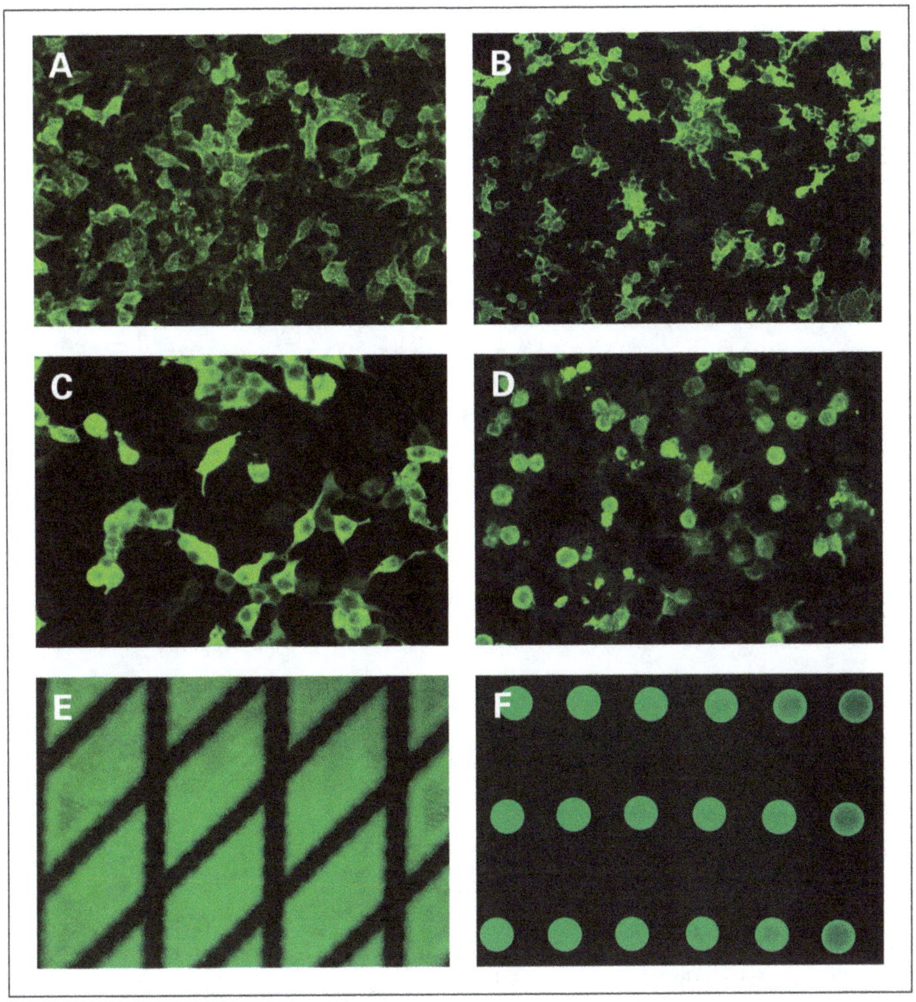

FIGURE 3 | Detection and differentiation of autoantibodies in autoimmune bullous dermatoses using monospecific substrates for BIOCHIP-based indirect immunofluorescence, reproduced (in part) from Gosink and Schlumberger, MEDLAB Magazine 2016 (1) and from Gosink, MEDLAB Magazine 2013 (148) with permission of MEDLAB Magazine. **(A–D)** Substrates based on human embryonic kidney (HEK293) cells expressing recombinant immunodominant antigen domains: **(A)** Dsg1 (ectodomain), **(B)** Dsg3 (ectodomain), **(C)** BP230gC (globular C-terminal domain), **(D)** type VII collagen (NC1 domain). **(E,F)** Substrates generated by spotting purified recombinant protein: **(E)** BP180-NC16A-4X (tetrameric NC16A domain), **(F)** GAF-3X (trimeric deamidated gliadin-analogous fusion peptide).

rare parameters, such as anti-laminin γ1 (162), anti-desmocollin (20, 33), anti-laminin 332 (71, 163), and anti-BP180 (various forms) (52, 164). The diagnostic performance of commercial and in-house ELISA systems has been examined in numerous studies (**Table 2**) and discussed in reviews by Tampoia et al. (190) and Horvath et al. (165).

Although being highly sensitive and specific, ELISA may produce positive results without clinical or other laboratory evidence.

Multiparametric ELISA

In order to further improve and accelerate the routine serological diagnosis of AIBD, two profile ELISA systems have been developed that enable multiparametric antigen-specific testing for autoantibodies in adjacent wells of a microplate. By simultaneous processing of the diagnostically most relevant antigens, multiplex ELISA offer an alternative to IIF as serological first-line approach and to a multi-step single testing strategy.

Horvath et al. analyzed the diagnostic performance of the MESACUP Anti-Skin Profile (MBL), which covers five target antigens: Dsgl, Dsg3, BP180, BP230, and type VII collagen. They reported a 88% concordance with data obtained from the respective individual ELISA systems (MBL), resulting in sensitivities of 92% (anti-Dsgl, PF), 93% (anti-Dsg3, PV), 66% (anti-BP180, BP), 62% (anti-BP230, BP), and 81% (anti-type VII collagen, EBA), and specificities of 98–100% (165).

van Beek et al. validated the Dermatology Profile ELISA (Euroimmun), comprising the same five parameters plus additional envoplakin. They demonstrated sensitivities of 95% (anti-Dsgl, PF), 100% (anti-Dsg3, PV), 95% (anti-BP180, BP), 60% (anti-BP230, BP), 93% (anti-type VII collagen, EBA), and 86% (anti-envoplakin, paraneoplastic pemphigus), and

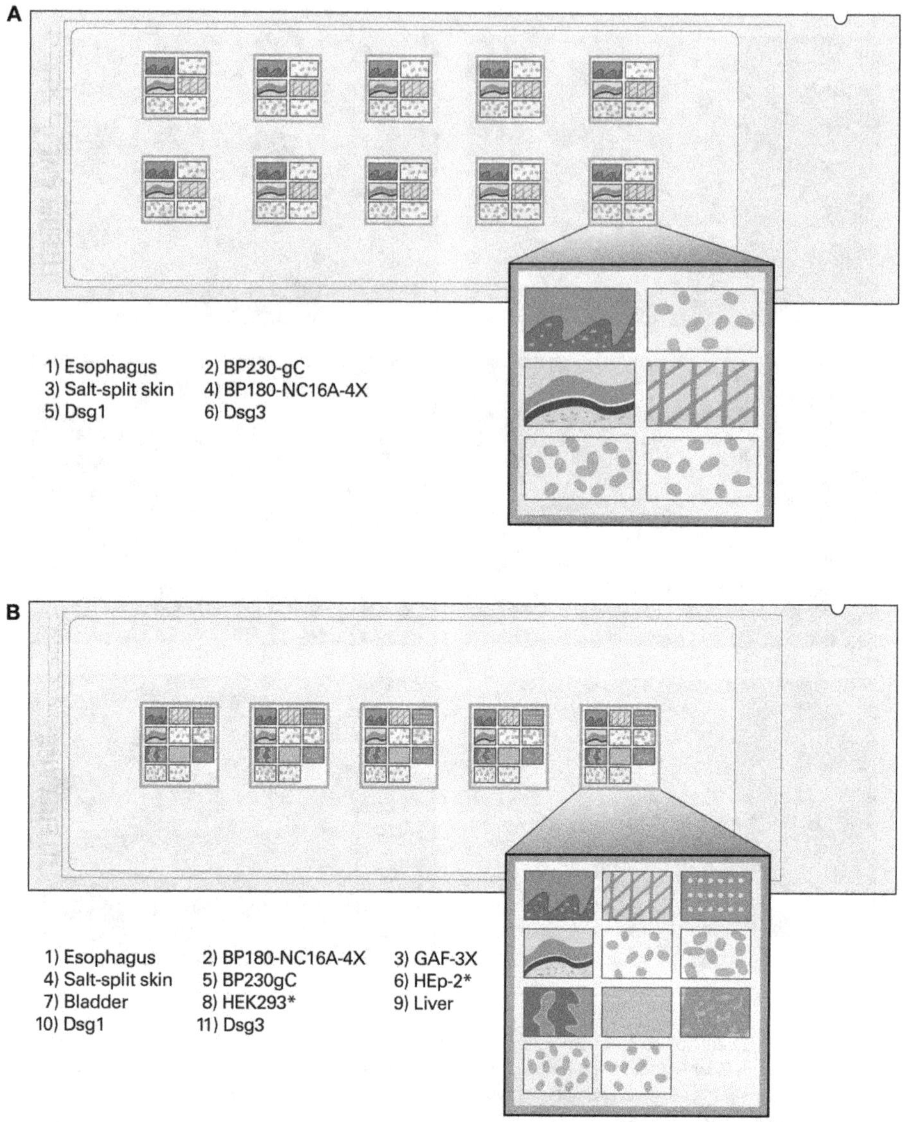

FIGURE 4 | BIOCHIP mosaics for simultaneous screening and monospecific confirmation of autoantibodies using indirect immunofluorescence, modified from Gosink, MEDLAB Magazine 2013 (148) with permission of MEDLAB Magazine. **(A)** "Dermatology Mosaic 7" (six substrates per reaction field). **(B)** "Dermatology Mosaic 11" (11 substrates per reaction field for extended analysis including paraneoplastic pemphigus and dermatitis herpetiformis). As indicated, the BIOCHIPs are coated with tissue sections (monkey esophagus, salt-split skin, liver, rat urinary bladder), HEK293 cells expressing recombinant antigens (Dsg1, Dsg3, BP230gC), or spots of purified recombinant antigen (BP180-NC16A-4X, GAF-3X). *HEp-2 and mock-transfected HEK293 cells serve as negative control substrates.

specificities in the range of 97–100% (114). These performance characteristics were also similar to those obtained with the individual ELISA (Euroimmun) (36, 54, 143, 147, 149). Comparison of the Dermatology Profile to the conventional multi-step approach yielded concordant results in 87%. Incongruent results were attributed to the lack of IgA detection and reactivity against antigens not included in the profile ELISA (114).

Immunoblotting

Immunoblotting and immunoprecipitation help to determine rather rare autoantibodies (e.g., anti-laminin γ1, anti-laminin 332, anti-LAD-1, anti-α6β4 integrin, anti-desmoplakin, anti-type VII collagen) and are based on recombinant proteins or cell extracts (e.g., epidermis, dermis, cultured keratinocytes) (28, 69, 80, 191–193). These tests, however, are time-consuming and available only as in-house assays in specialized laboratories. They allow for highly specific autoantibody detection, but have proven inadequate for targets with mainly conformational epitopes, such as Dsg1 and Dsg3 (127, 141, 194–196). Immunoblotting for anti-Dsg is thus not recommended in the diagnosis of PF/PV (97). In contrast, there are patients suspected of having pemphigoid disease who show positive DIF results in the absence of autoantibody reactivity by commercial ELISA systems. In such

TABLE 2 | Performance characteristics of reported ELISA systems for the detection of autoantibodies in autoimmune bullous dermatoses.

ELISA[a]	Disease	Sensitivity[b]	Specificity[b]	References
Anti-Dsg1[c]	Pemphigus foliaceus	96 – 100%	96–100%	(147, 159, 165–169)
Anti-Dsg3[c]	Pemphigus vulgaris	85–100%	96–100%	(147, 159, 165–173)
Anti-envoplakin[d]	Paraneoplastic pemphigus	63–83%	91–98%	(36–38)
Anti-periplakin	Paraneoplastic pemphigus	74%	96%	(36)
Anti-desmocollin	Paraneoplastic pemphigus	60%	NA	(33)
Anti-BP180[e]	Bullous pemphigoid	54–95%	90–100%	(50, 51, 53, 106, 143, 144, 160, 164, 165, 169, 173–181)
Anti-BP230[f]	Bullous pemphigoid	48–82%	65–99%	(50, 51, 53, 54, 106, 144, 165, 175–177, 182)
Anti-laminin 332	Mucous membrane pemphigoid	20–75%	84–96%	(71, 163)
Anti-laminin γ1	Anti-lamininγ1/p200 pemphigoid	69%	99%	(162)
Anti-type VII collagen[g]	Epidermolysis bullosa acquisita	86–100%	98–100%	(114, 149, 161, 183–186)
Anti-deamidated gliadin	Dermatitis herpetiformis, coeliac disease	84–95% (IgA) 80–99% (IgG)	86–93% (IgA) 93–94% (IgG)	(92, 145)
Anti-tissue transglutaminase	Dermatitis herpetiformis, coeliac disease	78–98%	96–99%	(92, 94, 145, 187–189)

[a] *Parameters for which commercial ELISA systems are not available are indicated in italics.*
[b] *Including performance data reported for commercial and in-house assays.*
[c] *Commercial assays employ the ectodomains of Dsg1 and Dsg3 after recombinant expression in baculovirus (MBL) or HEK293 cells (Euroimmun).*
[d] *Commercial assay based on the N-terminal envoplakin 1–481 fragment (Euroimmun).*
[e] *Commercial assays employ a single recombinant NC16A domain (MBL) or a tetramer of four NC16A domains to increase epitope exposure (BP180-NC16A-4X, Euroimmun).*
[f] *Commercial assays employ recombinant protein of both N- and C-terminal parts of BP230 (MBL) or only a fragment of the C-terminal domain ($BP230_{2326-2649}$, Euroimmun).*
[g] *Commercial assays employ the NC1 and NC2 domains of type VII collagen (MBL) or only NC1 (Euroimmun).*

cases, immunoblotting using antigenic fragments outside the immunodominant domains may provide diagnostically relevant information on the autoantibodies' target.

IMMUNOLOGICAL MONITORING

Autoantibodies in several AIBD entities are directly pathogenic (4, 197–205). Their titers correlate with the disease activity over time, as reported for anti-Dsgl, anti-Dsg3 (147, 159, 166, 170, 206–209), anti-BP180 (51, 52, 143, 160, 210–214), and anti-type VII collagen (161, 183, 184, 215). By contrast, anti-BP230 reactivity appears not to fluctuate with changes in the clinical course of BP patients or only in a small subset of cases (50–52).

IIF evaluation is subjective and produces only semiquantitative data, based on serial serum dilutions, with titers depending on the type of substrate due to variable antigen expression levels. As opposed to this, ELISA provide objective and quantitative scores, which tend to reflect the disease activity better than IIF titers (130, 160). Therefore, ELISA testing is routinely used in many laboratories for the monitoring of disease activity. However, the relationship is not always perfect as there are cases of active disease with negative ELISA results and vice versa, as well as cases where antibody levels do not fluctuate in correlation with clinical activity (116, 209).

As an adjunct to the paramount clinical assessment, the follow-up of autoantibody titers has relevance for disease monitoring and can be helpful in therapeutic decisions, such as adjusting the dose of immunosuppressants. For example, when lesions have healed, decreasing or undetectable autoantibody levels may indicate dosage reduction or omission, respectively. In addition, relapses may be anticipated by the detection of increased autoantibody levels (99). However, the clinical judgement and the above-mentioned imperfections of the assays should always be taken into consideration (97, 116).

PREDICTIVE BIOMARKERS FOR DISEASE PROGRESSION

Several molecules involved in, e.g., autoimmune and inflammatory responses in AIBD have recently been identified as potential biomarkers for disease development and outcome. The measurement of these biomarkers could help to adapt the duration and intensity of treatment in order to prevent the occurrence of relapses. The relevance of stratifying patients at risk of relapse, preferably at initiation of treatment, is reflected by a rate of about 30% of clinical relapses within the first year of treatment in patients with BP (216).

In BP patients, the value of monitoring anti-BP180 autoantibodies as a potential risk factor for relapse has been demonstrated. It was found that anti-BP180 IgG levels are significantly higher at baseline in patients who experience a relapse compared to non-relapse cases, whereas no such association was observed for anti-BP230 IgG, serum IgE, and peripheral eosinophils (217, 218). A multicenter prospective study demonstrated that the decrease in anti-BP180 titers during the first 60 days of treatment is lower in patients with relapse than in patients with ongoing remission. In addition, high anti-BP180 levels at day 150 provide high sensitivity for a relapse between days 150–360 of treatment (219). Cai et al. confirmed that increasing anti-BP180 IgG titers are associated with a decreasing remission rate (220). Along with anti-BP180, the detection of autoantibodies against type VII collagen may help to stratify BP patients based on the observation that about

40% of relapsing cases display positive and increasing anti-type VII collagen serum levels at the time of relapse (221).

In addition, the follow-up of molecules involved in inflammatory mechanisms can contribute to the prediction of BP outcome. Amongst others, this pertains to serum concentrations of the cytokines interleukin 17 (IL-17) and IL-23. The former shows significant decreases in patients with ongoing remission as well as constantly elevated levels prior to relapse, whereas the latter increases in early treatment stages in patients who later relapse (222). Similarly, an increased release of the chemokine CXCL10 favors BP relapse within the first year of treatment (223). These three inflammatory biomarkers all upregulate the secretion by leukocytes of matrix-metalloproteinase-9 (MMP-9), which was shown to decrease over time upon remission and to remain elevated in patients who relapse. Consequently, the follow-up of protease MMP-9 expression is regarded as another promising tool for the prediction of relapse in BP (222, 223). Also the serum concentrations of eosinophil cationic protein (ECP), as a measure of eosinophil activation, may help to predict a relapse as indicated by the absence of ECP alterations under treatment (224).

Moreover, an increased expression of the glucocorticoid receptor-beta in skin epithelial cells was suggested to be predictive of reduced treatment efficacy and increased risk of BP relapse (225). The presence of extensive disease (more than ten new blisters daily) at baseline and of neurological conditions associated with BP (e.g., dementia) may also play a role in the prediction of BP outcome (219).

In patients with PV, anti-Dsg3 positivity and, to a lesser extent, positive DIF results are predictors of relapse (226). Positivity for anti-Dsg1 and anti-Dsg3 was shown to provide high predictive values for the occurrence of relapses following treatment (209, 227). In addition, B-cell repopulation and low CD4+ T-cell count are associated with relapses in patients with pemphigus (227).

Altogether, this relatively new field warrants further investigation and holds the potential to benefit both clinicians and patients. In particular, to link cytokine/chemokine variations to clinical practice, large prospective studies will have to confirm the findings to date.

PERSPECTIVES

Accurate diagnosis and discrimination of the different AIBD forms is crucial for therapeutic decisions and prognosis. Owing to highly sensitive and specific assays, it is estimated that a serological diagnosis can be made in about 90% of patients, subject to clinical expression (99, 112). Both the increasingly aging population and the constantly improved diagnostics cause a steady growth in the incidence of AIBD. In Germany, the annual incidence doubled within a decade, meanwhile amounting to about 25–30 cases per million inhabitants (112, 228). Hence, the continuous development and application of serological assays for known and yet unknown parameters will play a crucial role in the future. Patient management will further benefit from ongoing basic research on pathophysiological mechanisms and from clinical trials on forthcoming treatment options (229). For example, there is a growing number of data regarding the potential pathogenic role of IgE class autoantibodies in BP and the option of anti-IgE treatment (230–233).

AUTHOR CONTRIBUTIONS

SS performed the literature research, acquired and modified the figures, and wrote the first manuscript draft. IK, LK, CP, CD, KF, WSt, and WSc critically revised the manuscript. All authors have made a substantial, direct and intellectual contribution to the work, and approved it for publication.

REFERENCES

1. Gosink J, Schlumberger W. Multiplex serological diagnostics in autoimmune skin-blistering diseases. *MEDLAB Magazine.* (2016) 4:28–30.
2. Kasperkiewicz M, Ellebrecht CT, Takahashi H, Yamagami J, Zillikens D, Payne AS, et al. Pemphigus. *Nat Rev Dis Primers.* (2017) 3:17026. doi: 10.1038/nrdp.2017.27
3. Schmidt E, Zillikens D. Pemphigoid diseases. *Lancet Lond Engl.* (2013) 381:320–32. doi: 10.1016/S0140-6736(12)61140-4
4. Spindler V, Eming R, Schmidt E, Amagai M, Grando S, Jonkman MF, et al. Mechanisms causing loss of keratinocyte cohesion in pemphigus. *J Invest Dermatol.* (2018) 138:32–7. doi: 10.1016/j.jid.2017.06.022
5. Di Zenzo G, Amber KT, Sayar BS, Muller EJ, Borradori L. Immune response in pemphigus and beyond: progresses and emerging concepts. *Semin Immunopathol.* (2016) 38:57–74. doi: 10.1007/s00281-015-0541-1
6. Amagai M, Koch PJ, Nishikawa T, Stanley JR. Pemphigus vulgaris antigen (desmoglein 3) is localized in the lower epidermis, the site of blister formation in patients. *J Invest Dermatol.* (1996) 106:351–5. doi: 10.1111/1523-1747.ep12343081
7. Amagai M. Pemphigus as a paradigm of autoimmunity and cell adhesion. *Keio J Med.* (2002) 51:133–9. doi: 10.2302/kjm.51.133
8. Shirakata Y, Amagai M, Hanakawa Y, Nishikawa T, Hashimoto K. Lack of mucosal involvement in pemphigus foliaceus may be due to low expression of desmoglein 1. *J Invest Dermatol.* (1998) 110:76–8. doi: 10.1046/j.1523-1747.1998.00085.x
9. Amagai M, Tsunoda K, Zillikens D, Nagai T, Nishikawa T. The clinical phenotype of pemphigus is defined by the anti-desmoglein autoantibody profile. *J Am Acad Dermatol.* (1999) 40:167–70. doi: 10.1016/S0190-9622(99)70183-0
10. Ding X, Aoki V, Mascaro JM Jr, Lopez-Swiderski A, Diaz LA, Fairley JA. Mucosal and mucocutaneous (generalized) pemphigus vulgaris show distinct autoantibody profiles. *J Invest Dermatol.* (1997) 109:592–6. doi: 10.1111/1523-1747.ep12337524
11. Mahoney MG, Wang Z, Rothenberger K, Koch PJ, Amagai M, Stanley JR. Explanations for the clinical and microscopic localization of lesions in pemphigus foliaceus and vulgaris. *J Clin Invest.* (1999) 103:461–8. doi: 10.1172/JCI5252
12. Kalantari-Dehaghi M, Anhalt GJ, Camilleri MJ, Chernyavsky AI, Chun S, Felgner PL, et al. Pemphigus vulgaris autoantibody profiling by proteomic technique. *PLoS ONE.* (2013) 8:e57587. doi: 10.1371/journal.pone.0057587
13. Amber KT, Valdebran M, Grando SA. Non-desmoglein antibodies in patients with pemphigus vulgaris. *Front Immunol.* (2018) 9:1190. doi: 10.3389/fimmu.2018.01190

14. Ahmed AR, Carrozzo M, Caux F, Cirillo N, Dmochowski M, Alonso AE, et al. Monopathogenic vs multipathogenic explanations of pemphigus pathophysiology. *Exp Dermatol.* (2016) 25:839–46. doi: 10.1111/exd.13106
15. Lakshmi MJD, Jaisankar TJ, Rajappa M, Thappa DM, Chandrashekar L, Divyapriya D, et al. Correlation of antimuscarinic acetylcholine receptor antibody titers and antidesmoglein antibody titers with the severity of disease in patients with pemphigus. *J Am Acad Dermatol.* (2017) 76:895–902. doi: 10.1016/j.jaad.2016.11.039
16. Tsuruta D, Ishii N, Hamada T, Ohyama B, Fukuda S, Koga H, et al. IgA pemphigus. *Clin Dermatol.* (2011) 29:437–42. doi: 10.1016/j.clindermatol.2011.01.014
17. Tsuruta D. Intercellular IgA dermatosis. *Br J Dermatol.* (2017) 176:13–4. doi: 10.1111/bjd.15034
18. Hisamatsu Y, Amagai M, Garrod DR, Kanzaki T, Hashimoto T. The detection of IgG and IgA autoantibodies to desmocollins 1–3 by enzyme-linked immunosorbent assays using baculovirus-expressed proteins, in atypical pemphigus but not in typical pemphigus. *Br J Dermatol.* (2004) 151:73–83. doi: 10.1111/j.1365-2133.2004.05995.x
19. Hashimoto T, Kiyokawa C, Mori O, Miyasato M, Chidgey MA, Garrod DR, et al. Human desmocollin 1 (Dsc1) is an autoantigen for the subcorneal pustular dermatosis type of IgA pemphigus. *J Invest Dermatol.* (1997) 109:127–31. doi: 10.1111/1523-1747.ep12319025
20. Muller R, Heber B, Hashimoto T, Messer G, Mullegger R, Niedermeier A, et al. Autoantibodies against desmocollins in European patients with pemphigus. *Clin Exp Dermatol.* (2009) 34:898–903. doi: 10.1111/j.1365-2230.2009.03241.x
21. Teye K, Numata S, Ohzono A, Ohyama B, Tsuchisaka A, Koga H, et al. Establishment of IgA ELISAs of mammalian recombinant proteins of human desmocollins 1–3. *J Dermatol Sci.* (2016) 83:75–7. doi: 10.1016/j.jdermsci.2016.04.001
22. Anhalt GJ. Paraneoplastic pemphigus. *J Investig Dermatol Symp Proc.* (2004) 9:29–33. doi: 10.1111/j.1087-0024.2004.00832.x
23. Kim JH, Kim SC. Paraneoplastic pemphigus: paraneoplastic autoimmune disease of the skin and mucosa. *Front Immunol.* (2019) 10:1259 doi: 10.3389/fimmu.2019.01259
24. Ohzono A, Sogame R, Li X, Teye K, Tsuchisaka A, Numata S, et al. Clinical and immunological findings in 104 cases of paraneoplastic pemphigus. *Br J Dermatol.* (2015) 173:1447–52. doi: 10.1111/bjd.14162
25. Schepens I, Jaunin F, Begre N, Laderach U, Marcus K, Hashimoto T, et al. The protease inhibitor alpha-2-macroglobulin-like-1 is the p170 antigen recognized by paraneoplastic pemphigus autoantibodies in human. *PLoS ONE.* (2010) 5:e12250. doi: 10.1371/journal.pone.0012250
26. Wieczorek M, Czernik A. Paraneoplastic pemphigus: a short review. *Clin Cosmet Investig Dermatol.* (2016) 9:291–5. doi: 10.2147/CCID.S100802
27. Gallo E, Garcia-Martin P, Fraga J, Teye K, Koga H, Hashimoto T, et al. Paraneoplastic pemphigus with eosinophilic spongiosis and autoantibodies against desmocollins 2 and 3. *Clin Exp Dermatol.* (2014) 39:323–6. doi: 10.1111/ced.12296
28. Oursler JR, Labib RS, riss-Abdo L, Burke T, O'Keefe EJ, Anhalt GJ. Human autoantibodies against desmoplakins in paraneoplastic pemphigus. *J Clin Invest.* (1992) 89:1775–82. doi: 10.1172/JCI115781
29. Amagai M, Nishikawa T, Nousari HC, Anhalt GJ, Hashimoto T. Antibodies against desmoglein 3 (pemphigus vulgaris antigen) are present in sera from patients with paraneoplastic pemphigus and cause acantholysis *in vivo* in neonatal mice. *J Clin Invest.* (1998) 102:775–82. doi: 10.1172/JCI3647
30. Kiyokawa C, Ruhrberg C, Nie Z, Karashima T, Mori O, Nishikawa T, et al. Envoplakin and periplakin are components of the paraneoplastic pemphigus antigen complex. *J Invest Dermatol.* (1998) 111:1236–8. doi: 10.1046/j.1523-1747.1998.00449.x
31. Aho S, Mahoney MG, Uitto J. Plectin serves as an autoantigen in paraneoplastic pemphigus. *J Invest Dermatol.* (1999) 113:422–3. doi: 10.1046/j.1523-1747.1999.00695.x
32. Brandt O, Rafei D, Podstawa E, Niedermeier A, Jonkman MF, Terra JB, et al. Differential IgG recognition of desmoglein 3 by paraneoplastic pemphigus and pemphigus vulgaris sera. *J Invest Dermatol.* (2012) 132:1738–41. doi: 10.1038/jid.2012.1
33. Ishii N, Teye K, Fukuda S, Uehara R, Hachiya T, Koga H, et al. Anti-desmocollin autoantibodies in nonclassical pemphigus. *Br J Dermatol.* (2015) 173:59–68. doi: 10.1111/bjd.13711
34. Zimmermann J, Bahmer F, Rose C, Zillikens D, Schmidt E. Clinical and immunopathological spectrum of paraneoplastic pemphigus. *J Dtsch Dermatol Ges.* (2010) 8:598–606. doi: 10.1111/j.1610-0387.2010.07380.x
35. Joly P, Richard C, Gilbert D, Courville P, Chosidow O, Roujeau JC, et al. Sensitivity and specificity of clinical, histologic, and immunologic features in the diagnosis of paraneoplastic pemphigus. *J Am Acad Dermatol.* (2000) 43:619–26. doi: 10.1067/mjd.2000.107488
36. Probst C, Schlumberger W, Stocker W, Recke A, Schmidt E, Hashimoto T, et al. Development of ELISA for the specific determination of autoantibodies against envoplakin and periplakin in paraneoplastic pemphigus. *Clin Chim Acta.* (2009) 410:13–8. doi: 10.1016/j.cca.2009.08.022
37. Powell JG, Grover RK, Plunkett RW, Seiffert-Sinha K, Sinha AA. Evaluation of a newly available ELISA for envoplakin autoantibodies for the diagnosis of paraneoplastic pemphigus. *J Drugs Dermatol.* (2015) 14:1103–6.
38. Poot AM, Diercks GF, Kramer D, Schepens I, Klunder G, Hashimoto T, et al. Laboratory diagnosis of paraneoplastic pemphigus. *Br J Dermatol.* (2013) 169:1016–24. doi: 10.1111/bjd.12479
39. Mergler R, Kerstan A, Schmidt E, Goebeler M, Benoit S. Atypical clinical and serological manifestation of pemphigus vegetans: a case report and review of the literature. *Case Rep Dermatol.* (2017) 9:121–30. doi: 10.1159/000468919
40. Perez-Perez ME, valos-Diaz E, Herrera-Esparza R. Autoantibodies in senear-usher syndrome: cross-reactivity or multiple autoimmunity? *Autoimmune Dis.* (2012) 2012:296214. doi: 10.1155/2012/296214
41. Amerian ML, Ahmed AR. Pemphigus erythematosus. Senear-Usher syndrome. *Int J Dermatol.* (1985) 24:16–25. doi: 10.1111/j.1365-4362.1985.tb05349.x
42. Kasperkiewicz M, Kowalewski C, Jablonska S. Pemphigus herpetiformis: from first description until now. *J Am Acad Dermatol.* (2014) 70:780–7. doi: 10.1016/j.jaad.2013.11.043
43. Aoki V, Rivitti EA, Diaz LA. Update on fogo selvagem, an endemic form of pemphigus foliaceus. *J Dermatol.* (2015) 42:18–26. doi: 10.1111/1346-8138.12675
44. Brenner S, Bialy-Golan A, Ruocco V. Drug-induced pemphigus. *Clin Dermatol.* (1998) 16:393–7. doi: 10.1016/S0738-081X(98)00010-8
45. Yoshimura K, Ishii N, Hamada T, Abe T, Ono F, Hashikawa K, et al. Clinical and immunological profiles in 17 Japanese patients with drug-induced pemphigus studied at Kurume University. *Br J Dermatol.* (2014) 171:544–53. doi: 10.1111/bjd.12925
46. Goletz S, Zillikens D, Schmidt E. Structural proteins of the dermal-epidermal junction targeted by autoantibodies in pemphigoid diseases. *Exp Dermatol.* (2017) 26:1154–62. doi: 10.1111/exd.13446
47. Kridin K, Ludwig RJ. The growing incidence of bullous pemphigoid: overview and potential explanations. *Front Med.* (2018) 5:220. doi: 10.3389/fmed.2018.00220
48. Zillikens D, Rose PA, Balding SD, Liu Z, Olague-Marchan M, Diaz LA, et al. Tight clustering of extracellular BP180 epitopes recognized by bullous pemphigoid autoantibodies. *J Invest Dermatol.* (1997) 109:573–9. doi: 10.1111/1523-1747.ep12337492
49. Skaria M, Jaunin F, Hunziker T, Riou S, Schumann H, Bruckner-Tuderman L, et al. IgG autoantibodies from bullous pemphigoid patients recognize multiple antigenic reactive sites located predominantly within the B and C subdomains of the COOH-terminus of BP230. *J Invest Dermatol.* (2000) 114:998–1004. doi: 10.1046/j.1523-1747.2000.00893.x
50. Yoshida M, Hamada T, Amagai M, Hashimoto K, Uehara R, Yamaguchi K, et al. Enzyme-linked immunosorbent assay using bacterial recombinant proteins of human BP230 as a diagnostic tool for bullous pemphigoid. *J Dermatol Sci.* (2006) 41:21–30. doi: 10.1016/j.jdermsci.2005.11.002
51. Charneux J, Lorin J, Vitry F, Antonicelli F, Reguiai Z, Barbe C, et al. Usefulness of BP230 and BP180-NC16a enzyme-linked immunosorbent assays in the initial diagnosis of bullous pemphigoid: a retrospective study of 138 patients. *Arch Dermatol.* (2011) 147:286–91. doi: 10.1001/archdermatol.2011.23
52. Di Zenzo G., Thoma-Uszynski S, Fontao L, Calabresi V, Hofmann SC, Hellmark T, et al. Multicenter prospective study of the humoral autoimmune response in bullous pemphigoid. *Clin Immunol.* (2008) 128:415–26. doi: 10.1016/j.clim.2008.04.012

53. Roussel A, Benichou J, Randriamanantany ZA, Gilbert D, Drenovska K, Houivet E, et al. Enzyme-linked immunosorbent assay for the combination of bullous pemphigoid antigens 1 and 2 in the diagnosis of bullous pemphigoid. *Arch Dermatol.* (2011) 147:293–8. doi: 10.1001/archdermatol.2011.21
54. Blocker IM, Dahnrich C, Probst C, Komorowski L, Saschenbrecker S, Schlumberger W, et al. Epitope mapping of BP230 leading to a novel enzyme-linked immunosorbent assay for autoantibodies in bullous pemphigoid. *Br J Dermatol.* (2012) 166:964–70. doi: 10.1111/j.1365-2133.2012.10820.x
55. Di Zenzo G, Grosso F, Terracina M, Mariotti F, De Pita O, Owaribe K, et al. Characterization of the anti-BP180 autoantibody reactivity profile and epitope mapping in bullous pemphigoid patients. *J Invest Dermatol.* (2004) 122:103–10. doi: 10.1046/j.0022-202X.2003.22126.x
56. Sitaru C, Powell J, Messer G, Brocker EB, Wojnarowska F, Zillikens D. Immunoblotting and enzyme-linked immunosorbent assay for the diagnosis of pemphigoid gestationis. *Obstet Gynecol.* (2004) 103:757–63. doi: 10.1097/01.AOG.0000115506.76104.ad
57. Di Zenzo G, Calabresi V, Grosso F, Caproni M, Ruffelli M, Zambruno G. The intracellular and extracellular domains of BP180 antigen comprise novel epitopes targeted by pemphigoid gestationis autoantibodies. *J Invest Dermatol.* (2007) 127:864–73. doi: 10.1038/sj.jid.5700594
58. Zone JJ, Taylor TB, Kadunce DP, Meyer LJ. Identification of the cutaneous basement membrane zone antigen and isolation of antibody in linear immunoglobulin A bullous dermatosis. *J Clin Invest.* (1990) 85:812–20. doi: 10.1172/JCI114508
59. Marinkovich MP, Taylor TB, Keene DR, Burgeson RE, Zone JJ. LAD-1, the linear IgA bullous dermatosis autoantigen, is a novel 120-kDa anchoring filament protein synthesized by epidermal cells. *J Invest Dermatol.* (1996) 106:734–8. doi: 10.1111/1523-1747.ep12345782
60. Fortuna G, Marinkovich MP. Linear immunoglobulin A bullous dermatosis. *Clin Dermatol.* (2012) 30:38–50. doi: 10.1016/j.clindermatol.2011.03.008
61. Hirako Y, Nishizawa Y, Sitaru C, Opitz A, Marcus K, Meyer HE, et al. The 97-kDa (LABD97) and 120-kDa (LAD-1) fragments of bullous pemphigoid antigen 180/type XVII collagen have different N-termini. *J Invest Dermatol.* (2003) 121:1554–6. doi: 10.1046/j.1523-1747.2003.12607.x
62. Zillikens D, Herzele K, Georgi M, Schmidt E, Chimanovitch I, Schumann H, et al. Autoantibodies in a subgroup of patients with linear IgA disease react with the NC16A domain of BP1801. *J Invest Dermatol.* (1999) 113:947–53. doi: 10.1046/j.1523-1747.1999.00808.x
63. Arechalde A, Braun RP, Calza AM, Hertl M, Didierjean L, Saurat JH, et al. Childhood bullous pemphigoid associated with IgA antibodies against BP180 or BP230 antigens. *Br J Dermatol.* (1999) 140:112–8. doi: 10.1046/j.1365-2133.1999.02618.x
64. Ghohestani RF, Nicolas JF, Kanitakis J, Claudy A. Linear IgA bullous dermatosis with IgA antibodies exclusively directed against the 180- or 230-kDa epidermal antigens. *J Invest Dermatol.* (1997) 108:854–8. doi: 10.1111/1523-1747.ep12292581
65. Kamaguchi M, Iwata H. The diagnosis and blistering mechanisms of mucous membrane pemphigoid. *Front Immunol.* (2019) 10:34. doi: 10.3389/fimmu.2019.00034
66. Balding SD, Prost C, Diaz LA, Bernard P, Bedane C, Aberdam D, et al. Cicatricial pemphigoid autoantibodies react with multiple sites on the BP180 extracellular domain. *J Invest Dermatol.* (1996) 106:141–6. doi: 10.1111/1523-1747.ep12329728
67. Bedane C, McMillan JR, Balding SD, Bernard P, Prost C, Bonnetblanc JM, et al. Bullous pemphigoid and cicatricial pemphigoid autoantibodies react with ultrastructurally separable epitopes on the BP180 ectodomain: evidence that BP180 spans the lamina lucida. *J Invest Dermatol.* (1997) 108:901–7. doi: 10.1111/1523-1747.ep12292701
68. Oyama N, Setterfield JF, Powell AM, Sakuma-Oyama Y, Albert S, Bhogal BS, et al. Bullous pemphigoid antigen II (BP180) and its soluble extracellular domains are major autoantigens in mucous membrane pemphigoid: the pathogenic relevance to HLA class II alleles and disease severity. *Br J Dermatol.* (2006) 154:90–8. doi: 10.1111/j.1365-2133.2005.06998.x
69. Schmidt E, Skrobek C, Kromminga A, Hashimoto T, Messer G, Brocker EB, et al. Cicatricial pemphigoid: IgA and IgG autoantibodies target epitopes on both intra- and extracellular domains of bullous pemphigoid antigen 180. *Br J Dermatol.* (2001) 145:778–83. doi: 10.1046/j.1365-2133.2001.04471.x
70. Lazarova Z, Salato VK, Lanschuetzer CM, Janson M, Fairley JA, Yancey KB. IgG anti-laminin-332 autoantibodies are present in a subset of patients with mucous membrane, but not bullous, pemphigoid. *J Am Acad Dermatol.* (2008) 58:951–8. doi: 10.1016/j.jaad.2008.02.035
71. Bekou V, Thoma-Uszynski S, Wendler O, Uter W, Schwietzke S, Hunziker T, et al. Detection of laminin 5-specific auto-antibodies in mucous membrane and bullous pemphigoid sera by ELISA. *J Invest Dermatol.* (2005) 124:732–40. doi: 10.1111/j.0022-202X.2005.23646.x
72. Goletz S, Probst C, Komorowski L, Schlumberger W, Fechner K, van BN, et al. A sensitive and specific assay for the serological diagnosis of antilaminin 332 mucous membrane pemphigoid. *Br J Dermatol.* (2019) 180:149–56. doi: 10.1111/bjd.17202
73. Egan CA, Lazarova Z, Darling TN, Yee C, Cote T, Yancey KB. Anti-epiligrin cicatricial pemphigoid and relative risk for cancer. *Lancet.* (2001) 357:1850–1. doi: 10.1016/S0140-6736(00)04971-0
74. Bernard P, Prost C, Lecerf V, Intrator L, Combemale P, Bedane C, et al. Studies of cicatricial pemphigoid autoantibodies using direct immunoelectron microscopy and immunoblot analysis. *J Invest Dermatol.* (1990) 94:630–5. doi: 10.1111/1523-1747.ep12876206
75. Leverkus M, Bhol K, Hirako Y, Pas H, Sitaru C, Baier G, et al. Cicatricial pemphigoid with circulating autoantibodies to beta4 integrin, bullous pemphigoid 180 and bullous pemphigoid 230. *Br J Dermatol.* (2001) 145:998–1004. doi: 10.1046/j.1365-2133.2001.04543.x
76. Bhol KC, Dans MJ, Simmons RK, Foster CS, Giancotti FG, Ahmed AR. The autoantibodies to alpha 6 beta 4 integrin of patients affected by ocular cicatricial pemphigoid recognize predominantly epitopes within the large cytoplasmic domain of human beta 4. *J Immunol.* (2000) 165:2824–9. doi: 10.4049/jimmunol.165.5.2824
77. Li X, Qian H, Sogame R, Hirako Y, Tsuruta D, Ishii N, et al. Integrin beta4 is a major target antigen in pure ocular mucous membrane pemphigoid. *Eur J Dermatol.* (2016) 26:247–53. doi: 10.1684/ejd.2016.2772
78. Amber KT, Murrell DF, Schmidt E, Joly P, Borradori L. Autoimmune subepidermal bullous diseases of the skin and mucosae: clinical features, diagnosis, and management. *Clin Rev Allergy Immunol.* (2018) 54:26–51. doi: 10.1007/s12016-017-8633-4
79. Dilling A, Rose C, Hashimoto T, Zillikens D, Shimanovich I. Anti-p200 pemphigoid: a novel autoimmune subepidermal blistering disease. *J Dermatol.* (2007) 34:1–8. doi: 10.1111/j.1346-8138.2007.00208.x
80. Zillikens D, Kawahara Y, Ishiko A, Shimizu H, Mayer J, Rank CV, et al. A novel subepidermal blistering disease with autoantibodies to a 200-kDa antigen of the basement membrane zone. *J Invest Dermatol.* (1996) 106:1333–8. doi: 10.1111/1523-1747.ep12349283
81. Dainichi T, Koga H, Tsuji T, Ishii N, Ohyama B, Ueda A, et al. From anti-p200 pemphigoid to anti-laminin gamma1 pemphigoid. *J Dermatol.* (2010) 37:231–8. doi: 10.1111/j.1346-8138.2009.00793.x
82. Hubner F, Langan EA, Recke A. Lichen planus pemphigoides: from lichenoid inflammation to autoantibody-mediated blistering. *Front Immunol.* (2019) 10:1389. doi: 10.3389/fimmu.2019.01389
83. Tamada Y, Yokochi K, Nitta Y, Ikeya T, Hara K, Owaribe K. Lichen planus pemphigoides: identification of 180 kd hemidesmosome antigen. *J Am Acad Dermatol.* (1995) 32:883–7. doi: 10.1016/0190-9622(95)91554-0
84. Zillikens D, Caux F, Mascaro JM, Wesselmann U, Schmidt E, Prost C, et al. Autoantibodies in lichen planus pemphigoides react with a novel epitope within the C-terminal NC16A domain of BP180. *J Invest Dermatol.* (1999) 113:117–21. doi: 10.1046/j.1523-1747.1999.00618.x
85. Mehren CR, Gniadecki R. Epidermolysis bullosa acquisita: current diagnosis and therapy. *Dermatol Rep.* (2011) 3:e38. doi: 10.4081/dr.2011.e38
86. Koga H, Prost-Squarcioni C, Iwata H, Jonkman MF, Ludwig RJ, Bieber K. Epidermolysis bullosa acquisita: the 2019 update. *Front Med.* (2018) 5:362. doi: 10.3389/fmed.2018.00362
87. Ishii N, Hamada T, Dainichi T, Karashima T, Nakama T, Yasumoto S, et al. Epidermolysis bullosa acquisita: what's new? *J Dermatol.* (2010) 37:220–30. doi: 10.1111/j.1346-8138.2009.00799.x
88. Woodley DT, Briggaman RA, O'Keefe EJ, Inman AO, Queen LL, Gammon WR. Identification of the skin basement-membrane autoantigen

in epidermolysis bullosa acquisita. *N Engl J Med.* (1984) 310:1007–13. doi: 10.1056/NEJM198404193101602

89. Jones DA, Hunt SW III, Prisayanh PS, Briggaman RA, Gammon WR. Immunodominant autoepitopes of type VII collagen are short, paired peptide sequences within the fibronectin type III homology region of the noncollagenous (NC1) domain. *J Invest Dermatol.* (1995) 104:231–5. doi: 10.1111/1523-1747.ep12612780
90. Lapiere JC, Woodley DT, Parente MG, Iwasaki T, Wynn KC, Christiano AM, et al. Epitope mapping of type VII collagen. Identification of discrete peptide sequences recognized by sera from patients with acquired epidermolysis bullosa. *J Clin Invest.* (1993) 92:1831–9. doi: 10.1172/JCI116774
91. Chorzelski TP, Beutner EH, Sulej J, Tchorzewska H, Jablonska S, Kumar V, et al. IgA anti-endomysium antibody. A new immunological marker of dermatitis herpetiformis and coeliac disease. *Br J Dermatol.* (1984) 111:395–402. doi: 10.1111/j.1365-2133.1984.tb06601.x
92. Kasperkiewicz M, Dahnrich C, Probst C, Komorowski L, Stocker W, Schlumberger W, et al. Novel assay for detecting celiac disease-associated autoantibodies in dermatitis herpetiformis using deamidated gliadin-analogous fusion peptides. *J Am Acad Dermatol.* (2012) 66:583–8. doi: 10.1016/j.jaad.2011.02.025
93. Dieterich W, Ehnis T, Bauer M, Donner P, Volta U, Riecken EO, et al. Identification of tissue transglutaminase as the autoantigen of celiac disease. *Nat Med.* (1997) 3:797–801. doi: 10.1038/nm0797-797
94. Rose C, Armbruster FP, Ruppert J, Igl BW, Zillikens D, Shimanovich I. Autoantibodies against epidermal transglutaminase are a sensitive diagnostic marker in patients with dermatitis herpetiformis on a normal or gluten-free diet. *J Am Acad Dermatol.* (2009) 61:39–43. doi: 10.1016/j.jaad.2008.12.037
95. Sardy M, Karpati S, Merkl B, Paulsson M, Smyth N. Epidermal transglutaminase (TGase 3) is the autoantigen of dermatitis herpetiformis. *J Exp Med.* (2002) 195:747–57. doi: 10.1084/jem.20011299
96. Villalta D, Tonutti E, Prause C, Koletzko S, Uhlig HH, Vermeersch P, et al. IgG antibodies against deamidated gliadin peptides for diagnosis of celiac disease in patients with IgA deficiency. *Clin Chem.* (2010) 56:464–8. doi: 10.1373/clinchem.2009.128132
97. Schmidt E, Goebeler M, Hertl M, Sardy M, Sitaru C, Eming R, et al. S2k guideline for the diagnosis of pemphigus vulgaris/foliaceus and bullous pemphigoid. *J Dtsch Dermatol Ges.* (2015) 13:713–27. doi: 10.1111/ddg.12612
98. Kneisel A, Hertl M. Autoimmune bullous skin diseases. Part 2: diagnosis and therapy. *J Dtsch Dermatol Ges.* (2011) 9:927–47. doi: 10.1111/j.1610-0387.2011.07809.x
99. Schmidt E, Zillikens D. Modern diagnosis of autoimmune blistering skin diseases. *Autoimmun Rev.* (2010) 10:84–9. doi: 10.1016/j.autrev.2010.08.007
100. van Beek N, Zillikens D, Schmidt E. Diagnosis of autoimmune bullous diseases. *J Dtsch Dermatol Ges.* (2018) 16:1077–91. doi: 10.1111/ddg.13637
101. Prost-Squarcioni C, Caux F, Schmidt E, Jonkman MF, Vassileva S, Kim SC, et al. International Bullous Diseases Group: consensus on diagnostic criteria for epidermolysis bullosa acquisita. *Br J Dermatol.* (2018) 179:30–41. doi: 10.1111/bjd.16138
102. Murrell DF, Peña S, Joly P, Marinovic B, Hashimoto T, Diaz LA, et al. Diagnosis and Management of Pemphigus: recommendations by an International Panel of Experts. *J Am Acad Dermatol.* (2018). doi: 10.1016/j.jaad.2018.02.021. [Epub ahead of print].
103. Witte M, Zillikens D, Schmidt E. Diagnosis of Autoimmune Blistering Diseases. *Front Med.* (2018) 5:296. doi: 10.3389/fmed.2018.00296
104. Hashimoto T, Tsuruta D, Koga H, Fukuda S, Ohyama B, Komai A, et al. Summary of results of serological tests and diagnoses for 4774 cases of various autoimmune bullous diseases consulted to Kurume University. *Br J Dermatol.* (2016) 175:953–65. doi: 10.1111/bjd.14692
105. Kneisel A, Hertl M. Autoimmune bullous skin diseases. Part 1: clinical manifestations. *J Dtsch Dermatol Ges.* (2011) 9:844–56. doi: 10.1111/j.1610-0387.2011.07793.x
106. Sardy M, Kostaki D, Varga R, Peris K, Ruzicka T. Comparative study of direct and indirect immunofluorescence and of bullous pemphigoid 180 and 230 enzyme-linked immunosorbent assays for diagnosis of bullous pemphigoid. *J Am Acad Dermatol.* (2013) 69:748–53. doi: 10.1016/j.jaad.2013.07.009
107. Inchara YK, Rajalakshmi T. Direct immunofluorescence in cutaneous vesiculobullous lesions. *Indian J Pathol Microbiol.* (2007) 50:730–2.
108. Chan YC, Sun YJ, Ng PP, Tan SH. Comparison of immunofluorescence microscopy, immunoblotting and enzyme-linked immunosorbent assay methods in the laboratory diagnosis of bullous pemphigoid. *Clin Exp Dermatol.* (2003) 28:651–6. doi: 10.1046/j.1365-2230.2003.01419.x
109. Giurdanella F, Diercks GF, Jonkman MF, Pas HH. Laboratory diagnosis of pemphigus: direct immunofluorescence remains the gold standard. *Br J Dermatol.* (2016) 175:185–6. doi: 10.1111/bjd.14408
110. Kamaguchi M, Iwata H, Ujiie I, Ujiie H, Sato J, Kitagawa Y, et al. Direct immunofluorescence using non-lesional buccal mucosa in mucous membrane pemphigoid. *Front Med.* (2018) 5:20. doi: 10.3389/fmed.2018.00020
111. Meijer JM, Atefi I, Diercks GFH, Vorobyev A, Zuiderveen J, Meijer HJ, et al. Serration pattern analysis for differentiating epidermolysis bullosa acquisita from other pemphigoid diseases. *J Am Acad Dermatol.* (2018) 78:754–9. doi: 10.1016/j.jaad.2017.11.029
112. Schmidt E, Zillikens D. The diagnosis and treatment of autoimmune blistering skin diseases. *Dtsch Arztebl Int.* (2011) 108:399-III. doi: 10.3238/arztebl.2011.0399
113. van Beek N, Rentzsch K, Probst C, Komorowski L, Kasperkiewicz M, Fechner K, et al. Serological diagnosis of autoimmune bullous skin diseases: prospective comparison of the BIOCHIP mosaic-based indirect immunofluorescence technique with the conventional multi-step single test strategy. *Orphanet J Rare Dis.* (2012) 7:49. doi: 10.1186/1750-1172-7-49
114. van Beek N, Dahnrich C, Johannsen N, Lemcke S, Goletz S, Hubner F, et al. Prospective studies on the routine use of a novel multivariant enzyme-linked immunosorbent assay for the diagnosis of autoimmune bullous diseases. *J Am Acad Dermatol.* (2017) 76:889–94. doi: 10.1016/j.jaad.2016.11.002
115. Giurdanella F, Nijenhuis AM, Diercks GFH, Jonkman MF, Pas HH. Keratinocyte binding assay identifies anti-desmosomal pemphigus antibodies where other tests are negative. *Front Immunol.* (2018) 9:839. doi: 10.3389/fimmu.2018.00839
116. Harman KE, Brown D, Exton LS, Groves RW, Hampton PJ, Mohd Mustapa MF, et al. British Association of Dermatologists' guidelines for the management of pemphigus vulgaris 2017. *Br J Dermatol.* (2017) 177:1170–201. doi: 10.1111/bjd.15930
117. Kasperkiewicz M, Schmidt E, Zillikens D. Current therapy of the pemphigus group. *Clin Dermatol.* (2012) 30:84–94. doi: 10.1016/j.clindermatol.2011.03.014
118. Martin LK, Werth VP, Villaneuva EV, Murrell DF. A systematic review of randomized controlled trials for pemphigus vulgaris and pemphigus foliaceus. *J Am Acad Dermatol.* (2011) 64:903–8. doi: 10.1016/j.jaad.2010.04.039
119. Joly P, Roujeau JC, Benichou J, Delaporte E, D'Incan M, Dreno B, et al. A comparison of two regimens of topical corticosteroids in the treatment of patients with bullous pemphigoid: a multicenter randomized study. *J Invest Dermatol.* (2009) 129:1681–7. doi: 10.1038/jid.2008.412
120. Behzad M, Mobs C, Kneisel A, Moller M, Hoyer J, Hertl M, et al. Combined treatment with immunoadsorption and rituximab leads to fast and prolonged clinical remission in difficult-to-treat pemphigus vulgaris. *Br J Dermatol.* (2012) 166:844–52. doi: 10.1111/j.1365-2133.2011.10732.x
121. Eming R, Hertl M. Immunoadsorption in pemphigus. *Autoimmunity.* (2006) 39:609–16. doi: 10.1080/08916930600972040
122. Arin MJ, Engert A, Krieg T, Hunzelmann N. Anti-CD20 monoclonal antibody (rituximab) in the treatment of pemphigus. *Br J Dermatol.* (2005) 153:620–5. doi: 10.1111/j.1365-2133.2005.06651.x
123. Hertl M, Zillikens D, Borradori L, Bruckner-Tuderman L, Burckhard H, Eming R, et al. Recommendations for the use of rituximab (anti-CD20 antibody) in the treatment of autoimmune bullous skin diseases. *J Dtsch Dermatol Ges.* (2008) 6:366–73. doi: 10.1111/j.1610-0387.2007.06602.x
124. Amagai M, Hashimoto T, Shimizu N, Nishikawa T. Absorption of pathogenic autoantibodies by the extracellular domain of pemphigus vulgaris antigen (Dsg3) produced by baculovirus. *J Clin Invest.* (1994) 94:59–67. doi: 10.1172/JCI117349
125. Anhalt GJ, Kim SC, Stanley JR, Korman NJ, Jabs DA, Kory M, et al. Paraneoplastic pemphigus. An autoimmune mucocutaneous disease associated with neoplasia. *N Engl J Med.* (1990) 323:1729–35. doi: 10.1056/NEJM199012203232503

126. Harman KE, Gratian MJ, Bhogal BS, Challacombe SJ, Black MM. The use of two substrates to improve the sensitivity of indirect immunofluorescence in the diagnosis of pemphigus. *Br J Dermatol.* (2000) 142:1135–9. doi: 10.1046/j.1365-2133.2000.03538.x
127. Jiao D, Bystryn JC. Sensitivity of indirect immunofluorescence, substrate specificity, and immunoblotting in the diagnosis of pemphigus. *J Am Acad Dermatol.* (1997) 37:211–6. doi: 10.1016/S0190-9622(97)80127-2
128. Hahn K, Kippes W, Amagai M, Rzany B, Brocker EB, Zillikens D. [Clinical aspects and immunopathology in 48 patients with pemphigus]. *Hautarzt.* (2000) 51:670–7. doi: 10.1007/s001050051193
129. Zagorodniuk I, Weltfriend S, Shtruminger L, Sprecher E, Kogan O, Pollack S, et al. A comparison of anti-desmoglein antibodies and indirect immunofluorescence in the serodiagnosis of pemphigus vulgaris. *Int J Dermatol.* (2005) 44:541–4. doi: 10.1111/j.1365-4632.2004.02541.x
130. Ng PP, Thng ST, Mohamed K, Tan SH. Comparison of desmoglein ELISA and indirect immunofluorescence using two substrates (monkey oesophagus and normal human skin) in the diagnosis of pemphigus. *Australas J Dermatol.* (2005) 46:239–41. doi: 10.1111/j.1440-0960.2005.00191.x
131. Sabolinski ML, Beutner EH, Krasny S, Kumar V, Huang J, Chorzelski TP, et al. Substrate specificity of anti-epithelial antibodies of pemphigus vulgaris and pemphigus foliaceus sera in immunofluorescence tests on monkey and guinea pig esophagus sections. *J Invest Dermatol.* (1987) 88:545–9. doi: 10.1111/1523-1747.ep12470131
132. Kridin K, Bergman R. The usefulness of indirect immunofluorescence in pemphigus and the natural history of patients with initial false-positive results: a Retrospective Cohort Study. *Front Med.* (2018) 5:266. doi: 10.3389/fmed.2018.00266
133. Kippes W, Schmidt E, Roth A, Rzany B, Brocker EB, Zillikens D. [Immunopathologic changes in 115 patients with bullous pemphigoid]. *Hautarzt.* (1999) 50:866–72. doi: 10.1007/s001050051001
134. Lee FJ, Silvestrini R, Fulcher DA. False-positive intercellular cement substance antibodies due to group A/B red cell antibodies: frequency and approach. *Pathology.* (2010) 42:574–7. doi: 10.3109/00313025.2010.508792
135. Ghohestani RF, Nicolas JF, Rousselle P, Claudy AL. Diagnostic value of indirect immunofluorescence on sodium chloride-split skin in differential diagnosis of subepidermal autoimmune bullous dermatoses. *Arch Dermatol.* (1997) 133:1102–7. doi: 10.1001/archderm.133.9.1102
136. Gammon WR, Fine JD, Forbes M, Briggaman RA. Immunofluorescence on split skin for the detection and differentiation of basement membrane zone autoantibodies. *J Am Acad Dermatol.* (1992) 27:79–87. doi: 10.1016/0190-9622(92)70161-8
137. Ghohestani R, Kanitakis J, Nicolas JF, Cozzani E, Claudy A. Comparative sensitivity of indirect immunofluorescence to immunoblot assay for the detection of circulating antibodies to bullous pemphigoid antigens 1 and 2. *Br J Dermatol.* (1996) 135:74–9. doi: 10.1111/j.1365-2133.1996.tb03611.x
138. Lau I, Goletz S, Holtsche MM, Zillikens D, Fechner K, Schmidt E. Anti-p200 pemphigoid is the most common pemphigoid disease with serum antibodies against the dermal side by indirect immunofluorescence microscopy on human salt-split skin. *J Am Acad Dermatol.* (2019). doi: 10.1016/j.jaad.2019.03.077. [Epub ahead of print].
139. Liu AY, Valenzuela R, Helm TN, Camisa C, Melton AL, Bergfeld WF. Indirect immunofluorescence on rat bladder transitional epithelium: a test with high specificity for paraneoplastic pemphigus. *J Am Acad Dermatol.* (1993) 28:696–9. doi: 10.1016/0190-9622(93)70095-B
140. Vainio E, Kalimo K, Reunala T, Viander M, Palosuo T. Circulating IgA- and IgG-class antigliadin antibodies in dermatitis herpetiformis detected by enzyme-linked immunosorbent assay. *Arch Dermatol Res.* (1983) 275:15–8. doi: 10.1007/BF00516548
141. Wandinger KP, Probst C, Komorowski L, Saschenbrecker S, Rosemann A, Mothes T, et al. Novel recombinant antigenic targets for the determination of (auto)antibodies in autoimmune dermatoses, neurological disorders and gastrointestinal diseases. In: Conrad K, Chan EKL, Fritzler MJ, Humbel RL, von Landenberg P, Shoenfeld Y, editors. *From Pathogenesis to Therapy of Autoimmune Diseases.* Lengerich: Pabst Science Publishers (2009). p 179–90.
142. Schwertz E, Kahlenberg F, Sack U, Richter T, Stern M, Conrad K, et al. Serologic assay based on gliadin-related nonapeptides as a highly sensitive and specific diagnostic aid in celiac disease. *Clin Chem.* (2004) 50:2370–5. doi: 10.1373/clinchem.2004.036111
143. Sitaru C, Dahnrich C, Probst C, Komorowski L, Blocker I, Schmidt E, et al. Enzyme-linked immunosorbent assay using multimers of the 16th non-collagenous domain of the BP180 antigen for sensitive and specific detection of pemphigoid autoantibodies. *Exp Dermatol.* (2007) 16:770–7. doi: 10.1111/j.1600-0625.2007.00592.x
144. Damoiseaux J, van Rijsingen M, Warnemunde N, Dahnrich C, Fechner K, Tervaert JW. Autoantibody detection in bullous pemphigoid: clinical evaluation of the EUROPLUS Dermatology Mosaic. *J Immunol Methods.* (2012) 382:76–80. doi: 10.1016/j.jim.2012.05.007
145. Prause C, Ritter M, Probst C, Daehnrich C, Schlumberger W, Komorowski L, et al. Antibodies against deamidated gliadin as new and accurate biomarkers of childhood coeliac disease. *J Pediatr Gastroenterol Nutr.* (2009) 49:52–8. doi: 10.1097/MPG.0b013e318195dae3
146. Stöcker W. [Rational histochemistry using a new microanalytic technic]. *Acta Histochem Suppl.* (1985) 31:269–81.
147. Schmidt E, Dahnrich C, Rosemann A, Probst C, Komorowski L, Saschenbrecker S, et al. Novel ELISA systems for antibodies to desmoglein 1 and 3: correlation of disease activity with serum autoantibody levels in individual pemphigus patients. *Exp Dermatol.* (2010) 19:458–63. doi: 10.1111/j.1600-0625.2010.01069.x
148. Gosink J. Autoantibody diagnostics in skin-blistering diseases. *MEDLAB Magazine.* (2013) 4:16–8.
149. Komorowski L, Muller R, Vorobyev A, Probst C, Recke A, Jonkman MF, et al. Sensitive and specific assays for routine serological diagnosis of epidermolysis bullosa acquisita. *J Am Acad Dermatol.* (2013) 68:e89–95. doi: 10.1016/j.jaad.2011.12.032
150. Xuan RR, Yang A, Murrell DF. New biochip immunofluorescence test for the serological diagnosis of pemphigus vulgaris and foliaceus: a review of the literature. *Int J Womens Dermatol.* (2018) 4:102–8. doi: 10.1016/j.ijwd.2017.10.001
151. Yang A, Xuan R, Murrell DF. A new indirect immunofluorescence BIOCHIP method for the serological diagnosis of bullous pemphigoid: a review of literature. *Australas J Dermatol.* (2019) 60:e173–7. doi: 10.1111/ajd.13034
152. Özkesici B, Mutlu D, Donmez L, Uzun S. The value of the BIOCHIP mosaic-based indirect immunofluorescence technique in the diagnosis of pemphigus and bullous pemphigoid in Turkish patients. *Acta Dermatovenerol Croat.* (2017) 25:202–9.
153. Russo I, Saponeri A, Peserico A, Alaibac M. The use of biochip immunofluorescence microscopy for the diagnosis of Pemphigus vulgaris. *Acta Histochem.* (2014) 116:713–6. doi: 10.1016/j.acthis.2013.12.012
154. Tampoia M, Zucano A, Villalta D, Antico A, Bizzaro N. Anti-skin specific autoantibodies detected by a new immunofluorescence multiplex biochip method in patients with autoimmune bullous diseases. *Dermatology.* (2012) 225:37–44. doi: 10.1159/000339776
155. Zarian H, Saponeri A, Michelotto A, Zattra E, Belloni-Fortina A, Alaibac M. Biochip technology for the serological diagnosis of bullous pemphigoid. *ISRN Dermatol.* (2012) 2012:237802. doi: 10.5402/2012/237802
156. Schmidt E, Zillikens D. Diagnosis and treatment of patients with autoimmune bullous disorders in Germany. *Dermatol Clin.* (2011) 29:663–71. doi: 10.1016/j.det.2011.06.007
157. Sadik CD, Pas HH, Bohlmann MK, Mousavi S, Benoit S, Sardy M, et al. Value of BIOCHIP technology in the serological diagnosis of pemphigoid gestationis. *Acta Derm Venereol.* (2017) 97:128–30. doi: 10.2340/00015555-2460
158. Mindorf S, Dettmann IM, Kruger S, Fuhrmann T, Rentzsch K, Karl I, et al. Routine detection of serum antidesmocollin autoantibodies is only useful in patients with atypical pemphigus. *Exp Dermatol.* (2017) 26:1267–70. doi: 10.1111/exd.13409
159. Ishii K, Amagai M, Hall RP, Hashimoto T, Takayanagi A, Gamou S, et al. Characterization of autoantibodies in pemphigus using antigen-specific enzyme-linked immunosorbent assays with baculovirus-expressed recombinant desmogleins. *J Immunol.* (1997) 159:2010–7.
160. Kobayashi M, Amagai M, Kuroda-Kinoshita K, Hashimoto T, Shirakata Y, Hashimoto K, et al. BP180 ELISA using bacterial recombinant NC16a protein as a diagnostic and monitoring tool for bullous pemphigoid. *J Dermatol Sci.* (2002) 30:224–32. doi: 10.1016/S0923-1811(02)00109-3
161. Marzano AV, Cozzani E, Fanoni D, De PO, Vassallo C, Berti E, et al. Diagnosis and disease severity assessment of epidermolysis bullosa acquisita by ELISA

for anti-type VII collagen autoantibodies: an Italian multicentre study. *Br J Dermatol.* (2013) 168:80–4. doi: 10.1111/bjd.12011

162. Groth S, Recke A, Vafia K, Ludwig RJ, Hashimoto T, Zillikens D, et al. Development of a simple enzyme-linked immunosorbent assay for the detection of autoantibodies in anti-p200 pemphigoid. *Br J Dermatol.* (2011) 164:76–82. doi: 10.1111/j.1365-2133.2010.10056.x
163. Bernard P, Antonicelli F, Bedane C, Joly P, Le Roux-Villet C, Duvert-Lehembre S, et al. Prevalence and clinical significance of anti-laminin 332 autoantibodies detected by a novel enzyme-linked immunosorbent assay in mucous membrane pemphigoid. *JAMA Dermatol.* (2013) 149:533–40. doi: 10.1001/jamadermatol.2013.1434
164. Hofmann S, Thoma-Uszynski S, Hunziker T, Bernard P, Koebnick C, Stauber A, et al. Severity and phenotype of bullous pemphigoid relate to autoantibody profile against the NH2- and COOH-terminal regions of the BP180 ectodomain. *J Invest Dermatol.* (2002) 119:1065–73. doi: 10.1046/j.1523-1747.2002.19529.x
165. Horvath ON, Varga R, Kaneda M, Schmidt E, Ruzicka T, Sardy M. Diagnostic performance of the "MESACUP anti-Skin profile TEST". *Eur J Dermatol.* (2016) 26:56–63. doi: 10.1684/ejd.2015.2692
166. Amagai M, Komai A, Hashimoto T, Shirakata Y, Hashimoto K, Yamada T, et al. Usefulness of enzyme-linked immunosorbent assay using recombinant desmogleins 1 and 3 for serodiagnosis of pemphigus. *Br J Dermatol.* (1999) 140:351–7. doi: 10.1046/j.1365-2133.1999.02752.x
167. Harman KE, Gratian MJ, Seed PT, Bhogal BS, Challacombe SJ, Black MM. Diagnosis of pemphigus by ELISA: a critical evaluation of two ELISAs for the detection of antibodies to the major pemphigus antigens, desmoglein 1 and 3. *Clin Exp Dermatol.* (2000) 25:236–40. doi: 10.1046/j.1365-2230.2000.00624.x
168. Huang CH, Chen CC, Wang CJ, Chang YT, Liu HN. Using desmoglein 1 and 3 enzyme-linked immunosorbent assay as an adjunct diagnostic tool for pemphigus. *J Chin Med Assoc.* (2007) 70:65–70. doi: 10.1016/S1726-4901(09)70304-1
169. D'Agosto G, Latini A, Carducci M, Mastroianni A, Vento A, Fei PC. Evaluation of recombinant antigen-based assays for diagnosis of bullous autoimmune diseases. *Clin Diagn Lab Immunol.* (2004) 11:762–5. doi: 10.1128/CDLI.11.4.762-765.2004
170. Daneshpazhooh M, Chams-Davatchi C, Khamesipour A, Mansoori P, Taheri A, Firooz A, et al. Desmoglein 1 and 3 enzyme-linked immunosorbent assay in Iranian patients with pemphigus vulgaris: correlation with phenotype, severity, and disease activity. *J Eur Acad Dermatol Venereol.* (2007) 21:1319–24. doi: 10.1111/j.1468-3083.2007.02254.x
171. Hallaji Z, Mortazavi H, Lajevardi V, Tamizifar B, AmirZargar A, Daneshpazhooh M, et al. Serum and salivary desmoglein 1 and 3 enzyme-linked immunosorbent assay in pemphigus vulgaris: correlation with phenotype and severity. *J Eur Acad Dermatol Venereol.* (2010) 24:275–80. doi: 10.1111/j.1468-3083.2009.03408.x
172. Sharma VK, Prasad HR, Khandpur S, Kumar A. Evaluation of desmoglein enzyme-linked immunosorbent assay (ELISA) in Indian patients with pemphigus vulgaris. *Int J Dermatol.* (2006) 45:518–22. doi: 10.1111/j.1365-4632.2006.02593.x
173. Atzori L, Deidda S, Aste N. Enzyme-linked immunosorbent assay in autoimmune blistering diseases: preliminary experience of the Dermatology Department of Cagliari. *G Ital Dermatol Venereol.* (2008) 143:1–8.
174. Zillikens D, Mascaro JM, Rose PA, Liu Z, Ewing SM, Caux F, et al. A highly sensitive enzyme-linked immunosorbent assay for the detection of circulating anti-BP180 autoantibodies in patients with bullous pemphigoid. *J Invest Dermatol.* (1997) 109:679–83. doi: 10.1111/1523-1747.ep12338088
175. Keller JJ, Kittridge AL, Debanne SM, Korman NJ. Evaluation of ELISA testing for BP180 and BP230 as a diagnostic modality for bullous pemphigoid: a clinical experience. *Arch Dermatol Res.* (2016) 308:269–72. doi: 10.1007/s00403-016-1631-1
176. Tampoia M, Lattanzi V, Zucano A, Villalta D, Filotico R, Fontana A, et al. Evaluation of a new ELISA assay for detection of BP230 autoantibodies in bullous pemphigoid. *Ann N Y Acad Sci.* (2009) 1173:15–20. doi: 10.1111/j.1749-6632.2009.04630.x
177. Thoma-Uszynski S, Uter W, Schwietzke S, Hofmann SC, Hunziker T, Bernard P, et al. BP230- and BP180-specific auto-antibodies in bullous pemphigoid. *J Invest Dermatol.* (2004) 122:1413–22. doi: 10.1111/j.0022-202X.2004.22603.x
178. Sakuma-Oyama Y, Powell AM, Oyama N, Albert S, Bhogal BS, Black MM. Evaluation of a BP180-NC16a enzyme-linked immunosorbent assay in the initial diagnosis of bullous pemphigoid. *Br J Dermatol.* (2004) 151:126–31. doi: 10.1111/j.1365-2133.2004.06082.x
179. Mariotti F, Grosso F, Terracina M, Ruffelli M, Cordiali-Fei P, Sera F, et al. Development of a novel ELISA system for detection of anti-BP180 IgG and characterization of autoantibody profile in bullous pemphigoid patients. *Br J Dermatol.* (2004) 151:1004–10. doi: 10.1111/j.1365-2133.2004.06245.x
180. Barnadas MA, Rubiales MV, Gonzalez MJ, Puig L, Garcia P, Baselga E, et al. Enzyme-linked immunosorbent assay (ELISA) and indirect immunofluorescence testing in a bullous pemphigoid and pemphigoid gestationis. *Int J Dermatol.* (2008) 47:1245–9. doi: 10.1111/j.1365-4632.2008.03824.x
181. Messingham KA, Noe MH, Chapman MA, Giudice GJ, Fairley JA. A novel ELISA reveals high frequencies of BP180-specific IgE production in bullous pemphigoid. *J Immunol Methods.* (2009) 346:18–25. doi: 10.1016/j.jim.2009.04.013
182. Kromminga A, Sitaru C, Hagel C, Herzog S, Zillikens D. Development of an ELISA for the detection of autoantibodies to BP230. *Clin Immunol.* (2004) 111:146–52. doi: 10.1016/j.clim.2003.12.007
183. Schmidt T, Hoch M, Lotfi Jad SS, Solimani F, Di ZG, Marzano AV, et al. Serological diagnostics in the detection of IgG autoantibodies against human collagen VII in epidermolysis bullosa acquisita: a multicentre analysis. *Br J Dermatol.* (2017) 177:1683–92. doi: 10.1111/bjd.15800
184. Saleh MA, Ishii K, Kim YJ, Murakami A, Ishii N, Hashimoto T, et al. Development of NC1 and NC2 domains of type VII collagen ELISA for the diagnosis and analysis of the time course of epidermolysis bullosa acquisita patients. *J Dermatol Sci.* (2011) 62:169–75. doi: 10.1016/j.jdermsci.2011.03.003
185. Kim JH, Kim YH, Kim S, Noh EB, Kim SE, Vorobyev A, et al. Serum levels of anti-type VII collagen antibodies detected by enzyme-linked immunosorbent assay in patients with epidermolysis bullosa acquisita are correlated with the severity of skin lesions. *J Eur Acad Dermatol Venereol.* (2013) 27:e224–30. doi: 10.1111/j.1468-3083.2012.04617.x
186. Chen M, Chan LS, Cai X, O'Toole EA, Sample JC, Woodley DT. Development of an ELISA for rapid detection of anti-type VII collagen autoantibodies in epidermolysis bullosa acquisita. *J Invest Dermatol.* (1997) 108:68–72. doi: 10.1111/1523-1747.ep12285634
187. Sardy M, Odenthal U, Karpati S, Paulsson M, Smyth N. Recombinant human tissue transglutaminase ELISA for the diagnosis of gluten-sensitive enteropathy. *Clin Chem.* (1999) 45:2142–9.
188. Sardy M, Karpati S, Peterfy F, Rasky K, Tomsits E, Zagoni T, et al. Comparison of a tissue transglutaminase ELISA with the endomysium antibody test in the diagnosis of gluten-sensitive enteropathy. *Z Gastroenterol.* (2000) 38:357–64. doi: 10.1055/s-2000-14883
189. Mankai A, Sakly W, Landolsi H, Gueddah L, Sriha B, Ayadi A, et al. Tissue transglutaminase antibodies in celiac disease, comparison of an enzyme linked immunosorbent assay and a dot blot assay. *Pathol Biol.* (2005) 53:204–9. doi: 10.1016/j.patbio.2004.07.022
190. Tampoia M, Giavarina D, Di GC, Bizzaro N. Diagnostic accuracy of enzyme-linked immunosorbent assays (ELISA) to detect anti-skin autoantibodies in autoimmune blistering skin diseases: a systematic review and meta-analysis. *Autoimmun Rev.* (2012) 12:121–6. doi: 10.1016/j.autrev.2012.07.006
191. Hisamatsu Y, Nishiyama T, Amano S, Matsui C, Ghohestani R, Hashimoto T. Usefulness of immunoblotting using purified laminin 5 in the diagnosis of anti-laminin 5 cicatricial pemphigoid. *J Dermatol Sci.* (2003) 33:113–9. doi: 10.1016/S0923-1811(03)00158-0
192. Mignogna M, Lanza A, Rossiello L, Ruocco V, Ahmed AR. Comparison of reactivity and epitope recognition between sera from American and Italian patients with oral pemphigoid. *Clin Exp Immunol.* (2006) 145:28–35. doi: 10.1111/j.1365-2249.2006.03103.x
193. Ishii N, Yoshida M, Hisamatsu Y, Ishida-Yamamoto A, Nakane H, Iizuka H, et al. Epidermolysis bullosa acquisita sera react with distinct epitopes on the NC1 and NC2 domains of type VII collagen: study using immunoblotting of domain-specific recombinant proteins and postembedding immunoelectron microscopy. *Br J Dermatol.* (2004) 150:843–51. doi: 10.1111/j.1365-2133.2004.05933.x

194. Futei Y, Amagai M, Sekiguchi M, Nishifuji K, Fujii Y, Nishikawa T. Use of domain-swapped molecules for conformational epitope mapping of desmoglein 3 in pemphigus vulgaris. *J Invest Dermatol.* (2000) 115:829–34. doi: 10.1046/j.1523-1747.2000.00137.x

195. Amagai M, Ishii K, Hashimoto T, Gamou S, Shimizu N, Nishikawa T. Conformational epitopes of pemphigus antigens (Dsgl and Dsg3) are calcium dependent and glycosylation independent. *J Invest Dermatol.* (1995) 105:243–7. doi: 10.1111/1523-1747.ep12317587

196. Kowalczyk AP, Anderson JE, Borgwardt JE, Hashimoto T, Stanley JR, Green KJ. Pemphigus sera recognize conformationally sensitive epitopes in the amino-terminal region of desmoglein-1. *J Invest Dermatol.* (1995) 105:147–52. doi: 10.1111/1523-1747.ep12316680

197. Bieber K, Sun S, Ishii N, Kasperkiewicz M, Schmidt E, Hirose M, et al. Animal models for autoimmune bullous dermatoses. *Exp Dermatol.* (2010) 19:2–11. doi: 10.1111/j.1600-0625.2009.00948.x

198. Culton DA, Qian Y, Li N, Rubenstein D, Aoki V, Filhio GH, et al. Advances in pemphigus and its endemic pemphigus foliaceus (Fogo Selvagem) phenotype: a paradigm of human autoimmunity. *J Autoimmun.* (2008) 31:311–24. doi: 10.1016/j.jaut.2008.08.003

199. Liu Z, Sui W, Zhao M, Li Z, Li N, Thresher R, et al. Subepidermal blistering induced by human autoantibodies to BP180 requires innate immune players in a humanized bullous pemphigoid mouse model. *J Autoimmun.* (2008) 31:331–8. doi: 10.1016/j.jaut.2008.08.009

200. Schiltz JR, Michel B. Production of epidermal acantholysis in normal human skin *in vitro* by the IgG fraction from pemphigus serum. *J Invest Dermatol.* (1976) 67:254–60. doi: 10.1111/1523-1747.ep12513454

201. Anhalt GJ, Labib RS, Voorhees JJ, Beals TF, Diaz LA. Induction of pemphigus in neonatal mice by passive transfer of IgG from patients with the disease. *N Engl J Med.* (1982) 306:1189–96. doi: 10.1056/NEJM198205203062001

202. Lazarova Z, Hsu R, Yee C, Yancey KB. Human anti-laminin 5 autoantibodies induce subepidermal blisters in an experimental human skin graft model. *J Invest Dermatol.* (2000) 114:178–84. doi: 10.1046/j.1523-1747.2000.00829.x

203. Woodley DT, Chang C, Saadat P, Ram R, Liu Z, Chen M. Evidence that anti-type VII collagen antibodies are pathogenic and responsible for the clinical, histological, and immunological features of epidermolysis bullosa acquisita. *J Invest Dermatol.* (2005) 124:958–64. doi: 10.1111/j.0022-202X.2005.23702.x

204. Ludwig RJ, Vanhoorelbeke K, Leypoldt F, Kaya Z, Bieber K, McLachlan SM, et al. Mechanisms of autoantibody-induced pathology. *Front Immunol.* (2017) 8:603. doi: 10.3389/fimmu.2017.00603

205. Genovese G, Di Zenzo G, Cozzani E, Berti E, Cugno M, Marzano AV. New insights into the pathogenesis of bullous pemphigoid: 2019 update. *Front Immunol.* (2019) 10:1506. doi: 10.3389/fimmu.2019.01506

206. Pfutze M, Eming R, Kneisel A, Kuhlmann U, Hoyer J, Hertl M. Clinical and immunological follow-up of pemphigus patients on adjuvant treatment with immunoadsorption or rituximab. *Dermatology.* (2009) 218:237–45. doi: 10.1159/000187431

207. Cheng SW, Kobayashi M, Kinoshita-Kuroda K, Tanikawa A, Amagai M, Nishikawa T. Monitoring disease activity in pemphigus with enzyme-linked immunosorbent assay using recombinant desmogleins 1 and 3. *Br J Dermatol.* (2002) 147:261–5. doi: 10.1046/j.1365-2133.2002.04838.x

208. Harman KE, Seed PT, Gratian MJ, Bhogal BS, Challacombe SJ, Black MM. The severity of cutaneous and oral pemphigus is related to desmoglein 1 and 3 antibody levels. *Br J Dermatol.* (2001) 144:775–80. doi: 10.1046/j.1365-2133.2001.04132.x

209. Abasq C, Mouquet H, Gilbert D, Tron F, Grassi V, Musette P, et al. ELISA testing of anti-desmoglein 1 and 3 antibodies in the management of pemphigus. *Arch Dermatol.* (2009) 145:529–35. doi: 10.1001/archdermatol.2009.9

210. Schmidt E, Obe K, Brocker EB, Zillikens D. Serum levels of autoantibodies to BP180 correlate with disease activity in patients with bullous pemphigoid. *Arch Dermatol.* (2000) 136:174–8. doi: 10.1001/archderm.136.2.174

211. Tsuji-Abe Y, Akiyama M, Yamanaka Y, Kikuchi T, Sato-Matsumura KC, Shimizu H. Correlation of clinical severity and ELISA indices for the NC16A domain of BP180 measured using BP180 ELISA kit in bullous pemphigoid. *J Dermatol Sci.* (2005) 37:145–9. doi: 10.1016/j.jdermsci.2004.10.007

212. Feng S, Wu Q, Jin P, Lin L, Zhou W, Sang H, et al. Serum levels of autoantibodies to BP180 correlate with disease activity in patients with bullous pemphigoid. *Int J Dermatol.* (2008) 47:225–8. doi: 10.1111/j.1365-4632.2008.03473.x

213. Amo Y, Ohkawa T, Tatsuta M, Hamada Y, Fujimura T, Katsuoka K, et al. Clinical significance of enzyme-linked immunosorbent assay for the detection of circulating anti-BP180 autoantibodies in patients with bullous pemphigoid. *J Dermatol Sci.* (2001) 26:14–8. doi: 10.1016/S0923-1811(00)00149-3

214. Zone JJ, Taylor T, Hull C, Schmidt L, Meyer L. IgE basement membrane zone antibodies induce eosinophil infiltration and histological blisters in engrafted human skin on SCID mice. *J Invest Dermatol.* (2007) 127:1167–74. doi: 10.1038/sj.jid.5700681

215. Terra JB, Jonkman MF, Diercks GF, Pas HH. Low sensitivity of type VII collagen enzyme-linked immunosorbent assay in epidermolysis bullosa acquisita: serration pattern analysis on skin biopsy is required for diagnosis. *Br J Dermatol.* (2013) 169:164–7. doi: 10.1111/bjd.12300

216. Giusti D, Le Jan S, Gatouillat G, Bernard P, Pham BN, Antonicelli F. Biomarkers related to bullous pemphigoid activity and outcome. *Exp Dermatol.* (2017) 26:1240–7. doi: 10.1111/exd.13459

217. Koga H, Teye K, Ishii N, Ohata C, Nakama T. High index values of enzyme-linked immunosorbent assay for BP180 at baseline predict relapse in patients with bullous pemphigoid. *Front Med.* (2018) 5:139. doi: 10.3389/fmed.2018.00139

218. Bernard P, Reguiai Z, Tancrede-Bohin E, Cordel N, Plantin P, Pauwels C, et al. Risk factors for relapse in patients with bullous pemphigoid in clinical remission: a multicenter, prospective, cohort study. *Arch Dermatol.* (2009) 145:537–42. doi: 10.1001/archdermatol.2009.53

219. Fichel F, Barbe C, Joly P, Bedane C, Vabres P, Truchetet F, et al. Clinical and immunologic factors associated with bullous pemphigoid relapse during the first year of treatment: a multicenter, prospective study. *JAMA Dermatol.* (2014) 150:25–33. doi: 10.1001/jamadermatol.2013.5757

220. Cai SC, Lim YL, Li W, Allen JC, Chua SH, Tan SH, et al. Anti-BP180 NC16A IgG titres as an indicator of disease activity and outcome in asian patients with bullous pemphigoid. *Ann Acad Med Singapore.* (2015) 44:119–26.

221. Giusti D, Gatouillat G, Le Jan S, Plee J, Bernard P, Antonicelli F, et al. Anti-type VII collagen antibodies are identified in a subpopulation of bullous pemphigoid patients with relapse. *Front Immunol.* (2018) 9:570. doi: 10.3389/fimmu.2018.00570

222. Plee J, Le Jan S, Giustiniani J, Barbe C, Joly P, Bedane C, et al. Integrating longitudinal serum IL-17 and IL-23 follow-up, along with autoantibodies variation, contributes to predict bullous pemphigoid outcome. *Sci Rep.* (2015) 5:18001. doi: 10.1038/srep18001

223. Riani M, Le Jan S, Plee J, Durlach A, Le Naour R, Haegeman G, et al. Bullous pemphigoid outcome is associated with CXCL10-induced matrix metalloproteinase 9 secretion from monocytes and neutrophils but not lymphocytes. *J Allergy Clin Immunol.* (2017) 139:863–72. doi: 10.1016/j.jaci.2016.08.012

224. Giusti D, Gatouillat G, Le Jan S, Plee J, Bernard P, Antonicelli F, et al. Eosinophil Cationic Protein (ECP), a predictive marker of bullous pemphigoid severity and outcome. *Sci Rep.* (2017) 7:4833. doi: 10.1038/s41598-017-04687-5

225. Brulefert A, Le Jan S, Plee J, Durlach A, Bernard P, Antonicelli F, et al. Variation of the epidermal expression of glucocorticoid receptor-beta as potential predictive marker of bullous pemphigoid outcome. *Exp Dermatol.* (2017) 26:1261–6. doi: 10.1111/exd.13444

226. Daneshpazhooh M, Zafarmand Sedigh V, Balighi K, Hosseini SH, Ramezani A, Kalantari MS, et al. Immunologic prediction of relapse in patients with pemphigus vulgaris (PV) in clinical remission. *J Am Acad Dermatol.* (2016) 74:1160–5. doi: 10.1016/j.jaad.2015.10.051

227. Albers LN, Liu Y, Bo N, Swerlick RA, Feldman RJ. Developing biomarkers for predicting clinical relapse in pemphigus patients treated with rituximab. *J Am Acad Dermatol.* (2017) 77:1074–82. doi: 10.1016/j.jaad.2017.07.012

228. Schmidt E, Eming R. [Autoimmune bullous dermatoses : update on treatments and rare forms]. *Hautarzt.* (2019) 70:234–5. doi: 10.1007/s00105-019-4391-y

229. Izumi K, Bieber K, Ludwig RJ. Current clinical trials in pemphigus and pemphigoid. *Front Immunol.* (2019) 10:978. doi: 10.3389/fimmu.2019.00978
230. Hashimoto T, Ohzono A, Teye K, Numata S, Hiroyasu S, Tsuruta D, et al. Detection of IgE autoantibodies to BP180 and BP230 and their relationship to clinical features in bullous pemphigoid. *Br J Dermatol.* (2017) 177:141–51. doi: 10.1111/bjd.15114
231. van Beek N, Schulze FS, Zillikens D, Schmidt E. IgE-mediated mechanisms in bullous pemphigoid and other autoimmune bullous diseases. *Expert Rev Clin Immunol.* (2016) 12:267–77. doi: 10.1586/1744666X.2016.1123092
232. Fairley JA, Baum CL, Brandt DS, Messingham KA. Pathogenicity of IgE in autoimmunity: successful treatment of bullous pemphigoid with omalizumab. *J Allergy Clin Immunol.* (2009) 123:704–5. doi: 10.1016/j.jaci.2008.11.035
233. Dopp R, Schmidt E, Chimanovitch I, Leverkus M, Brocker EB, Zillikens D. IgG4 and IgE are the major immunoglobulins targeting the NC16A domain of BP180 in Bullous pemphigoid: serum levels of these immunoglobulins reflect disease activity. *J Am Acad Dermatol.* (2000) 42:577–83. doi: 10.1067/mjd.2000.103986

4

Anti-p200 Pemphigoid: A Systematic Review

Khalaf Kridin[1] *and A. Razzaque Ahmed*[2*]

[1] *Department of Dermatology, Rambam Health Care Campus, Haifa, Israel,* [2] *Department of Dermatology, Center for Blistering Diseases, Tufts University School of Medicine, Boston, MA, United States*

***Correspondence:**
A. Razzaque Ahmed
arahmedmd@msn.com

The many clinical aspects of anti-p200 pemphigoid are not well-characterized. We aimed to analyze and correlate known existing data on the epidemiological, clinical, histological, and immunological features of anti-p200 pemphigoid. We performed a review using Medline, Embase, and Web of Science databases (1900–2018). Case reports and series of patients were included. A total of 68 eligible studies that comprised 113 anti-p200 pemphigoid patients were included in the qualitative analysis, where there was a mean age of onset of 65.5 years. All patients presented with bullae/vesicles, and 54.3% had urticarial plaques. A similarity to bullous pemphigoid was reported in 66.1% of cases, but palmoplantar (51.4%), cephalic (40.3%), and mucosal (38.5%) involvement, besides frequent development of scars/milia (15.7%), were reported. Autoantibodies against recombinant laminin γ1 were detected in the sera of 73.1% of patients. Psoriasis was present in 28.3% of anti-p200 pemphigoid patients, particularly among Japanese patients (56.4%). The incidence of pustular psoriasis in this subgroup, was significantly greater than in the normal population. In conclusion, the diagnosis of anti-p200 pemphigoid may be suspected when a subepidermal autoimmune blistering disease develops in a younger age group, along with significant acral and cephalic distribution and mucosal involvement.

Keywords: anti-p200 pemphigoid, anti-laminin gamma-1 pemphigoid, IIF of salt-split skin, immunoblotting, ELISA, BMZ autoantibodies, mucosal disease, psoriasis

INTRODUCTION

Anti-p200 pemphigoid is a rare subepidermal autoimmune bullous disease (AIBD) initially described in 1996 (1, 2). This novel disease, presumed to be a subset of pemphigoid, was characterized by autoantibodies targeting a 200-kDa protein localized within the lower lamina lucida of the basement membrane zone (BMZ). Their sera bound to the dermal side of salt-split skin by indirect immunofluorescence (IIF) microscopy (3). Subsequent studies demonstrated that sera from 90% of anti-p200 pemphigoid patients recognized laminin γ1, which C-terminus was identified as an immunodominant region and utilized for immunoblotting and ELISA for diagnosis (4, 5). In outstanding research by German and Japanese investigators, using human foreskin and various mouse strains, the investigators clearly demonstrated that autoantibodies in anti-p200 pemphigoid sera are pathogenic, but their pathogenicity is not entirely mediated by autoantibodies against laminin γ1. The specific or precise role for laminin γ1 in pathogenesis requires further study, as *ex vivo* and *in vivo* studies did not show evidence of a direct pathogenic role of anti-laminin γ1 antibodies, leaving the true molecular identity of the pathogenic 200 kDa autoantigen yet to be fully characterized (6, 7). To elaborate, in two different mouse animal models for anti-laminin γ1 pemphigoid, although murine IgG of the recombinant laminin γ1 C-terminus bound to the epidermal basement membrane zone in the passive transfer model, no obvious blister formation was seen (7). In an earlier *ex vivo* model of autoantibody-mediated leukocyte-dependent neutrophil activation, human and rabbit IgG from the C-terminus of laminin γ1 failed to attract neutrophils at the dermal-epidermal-junction and to induce dermal-epidermal separation (6).

The clinical presentation of anti-p200 is polymorphic and may mimic bullous pemphigoid (BP), mucous membrane pemphigoid (MMP), and other subepidermal AIBD (8). However, data on its morphological features and the clinical course are limited, primarily because of the small number of reported cases and the lack of a large cohort of patients studied in detail with long-term follow-up.

We did not focus on therapy because it was considered beyond the scope of this analysis due to lack of uniformity, cohesive information, defined protocol, and outcome data. The aim of the current study was to perform a review of the available epidemiological, clinical, histological, and immunopathological data and the major comorbidities in patients with anti-p200 pemphigoid. The purpose was to help clinicians recognize this newly described clinical entity. This could result in early therapy and better prognosis.

MATERIALS AND METHODS

Data Collection

The literature review was conducted using Ovid-Medline (1946–present), Embase (1947–present), and Web of Science (1900–present) to identify eligible articles. Publications until August 9th 2018, were searched. The search strategies are detailed in **Supplementary Table 1**.

Selection of Articles

All publications reporting on one or multiple cases of anti-p200 pemphigoid were included. All cases were defined by the authors of the respective publications as anti-p200 pemphigoid based on the following three mandatory criteria: (i) clinical profile suggestive of subepidermal AIBD; (ii) reactivity to the 200 kDa protein or to the recombinant C-terminus of laminin γ1 by immunoblot analysis; and (iii) exclusion of other subepidermal AIBDs. Additionally, at least one of the following two minor criteria was required to establish the diagnosis of anti-p200 pemphigoid: (i) subepidermal cleft on histology; (ii) and direct immunofluorescence (DIF), demonstrating linear deposition of IgG and/or C3. Publications lacking these criteria were excluded.

Data Extraction

The following information was obtained when authors provided it: age at onset, sex, ethnicity, morphological features of the mucocutaneous manifestation and their anatomic distribution, histopathology, immunopathology, comorbidities, and triggering factors (if known). All statistical analysis was performed using SPSS software, version 23 (SPSS, Chicago, IL, USA).

TABLE 1 | Demographic characteristics of the patients reported with anti-p200 pemphigoid.

Male patients, *n* (%)	85 (75.2%)
Age at diagnosis	
Mean (±SD)*	65.5 (15.9)
Median (range)	69 (5-94)
Mean age of male patients (±SD)*	66.0 (14.0)
Mean age of female patients (±SD)*	63.4 (20.8)
Ethnicity of reported patients, *n* (%)	
Asian	57 (50.4%)
Caucasians	22 (19.5%)
Jews	1 (0.9%)
African American	1 (0.9%)
Not reported	32 (28.3%)
Geographical distribution of reported cases, % (*n*)	
Japan	50 (44.2%)
France	18 (15.9%)
Germany	13 (11.5%)
Netherlands	12 (10.6%)
USA	7 (6.2%)
India	3 (2.7)
Poland	2 (1.8%)
Spain	2 (1.8%)
China	1 (0.9%)
UK	1 (0.9%)
Israel	1 (0.9%)
Croatia	1 (0.9%)
Greece	1 (0.9%)
Austria	1 (0.9%)
Korea	1 (0.9%)

n, number; SD, standard deviation; USA, United States of America; UK, United Kingdom.
Excluding the study of Meijer et al. (3) which did not report standard deviation.

RESULTS

After a full-text review, 68 articles fulfilled the inclusion criteria, thereby providing 113 patients from 15 different countries that were included in the qualitative synthesis. Between 1996 and 2018, 50 cases (44.2%) were reported from Japan (**Table 1**).

Clinical Characteristics

The mean age at onset was 65.5 years (range 5–94) (9, 10). The majority of the patients were males ($n = 85$; 75.2%) and of Asian ancestry ($n = 57$, 50.4%; **Table 1**).

The clinical presentation was described as resembling other subepidermal AIBD and inflammatory dermatoses by authors in 68 (60.2%) patients. The leading similar condition was BP ($n = 45$; 66.2%), followed by linear IgA bullous dermatosis (LABD; $n = 5$; 7.4%) (9, 11–14), epidermolysis bullosa acquisita (EBA; $n = 3$; 4.4%) (15–17), dermatitis herpetiformis (DH; $n = 3$; 4.4%) (18–20), mucous membrane pemphigoid ($n = 3$; 4.4%) (21–23), and others (**Table 2**). In the remaining 45 patients, a similarity to a distinct clinical entity was not mentioned.

TABLE 2 | Clinical and morphological characteristics of the reported patients with anti-p200 pemphigoid.

		Number of reported cases
Similar condition, *n* (%)-reported in 68 cases		
Bullous pemphigoid	45 (66.2%)	68
Linear IgA bullous dermatosis	5 (7.4%)	68
Vesicular pemphigoid	4 (5.9%)	68
Epidermolysis bullosa acquisita	3 (4.4%)	68
Dermatitis herpetiformis	3 (4.4%)	68
Mucous membrane pemphigoid	3 (4.4%)	68
Erythema gyratum repens	2 (2.9%)	68
Pemphigus	1 (1.5%)	68
Pompholyx	1 (1.5%)	68
Morphology of cutaneous lesions, *n* (%)		
Bullae/vesicles	113 (100%)	113
Urticarial plaques	50 (54.3%)	92
Scars/milia	16 (15.7%)	102
Anatomical distribution of cutaneous lesions, *n* (%)		
Extremities	78 (95.1%)	82
Trunk	58 (70.7%)	82
Palms and soles	38 (51.4%)	74
Head and neck	29 (40.3%)	72
Mucosal involvement	37 (38.5%)	96
Mucosal involvement, *n* (%)		
One mucosal surface	29 (30.2%)	96
Two mucosal surfaces concomitantly	6 (6.3%)	96
Three mucosal surfaces concomitantly	2 (2.1%)	96
Oral mucosa	31 (32.3%)	96
Anogenital mucosa	12 (12.5%)	96
Conjunctival mucosa	2 (2.1%)	96

n, number. The right column represents the number of cases where the variable was reported or could be concluded. The ratios represent number of positive cases out of the number of reported cases.

TABLE 3 | Immunopathological and immunological characteristics of the reported patients with anti-p200 pemphigoid.

		Number of reported cases
Direct immunofluorescence, *n* (%)		
Linear deposition along the BMZ	113 (100%)	113
Linear deposition of IgG and C3	77 (78.6%)	98
Linear deposition of IgG, IgA, and C3	10 (10.2%)	98
Linear deposition of C3 alone	4 (4.1%)	98
Linear deposition of IgG, IgA, IgM, and C3	2 (2.0%)	98
Linear deposition of IgG alone	2 (2.0%)	98
N-serration deposition pattern	11 (84.6%)	13
U-serration deposition pattern	0 (0%)	13
Undetermined deposition pattern	2 (15.4%)	13
NaCl-split indirect immunofluorescence deposition, *n* (%)		
Dermal side	90 (83.3%)	108
Both dermal and epidermal sides (more prominently in the dermal side)	16 (14.8%)	108
Epidermal side	1 (0.9%)	108
Negative	1 (0.9%)	108
Immunoblot analysis, *n* (%)		
200-kDa dermal protein	111 (100%)	111
Recombinant C-terminus of laminin γ1	19 (73.1%)	26
ELISA detecting recombinant monomeric C-terminal fragment of human laminin γ1, *n* (%)		
	10 (100%)	10

n, number; BMZ, basement membrane zone; Ig, immunoglobulin; ELISA, enzyme-linked immunosorbent assay. The right column represents the number of cases where the variable was reported or could be concluded. The ratios represent the number of positive cases out of the number of reported cases.

All patients presented with bullae and/or vesicles, 54.3% (50/92) had urticarial plaques, 15.7% (16/102) had scars and/or milia (**Table 2**).

The distribution of cutaneous lesions was reported in 72 patients. The extremities were the most frequently involved (95.1%), the trunk in 70.7%, and palmoplantar and cephalic involvement in 51.4 and 40.3% of patients, respectively. Generalized involvement was reported in 41.5% of patients. Mucosal involvement was reported in 38.5% of patients, with the oral mucosa (32.3%) being the most frequently involved. None of the patients had exclusively mucosal diseases (**Table 2**). Of great interest, the prevalence of mucosal involvement among Japanese patients (22.5%) was significantly lower when compared to the remaining patients (48.2%; $P < 0.001$).

Histological Characteristics

Histology data was available on 100 (88.5%) patients. A subepidermal blistering was observed in all patients, along with mild to dense inflammatory infiltrates in the upper dermis composed of neutrophils and eosinophils in 41 (41.0%) and 15 (15.0%) patients, respectively. A mixed infiltrate of neutrophils and eosinophils was seen in 40 (40.0%) of patients. In two patients, an exclusively lymphocytic infiltrate was observed (24, 25); papillary microabscesses were observed in 11 (11.0%) patients, a predominantly neutrophilic infiltrate in 10 patients (2, 14, 18–20, 26–29) and a mixed infiltrate in one patient (3). Eosinophilic spongiosis was observed in two patients (3, 27) and ruptured secondary milia with inflammatory granulomatous in one patient (16).

Immunopathological Characteristics

DIF microscopy of perilesional skin was reported in 98 (88.1%) patients. Deposition of IgG and C3 was observed in 77 (78.6%), whereas the simultaneous deposition of IgG, IgA, and C3 was observed in 10 (10.2%) patients (3, 9, 12, 14, 20, 30). Deposition of IgG or C3 alone was observed in two (2.0%) (16, 31) and four (4.1%) patients (22, 32–34), respectively. N-serration deposition pattern from a BMZ immunoreactant was shown in 11 of 13 (84.6%) patients, whereas this pattern was undetermined in the remaining two (15.4%) patients (3, 35, 36) (**Table 3**).

On salt-split skin, binding to the dermal side of the split was reported in 90 patients (83.3%) and binding to both the dermal and epidermal sides in 16 patients (14.8%) (**Table 3**). Immunoblot analysis demonstrated reactivity to the 200 kDa protein in all 111 patients tested using human dermal extract ($n = 108$), epidermal extracts ($n = 11$) (10, 37) and keratinocytes extracts ($n = 2$) (32). Sera of several patients were tested on multiple extracts, and 10 of the 11 patients reacting to the epidermal extract were also seropositive on dermal extracts (10). In the remaining two patients, immunoblotting showed reactivity only to the recombinant C-terminus of laminin γ1 (38, 39). Of significant interest is that the sera of patients who were positive for antibodies when tested using immunoblot analysis with the recombinant C-terminus of laminin γ1 was positive in 17 of 24, with a 70.8% sensitivity (3, 9, 31, 38–43). Sera of 10 patients was tested by ELISA bound to a recombinant monomeric C-terminal fragment of human laminin γ1 (10, 44, 45) (**Table 3**).

Autoantibodies targeting other antigens were detected in 20 (17.7%). Autoantibodies against BP-180 alone, BP-230 alone and both BP-180 and BP-230 were identified in two (1.8%) (19, 46), four (3.5%) (2, 36, 47), and three (2.7%) patients (10, 48), respectively. Antibodies to Type-VII collagen were found in three (2.7%) patients (15, 16, 49), whereas autoantibodies against different subunits of laminin 332 were detected in 7 (6.2%) patients (21, 22, 34, 44, 50–52).

Associated Comorbidities

An association with psoriasis was reported in 32 patients (28.3%). Psoriasis preceded the diagnosis of anti-p200 pemphigoid in all patients by a mean of 15.1 ± 10.4 years (median, 18 years; range, 0.1–30 years). Four (12.5%) patients had developed bullous disease with pustular psoriasis simultaneously (33, 35, 53, 54). The onset of anti-p200 pemphigoid was associated with erythrodermic psoriasis in one (3.1%) patient (55). The remaining patients (84.4%) had psoriasis vulgaris. Of interest, 28 (87.5%) patients with psoriasis were Japanese, whereas the remaining four (12.5%) were Europeans (10, 27, 56, 57).

Taken together, the prevalence of psoriasis in anti-p200 pemphigoid Japanese patients was 56.0% (95% CI, 42.3–68.8%) as compared to only 6.4% (95% CI, 2.5–15.2%) among non-Japanese patients ($P < 0.001$). There was a slightly higher frequency of males among anti-p200 pemphigoid patients with psoriasis compared to those without psoriasis (87.5 vs. 70.4%; $P = 0.058$). The age of presentation was comparable in the two subgroups (data not shown).

Concomitant malignancies were reported in three female patients. One had metastatic clear cell carcinoma of the ovary (21), one had uterine adenocarcinoma (58), and the other had metastatic esophageal adenocarcinoma (38). Other comorbidities reported included: end-stage kidney disease due to IgA nephropathy and glomerulonephritis ($n = 2$) (22, 34), ulcerative colitis ($n = 1$) (50), esophagitis ($n = 1$) (15), polyarteritis nodosa ($n = 1$) (59), and autosomal recessive congenital ichthyosis ($n = 1$) (36). Unproven trigger factors included scabies ($n = 2$) (60, 61) and use of penicillin ($n = 1$) (62).

DISCUSSION

This review highlights the multiple aspects of a recently described interesting subset of pemphigoid. Based on the current information, its main focus is the clinical features. Many of the unique characteristics and associations could be important to cutaneous biology and the pathogenesis of autoimmunity. A heterogeneous clinical profile that mimicked BP was present in the majority of patients, accompanied by a high prevalence of cephalic, palmoplantar and mucosal involvement. Autoantibodies against the recombinant C-terminus of laminin γ1 were detected by immunoblotting in 73.1% of patients. The prevalence of coexistent psoriasis was significantly higher than in the general population. Interestingly, the presence of psoriasis was very significantly higher in Japanese than non-Japanese patients (56.0 vs. 6.4%, respectively).

Palmoplantar lesions and mucosal involvement in BP has been reported in up to 20% of patients (63–65), and these regions were affected in 51.4 and 38.5% of patients with anti-p200 pemphigoid, respectively. Interestingly, scars and milia were reported in 3.4% of patients with BP (63) but in 15.7% of patients with anti-p200 pemphigoid. In the clinical criteria suggested by Vaillant et al. (66), which yield a positive predictive value of 95% for a clinical diagnosis of BP, it is the absence of each of the three aforementioned features that has been identified as an independent predictive criterion for the diagnosis of BP.

The age at onset of patients with anti-p200 pemphigoid (65.5 years) is younger than many with BP, where it commonly occurs in those older than 70 (67–69). An overwhelming preponderance of males (75.2%) were reported with anti-p200 pemphigoid, which contrasts with the female-to-male ratio ranges between 1.04 and 5.1 in different cohorts of BP (69).

In 2009, Dainichi et al. (4) found that 90% of sera tested from anti-p200 pemphigoid patients reacted to the C-terminus of recombinant laminin γ1, using an immunoblot assay. This observation has been confirmed by Groth et al. (5). This analysis demonstrates that sera from 73.1% of the patients reported reacting to the C-terminus of recombinant laminin γ1 protein using the immunoblotting assay. With respect to the ELISA using a monomeric C-terminal fragment of human laminin, the sensitivity was estimated at 68.6% (5).

The incidence of anti-p200 pemphigoid is considerably low amongst AIBD (70). In a cohort of 145 Japanese patients with various AIBDs, anti-p200 pemphigoid was the second most prevalent AIBD (37.2%). The prevalence of psoriasis among non-Japanese anti-p200 pemphigoid patients (6.4%) was greater than its incidence in the general population of the world (71, 72). The pathomechanism of this ethnic association is yet to be established (70). Pustular psoriasis was present in 12.5% of p-200 pemphigoid patients. This incidence is significantly higher than the 1.3% reported in a cohort of 104,669 patients with different variants of psoriasis ($P < 0.001$) (73). This observation confirmed an earlier Japanese study which reported that 53.8% of patients with pustular psoriasis and AIBD had anti-p200 pemphigoid (70). The molecular basis for this rare and unique combination of clinical entities has not been clearly defined and warrants attention. Senescence was suggested to alter the distribution and amount of proteins in the BMZ, thus increasing its antigenicity and raising the risk of the development of an autoimmune response against its components (74). Since the cell cycle and turnover of the epidermal keratinocytes are extremely accelerated in psoriasis, it was recently assumed that the extracellular matrix in psoriatic skin may simulate the senescent extracellular matrix and contribute to the development of BP and other AIBDs that were found to be associated with psoriasis (75).

Our current knowledge of anti-p-200 pemphigoid brings into focus several important and interesting issues. Traditionally, pemphigoid is divided into BP and mucous membrane pemphigoid. It is possible that because anti-p200 pemphigoid has certain features of both conditions, it could be the bridge or missing link between them. Some anti-p200 pemphigoid also has features of other AIBD, since their sera contain autoantibodies associated with them. It would be interesting to speculate whether this was due to epitope spreading (76). Patients with systemic lupus erythematosus have multiple pathogenic autoantibodies per patient (77), including multiple phenotypes and symptomatologies.

An additional unsolved question is whether anti-p-200 pemphigoid is truly rare or whether it is rather underdiagnosed worldwide. In the US, tests for detecting autoantibodies to laminin γ1 are commercially unavailable, though they are available in Germany and Japan. Moreover, investigators in those countries, whose laboratories are equipped to perform these assays, provide them to their colleagues. The majority of patients are thus reported from Japan and Europe. Unless there are very specific unidentified reasons, there are generally no reasons to believe that it cannot not be as prevalent in other countries. Unless more patients are studied, serologically characterized and followed up for several years, this challenging variant of pemphigoid will remain less well-studied and understood. This would be tragic, because it could help advance our knowledge.

The main limitations of this review are that it was based on case reports and small case series and that it is retrospective. Some of the variables were not provided by some authors. Data on treatment were scarce, limited and not comprehensive. Limited follow-up did not provide a clear clinical course or an overview of the impact of treatment on clinical course. The universal lack of the ELISAs makes it impossible to assess its global presence. Since psoriasis is present universally, its relationship could not be accurately assessed.

In conclusion, this new subset provides, to clinicians and scientists alike, a unique opportunity to study several new frontiers of cutaneous biology, inflammation, immunology, scar formation and disease pathogenesis. The location of laminin γ1 provides the opportunity to study interactions amongst other BMZ proteins. An association with psoriasis provides a playground to study what influences neutrophils to cause different pathologies and clinical profiles. The presence of scarring in mucosal tissues of some patients and not in others could provide important leads into what thrusts patients into one direction or the other. This opportunity, provided by nature, should not be missed but utilized to the advantage of our patients and the progress of our specialty.

AUTHOR CONTRIBUTIONS

AA and KK contributed to the concept, content, and writing of the manuscript.

REFERENCES

1. Zillikens D, Kawahara Y, Ishiko A, Shimizu H, Mayer J, Rank CV, et al. A novel subepidermal blistering disease with autoantibodies to a 200-kDa antigen of the basement membrane zone. *J Invest Dermatol.* (1996) 106:1333–8. doi: 10.1111/1523-1747.ep12349283
2. Chen KR, Shimizu S, Miyakawa S, Ishiko A, Shimizu H, Hashimoto T. Coexistence of psoriasis and an unusual IgG-mediated subepidermal bullous dermatosis: identification of a novel 200-kDa lower lamina lucida target antigen. *Br J Dermatol.* (1996) 134:340–6. doi: 10.1111/j.1365-2133.1996.tb07625.x
3. Meijer JM, Diercks GFH, Schmidt E, Pas HH, Jonkman MF. Laboratory diagnosis and clinical profile of anti-p200 pemphigoid. *JAMA Dermatol.* (2016) 152:897–904. doi: 10.1001/jamadermatol.2016.1099
4. Dainichi T, Kurono S, Ohyama B, Ishii N, Sanzen N, Hayashi M, et al. Anti-laminin gamma-1 pemphigoid. *Proc Natl Acad Sci USA.* (2009) 106:2800–5. doi: 10.1073/pnas.0809230106
5. Groth S, Recke A, Vafia K, Ludwig RJ, Hashimoto T, Zillikens D, et al. Development of a simple enzyme-linked immunosorbent assay for the detection of autoantibodies in anti-p200 pemphigoid. *Br J Dermatol.* (2011) 164:76–82. doi: 10.1111/j.1365-2133.2010.10056.x
6. Vafia K, Groth S, Beckmann T, Hirose M, Dworschak J, Recke A, et al. Pathogenicity of autoantibodies in anti-p200 pemphigoid. *PLoS ONE.* (2012) 7:e41769. doi: 10.1371/journal.pone.0041769
7. Koga H, Ishii N, Dainichi T, Tsuruta D, Hamada T, Ohata C, et al. An attempt to develop mouse model for anti-laminin gamma 1 pemphigoid. *J Dermatol Sci.* (2013) 70:108–15. doi: 10.1016/j.jdermsci.2013.01.001
8. Goletz S, Hashimoto T, Zillikens D, Schmidt E. Anti-p200 pemphigoid. *J Am Acad Dermatol.* (2014) 71:185–91. doi: 10.1016/j.jaad.2014.02.036
9. Patsatsi A, Meltzanidou P, Katafigiotis S, Sotiriadis D, Schmidt E, Lambropoulos A. Chronic bullous disease of childhood with IgG reactivity to p200 antigen. *Int J Dermatol.* (2017) 56:773–5. doi: 10.1111/ijd.13616
10. Commin MH, Schmidt E, Duvert-Lehembre S, Lasek A, Morice C, Estival JL, et al. Clinical and immunological features and outcome of anti-p200 pemphigoid. *Br J Dermatol.* (2016) 175:776–81. doi: 10.1111/bjd.14629
11. Myers DJ, Unwala RD, Xia L, Groth S, Zillikens D, Stratman EJ. Generalized annular bullous eruption–quiz case. Anti-laminin gamma1 pemphigoid with a linear IgA bullous dermatosis-like presentation. *Arch Dermatol.* (2011) 147:109–14. doi: 10.1001/archdermatol.2010.404-a
12. Kawahara Y, Matsuo Y, Hashimoto T, Nishikawa T. A case of unique subepidermal blistering disease with autoantibodies against a novel dermal 200-kD antigen. *Dermatology.* (1998) 196:213–6. doi: 10.1159/000017901
13. Goto-Ohguchi Y, Nishie W, Akiyama M, Tateishi Y, Aoyagi S, Tsuji-Abe Y, et al. A severe and refractory case of anti-p200 pemphigoid resulting in multiple skin ulcers and scar formation. *Dermatology.* (2009) 218:265–71. doi: 10.1159/000182268
14. Watanabe M, Tsunoda T, Tagami H. A subepidermal blistering dermatosis associated with coexistent IgG and IgA anti-dermal basement membrane zone antibodies; demonstration of IgG antibodies reactive against a 200-kDa dermal antigen. *Eur J Dermatol.* (2002) 12:603–6.
15. Yamada T, Suzuki M, Koike Y, Kida K, Murata S, Ishii N, et al. A case of epidermolysis bullosa acquisita with autoantibody to anti-p200 pemphigoid antigen and exfoliative esophagitis. *Dermatology.* (2006) 212:381–

4. doi: 10.1159/000092292
16. Pastar Z, Rados J, Lipozencic J, Dobric I, Marinovic B, Ishii N, et al. Case of concurrent epidermolysis bullosa acquisita and anti-p200 pemphigoid - How to treat it? *Int J Dermatol.* (2007) 46:295–8. doi: 10.1111/j.1365-4632.2006.02969.x
17. Umemoto N, Demitsu T, Toda S, Noguchi T, Suzuki SI, Kakurai M, et al. A case of anti-p200 pemphigoid clinically mimicking inflammatory epidermolysis bullosa acquisita [1]. *Br J Dermatol.* (2003) 148:1058–60. doi: 10.1046/j.1365-2133.2003.05312.x
18. Wozniak K, Hashimoto T, Fukuda S, Ohyama B, Ishii N, Koga H, et al. IgA anti-p200 pemphigoid. *Arch Dermatol.* (2011) 147:1306–10. doi: 10.1001/archdermatol.2011.303
19. Salmhofer W, Kawahara Y, Soyer HP, Kerl H, Nishikawa T, Hashimoto T. A subepidermal blistering disease with histopathological features of dermatitis herpetiformis and immunofluorescence characteristics of bullous pemphigoid: a novel subepidermal blistering disease or a variant of bullous pemphigoid? *Br J Dermatol.* (1997) 137:599–604. doi: 10.1111/j.1365-2133.1997.tb03794.x
20. Yasuda H, Tomita Y, Shibaki A, Hashimoto T. Two cases of subepidermal blistering disease with anti-p200 or 180-kd bullous pemphigoid antigen associated with psoriasis. *Dermatology.* (2004) 209:149–55. doi: 10.1159/000079602
21. Mitsuya J, Hara H, Ito K, Ishii N, Hashimoto T, Terui T. Metastatic ovarian carcinoma-associated subepidermal blistering disease with autoantibodies to both the p200 dermal antigen and the γ2 subunit of laminin 5 showing unusual clinical features. *Br J Dermatol.* (2008) 158:1354–7. doi: 10.1111/j.1365-2133.2008.08483.x
22. Mitate E, Kawano S, Nakao Y, Goto Y, Kobayashi I, Onozawa K, et al. Concurrence of autoantibodies to both laminin γ1 and γ2 subunits in a patient with kidney rejection response. *Acta Derm Venereol.* (2013) 93:114–5. doi: 10.2340/00015555-1395
23. Zhiliang L, Xiaodong Z, Peiying J, Suying F, Baoxi W. A case of refractory antilaminin γ1 pemphigoid successfully treated with dexamethasone and mycophenolate mofetil. *Int J Dermatol.* (2015) 54:e194–6. doi: 10.1111/ijd.12763
24. Waki Y, Kamiya K, Komine M, Maekawa T, Murata S, Ishii N, et al. A case of anti-laminin gamma1 (p200) pemphigoid with psoriasis vulgaris successfully treated with apremilast. *Eur J Dermatol.* (2018) 28:413–4. doi: 10.1684/ejd.2018.3280
25. Majima Y, Yagi H, Tateishi C, Groth S, Schmidt E, Zillikens D, et al. A successful treatment with ustekinumab in a case of antilaminin-gamma1 pemphigoid associated with psoriasis. *Br J Dermatol.* (2013) 168:1367–9. doi: 10.1111/bjd.12163
26. Mascaro JMJ, Zillikens D, Giudice GJ, Caux F, Fleming MG, Katz HM, et al. A subepidermal bullous eruption associated with IgG autoantibodies to a 200 kd dermal antigen: the first case report from the United States. *J Am Acad Dermatol.* (2000) 42:309–15. doi: 10.1016/S0190-9622(00)90101-4
27. García-Díez I, Martínez-Escala ME, Ishii N, Hashimoto T, Mascaró Galy JM, Pujol RM, et al. Usefulness of a simple immunohistochemical staining technique to differentiate anti-p200 pemphigoid from other autoimmune blistering diseases: a report of 2 cases. *Actas Dermosifiliogr.* (2016) 108:e1–5. doi: 10.1016/j.adengl.2016.11.018
28. Rose C, Weyers W, Denisjuk N, Hillen U, Zillikens D, Shimanovich I. Histopathology of anti-p200 pemphigoid. *Am J Dermatopathol.* (2007) 29:119–24. doi: 10.1097/DAD.0b013e31803326e6
29. Egan CA, Yee C, Zillikens D, Yancey KB. Anti-p200 pemphigoid: diagnosis and treatment of a case presenting as an inflammatory subepidermal blistering disease. *J Am Acad Dermatol.* (2002) 46:786–9. doi: 10.1067/mjd.2002.120923
30. Kingsbery MY, Grossman ME, Nguyen H. Consider antilaminin gamma-1 pemphigoid when faced with conflicting histopathology and immunofluorescence results. *J Am Acad Dermatol.* (2013) 68:e60–1. doi: 10.1016/j.jaad.2012.08.038
31. Iikawa M, Muroi E, Ishii Y, Mochid AK, Setoyama M, Kurokawa M, et al. A case of anti-laminin gamma; 1 pemphigoid with cutaneous polyarteritis nodosa. *Nishi Nihon Hifuka.* (2013) 75:7–10. doi: 10.2336/nishinihonhifu.75.7
32. Hofmann SC, Voith U, Sasaki TS, Trueeb RM, Nischt RN, Bruckner-Tuderman L. Evidence for synthesis of p200, the autoantigen in anti-p200 pemphigoid, by keratinocytes and fibroblasts. *J Invest Dermatol.* (2007) 127:S73. doi: 10.1038/sj.jid.5700952
33. Miyakura T, Yamamoto T, Tashiro A, Okubo Y, Oyama B, Ishii N, et al. Anti-p200 pemphigoid associated with annular pustular psoriasis. *Eur J Dermatology.* (2008) 18:481–2. doi: 10.1684/ejd.2008.0465
34. Kamata M, Fujita H, Hamanaka T, Takahashi K, Koga H, Hashimoto T, et al. Anti-laminin gamma1 pemphigoid accompanied by autoantibodies to laminin alpha3 and gamma2 subunits of laminin-332. *JAMA Dermatol.* (2013) 149:1437–9. doi: 10.1001/jamadermatol.2013.5358
35. Igarashi M, Tsunemi Y, Koga H, Hashimoto T, Tateishi C, Tsuruta D, et al. Anti-laminin gamma1 pemphigoid associated with pustular psoriasis. *Eur J Dermatol.* (2014) 24:629–30. doi: 10.1684/ejd.2014.2419
36. Ohzone A, Numata S, Hamada T, Fukuda S, Teye K, Shirakashi Y, et al. Anti-laminin-gamma 1 pemphigoid developed in a case of autosomal recessive congenital ichthyosis. *Acta Derm Venereol.* (2015) 95:93–4. doi: 10.2340/00015555-1875
37. Munsch C, Prey S, Joly P, Meyer N, Lamant L, Livideanu C, et al. [Anti-p200 pemphigoid: a spectacular response to dapsone]. *Ann Dermatol Venereol.* (2011) 138:739–42. doi: 10.1016/j.annder.2011.05.024
38. Goetze S, Dumke A-K, Zillikens D, Hipler UC, Elsner P. Anti-p200/laminin gamma1 pemphigoid associated with metastatic oesophageal cancer. *J Eur Acad Dermatol Venereol.* (2017) 31:e219–21. doi: 10.1111/jdv.13983
39. Tatsumi M, Kamei R, Nakai D, Mabuchi E, Ikegami E, Fukuda S, et al. Complicated case of anti-laminin gamma-1 pemphigoid in psoriasis. *Ski Res.* (2012) 11:75–81. doi: 10.11340/skinresearch.11.1_75
40. McCarty M, Zillikens D, Fivenson D. Anti-p200 pemphigoid (anti-laminin-gamma1 pemphigoid) demonstrating pathergy. *Int J Women Dermatol.* (2015) 1:173–4. doi: 10.1016/j.ijwd.2015.09.002
41. Alloo A, Strazzula L, Rothschild B, Hawryluk E, Levine D, Hoang MP, et al. Refractory antilaminin γ1 pemphigoid successfully treated with intravenous immunoglobulin and mycophenolate mofetil. *J Eur Acad Dermatology Venereol.* (2014) 28:1401–3. doi: 10.1111/jdv.12352
42. Goyal N, Rao R, Shenoi S, Pai S, Kumar P, Bhogal B, et al. Epidermolysis bullosa acquisita and anti-p200 pemphigoid as major subepidermal autoimmune bullous diseases diagnosed by floor binding on indirect immunofluorescence microscopy using human salt-split skin. *Indian J Dermatol Venereol Leprol.* (2017) 83:550–5. doi: 10.4103/ijdvl.IJDVL_678_16
43. Geller S, Gat A, Zeeli T, Schmidt E, Ishii N, Hashimoto T, et al. A refractory, cutaneous, subepidermal bullous disease. *Clin Exp Dermatol.* (2016) 41:573–5. doi: 10.1111/ced.12823
44. Monshi B, Groth S, Richter L, Schmidt E, Zillikens D, Rappersberger K. A long-term study of a patient with anti-p200 pemphigoid: correlation of autoantibody levels with disease activity and an example of epitope spreading. *Br J Dermatol.* (2012) 167:1179–83. doi: 10.1111/j.1365-2133.2012.11076.x
45. Ishida S, Takahashi K, Kanaoka M, Okawa T, Tateishi C, Yasukochi A, et al. Case of subepidermal autoimmune bullous disease with psoriasis vulgaris reacting to both BP180 C-terminal domain and laminin gamma-1. *J Dermatol.* (2015) 42:391–3. doi: 10.1111/1346-8138.12801
46. Ansai S-I, Hashizume S, Kawana S, Tateishi C, Koga H, Hashimoto T. Case of anti-laminin gamma-1 pemphigoid with antibody against C-terminal domain of BP180 in a patient with psoriasis vulgaris. *J Dermatol.* (2014) 41:1031–3. doi: 10.1111/1346-8138.12625
47. Kawahara Y, Zillikens D, Yancey KB, Marinkovich MP, Nie Z, Hashimoto T, et al. Subepidermal blistering disease with autoantibodies against a novel dermal 200-kDa antigen. *J Dermatol Sci.* (2000) 23:93–102. doi: 10.1016/S0923-1811(99)00093-6
48. Imanishi A, Tateishi C, Imanishi H, Sowa-Osako J, Koga H, Tsuruta D, et al. Pemphigoid with antibodies to laminin gamma 1, BP180 and BP230, associated with psoriasis vulgaris: Successful disease control with cyclosporin. *J Dermatol.* (2015) 42:394–7. doi: 10.1111/1346-8138.12798
49. Furukawa H, Miura T, Takahashi M, Nakamura K, Kaneko F, Ishii F, et al. A case of anti-p200 pemphigoid with autoantibodies against both a novel 200-kD dermal antigen and the 290-kD epidermolysis bullosa acquisita antigen. *Dermatology.* (2004) 209:145–8. doi: 10.1159/000079601
50. Akasaka E, Nakano H, Korekawa A, Fukui T, Kaneko T, Koga H, et al. Anti-laminin γ1 pemphigoid associated with ulcerative colitis and psoriasis vulgaris showing autoantibodies to laminin γ1, type XVII collagen and laminin-332. *Eur J Dermatol.* (2015) 25:198–9. doi: 10.1684/ejd.2014.2499

51. Shimanovich I, Petersen EE, Weyers W, Sitaru C, Zillikens D. Subepidermal blistering disease with autoantibodies to both the p200 autoantigen and the alpha3 chain of laminin 5. (2005) 52:S90–2. doi: 10.1016/j.jaad.2004.07.036
52. Li X, Qian H, Ishii N, Yamaya M, Fukuda H, Mukai H, et al. A case of concurrent antilaminin gamma 1 pemphigoid and antilaminin-332-type mucous membrane pemphigoid. *Br J Dermatol.* (2014) 171:1257–9. doi: 10.1111/bjd.13107
53. Fujimura Y, Natsuga K, Hamade Y, Nomura Y, Kaku Y, Muramatsu R, et al. Anti-laminin-gamma 1 pemphigoid with generalized pustular psoriasis and psoriasis vulgaris. *Acta Derm Venereol.* (2016) 96:120–1. doi: 10.2340/00015555-2168
54. Saeki H, Hayashi N, Komine M, Soma Y, Shimada S, Watanabe K, et al. A case of generalized pustular psoriasis followed by bullous disease: an atypical case of bullous pemphigoid or a novel bullous disease? *Br J Dermatol.* (1996) 134:152–5. doi: 10.1046/j.1365-2133.1996.d01-758.x
55. Kaminaka C, Kanazawa N, Furukawa F, Hashimoto T. Case of anti-laminin-γ1 pemphigoid associated with psoriatic erythroderma. *J Dermatol.* (2010) 37:272–5. doi: 10.1111/j.1346-8138.2009.00790.x
56. Morris SD, Mallipeddi R, Oyama N, Gratian MJ, Harman KE, Bhogal BS, et al. Psoriasis bullosa acquisita. *Clin Exp Dermatol.* (2002) 27:665–9. doi: 10.1046/j.1365-2230.2002.01100.x
57. Gawaz A, Metzler G, Hertl M, Hashimoto T, Schaller M. Treatment of anti-laminin γ1 pemphigoid with mycophenolate mofetil. *J Dtsch Dermatol Ges.* (2015) 13:696–7. doi: 10.1111/ddg.12564
58. Hayashi M, Okamura K, Ujiie H, Iwata H, Suzuki T. Case of anti-p200 pemphigoid accompanying uterine malignancy. *J Dermatol.* (2018) 45:e341–2. doi: 10.1111/1346-8138.14473
59. Mai Y, Nishie W, Izumi K, Toyonaga E, Ikawa H, Mori T, et al. Detection of major epitopes for autoantibodies in dipeptidyl peptidase IV inhibitors-associated bullous pemphigoid. *J Invest Dermatol.* (2018) 138:S53. doi: 10.1016/j.jid.2018.03.319
60. Iijima S, Okazaki Y, Watanabe S, Tsuruta D, Tateishi C, Ishii N, et al. Case of concurrence of anti-laminin gamma-1 pemphigoid and scabies. *J Dermatol.* (2015) 42:1024–6. doi: 10.1111/1346-8138.13020
61. Ogata M, Misago N, Inoue T, Hirashima N, Narisawa Y, Ishii N, et al. A case of anti-p200 pemphigoid-discussion of association with scabies. *Nishi Nihon Hifuka.* (2006) 68:375–9. doi: 10.2336/nishinihonhifu.68.375
62. Wozniak K, Kowalewski C, Hashimoto T, Ishii N, Glinska-Wielochowska M, Schwartz RA. Penicillin-induced anti-p200 pemphigoid: an unusual morphology. *Acta Derm Venereol.* (2006) 86:443–6. doi: 10.2340/00015555-0117
63. Della Torre R, Combescure C, Cortés B, Marazza G, Beltraminelli H, Naldi L, et al. Clinical presentation and diagnostic delay in bullous pemphigoid: a prospective nationwide cohort. *Br J Dermatol.* (2012) 167:1111–7. doi: 10.1111/j.1365-2133.2012.11108.x
64. Clapé A, Muller C, Gatouillat G, Le Jan S, Barbe C, Pham B-N, et al. Mucosal involvement in bullous pemphigoid is mostly associated with disease severity and to absence of anti-BP230 autoantibody. *Front Immunol.* (2018) 9:479. doi: 10.3389/fimmu.2018.00479
65. Di Zenzo G, Thoma-Uszynski S, Fontao L, Calabresi V, Hofmann SC, Hellmark T, et al. Multicenter prospective study of the humoral autoimmune response in bullous pemphigoid. *Clin Immunol.* (2008) 128:415–26. doi: 10.1016/j.clim.2008.04.012
66. Vaillant L, Bernard P, Joly P, Prost C, Labeille B, Bedane C, et al. Evaluation of clinical criteria for diagnosis of bullous pemphigoid. French Bullous Study Group. *Arch Dermatol.* (1998) 134:1075–80. doi: 10.1001/archderm.134.9.1075
67. Joly P, Baricault S, Sparsa A, Bernard P, Bédane C, Duvert-Lehembre S, et al. Incidence and mortality of bullous pemphigoid in France. *J Invest Dermatol.* (2012) 132:1998–2004. doi: 10.1038/jid.2012.35
68. Kridin K, Bergman R. Ethnic variations in the epidemiology of bullous pemphigoid in Israel. *Int J Dermatol.* (2017) 57:34–9. doi: 10.1111/ijd.13813
69. Kridin K. Subepidermal autoimmune bullous diseases: overview, epidemiology, and associations. *Immunol Res.* (2018) 66:6–17. doi: 10.1007/s12026-017-8975-2
70. Ohata C, Ishii N, Koga H, Fukuda S, Tateishi C, Tsuruta D, et al. Coexistence of autoimmune bullous diseases (AIBDs) and psoriasis: a series of 145 cases. *J Am Acad Dermatol.* (2015) 73:50–5. doi: 10.1016/j.jaad.2015.03.016
71. Michalek IM, Loring B, John SM. A systematic review of worldwide epidemiology of psoriasis. *J Eur Acad Dermatol Venereol.* (2017) 31:205–12. doi: 10.1111/jdv.13854
72. Parisi R, Symmons DPM, Griffiths CEM, Ashcroft DM. Global epidemiology of psoriasis: a systematic review of incidence and prevalence. *J Invest Dermatol.* (2012) 133:377–85. doi: 10.1038/jid.2012.339
73. Takahashi H, Nakamura K, Kaneko F, Nakagawa H, Iizuka H. Analysis of psoriasis patients registered with the Japanese Society for Psoriasis Research from 2002-2008. *J Dermatol.* (2011) 38:1125–9. doi: 10.1111/j.1346-8138.2010.01145.x
74. Watanabe M, Natsuga K, Nishie W, Kobayashi Y, Donati G, Suzuki S, et al. Type XVII collagen coordinates proliferation in the interfollicular epidermis. *Elife.* (2017) 6:e26635. doi: 10.7554/eLife.26635
75. Dainichi T, Kabashima K. Interaction of psoriasis and bullous diseases. *Front Med.* (2018) 5:222. doi: 10.3389/fmed.2018.00222
76. Chan LS, Vanderlugt CJ, Hashimoto T, Nishikawa T, Zone JJ, Black MM, et al. Epitope spreading: lessons from autoimmune skin diseases. *J Invest Dermatol.* (1998) 110:103–9. doi: 10.1046/j.1523-1747.1998.00107.x
77. Ippolito A, Wallace DJ, Gladman D, Fortin PR, Urowitz M, Werth V, et al. Autoantibodies in systemic lupus erythematosus: comparison of historical and current assessment of seropositivity. *Lupus.* (2011) 20:250–5. doi: 10.1177/0961203310385738

5

Adaptive and Innate Immunity in Psoriasis and Other Inflammatory Disorders

*Michael P. Schön**

Department of Dermatology, Venereology and Allergology, University Medical Center Göttingen, Göttingen, Germany

***Correspondence:**
Michael P. Schön
michael.schoen@med.uni-goettingen.de
orcid.org/0000-0002-0698-4130

Over the past three decades, a considerable body of evidence has highlighted T cells as pivotal culprits in the pathogenesis of psoriasis. This includes the association of psoriasis with certain MHC (HLA) alleles, oligoclonal expansion of T cells in some cases, therapeutic response to T cell-directed immunomodulation, the onset of psoriasis following bone marrow transplantation, or induction of psoriasis-like inflammation by T cells in experimental animals. There is accumulating clinical and experimental evidence suggesting that both autoimmune and autoinflammatory mechanisms lie at the core of the disease. Indeed, some studies suggested antigenic functions of structural proteins, and complexes of self-DNA with cathelicidin (LL37) or melanocytic ADAMTSL5 have been proposed more recently as actual auto-antigens in some cases of psoriasis. These findings are accompanied by various immunoregulatory mechanisms, which we increasingly understand and which connect innate and adaptive immunity. Specific adaptive autoimmune responses, together with our current view of psoriasis as a systemic inflammatory disorder, raise the question of whether psoriasis may have connections to autoimmune or autoinflammatory disorders elsewhere in the body. While such associations have been suspected for many years, compelling mechanistic evidence in support of this notion is still scant. This review sets into context the current knowledge about innate and adaptive immunological processes in psoriasis and other autoimmune or autoinflammatory diseases.

Keywords: psoriasis, adaptive immunity, innate immunity, autoimmune disease, skin—immunology

SETTING THE STAGE: PSORIASIS AS AN IMMUNE-MEDIATED DISORDER

If I was to name diseases that in recent years have increased our understanding of both adaptive and innate immune mechanisms on the one hand and have contributed decisively to the development of modern biological therapies on the other, then psoriasis would certainly occupy one of the top ranks. Psoriasis is currently viewed as a systemic chronic inflammatory disease with an immunogenetic basis that can be triggered extrinsically or intrinsically (1, 2). Research into its pathophysiology has led to impressive therapeutic improvements (3, 4). The disease is based on close interactions between components of the adaptive and the innate branches of the immune system (3, 5–9) (**Figure 1**). Since it was shown in the late 1970s that psoriasis can be ameliorated by cyclosporin A (10), it can no longer be seriously denied that T lymphocytes play a central role in the pathogenesis of this disease. This view is substantiated by numerous subsequent observations

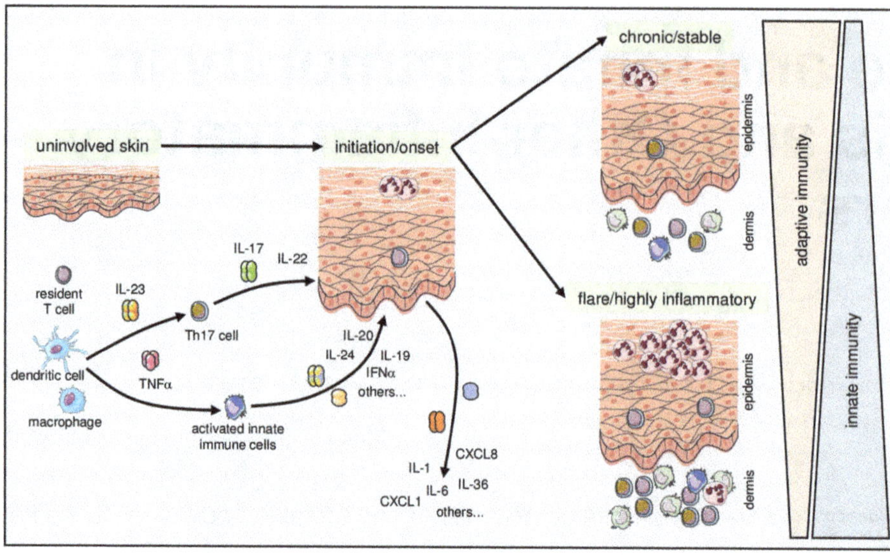

FIGURE 1 | Complex fine-tuning of innate and adaptive immune mechanisms determines onset, course, and activity of psoriasis. As detailed in the text, intricate interactions between components of the innate (exemplified here by dendritic cells and macrophages) with components of the adaptive immune system (exemplified here by T cells) lie at the core of the pathophysiology of psoriasis. Once established, the relative contribution and fine-tuning of various mediators of adaptive and innate immunity determine the clinical manifestation toward chronic stable vs. highly inflammatory and/or pustular psoriasis.

over the past four decades: psoriasis can be precipitated by bone marrow transplantation (11) and, similar to other autoinflammatory diseases, the disease is frequently associated with certain HLA expression patterns (7, 12–14). Drugs that specifically inhibit the function of T lymphocytes (such as CD2 blockade in the early days of biologics) can improve psoriasis (15). A therapeutic effect can also be achieved by interleukin (IL)-4, which pushes the cytokine milieu toward a T-helper (Th) cell 2-dominated immune response (16), probably through attenuation of Th17 function following diminished IL-23 production in antigen-presenting cells (17) and through induction of the transcription factor GATA3 (18, 19). IL-10 can also ameliorate psoriatic symptoms by modulating T cell functions (20). In addition, psoriasis-like skin inflammation in animal models can be initiated by certain CD4+ T cells (21–24), and T cells can induce psoriatic lesions in human skin xenografts (25, 26). Finally, the more recent discoveries that complexes of the antimicrobial peptide LL37 (a 37 amino acid C-terminal cleavage product of the antimicrobial peptide, cathelicidin) with own DNA or the melanocytic antigen ADAMTSL5 may function as autoantigens (27, 28), support the central role of T cells in the pathogenesis of psoriasis (29, 30).

AUTOIMMUNE PROCESSES IN PSORIASIS

The Plot Thickens: Actual Auto-Antigens in Psoriasis

Pathogenic T cells in psoriatic skin lesions facilitate hyperproliferation of keratinocytes, influx of neutrophilic granulocytes, as well as production of other inflammatory cytokines, chemokines and antimicrobial peptides. They feature a Th17 signature, i.e., they express IL-17A, IL-22, and IFN-γ (3, 31, 32) (**Figure 2**). Dendritic cells maintain activation and differentiation of lesional Th17 cells primarily through secretion of IL-23 [reviewed in (8)].

In general, both HLA restriction and peptide specificity of a given T cell are determined by its T cell receptor (TCR) repertoire (33). Activation and clonal expansion of T cells occur upon antigenic stimulation. In the absence of foreign antigens, clonal T cell expansion is highly suggestive for autoimmunity in inflammatory diseases (34). Indeed, oligoclonal T cell expansion has been identified in psoriatic lesions in early well-designed studies (35–40) as well as in more recent investigations (41). It has been interpreted as an indicator for antigen-specific immune responses.

In psoriasis, oligoclonality of cutaneous T-cell populations is usually confined to lesional skin. This suggests that psoriasis is driven by locally presented antigens (35, 42–46). Likewise, the clonal TCRs arguably mark T cells which mediate the disease process. Several landmark publications during the past years lent support to this notion through identification of putative autoantigens in psoriasis.

Early concepts of autoimmune processes in psoriasis stemmed from the recognition of sequence homologies between keratinocyte structural proteins and streptococcal antigens (*S. pyogenes* in particular) (47–51). Mechanistic proof, however, is still lacking.

It was previously known that complexes of LL37 and self-DNA can activate dermal plasmacytoid dendritic cells (pDC) through toll-like receptor (TLR) signaling (52–54). These stimulate pDC then facilitate the psoriatic inflammatory cascade (52, 53, 55),

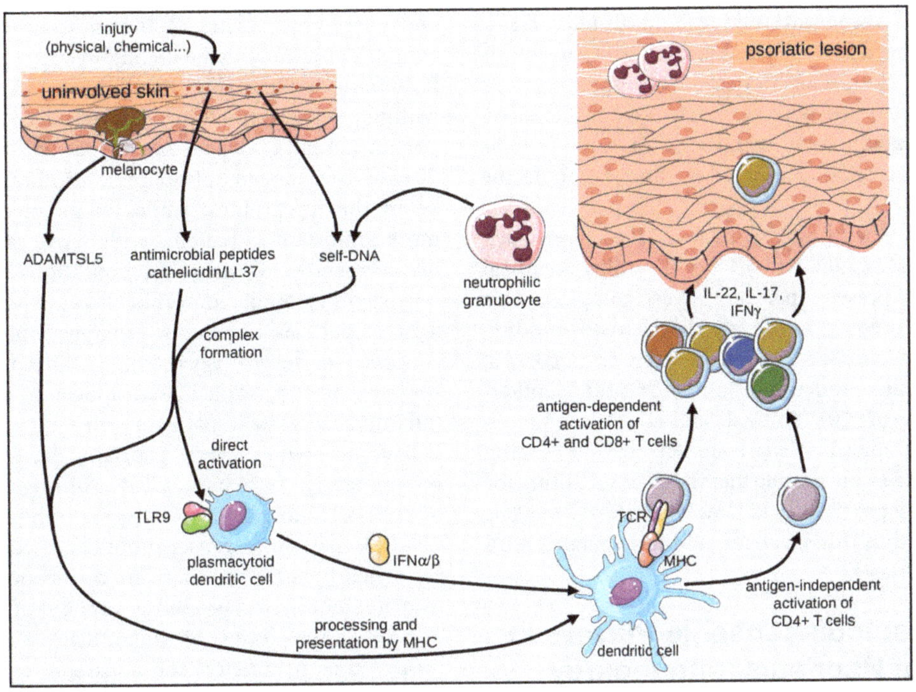

FIGURE 2 | Initiation of psoriasis by antigen-dependent and antigen-independent immune mechanisms. Complexes of self-DNA with fragments of the antimicrobial peptide, cathelicidin, can stimulate plasmacytoid dendritic cells through TLR9. They can also be presented by HLA-C*06:02 molecules and specifically activate T cells through their TCR. Likewise, the melanocyte-derived ADAMTSL5 can activate pathogenic CD8+ T cells after presentation by HLA-C*06:02.

a mechanism that is alluded to in more detail below. The activation *via* innate immune mechanisms was extended later by the finding that complexes of self-DNA and LL37 can also induce adaptive antigen-specific immune responses. Indeed, LL37 can trigger profound TCR and MHC (*HLA-C*06:02*)-dependent T-cell responses (28). It remains to be confirmed, however, that the LL37-related candidate peptides can be derived from the parent protein by antigen processing within the antigen presenting cell and then be presented by HLA-class I-molecules.

A more recent strategy to identify potential targets of pathogenic T-cells in psoriasis was based on the generation of T-cell hybridomas expressing the paired Vα3S1/Vβ13S1 TCR of clonal $CD8^+$ psoriatic T cells of an *HLA-C*06:02*-expressing psoriasis patient (27). This elegant approach identified melanocytes as target cells of the psoriatic immune response (27). A peptide derived from ADAMTS-like protein 5 (ADAMTSL5) by proteasomal cleavage and post-cleavage trimming induced the specific immune response. The auto-antigenic function of melanocytic ADAMTSL5 was then confirmed by mutation and knock-down experiments. Moreover, peripheral lymphocytes of the majority of psoriasis patients but not individuals without psoriasis responded to ADAMTSL5 with production of IL-17 or IFNγ (27) (**Figure 2**). In contrast to LL37, which has been shown to activate both $CD8^+$ cytotoxic T cells and $CD4^+$ T helper cells, ADAMTSL5 appears to activate preferentially $CD8^+$ T cells. Of note, both antigens are recognized by T cells when being presented by HLA-C*06:02, i.e., the most prominent psoriasis risk gene in the genome [located on PSORS1 (psoriasis susceptibility locus 1) on chromosome 6p21.3].

While the role of cellular adaptive immunity is becoming increasingly plausible, only recently autoantibodies, i.e., elements of humoral adaptive immunity, have been described in patients with psoriasis and psoriatic arthritis. Interestingly, these IgG are directed against (carbamylated/citrullinated) LL37 or ADAMTSL5 (56, 57). Since the serum concentrations of these antibodies were associated with the severity of psoriasis and since patients with psoriatic arthritis had higher serum levels, it is conceivable that a causal pathogenetic relationship and a contribution to systemic inflammation exist (56). It is also possible that the respective autoantibodies exert protective functions through scavenging autoantigens. However, their roles need to be clarified in future studies.

The Other Side: Antigen Presentation by HLA Molecules in Psoriasis

While most, if not all, autoimmune diseases are linked with certain HLA alleles (58–60), *HLA-C*06:02* is the predominant psoriasis risk gene (61–63). HLA class I molecules present short peptide antigens (8–10 amino acids) to αβ TCRs of CD8+ T cells. Such antigenic peptides are usually derived within the antigen presenting cell from (intracellular) parent proteins by proteasomal cleavage and loaded onto HLA-class I molecules. The HLA/peptide complex is then transported to the cell membrane where it can be recognized by CD8+ T cells (64, 65). Thus, HLA-class I-restricted immune responses are usually directed against target cells which produce the antigenic peptide.

HLA-C*06:02-presented non-apeptides (9 amino acids long) possess anchor amino acids at residues 2 (arginine) and 9 (leucine, valine, and less frequently methionine and isoleucine), along with a putative anchor at residue 7 (arginine). HLA-C*06:02 features very negatively charged pockets and thus binds to distinct positively charged peptides. Given that between 1,000 and 3,000 different self-peptides have been detected on HLA-C*06:02 under experimental conditions, multiple cellular proteins should be, in principle, presented by this HLA molecule and recognizable by CD8+ T cells (66, 67).

*HLA-C*06:02,* and other psoriasis-related HLA types such as *HLA-C*07:01*, *HLA-C*07:02*, and *HLA-B*27* utilize identical anchor residues and present partially overlapping peptide residues (66, 67). Moreover, a negatively charged binding pocket is shared with another risk allele, *HLA-C*12:03* (68, 69), resulting in similar functional domains and peptide-binding characteristics (67, 70). Thus, several HLA-class I types implicated in psoriasis appear to share similar peptide-binding properties. It is, therefore, conceivable that they can substitute for each other in conferring psoriasis risk. However, *HLA-C*06:02* is the prototype allele within this spectrum and is associated with the highest risk for psoriasis.

Supporting Acts: Indispensable Players in the Ensemble of Psoriasis Immunology

Autoantigen presentation alone does not suffice to induce the psoriatic cascade in genetically predisposed individuals. Rather, costimulatory effects of various gene products orchestrate the activation of the actual autoimmune response. Such risk gene variants modulate inflammatory signaling pathways (e.g., the IL-23 pathway), peptide epitope processing and/or Th/c17 differentiation (a selection of important factors is summarized in **Table 1**).

These genetic variations create costimulatory signals which modulate innate and adaptive immune mechanisms and shape the proinflammatory environment. In sum and in conjunction with the appropriate HLA molecules and autoantigens, they may eventually exceed the thresholds for activation and maintenance of pathogenic autoimmune and autoinflammatory responses in psoriasis (29, 71). Likewise, regulatory mechanisms involving programmed death (PD)-1 signals have emerged recently as modulators of chronic inflammation in psoriasis (72). However, the complex interactions of various players are by no means fully understood. Therefore, they are listed here only as a whole.

The autoantigens described so far cannot fully explain the genesis of psoriasis. To give just one example of the latter notion: Psoriatic lesions can also occur in vitiligo foci that do not contain melanocytes (73, 74). Alterations of resident cell types such as vascular endothelial cells or the cutaneous nervous system are also involved in the disease process (75–77). Further research is certainly needed here.

SHADES OF GRAY: CROSSTALK BETWEEN ADAPTIVE AND INNATE IMMUNITY IN PSORIASIS

In addition to the antigen-specific facilitation of inflammation in psoriasis, there are several strong connections to components of the innate immune system. The crosstalk between the innate and adaptive branches of the immune system in psoriasis is complex and can only be highlighted by a few selected examples. Its fine-tuning arguably determines the actual clinical correlate within the spectrum of the disease. Indeed, there is accumulating circumstantial evidence that in patients with stable and mild disease, mechanisms of adaptive immunity are more likely to be in the foreground, while innate mechanisms seem to be more important in patients with active severe disease, systemic involvement and comorbid conditions (78) (**Figure 1**). The impact on systemic comorbid diseases has been interpreted, at least in part, as a systemic "*spillover*" of innate inflammatory processes in severe psoriasis (78). Of course, such factors are not specific for psoriasis, but appear to account for a general inflammatory state in patients with severe psoriasis.

Patients with severe psoriasis have increased levels of inflammatory cytokines, CRP, fibrinogen, α2 macroglobulin or PAI-1 (plasminogen activator inhibitor-1) in the blood (79–81), they show transcriptomic, proteomic and metabolomic abnormalities (82) and there are connections with chronic stress (83) and biophysical properties of the skin (84).

The serum levels of inflammatory cytokines have been proposed as parameters for disease severity (85). Such general inflammatory markers are accompanied by increased numbers of Th1, Th17, and Th22 cells in patients with severe psoriasis (86, 87), which provides a direct link with autoimmune (adaptive) processes. Moreover, there is an increasing number of modulating factors, such as autoimmune reactivity to ribonucleoprotein A1 (HNRNPA1) (88), which impact on the course and severity of psoriasis.

One of the perhaps most vivid recent examples of how individual mediators influence the spectrum of psoriasis by shifting innate or adaptive immune processes comes from research on the interplay between IL-17- and IL-36-driven inflammation (89). The three IL-36 isoforms (IL-36α, β, and γ) belong to the IL-1 family and are upregulated in psoriatic skin (90, 91). They bind to the IL-36 receptor (IL-36R), thereby inducing transcription of several inflammatory mediators through NF-κβ activation. IL-36Ra (IL-1F9), an anti-inflammatory natural IL36R antagonist, is encoded by the *IL36RN* gene and is abundantly present in the skin of patients with psoriasis vulgaris, which may constitute part of the "*checks and balances*" that control the psoriatic inflammation (90, 92). Function-abrogating mutations in the *IL36RN* gene may result in unrestrained inflammatory effects of IL-36. Absence of IL-36Ra then leads to excessive neutrophil accumulation as observed in some cases of familial generalized pustular psoriasis (92–94). Palmoplantar pustular psoriasis, however, seems to be related to CARD14 variants rather than IL36RN mutations (95, 96).

While most cases of pustular psoriasis occur without such mutations (97), IL-36-related processes appear to contribute decisively to the actual clinical manifestation of specific psoriatic phenotypes: It has recently been shown elegantly that the skin of patients with psoriasis vulgaris differs significantly from that of patients with pustular psoriasis—in a sense, opposite ends of the spectrum of psoriasis: while in both forms numerous genes are expressed abnormally, these differentially expressed

TABLE 1 | Genetic factors implicated in psoriasis.

Pathogenic function	Psoriasis-associated gene locus
IL-23/IL-17A signaling	*IL23R*, interleukin-23 receptor
	IL12B, interleukin-12 subunit p40, also part of IL-23
	IL12RB, interleukin-12 receptor subunit beta 1, also termed IL-12Rβ1
	IL23A, interleukin-23 subunit alpha, p19
	IL23R, interleukin-23 receptor, a Janus kinase-2 associated type I cytokine receptor that activates STAT3 upon ligand binding
	TYK2, tyrosine-protein kinase 2, a Janus kinase family member, facilitates type I and II cytokine receptor and type I and III interferon signaling pathways, involved in innate and adaptive immune processes
	STAT3, signal transducer and activator of transcription 3, a central transcription factor in inflammatory processes
	STAT5A/B, signal transducer and activator of transcription 5A/B
	SOCS1, suppressor of cytokine signaling 1, a member of the STAT-induced STAT inhibitor family, negative regulator of cytokine signaling
	ETS1, a member of the E26 transformation-specific transcription factors, a negative regulator of Th17 cells
	TRAF3IP2, tumor necrosis factor receptor-associated factor 3-interacting protein-2, central role in response to inflammatory signals
	KLF4, Krüppel-like factor 4, influences NF-κB-mediated inflammatory pathways
	IF3, eukaryotic translation initiation factor 3
Effector T-cell function and differentiation	*ETS1*, E26 transformation-specific transcription factor 1, a negative regulator of Th17 cells
	RUNX3, runt-related transcription factor 3, a runt domain-containing transcription factor involved in regulation of many cellular processes
	TNFRSF9, tumor necrosis factor receptor superfamily member 9, CD137, costimulator of T cells
	MBD2, methyl-CpG-binding domain protein 2, binds to methylated DNA and regulates transcription from methylated gene promoters
	IRF4, interferon regulatory factor 4
Type I interferon and cytokine signaling	*ELMO1*, engulfment and cell motility protein 1
	TYK2, non-receptor tyrosine-protein kinase, a Janus kinase family member (see above)
	SOCS1, suppressor of cytokine signaling 1, a member of the STAT-induced STAT inhibitor family, negative regulator of cytokine signaling
	IFIH1/MDA5, Interferon-induced helicase C domain-containing protein 1/melanoma differentiation-associated protein 5, a CARD (caspase activation and recruitment domain) protein involved in IL-1 and IL-18 processing and in regulation of inflammation
	RNF114, ring finger protein 114, a ubiquitin ligase
	IRF4, interferon regulatory factor 4
	RIG1/DDX58, retinoic acid inducible gene I encoded by the DDX58 (DExD/H-Box Helicase 58) gene; contains a RNA helicase motif and a caspase recruitment domain (CARD), involved in regulation of immune responses
	IFNLR1/IL28RA, interferon lambda receptor 1, forms complex with IL10RB and interacts with IL-28A, IL-28B, and IL-29, involved in immune regulation
	IFNGR2, interferon gamma receptor 2, non-ligand-binding beta chain of the IFNγ chain
Regulation of NF-κB-associated inflammatory signaling pathways	*TNFAIP3*, TNFα induced protein 3, a ubiqitin-editing enzyme that inhibits NF-κB activation and TNF-mediated apoptosis; involved in the cytokine-mediated inflammatory responses
	TNIP1, TNFAIP3 interacting protein 1, a regulator of NF-κB activation
	TYK2, non-receptor tyrosine-protein kinase, a Janus kinase family member (see above)
	REL, reticuloendotheliosis oncogene, a NF-κB subunit (c-Rel) involved in apoptosis, inflammation and immune responses, SNPs are also associated with ulcerative colitis and rheumatoid arthritis
	NFkBIA, NF-κB inhibitor α, interacts with NF-κB/c-Rel involved in inflammatory responses.
	CARD14, caspase recruitment domain family member 14, a scaffold protein involved in cell adhesion, signal transduction and cell polarity, involved in NF-κB activation.
	CARM1, coactivator associated arginine methyltransferase 1, catalyzes methylation of histones and other chromatin-associated proteins, involved in regulation of gene expression
	UBE2L3, ubiquitin conjugating enzyme E2 L3, an E2 ubiquitin-conjugating enzyme, participates in ubiquitination of the p105 NF-κB precursor
	FBXL19, F-box and leucine rich repeat protein 19, an E3 ubiquitin ligase, binds to interleukin 1 receptor-like 1 and regulates its ubiquitination, associated with pulmonary inflammation and psoriasis
Antigen processing (N-terminal trimming)	*ERAP1*, endoplasmic reticulum aminopeptidase 1, involved in trimming of HLA class I-binding precursors enabling them to be presented on MHC class I molecules

Most genetic associations have direct connections with immune functions implicated in the pathophysiology of psoriasis.

genes overlap only to a relatively small extent. In psoriasis vulgaris, genes involved in adaptive (T-cell-associated) immune processes predominate, whereas in pustular psoriasis processes of innate immunity (mainly neutrophil-associated) they are dysregulated. Interestingly, IL-36 seems to play an important role for the accumulation of neutrophilic granulocytes and a pustular phenotype of psoriasis (89). The balance between IL-36 and IL-17 seems to contribute—at least partially—to clinical symptoms of psoriasis vulgaris vs. psoriasis pustulosa. If this interpretation of the data is correct, then this would constitute a mechanism that regulates the fine-tuning between innate and adaptive immune processes.

THE IL-23/IL-17 PATHWAY CONNECTS INNATE AND ADAPTIVE IMMUNITY IN PSORIASIS

The notion of psoriasis featuring elements of both antigen-specific autoimmunity and non-specific autoinflammation needs to be considered a bit more closely, in particular downstream of innate and/or adaptive activation processes. As of today, interfering with IL-17A or IL-23 are the most efficient treatment modalities against psoriasis (98). Indeed, the IL-23/IL-17 axis seems to be particularly well-suited to exemplify the intricate crosstalk between adaptive and innate immunity in psoriasis.

Healthy human skin contains only a few IL-17-producing T cells (99), a population of $CD4^+$ T cells distinct from the "classical" Th1 and Th2 cells. They were eponymously named for their production of IL-17 (100). In psoriasis (31, 101, 102), palmoplantar pustulosis (103) and other inflammatory disorders (104, 105), Th17 lymphocytes are vastly expanded and are thought to contribute decisively to the pathogenesis of these conditions (**Figure 3**). The resulting imbalance between Th17 and regulatory T cells (Treg) favors inflammation (106). The IL-17 production of T lymphocytes is further stimulated by activated keratinocytes, thus creating a positive feedback loop (107). Th17 cells are controlled by regulatory T cells through IL-10 (108). In psoriatic skin, IL-17A is considered the most relevant of the six known isoforms (102). IL-17A is not only secreted by CD4+ Th17 cells, but also by CD8+ T cells (109) and certain cells of the innate immune system including neutrophilic granulocytes (110–112), thus further highlighting the tight connection of innate and adaptive immunity in psoriasis. The presentation of IL-17 by neutrophil extracellular traps (NETs), which are generated upon activation of neutrophils in a clearly defined manner (113) and are prominently present in both pustular and plaque-type psoriasis (114), may also play a role (115).

In this context it should be mentioned that so-called tissue resident memory cells (T_{rm} cells) in psoriatic skin remain in the long term even after resolution of the lesions, which contribute as mediators of the local adaptive immune response to renewed exacerbations. Although the role of these cells is not yet fully understood, there is growing evidence of their pathogenic role in psoriasis and other chronic inflammatory diseases (116–118). T_{rm} cells in psoriatic lesions are $CD8^+$ but lack CD49a

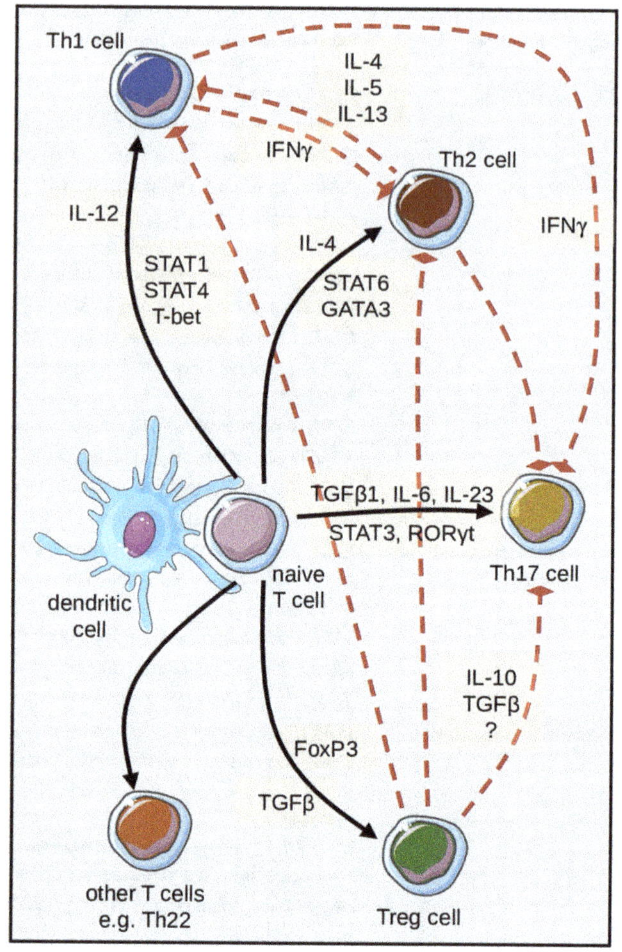

FIGURE 3 | Differentiation of pathogenic T cells in psoriasis is embedded in a complex regulatory network. Naïve T cells can differentiate into several directions; this is mainly determined by the cytokines and transcription factors depicted here. In addition, various regulatory feedback mechanisms exist, some of which are schematically highlighted here with particular reference to Th17 cell differentiation and function.

(α1 integrin) expression; they predominantly generate IL-17 responses that promote local inflammation (119).

In addition to Th17 cells, T cells which produce both IL-17 and IFNγ (termed Th17/Th1-T cells) and IL-22-producing T cells can also be detected in psoriatic skin (31). Naive T cells express several cytokine receptors including the IL-23 receptor. DC-derived TGFß1, IL-1ß, IL-6, and IL-23 facilitate priming and proliferation of Th17 cells (120–122), while IL-12 assumes these functions for Th1 cells, and IL-6 and TNFα contribute to the programming of Th22 cells.

The balance of Th17 cells and Th1 cells appears to be critical for the pathogenesis of psoriasis (123) and other related conditions (124). There are several exogenous factors such as ultraviolet light or vitamin D3 (125, 126), or other cytokines like IL-9 (127) that can modulate Th17-dependent inflammation. Of note, IL-17A can also be produced independent of IL-23, e.g., by γδ T lymphocytes or invariant natural killer (iNKT) cells (128–130). However, it is not clear yet whether this alternative pathway impacts on the accrual and course of inflammatory disorders or potential undesired effects of either IL-23 or IL-17 inhibition.

In any case, the IL-23/IL-17 axis in psoriasis clearly illuminates the close interaction of the innate immune system (represented by IL-23-producing myeloid cells) with cells of the adaptive immune system (in this case Th17- and IL17-expressing $CD8^+$ T-cells). Psoriasis could again serve as a "model disease" to clarify such relationships.

CONTRIBUTION OF RESIDENT SKIN CELLS TO IMMUNOLOGICAL PROCESSES IN PSORIASIS

Multiple genetic and environmental factors influence the immunopathology of psoriasis (131). The mechanisms leading to the first occurrence of psoriasis in predisposed individuals are only partly known. Infections with streptococci, medications such as lithium, antimalarials, or ß-blockers, or physical or chemical stress may trigger the disease. Minimal trauma can induce rapid immigration and activation of immune cells including T-cells and neutrophils (132), the so-called Köbner phenomenon (133, 134). Feedback loops between adaptive immune cells (T cells), innate immune cells (neutrophilic granulocytes, macrophages, dendritic cells), and resident skin cells (keratinocytes, endothelial cells) result in an amplification and chronification of the inflammatory response. Aspects of systemic inflammation in patients with severe psoriasis are thought to contribute to comorbid diseases (135).

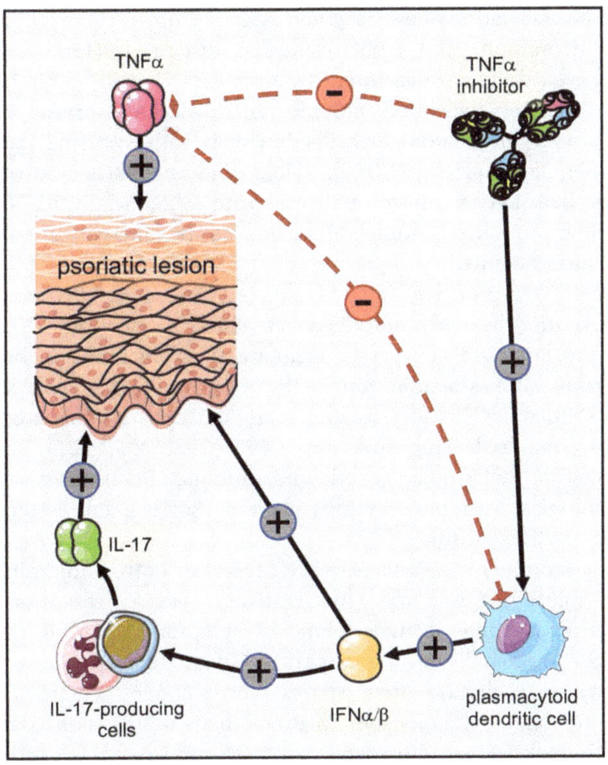

FIGURE 4 | Paradoxical psoriasis triggered by TNF inhibitors in predisposed individuals. Several cytokines contribute to the pathogenesis of psoriatic skin lesions, with TNFα and IL-17A playing prominent roles. However, TNFα also exerts an inhibitory effect on plasmacytoid dendritic cells. Upon therapeutic inhibition of TNFα, this inhibitory effect is abrogated and the resulting shift toward increased production of type I interferons fuels the secretion of IL-17. It is conceivable that additional mechanisms contribute to the shift of cytokines ultimately resulting in "paradoxical" psoriatic lesions.

Hyperproliferative keratinocytes in psoriatic plaques produce large amounts of antimicrobial peptides and proteins (AMP). These positively charged peptides, which have been termed alarmins, have strong proinflammatory properties. Most studies have addressed cathelicidin and its fragment, LL37, which is highly expressed psoriatic skin (136, 137). The positively charged LL37 can associate with negatively charged nucleic acids (DNA and RNA), thus forming immunostimulatory complexes. The free DNA required for such complexes probably comes from neutrophils (which form NETs) and damaged resident skin cells (e.g., traumatized keratinocytes). Plasmacytoid DC (pDC) and myeloid dendritic cells (DC) take up these complexes. Subsequently, RNA motifs stimulate toll-like receptors (TLR) 7 and 8, and DNA triggers TLR9 signaling (52, 138). Cytokines such as TNF, IL-23, and IL-12 are produced by TLR7/8-stimulated myeloid DC, while pDC make type I-interferons (IFNα), all of which fuel the psoriatic inflammation (131). A prominent role in psoriasis and other autoimmune diseases has been attributed to the so-called 6-sulfo LacNAc (slan) DC (139).

Several other skin-derived alarmins such as S100 proteins are inflammatory AMPs also implicated in the pathogenesis of psoriasis. Indeed, IL-17A induces the production of S100A7 (psoriasin) and S100A15 (koebnerisin) by keratinocytes (140, 141). Likewise, myeloid cells and keratinocytes produce the calgranulins, S100A8 and S100A9 [also termed myeloid-related protein (Mrp) 8 and Mrp14], both of which induce T-cell mediated autoimmune reactions and inflammatory changes in keratinocytes (142, 143). Similar to LL37, human ß-defensin (HBD) 2 and HBD4 bind DNA, trigger TLR9 and stimulate pDC (144). Innate immune sensing is also facilitated by IL-26 bound to self-DNA (145).

Activated DC in turn can program the differentiation of naive T into pathogenic T cells [reviewed in (8)]. Neutrophilic granulocytes, too, release AMP, inflammatory cytokines, proteases, free oxygen radicals, and NETs, all of which have been implicated in the inflammatory cascade in psoriasis (8, 114).

NOT ALONE: RELATIONS AND SIMILARITIES OF PSORIASIS WITH OTHER AUTOIMMUNE AND AUTOINFLAMMATORY DISORDERS

The highlights outlined so far show that both adaptive and innate immune processes contribute to psoriasis. Their balance and fine-tuning seem to determine the development of certain clinical forms of the disease, but also organ-specific manifestations. On the one hand, the outlined long-term systemic inflammatory processes probably contribute to the pathogenesis of important metabolic, cardiovascular, and mental concomitant diseases. In these areas, the evidence of a causal relationship is becoming increasingly clear and numerous publications prove this. A more detailed overview can be found elsewhere in this thematic focus. On the other hand, the contoured adaptive and innate immune mechanisms are not specific for psoriasis. Rather, many of them have been found—in varying degrees and weightings—in a whole range of other autoimmune and autoinflammatory diseases. In any case, although this interplay of different components of the immune system is certainly not yet fully understood, parallels with other chronic inflammatory and autoimmune diseases emerge that underpin our current view of psoriasis as a systemic disease.

Indeed, the prevalence of several autoimmune and/or autoinflammatory diseases including rheumatoid arthritis, celiac disease, Crohn's disease, multiple sclerosis, systemic lupus erythematosus, vitiligo, Sjögren's syndrome, alopecia areata, or autoimmune thyroiditis appears to be increased in patients with psoriasis compared to that in healthy controls (146, 147). Several other and more uncommon associations have also been reported (148). Such associations have been attributed to certain genetic and immunological similarities and "overlaps" (146, 149). Three such disease complexes associated with psoriasis, i.e., rheumatoid arthritis, Crohn's disease and systemic lupus erythematosus, will be briefly discussed as examples.

Psoriasis susceptibility 1 candidate gene 1 *(PSORS1C1)*, a gene thought to be involved in IL-17 and IL-1β regulation, is increased in immune cells from patients with rheumatoid arthritis (150). Moreover, aberrant expression of runt-related transcription factor 1 (*RUNX1*) has been implicated in defective regulation of sodium-hydrogen antiporter 3 regulator 1 (*SLC9A3R1*) and N-acetyltransferase 9 (*NAT9*) in both psoriasis and rheumatoid arthritis (151–153). Polymorphisms of the IL-23R gene have also been implicated in both diseases, which further underscores the general relevance of the IL-23/IL-17 axis (154). TNFα-induced protein 3 (*TNFAIP3*), which negatively regulates NF-κB signaling, is another gene thought to be involved in rheumatoid arthritis and psoriasis alike, but also in Crohn's disease, celiac disease, and systemic lupus erythematosus (155, 156).

Similar functional imbalances between Th17 and regulatory T cells (Tregs) as well as similar central cytokines including TNFα, IL-23, and IL-17A, but also IL-1β, IL-6, IL-17F, and IL-21 contribute to both diseases (131, 157–159). Such striking parallels result in the response of both disorders to the same therapies.

Similar to rheumatoid arthritis, Crohn's disease is significantly more prevalent in patients with psoriasis compared to healthy controls and *vice versa* (160–164). Moreover, considerable genetic overlap exists between both diseases as exemplified by seven mutual susceptibility loci (165). Genes involved in the same way include some relevant for the IL-23/I-17 axis such as *IL23R, IL12B,* and *TYK2* (166–169).

One of the first immunological parallels found between psoriasis and Crohn's disease was the central pathogenic role of TNFα (170–172). Hence, TNFα inhibitors ameliorate both disorders (172–175). Paradoxical induction of psoriasis in patients treated with TNFα inhibitors has been attributed to shifts within the balance of TNFα and type I interferons (IFNα) with impact on plasmacytoid dendritic cells (176–181) (**Figure 4**). The pathophysiology of such paradoxical reactions in other immunomodulating settings is less clear (182, 183). The composition of the inflammatory infiltrate (T cells, macrophages, dendritic cells and neutrophilic granulocytes) as well as inflammatory mediators (IFNγ, IL-12, IL-6, IL-17) are conspicuously similar in psoriasis and Crohn's disease (131, 184). A dysregulated balance between Th17 cells and CD4+CD25high Foxp3+ Tregs is thought to lie at the core of both diseases (101, 157, 185–187). In addition, there may even be IL-17 producing Tregs in lesions of both Crohn's disease and psoriasis (188, 189), suggesting differentiation of Tregs toward a pro-inflammatory phenotype. However, a putative protective role of IL-17 in Crohn's disease (190) may explain, at least in part, the worsening of gut inflammation in some cases upon inhibition of IL-17A (191).

Increased expression of IL-6 has been demonstrated in psoriatic plaques and inflamed intestinal mucosa alike (192, 193). IL-6 signaling induces STAT3 phosphorylation, which leads to relative resistance of effector T cells toward Tregs (194, 195).

The association of psoriasis and systemic lupus erythematosus is uncommon and controversially discussed (196, 197). However, dysfunctional interaction of RUNX1 with its binding site due to nucleotide polymorphisms links psoriasis not only with rheumatoid arthritis but also with systemic lupus erythematosus (153, 198, 199). RUNX1 binding on chromosome 2 is defective in some patients with SLE, while RUNX1 binding on chromosome 17 seems to be altered in some psoriasis patients.

TNF receptor-associated factor 3 Interacting Protein 2 (*TRAF3IP2*) has been described as a genetic susceptibility locus for psoriasis and appears to facilitate IL-17 signaling in both psoriasis and systemic lupus erythematosus (200–205). On the cellular level, psoriasis and systemic lupus erythematosus share impaired Treg functions (157, 192, 206, 207), thus suggesting that similar genetic and immune alterations govern pathological immune reactions in both psoriasis and systemic lupus erythematosus.

In summary, psoriasis shows elements of both autoimmune and autoinflammatory mechanisms, whose fine-tuning determines the actual clinical symptoms within the broad spectrum of the disease. Given that psoriasis is a systemic disease that shares conspicuous genetic and immunological similarities with other autoimmune and autoinflammatory disorders, it may serve as a model disorder for research into general mechanisms of such complex immunological regulations.

AUTHOR CONTRIBUTIONS

The author confirms being the sole contributor of this work and has approved it for publication.

REFERENCES

1. Boehncke WH, Sterry W. Psoriasis–a systemic inflammatory disorder: clinic, pathogenesis and therapeutic perspectives. *J Dtsch Dermatol Ges.* (2009) 7:946–52. doi: 10.1111/j.1610-0387.2009.07083.x
2. Schäkel K, Schön MP, Ghoreschi K. Pathogenesis of psoriasis. *Hautarzt.* (2016) 67:422–31. doi: 10.1007/s00105-016-3800-8
3. Boehncke WH, Schön MP. Psoriasis. *Lancet.* (2015) 386:983–94. doi: 10.1016/S0140-6736(14)61909-7
4. Volc S, Ghoreschi K. Pathophysiological basis of systemic treatments in psoriasis. *J Dtsch Dermatol Ges.* (2016) 14:557–72. doi: 10.1111/ddg.13050
5. Schön MP, Boehncke WH. Psoriasis. *N Engl J Med.* (2005) 352:1899–912. doi: 10.1056/NEJMra041320
6. Nestle FO, Kaplan DH, Barker J. Psoriasis. *N Engl J Med.* (2009) 361:496–509. doi: 10.1056/NEJMra0804595
7. Harden JL, Krueger JG, Bowcock AM. The immunogenetics of psoriasis: a comprehensive review. *J Autoimmun.* (2015) 64:66–73. doi: 10.1016/j.jaut.2015.07.008
8. Schön MP, Erpenbeck L. The Interleukin-23/Interleukin-17 axis links adaptive and innate immunity in psoriasis. *Front Immunol.* (2018) 9:1323. doi: 10.3389/fimmu.2018.01323
9. Prinz JC. Human leukocyte antigen-class I alleles and the autoreactive T cell response in psoriasis pathogenesis. *Front Immunol.* (2018) 9:954. doi: 10.3389/fimmu.2018.00954
10. Mueller W, Herrmann B. Cyclosporin A for psoriasis. *N Engl J Med.* (1979) 301:555. doi: 10.1056/NEJM197909063011015
11. Gardembas-Pain M, Ifrah N, Foussard C, Boasson M, Saint Andre JP, Verret JL. Psoriasis after allogeneic bone marrow transplantation. *Arch Dermatol.* (1990) 126:1523. doi: 10.1001/archderm.1990.01670350139033
12. Burden AD, Javed S, Bailey M, Hodgins M, Connor M, Tillman D. Genetics of psoriasis: paternal inheritance and a locus on chromosome 6p. *J Invest Dermatol.* (1998) 110:958–60. doi: 10.1046/j.1523-1747.1998.00213.x
13. Trembath RC, Clough RL, Rosbotham JL, Jones AB, Camp RD, Frodsham A, et al. Identification of a major susceptibility locus on chromosome 6p and evidence for further disease loci revealed by a two stage genome-wide search in psoriasis. *Hum Mol Genet.* (1997) 6:813–20. doi: 10.1093/hmg/6.5.813
14. Chen L, Tsai TF. HLA-Cw6 and psoriasis. *Br J Dermatol.* (2018) 178:854–62. doi: 10.1111/bjd.16083
15. Ellis CN, Krueger GG, Group. ACS. Treatment of chronic plaque psoriasis by selective targeting of memory effector T lymphocytes. *N Engl J Med.* (2001) 345:248–55. doi: 10.1056/NEJM200107263450403
16. Ghoreschi K, Thomas P, Breit S, Dugas M, Mailhammer R, van Eden W, et al. Interleukin-4 therapy of psoriasis induces Th2 responses and improves human autoimmune disease. *Nat Med.* (2003) 9:40–6. doi: 10.1038/nm804
17. Guenova E, Skabytska Y, Hoetzenecker W, Weindl G, Sauer K, Tham M, et al. IL-4 abrogates T(H)17 cell-mediated inflammation by selective silencing of IL-23 in antigen-presenting cells. *Proc Natl Acad Sci USA.* (2015) 112:2163–8. doi: 10.1073/pnas.1416922112
18. Onderdijk AJ, Baerveldt EM, Kurek D, Kant M, Florencia EF, Debets R, et al. IL-4 downregulates IL-1β and IL-6 and induces GATA3 in psoriatic epidermal cells: route of action of a Th2 cytokine. *J Immunol.* (2015) 195:1744–52. doi: 10.4049/jimmunol.1401740
19. Rácz E, Kurek D, Kant M, Baerveldt EM, Florencia E, Mourits S, et al. GATA3 expression is decreased in psoriasis and during epidermal regeneration; induction by narrow-band UVB and IL-4. *PLoS ONE.* (2011) 6:e19806. doi: 10.1371/journal.pone.0019806
20. Asadullah K, Sterry W, Stephanek K, Jasulaitis D, Leupold M, Audring H, et al. IL-10 is a key cytokine in psoriasis. Proof of principle by IL-10 therapy: a new therapeutic approach. *J Clin Invest.* (1998) 101:783–94. doi: 10.1172/JCI1476
21. Breban M, Hammer RE, Richardson JA, Taurog JD. Transfer of the inflammatory disease of HLA-B27 transgenic rats by bone marrow engraftment. *J Exp Med.* (1993) 178:1607–16. doi: 10.1084/jem.178.5.1607
22. Hammer RE, Maika SD, Richardson JA, Tang JP, Taurog JD. Spontaneous inflammatory disease in transgenic rats expressing HLA-B27 and human beta 2m: an animal model of HLA-B27-associated human disorders. *Cell.* (1990) 63:1099–112. doi: 10.1016/0092-8674(90)90512-D
23. Schön MP, Detmar M, Parker CM. Murine psoriasis-like disorder induced by naive CD4+ T cells. *Nat Med.* (1997) 3:183–8. doi: 10.1038/nm0297-183
24. Hong K, Chu A, Lúdvíksson BR, Berg EL, Ehrhardt RO. IL-12, independently of IFN-gamma, plays a crucial role in the pathogenesis of a murine psoriasis-like skin disorder. *J Immunol.* (1999) 162:7480–91.
25. Boehncke WH, Dressel D, Zollner TM, Kaufmann R. Pulling the trigger on psoriasis. *Nature.* (1996) 379:777. doi: 10.1038/379777a0
26. Wrone-Smith T, Nickoloff BJ. Dermal injection of immunocytes induces psoriasis. *J Clin Invest.* (1996) 98:1878–87. doi: 10.1172/JCI118989
27. Arakawa A, Siewert K, Stöhr J, Besgen P, Kim SM, Rühl G, et al. Melanocyte antigen triggers autoimmunity in human psoriasis. *J Exp Med.* (2015) 212:2203–12. doi: 10.1084/jem.20151093
28. Lande R, Botti E, Jandus C, Dojcinovic D, Fanelli G, Conrad C, et al. The antimicrobial peptide LL37 is a T-cell autoantigen in psoriasis. *Nat Commun.* (2014) 5:6595. doi: 10.1038/ncomms6621
29. Prinz JC. Autoimmune aspects of psoriasis: heritability and autoantigens. *Autoimmun Rev.* (2017) 16:970–9. doi: 10.1016/j.autrev.2017.07.011
30. Prinz JC. Melanocytes: target cells of an HLA-C*06:02-restricted autoimmune response in psoriasis. *J Invest Dermatol.* (2017) 137:2053–8. doi: 10.1016/j.jid.2017.05.023
31. Lowes MA, Kikuchi T, Fuentes-Duculan J, Cardinale I, Zaba LC, Haider AS, et al. Psoriasis vulgaris lesions contain discrete populations of Th1 and Th17 T cells. *J Invest Dermatol.* (2008) 128:1207–11. doi: 10.1038/sj.jid.5701213
32. Perera GK, Di Meglio P, Nestle FO. Psoriasis. *Annu Rev Pathol.* (2012) 7(385–422). doi: 10.1146/annurev-pathol-011811-132448
33. Davis MM, Bjorkman PJ. T-cell antigen receptor genes and T-cell recognition. *Nature.* (1988) 334:395–402. doi: 10.1038/334395a0
34. Woodsworth DJ, Castellarin M, Holt RA. Sequence analysis of T-cell repertoires in health and disease. *Genome Med.* (2013) 5:98. doi: 10.1186/gm502
35. Menssen A, Trommler P, Vollmer S, Schendel D, Albert E, Gürtler L, et al. Evidence for an antigen-specific cellular immune response in skin lesions of patients with psoriasis vulgaris. *J Immunol.* (1995) 155:4078–83.
36. Bour H, Puisieux I, Even J, Kourilsky P, Favrot M, Musette P, et al. T-cell repertoire analysis in chronic plaque psoriasis suggests an antigen-specific immune response. *Hum Immunol.* (1999) 60:665–76. doi: 10.1016/S0198-8859(99)00027-0
37. Prinz JC, Vollmer S, Boehncke WH, Menssen A, Laisney I, Trommler P. Selection of conserved TCR VDJ rearrangements in chronic psoriatic plaques indicates a common antigen in psoriasis vulgaris. *Eur J Immunol.* (1999) 29:3360–8.
38. Costello PJ, Winchester RJ, Curran SA, Peterson KS, Kane DJ, Bresnihan B, et al. Psoriatic arthritis joint fluids are characterized by CD8 and CD4 T cell clonal expansions appear antigen driven. *J Immunol.* (2001) 166:2878–86. doi: 10.4049/jimmunol.166.4.2878
39. Lin WJ, Norris DA, Achziger M, Kotzin BL, Tomkinson B. Oligoclonal expansion of intraepidermal T cells in psoriasis skin lesions. *J Invest Dermatol.* (2001) 117:1546–53. doi: 10.1046/j.0022-202x.2001.01548.x
40. Borgato L, Puccetti A, Beri R, Codella O, Frigo A, Simeoni S, et al. The T cell receptor repertoire in psoriatic synovitis is restricted and T lymphocytes expressing the same TCR are present in joint and skin lesions. *J Rheumatol.* (2002) 29:1914–9.
41. Matos TR, O'Malley JT, Lowry EL, Hamm D, Kirsch IR, Robins HS, et al. Clinically resolved psoriatic lesions contain psoriasis-specific IL-17-producing αβ T cell clones. *J Clin Invest.* (2017) 127:4031–41. doi: 10.1172/JCI93396
42. Conrad C, Boyman O, Tonel G, Tun-Kyi A, Laggner U, de Fougerolles A, et al. Alpha1beta1 integrin is crucial for accumulation of epidermal T cells and the development of psoriasis. *Nat Med.* (2007) 13:836–42. doi: 10.1038/nm1605
43. Di Meglio P, Villanova F, Navarini AA, Mylonas A, Tosi I, Nestle FO, et al. Targeting CD8(+) T cells prevents psoriasis development. *J Allergy Clin Immunol.* (2016) 138:274–6. doi: 10.1016/j.jaci.2015.10.046
44. Chang JC, Smith LR, Froning KJ, Schwabe BJ, Laxer JA, Caralli LL, et al. CD8+ T cells in psoriatic lesions preferentially use T-cell receptor V beta 3 and/or V beta 13.1 genes. *Proc Natl Acad Sci USA.* (1994) 91:9282–6. doi: 10.1073/pnas.91.20.9282

45. Diluvio L, Vollmer S, Besgen P, Ellwart JW, Chimenti S, Prinz JC. Identical TCR beta-chain rearrangements in streptococcal angina and skin lesions of patients with psoriasis vulgaris. *J Immunol.* (2006) 176:7104–11. doi: 10.4049/jimmunol.176.11.7104
46. Kim SM, Bhonsle L, Besgen P, Nickel J, Backes A, Held K, et al. Analysis of the paired TCR alpha- and beta-chains of single human T cells. *PLoS ONE.* (2012) 7:e7338. doi: 10.1371/journal.pone.0037338
47. Valdimarsson H, Thorleifsdottir RH, Sigurdardottir SL, Gudjonsson JE, Johnston A. Psoriasis–as an autoimmune disease caused by molecular mimicry. *Trends Immunol.* (2009) 30:494–501. doi: 10.1016/j.it.2009.07.008
48. Thorleifsdottir RH, Sigurdardottir SL, Sigurgeirsson B, Olafsson JH, Sigurdsson MI, Petersen H, et al. Improvement of psoriasis after tonsillectomy is associated with a decrease in the frequency of circulating T cells that recognize streptococcal determinants and homologous skin determinants. *J Immunol.* (2012) 188:5160–5. doi: 10.4049/jimmunol.1102834
49. Sigmundsdottir H, Sigurgeirsson B, Troye-Blomberg M, Good MF, Valdimarsson H, Jonsdottir I. Circulating T cells of patients with active psoriasis respond to streptococcal M-peptides sharing sequences with human epidermal keratins. *Scand J Immunol.* (1997) 45:688–97. doi: 10.1046/j.1365-3083.1997.d01-438.x
50. Besgen P, Trommler P, Vollmer S, Prinz JC. Ezrin, maspin, peroxiredoxin 2, heat shock protein 27: potential targets of a streptococcal-induced auto- immune response in psoriasis. *J Immunol.* (2010) 184:5392–402. doi: 10.4049/jimmunol.0903520
51. Gudmundsdottir AS, Sigmundsdottir H, Sigurgeirsson B, Good MF, Valdimarsson H, Jonsdottir I. Is an epitope on keratin 17 a major target for autoreactive T lymphocytes in psoriasis? *Clin Exp Immunol.* (1999) 117:580–6. doi: 10.1046/j.1365-2249.1999.01013.x
52. Lande R, Gregorio J, Facchinetti V, Chatterjee B, Wang YH, Homey B, et al. Plasmacytoid dendritic cells sense self-DNA coupled with antimicrobial peptide. *Nature.* (2007) 449:564–9. doi: 10.1038/nature06116
53. Nestle FO, Conrad C, Tun-Kyi A, Homey B, Gombert M, Boyman O, et al. Plasmacytoid predendritic cells initiate psoriasis through interferon-alpha production. *J Exp Med.* (2005) 202:135–43. doi: 10.1084/jem.20050500
54. Kahlenberg JM, Kaplan MJ. Little peptide, big effects: the role of LL-37 in inflammation and autoimmune disease. *J Immunol.* (2013) 191:4895–901. doi: 10.4049/jimmunol.1302005
55. Lande R, Ganguly D, Facchinetti V, Frasca L, Conrad C, Gregorio J, et al. Neutrophils activate plasmacytoid dendritic cells by releasing self-DNA-peptide complexes in systemic lupus erythematosus. *Sci Transl Med.* (2011) 3:73ra19. doi: 10.1126/scitranslmed.3001180
56. Frasca L, Palazzo R, Chimenti MS, Alivernini S, Tolusso B, Bui L, et al. Anti-LL37 antibodies are present in Psoriatic Arthritis (PsA) patients: new biomarkers in PsA. *Front Immunol.* (2018) 9:1936. doi: 10.3389/fimmu.2018.01936
57. Yuan Y, Qiu J, Lin ZT, Li W, Haley C, Mui UN, et al. Identification of novel autoantibodies associated with psoriatic arthritis. *Arthritis Rheumatol.* (2019) 71:941–951. doi: 10.1002/art.40830
58. De Bakker PI, Raychaudhuri S. Interrogating the major histocompatibility complex with high-throughput genomics. *Hum Mol Genet.* (2012) 21:R29–36. doi: 10.1093/hmg/dds384
59. Fernando MM, Stevens CR, Walsh EC, De Jager PL, Goyette P, Plenge RM, et al. Defining the role of the MHC in autoimmunity: a review and pooled analysis. *PLoS Genet.* (2008) 4:e1000024. doi: 10.1371/journal.pgen.1000024
60. Horton R, Wilming L, Rand V, Lovering RC, Bruford EA, Khodiyar VK, et al. Gene map of the extended human MHC. *Nat Rev Genet.* (2004) 5:889–99. doi: 10.1038/nrg1489
61. Nair RP, Stuart PE, Nistor I, Hiremagalore R, Chia NV, Jenisch S, et al. Sequence and haplotype analysis supports HLA-C as the psoriasis susceptibility 1 gene. *Am J Hum Genet.* (2006) 78:827–51. doi: 10.1086/503821
62. Tiilikainen A, Lassus A, Karvonen J, Vartiainen P, Julin M. Psoriasis and HLA-Cw6. *Br J Dermatol.* (1980) 102:179–84. doi: 10.1111/j.1365-2133.1980.tb05690.x
63. Zhou F, Cao H, Zuo X, Zhang T, Zhang X, Liu X, et al. Deep sequencing of the MHC region in the Chinese population contributes to studies of complex disease. *Nat Genet.* (2016) 48:740–6. doi: 10.1038/ng.3576
64. Blum JS, Wearsch PA, Cresswell P. Pathways of antigen processing. *Annu Rev Immunol.* (2013) 31:443–73. doi: 10.1146/annurev-immunol-032712-095910
65. Neefjes J, Jongsma ML, Paul P, Bakke O. Towards a systems understanding of MHC class I and MHC class II antigen presentation. *Nat Rev Immunol.* (2011) 11:823–36. doi: 10.1038/nri3084
66. Di Marco M, Schuster H, Backert L, Ghosh M, Rammensee HG, Stevanovic S. Unveiling the peptide motifs of HLA-C and HLA-G from naturally presented peptides and generation of binding prediction matrices. *J Immunol.* (2017) 199:2639–2651. doi: 10.4049/jimmunol.1700938
67. Mobbs JI, Illing PT, Dudek NL, Brooks AG, Baker DG, Purcell AW, et al. The molecular basis for peptide repertoire selection in the human leucocyte antigen (HLA) C*06:02 molecule. *J Biol Chem.* (2017) 292:17203–15. doi: 10.1074/jbc.M117.806976
68. Okada Y, Han B, Tsoi LC, Stuart PE, Ellinghaus E, Tejasvi T, et al. Fine mapping major histocompatibility complex associations in psoriasis and its clinical subtypes. *Am J Hum Genet.* (2014) 95:162–72. doi: 10.1016/j.ajhg.2014.07.002
69. Fitzgerald O, Haroon M, Giles JT, Winchester R. Concepts of pathogenesis in psoriatic arthritis: genotype determines clinical phenotype. *Arthritis Res Ther.* (2015) 17:115. doi: 10.1186/s13075-015-0640-3
70. Helms C, Saccone NL, Cao L, Daw JA, Cao K, Hsu TM, et al. Localization of PSORS1 to a haplotype block harboring HLA-C and distinct from corneodesmosin and HCR. *Hum Genet.* (2005) 118:466–76. doi: 10.1007/s00439-005-0048-2
71. Indhumathi S, Rajappa M, Chandrashekar L, Ananthanarayanan PH, Thappa DM, Negi VS. Polymorphisms in T helper 1 proinflammatory cytokine genes and the risk of psoriasis in a South Indian Tamil cohort. *J Dtsch Dermatol Ges.* (2017) 15:208–11. doi: 10.1111/ddg.13043
72. Geller S, Pulitzer M, Horwitz SM, Moskowitz AJ, Myskowski PL. Mycosis fungoides, Psoriasis and Anti-PD-1 - A New Aspect of Known Associations. *J Dtsch Dermatol Ges.* (2019) 17:186–8. doi: 10.1111/ddg.13715_g
73. Yazdanpanah MJ, Banihashemi M, Pezeshkpoor F, Moradifar M, Feli S, Esmaeili H. Evaluation between Association of Psoriasis and Vitiligo. *J Cutan Med Surg.* (2015) 19:140–3. doi: 10.2310/7750.2014.14074
74. Furue K, Ito T, Tsuji G, Kadono T, Nakahara T, Furue M. Autoimmunity and autoimmune co-morbidities in psoriasis. *Immunology.* (2018) 154:21–7. doi: 10.1111/imm.12891
75. Zibert JR, Wallbrecht K, Schön M, Mir LM, Jacobsen GK, Trochon-Joseph V, et al. Halting angiogenesis by non-viral somatic gene therapy alleviates psoriasis and murine psoriasiform skin lesions. *J Clin Invest.* (2011) 121:410–21. doi: 10.1172/JCI41295
76. Raychaudhuri SP, Sanyal M, Weltman H, Kundu-Raychaudhuri S. K252a, a high-affinity nerve growth factor receptor blocker, improves psoriasis: an *in vivo* study using the severe combined immunodeficient mouse-human skin model. *J Invest Dermatol.* (2004) 122:812–9. doi: 10.1111/j.0022-202X.2003.12602.x
77. Raychaudhuri SK, Raychaudhuri SP. NGF and its receptor system: a new dimension in the pathogenesis of psoriasis and psoriatic arthritis. *Ann N Y Acad Sci.* (2009) 1173:470–7. doi: 10.1111/j.1749-6632.2009.04652.x
78. Christophers E, van de Kerkhof PCM. Severity, heterogeneity and systemic inflammation in psoriasis. *J Eur Acad Dermatol Venereol.* (2019) 33:643–7. doi: 10.1111/jdv.15339
79. Rocha-Pereira P, Santos-Silva A, Rebelo I, Figueiredo A, Quintanilha A, Teixeira F. The inflammatory response in mild and in severe psoriasis. *Br J Dermatol.* (2004) 150:917–28. doi: 10.1111/j.1365-2133.2004.05984.x
80. Siegel D, Devaraj S, Mitra A, Raychaudhuri SP, Raychaudhuri SK, Jialal I. Inflammation, atherosclerosis, and psoriasis. *Clin Rev Allergy Immunol.* (2013) 44:194–204. doi: 10.1007/s12016-012-8308-0
81. Gisondi P, Malerba M, Malara G, Puglisi Guerra A, Sala R, Radaeli A, et al. C-reactive protein and markers for thrombophilia in patients with chronic plaque psoriasis. *Int J Immunopathol Pharmacol.* (2010) 23:1195–202. doi: 10.1177/039463201002300423
82. Jiang S, Hinchliffe TE, Wu T. Biomarkers of An autoimmune skin disease–psoriasis. *Genomics Proteomics Bioinformatics.* (2015) 13:224–33. doi: 10.1016/j.gpb.2015.04.002
83. Breuer K, Göldner FM, Jäger B, Werfel T, Schmid-Ott G. Relationship between chronic stress and CRP levels in women with psoriasis. *J Dtsch Dermatol Ges.* (2016) 14:528–30. doi: 10.1111/ddg.12850

84. Schmuth M, Blunder S, Dubrac S, Gruber R, Moosbrugger-Martinz V. Epidermal barrier in hereditary ichthyoses, atopic dermatitis, and psoriasis. *J Dtsch Dermatol Ges.* (2015) 13:1119–23. doi: 10.1111/ddg.12827
85. Jafri K, Bartels CM, Shin D, Gelfand JM, Ogdie A. Incidence and management of cardiovascular risk factors in psoriatic arthritis and rheumatoid arthritis: a population-based study. *Arthritis Care Res.* (2017) 69:51–7. doi: 10.1002/acr.23094
86. Kagami S, Rizzo HL, Lee JJ, Koguchi Y, Blauvelt A. Circulating Th17, Th22, and Th1 cells are increased in psoriasis. *J Invest Dermatol.* (2010) 130:1373–83. doi: 10.1038/jid.2009.399
87. Owczarczyk-Saczonek A, Placek W. Interleukin-17 as a factor linking the pathogenesis of psoriasis with metabolic disorders. *Int J Dermatol.* (2017) 56:260–8. doi: 10.1111/ijd.13420
88. Guarneri C, Aguennouz M, Guarneri F, Polito F, Benvenga S, Cannavò SP. Autoimmunity to heterogeneous nuclear ribonucleoprotein A1 in psoriatic patients and correlation with disease severity. *J Dtsch Dermatol Ges.* (2018) 16:1103–7. doi: 10.1111/ddg.13631
89. Johnston A, Xing X, Wolterink L, Barnes DH, Yin Z, Reingold L, et al. IL-1 and IL-36 are dominant cytokines in generalized pustular psoriasis. *J Allergy Clin Immunol.* (2017) 140:109–20. doi: 10.1016/j.jaci.2016.08.056
90. Johnston A, Xing X, Guzman AM, Riblett M, Loyd CM, Ward NL, et al. IL-1F5, -F6, -F8, -F9: a novel IL-1 family signaling system that is active in psoriasis and promotes keratinocyte antimicrobial peptide expression. *J Immunol.* (2011) 186:2613–22. doi: 10.4049/jimmunol.1003162
91. Muhr P, Zeitvogel J, Heitland I, Werfel T, Wittmann M. Expression of interleukin (IL)-1 family members upon stimulation with IL-17 differs in keratinocytes derived from patients with psoriasis and healthy donors. *Br J Dermatol.* (2011) 165:189–93. doi: 10.1111/j.1365-2133.2011.10302.x
92. Lowes MA, Russell CB, Martin DA, Towne JE, Krueger JG. The IL-23/ T17 pathogenic axis in psoriasis is amplified by keratinocyte responses. *Trends Immunol.* (2013) 34:174–81. doi: 10.1016/j.it.2012.11.005
93. Marrakchi S, Guigue P, Renshaw BR, Puel A, Pei XY, Fraitag S, et al. Interleukin-36-receptor antagonist deficiency and generalized pustular psoriasis. *N Engl J Med.* (2011) 365:620–8. doi: 10.1056/NEJMoa1013068
94. Ayala-Fontanez N, Soler DC, McCormick TS. Current knowledge on psoriasis and autoimmune diseases. *Psoriasis Targets Ther.* (2016) 6:7–32. doi: 10.2147/PTT.S64950
95. Mössner R, Frambach Y, Wilsmann-Theis D, Löhr S, Jacobi A, Weyergraf A, et al. Palmoplantar pustular psoriasis is associated with missense variants in CARD14, but not with loss-of-function mutations in IL36RN in European patients. *J Invest Dermatol.* (2015) 135:2538–41. doi: 10.1038/jid.2015.186
96. Sugiura K, Muto M, Akiyama M. CARD14 c.526G>C (p.Asp176His) is a significant risk factor for generalized pustular psoriasis with psoriasis vulgaris in the Japanese cohort. *J Invest Dermatol.* (2014) 134:1755–7. doi: 10.1038/jid.2014.46
97. Wilsmann-Theis D, Schnell LM, Ralser-Isselstein V, Bieber T, Schön MP, Hüffmeier U, et al. Successful treatment with interleukin-17A antagonists of generalized pustular psoriasis in patients without IL36RN mutations. *J Dermatol.* (2018) 45:850–4. doi: 10.1111/1346-8138.14318
98. Girolomoni G, Strohal R, Puig L, Bachelez H, Barker J, Boehncke WH, et al. The role of IL-23 and the IL-23/TH 17 immune axis in the pathogenesis and treatment of psoriasis. *J Eur Acad Dermatol Venereol.* (2017) 31:1616–26. doi: 10.1111/jdv.14433
99. Poot J, Thewissen M, Booi D, Nieuwhof C. Characterization of skin-resident T cells using a crawl-out method and flow cytometry. *Exp Dermatol.* (2013) 22:554–5. doi: 10.1111/exd.12191
100. Steinman L. A brief history of T(H)17, the first major revision in the T(H)1/T(H)2 hypothesis of T cell-mediated tissue damage. *Nat Med.* (2007) 13:139–45. doi: 10.1038/nm1551
101. Di Cesare A, Di Meglio P, Nestle FO. The IL-23/Th17 axis in the immunopathogenesis of psoriasis. *J Invest Dermatol.* (2009) 129:1339–50. doi: 10.1038/jid.2009.59
102. Lynde CW, Poulin Y, Vender R, Bourcier M, Khalil S. Interleukin 17A: toward a new understanding of psoriasis pathogenesis. *J Am Acad Dermatol.* (2014) 71:141–50. doi: 10.1016/j.jaad.2013.12.036
103. Murakami M, Hagforsen E, Morhenn V, Ishida-Yamamoto A, Iizuka H. Patients with palmoplantar pustulosis have increased IL-17 and IL-22 levels both in the lesion and serum. *Exp Dermatol.* (2011) 20:845–7. doi: 10.1111/j.1600-0625.2011.01325.x
104. Neurath MF. IL-23: a master regulator in Crohn disease. *Nat Med.* (2007) 13:26–8. doi: 10.1038/nm0107-26
105. Kebir H, Kreymborg K, Ifergan I, Dodelet-Devillers A, Cayrol R, Bernard M, et al. Human TH17 lymphocytes promote blood-brain barrier disruption and central nervous system inflammation. *Nat Med.* (2007) 13:1173–5. doi: 10.1038/nm1651
106. Chen X, Oppenheim JJ. Th17 cells and Tregs: unlikely allies. *J Leukoc Biol.* (2014) 95:723–31. doi: 10.1189/jlb.1213633
107. Muhr P, Renne J, Schaefer V, Werfel T, Wittmann M. Primary human keratinocytes efficiently induce IL-1-dependent IL-17 in CCR6+ T cells. *Exp Dermatol.* (2010) 19:1105–7. doi: 10.1111/j.1600-0625.2010.01134.x
108. Huber S, Gagliani N, Esplugues E, O'Connor WJ, Huber FJ, Chaudhry A, et al. Th17 cells express interleukin-10 receptor and are controlled by Foxp3? and Foxp3+ regulatory CD4+ T cells in an interleukin-10-dependent manner. *Immunity.* (2011) 34:554–65. doi: 10.1016/j.immuni.2011.01.020
109. Kryczek I, Bruce AT, Gudjonsson JE, Johnston A, Aphale A, Vatan L, et al. Induction of IL-17+ T cell trafficking and development by IFN-gamma: mechanism and pathological relevance in psoriasis. *J Immunol.* (2008) 181:4733–41. doi: 10.4049/jimmunol.181.7.4733
110. Keijsers RR, Joosten I, van Erp PE, Koenen HJ, van de Kerkhof PC. Cellular sources of IL-17 in psoriasis: a paradigm shift? *Exp Dermatol.* (2014) 23:799–803. doi: 10.1111/exd.12487
111. Dyring-Andersen B, Honoré TV, Madelung A, Bzorek M, Simonsen S, Clemmensen SN, et al. Interleukin (IL)-17A and IL-22-producing neutrophils in psoriatic skin. *Br J Dermatol.* (2017) 177:e321-e2. doi: 10.1111/bjd.15533
112. Schön MP. The plot thickens while the scope broadens: a holistic view on IL-17 in psoriasis and other inflammatory disorders. *Exp Dermatol.* (2017) 23:804–6. doi: 10.1111/exd.12541
113. Neubert E, Meyer D, Rocca F, Günay G, Kwaczala-Tessmann A, Grandke J, et al. Chromatin swelling drives neutrophil extracellular trap release. *Nat Commun.* (2018) 9:3767. doi: 10.1038/s41467-018-06263-5
114. Schön MP, Broekaert SM, Erpenbeck L. Sexy again: the renaissance of neutrophils in psoriasis. *Exp Dermatol.* (2017) 26:305–11. doi: 10.1111/exd.13067
115. Lin AM, Rubin CJ, Khandpur R, Wang JY, Riblett M, Yalavarthi S, et al. Mast cells and neutrophils release IL-17 through extracellular trap formation in psoriasis. *J Immunol.* (2011) 187:490–500. doi: 10.4049/jimmunol.1100123
116. Chemin K, Gerstner C, Malmström V. Effector functions of $CD4^+$ T cells at the site of local autoimmune inflammation-lessons from rheumatoid arthritis. *Front Immunol.* (2019) 10:353. doi: 10.3389/fimmu.2019.00353
117. Wu H, Liao W, Li Q, Long H, Yin H, Zhao M, et al. Pathogenic role of tissue-resident memory T cells in autoimmune diseases. *Autoimmun Rev.* (2018) 17:906–911. doi: 10.1016/j.autrev.2018.03.014
118. Pan Y, Kupper TS. Metabolic reprogramming and longevity of tissue-resident memory T cells. *Front Immunol.* (2018) 9:1347. doi: 10.3389/fimmu.2018.01347
119. Cheuk S, Schlums H, Gallais Sérézal I, Martini E, Chiang SC, Marquardt N, et al. CD49a expression defines tissue-resident $CD8^+$ T cells poised for cytotoxic function in human skin. *Immunity.* (2017) 46:287–300. doi: 10.1016/j.immuni.2017.01.009
120. McGeachy MJ, Chen Y, Tato CM, Laurence A, Joyce-Shaikh B, Blumenschein WM, et al. The interleukin 23 receptor is essential for the terminal differentiation of interleukin 17-producing effector T helper cells *in vivo*. *Nat Immunol.* (2009) 10:314–24. doi: 10.1038/ni.1698
121. Bettelli E, Korn T, Kuchroo VK. Th17: the third member of the effector T cell trilogy. *Curr Opin Immunol.* (2007) 19:652–7. doi: 10.1016/j.coi.2007.07.020
122. Stritesky GL, Yeh N, Kaplan MH. IL-23 promotes maintenance but not commitment to the Th17 lineage. *J Immunol.* (2008) 181:5948–55. doi: 10.4049/jimmunol.181.9.5948
123. Ghoreschi K, Weigert C, Röcken M. Immunopathogenesis and role of T cells in psoriasis. *Clin Dermatol.* (2007) 25:574–80. doi: 10.1016/j.clindermatol.2007.08.012

124. Boniface K, Blom B, Liu YJ, de Waal Malefyt R. From interleukin-23 to T-helper 17 cells: human T-helper cell differentiation revisited. *Immunol Rev.* (2008) 226:132–46. doi: 10.1111/j.1600-065X.2008.00714.x
125. Singh TP, Schön MP, Wallbrecht K, Michaelis K, Rinner B, Mayer G, et al. 8-methoxypsoralen plus ultraviolet A therapy acts via inhibition of the IL-23/Th17 axis and induction of Foxp3+ regulatory T cells involving CTLA4 signaling in a psoriasis-like skin disorder. *J Immunol.* (2010) 184:7257–67. doi: 10.4049/jimmunol.0903719
126. Drozdenko G, Heine G, M. W. Oral vitamin D increases the frequencies of CD38+ human B cells and ameliorates IL-17-producing T cells. *Exp Dermatol.* (2014) 23:107–12. doi: 10.1111/exd.12300
127. Singh TP, Schön MP, Wallbrecht K, Gruber-Wackernagel A, Wang XJ, Wolf P. Involvement of IL-9 in Th17-associated inflammation and angio- genesis of psoriasis. *PLoS ONE.* (2013) 8:e51752. doi: 10.1371/journal.pone.0051752
128. Cua DJ, Tato CM. Innate IL-17-producing cells: the sentinels of the immune system. *Nat Rev Immunol.* (2010) 10:479–89. doi: 10.1038/nri2800
129. Lee JS, Tato CM, Joyce-Shaikh B, Gulen MF, Cayatte C, Chen Y, et al. Interleukin-23-independent IL-17 production regulates intestinal epithelial permeability. *Immunity.* (2015) 43:727–38. doi: 10.1016/j.immuni.2015.09.003
130. Yoshiga Y, Goto D, Segawa S, Ohnishi Y, Matsumoto I, Ito S, et al. Invariant NKT cells produce IL-17 through IL-23-dependent and -independent pathways with potential modulation of Th17 response in collagen-induced arthritis. *Int J Mol Med.* (2008) 22:369–74. doi: 10.3892/ijmm_00000032
131. Lowes MA, Suarez-Farinas M, Krueger JG. Immunology of psoriasis. *Annu Rev Immunol.* (2014) 32:227–55. doi: 10.1146/annurev-immunol-032713-120225
132. Keijsers RR, Hendriks AGM, van Erp PE, van Cranenbroek B, van de Kerkhof PCM, Koenen HJ, et al. *In vivo* induction of cutaneous inflammation results in the accumulation of extracellular trap-forming neutrophils expressing RORγt and IL-17. *J Invest Dermatol.* (2014) 134:1276–84. doi: 10.1038/jid.2013.526
133. Wu CY, Lin FL. Hand-foot-and-mouth-disease-induced Koebner phenomenon in psoriasis. *J Dtsch Dermatol Ges.* (2019) 17:549–51. doi: 10.1111/ddg.13824
134. Elsner P, Darr-Foit S, Schliemann S. Occupational koebnerization of psoriasis caused by glyphosate. *J Dtsch Dermatol Ges.* (2018) 16:70–1. doi: 10.1111/ddg.13393
135. Wohlrab J, Fiedler G, Gerdes S, Nast A, Philipp S, Radtke MA, et al. Recommendations for detection of individual risk for comorbidities in patients with psoriasis. *Arch Dermatol Res.* (2013) 305:91–8. doi: 10.1007/s00403-013-1318-9
136. Frohm M, Agerberth B, Ahangari G, Ståhle-Bäckdahl M, Lidén S, Wigzell H, et al. The expression of the gene coding for the antibacterial peptide LL-37 is induced in human keratinocytes during inflammatory disorders. *J Biol Chem.* (1997) 272:15258–63. doi: 10.1074/jbc.272.24.15258
137. Morizane S, Yamasaki K, Mühleisen B, Kotol PF, Murakami M, Aoyama Y, et al. Cathelicidin antimicrobial peptide LL-37 in psoriasis enables keratinocyte reactivity against TLR9 ligands. *J Invest Dermatol.* (2012) 132:135–43. doi: 10.1038/jid.2011.259
138. Ganguly D, Chamilos G, Lande R, Gregorio J, Meller S, Facchinetti V, et al. Self-RNA-antimicrobial peptide complexes activate human dendritic cells through TLR7 and TLR8. *J Exp Med.* (2009) 206:1983–94. doi: 10.1084/jem.20090480
139. Döbel T, Schäkel K. The role of human 6-sulfo LacNAc dendritic cells (slanDCs) in autoimmunity and tumor diseases. *J Dtsch Dermatol Ges.* (2014) 12:874–80. doi: 10.1111/ddg.12439_suppl
140. Hegyi Z, Zwicker S, Bureik D, Peric M, Koglin S, Batycka-Baran A, et al. Vitamin D analog calcipotriol suppresses the Th17 cytokine-induced proinflammatory S100 "alarmins" psoriasin (S100A7) and koebnerisin (S100A15) in psoriasis. *J Invest Dermatol.* (2012) 132:1416–24. doi: 10.1038/jid.2011.486
141. Batycka-Baran A, Maj J, Wolf R, Szepietowski JC. The new insight into the role of antimicrobial proteins-alarmins in the immunopathogenesis of psoriasis. *J Immunol Res.* (2014) 2014:628289. doi: 10.1155/2014/628289
142. Lee Y, Jang S, Min JK, Lee K, Sohn KC, Lim JS, et al. S100A8 and S100A9 are messengers in the crosstalk between epidermis and dermis modulating a psoriatic milieu in human skin. *Biochem Biophys Res Commun.* (2012) 423:647–53. doi: 10.1016/j.bbrc.2012.05.162
143. Loser K, Vogl T, Voskort M, Lueken A, Kupas V, Nacken W, et al. The Toll-like receptor 4 ligands Mrp8 and Mrp14 are crucial in the development of autoreactive CD8+ T cells. *Nat Med.* (2010) 16:713–7. doi: 10.1038/nm.2150
144. Tewary P, de la Rosa G, Sharma N, Rodriguez LG, Tarasov SG, Howard OM, et al. β-Defensin 2 and 3 promote the uptake of self or CpG DNA, enhance IFN-α production by human plasmacytoid dendritic cells, promote inflammation. *J Immunol.* (2013) 191:865–74. doi: 10.4049/jimmunol.1201648
145. Meller S, Di Domizio J, Voo KS, Friedrich HC, Chamilos G, Ganguly D, et al. T(H)17 cells promote microbial killing and innate immune sensing of DNA via interleukin 26. *Nat Immunol.* (2015) 16:970–9. doi: 10.1038/ni.3211
146. Wu JJ, Nguyen TU, Poon KY, Herrinton LJ. The association of psoriasis with autoimmune diseases. *J Am Acad Dermatol.* (2012) 67:924–30. doi: 10.1016/j.jaad.2012.04.039
147. Hsu LN, Armstrong AW. Psoriasis and autoimmune disorders: a review of the literature. *J Am Acad Dermatol.* (2012) 67:1076–9. doi: 10.1016/j.jaad.2012.01.029
148. Claus S, Ziemer M, Simon JC, Treudler R. Coincidence of annular pustular psoriasis, pemphigus foliaceus, and leukocytoclastic vasculitis associated with chronic cholecystitis. *J Dtsch Dermatol Ges.* (2016) 14:830–1. doi: 10.1111/ddg.12619
149. Makredes M, Robinson DJ, Bala M, Kimball AB. The burden of autoimmune disease: a comparison of prevalence ratios in patients with psoriatic arthritis and psoriasis. *J Am Acad Dermatol.* (2009) 61:405–10. doi: 10.1016/j.jaad.2009.02.015
150. Sun H, Xia Y, Wang L, Wang Y, Chang X. PSORS1C1 may be involved in rheumatoid arthritis. *Immunol Lett.* (2013) 153:9–14. doi: 10.1016/j.imlet.2013.06.001
151. Alarcon-Riquelme ME. Role of RUNX in autoimmune diseases linking rheumatoid arthritis, psoriasis and lupus. *Arthritis Res Ther.* 204;6:169–73. doi: 10.1186/ar1203
152. Okuda T, Nishimura M, Nakao M, Fujita Y. RUNX1/AML1: a central player in hematopoiesis. *Int J Hematol.* (2001) 74:252–7. doi: 10.1007/BF02982057
153. Helms C, Cao L, Krueger JG, Wijsman EM, Chamian F, Gordon D, et al. A putative RUNX1 binding site variant between SLC9A3R1 and NAT9 is associated with susceptibility to psoriasis. *Nat Genet.* (2003) 35:349–56. doi: 10.1038/ng1268
154. Gregersen PK, Olsson LM. Recent advances in the genetics of autoimmune disease. *Annu Rev Immunol.* (2009) 27:363–91. doi: 10.1146/annurev.immunol.021908.132653
155. Vereecke L, Beyaert R, van Loo G. The ubiquitin-editing enzyme A20 (TNFAIP3) is a central regulator of immunopathology. *Trends Immunol.* (2009) 30:383–91. doi: 10.1016/j.it.2009.05.007
156. Wang F, Zhang X, Xia P, Zhang L, Zhang Z. Upregulation of tumor necrosis factor alpha-induced protein 3 interacting protein 1 mRNA in psoriasis vulgaris. *J Dtsch Dermatol Ges.* (2015) 13:159–61. doi: 10.1111/ddg.12462
157. Sugiyama H, Gyulai R, Toichi E, Garaczi E, Shimada S, Stevens SR, et al. Dysfunctional blood and target tissue CD4+CD25high regulatory T cells in psoriasis: mechanism underlying unrestrained pathogenic effector T cell proliferation. *J Immunol.* (2005) 174:164–73. doi: 10.4049/jimmunol.174.1.164
158. Hueber W, Patel DD, Dryja T, Wright AM, Koroleva I, Bruin G, et al. Effects of AIN457, a fully human antibody to interleukin-17A, on psoriasis, rheumatoid arthritis, and uveitis. *Sci Transl Med.* (2010) 2:52ra72. doi: 10.1126/scitranslmed.3001107
159. McInnes IB, Schett G. The pathogenesis of rheumatoid arthritis. *N Engl J Med.* (2011) 365:2205–19. doi: 10.1056/NEJMra1004965
160. Yates VM, Watkinson G, Kelman A. Further evidence for an associa- tion between psoriasis, Crohn's disease and ulcerative colitis. *Br J Dermatol.* (1982) 106:323–30. doi: 10.1111/j.1365-2133.1982.tb01731.x
161. Bernstein CN, Wajda A, Blanchard JF. The clustering of other chronic inflammatory diseases in inflammatory bowel disease: a population- based study. *Gastroenterology.* (2005) 129:827–36. doi: 10.1053/j.gastro.2005.06.021
162. Weng X, Liu L, Barcellos LF, Allison JE, Herrinton LJ. Clustering of inflammatory bowel disease with immune mediated diseases among

members of a northern california-managed care organization. *Am J Gastroenterol.* (2007) 102:1429–35. doi: 10.1111/j.1572-0241.2007.01215.x
163. Lee FI, Bellary SV, Francis C. Increased occurrence of psoriasis in patients with Crohn's disease and their relatives. *Am J Gastroenterol.* (1990) 85:962–3.
164. Scarpa R, Manguso F, D'Arienzo A, D'Armiento FP, Astarita C, Mazzacca G, et al. Microscopic inflammatory changes in colon of patients with both active psoriasis and psoriatic arthritis without bowel symptoms. *J Rheumatol.* (2000) 27:1241–6.
165. Ellinghaus D, Ellinghaus E, Nair RP, Stuart PE, Esko T, Metspalu A, et al. Combined analysis of genome-wide association studies for Crohn disease and psoriasis identifies seven shared susceptibility loci. *Am J Hum Genet.* (2012) 90:636–47. doi: 10.1016/j.ajhg.2012.02.020
166. Ferguson LR, Han DY, Fraser AG, Huebner C, Lam WJ, Morgan AR. IL23R and IL12B SNPs and haplotypes strongly associate with Crohn's disease risk in a New Zealand population. *Gastroenterol Res Pract.* (2010) 2010:539461. doi: 10.1155/2010/539461
167. Cargill M, Schrodi SJ, Chang M, Garcia VE, Brandon R, Callis KP, et al. A large-scale genetic association study confirms IL12B and leads to the identification of IL23R as psoriasis-risk genes. *Am J Hum Genet.* (2007) 80:273–90. doi: 10.1086/511051
168. Nair RP, Ruether A, Stuart PE, Jenisch S, Tejasvi T, Hiremagalore R, et al. Polymorphisms of the IL12B and IL23R genes are associated with psoriasis. *J Invest Dermatol.* (2008) 128:1653–61. doi: 10.1038/sj.jid.5701255
169. Genetic Analysis of Psoriasis Consortium & the Wellcome Trust Case Control Consortium 2, Strange A, Capon F, Spencer CC, Knight J, Weale ME, et al. A genome-wide association study identifies new psoriasis susceptibility loci and an interaction between HLA-C and ERAP1. *Nat Genet.* (2010) 42:985–90. doi: 10.1038/ng.694
170. Braegger CP, Nicholls S, Murch SH, Stephens S, MacDonald TT. Tumour necrosis factor alpha in stool as a marker of intestinal inflammation. *Lancet.* (1992) 339:89–91. doi: 10.1016/0140-6736(92)90999-J
171. Murch SH, Braegger CP, Walker-Smith JA, MacDonald TT. Location of tumour necrosis factor alpha by immunohistochemistry in chronic inflammatory bowel disease. *Gut.* (1993) 34:1705–9. doi: 10.1136/gut.34.12.1705
172. Oh CJ, Das KM, Gottlieb AB. Treatment with anti-tumor necrosis factor alpha (TNF-alpha) monoclonal antibody dramatically decreases the clinical activity of psoriasis lesions. *J Am Acad Dermatol.* (2000) 42(5 pt 1):829–30. doi: 10.1067/mjd.2000.105948
173. Chaudhari U, Romano P, Mulcahy LD, Dooley LT, Baker DG, Gottlieb AB. Efficacy and safety of infliximab monotherapy for plaque-type psoriasis: a randomised trial. *Lancet.* (2001) 357:1842–7. doi: 10.1016/S0140-6736(00)04954-0
174. Plevy SE, Landers CJ, Prehn J, Carramanzana NM, Deem RL, Shealy D, et al. A role for TNF-alpha and mucosal T helper-1 cytokines in the pathogenesis of Crohn's disease. *J Immunol.* (1997) 159:6276–82.
175. Targan SR, Hanauer SB, van Deventer SJ, Mayer L, Present DH, Braakman T, et al. A short-term study of chimeric monoclonal antibody cA2 to tumor necrosis factor alpha for Crohn's disease. Crohn's Disease cA2 Study Group. *N Engl J Med.* (1997) 337:1029–35. doi: 10.1056/NEJM199710093371502
176. Amschler K, Broekaert SMC, Mohr J, Schön MP, Mössner R. Persistent neutrophilic scarring alopecia triggered by anti-TNF blockade for Crohn's disease. *Eur J Dermatol.* (2018) 28:403–5. doi: 10.1684/ejd.2018.3270
177. Angelucci E, Cocco A, Viscido A, Vernia P, Caprilli R. Another paradox in Crohn's disease: new onset of psoriasis in a patient receiving tumor necrosis factor-alpha antagonist. *Inflamm Bowel Dis.* (2007) 13:1059–61. doi: 10.1002/ibd.20137
178. Cottone M, Sapienza C, Macaluso FS, Cannizzaro M. Psoriasis and Inflammatory Bowel Disease. *Dig Dis.* (2019) 10:1–7. doi: 10.1159/000500116
179. Fiorino G, Allez M, Malesci A, Danese S. Review article: anti TNF- alpha induced psoriasis in patients with inflammatory bowel disease. *Aliment Pharmacol Ther.* (2009) 29:921–7. doi: 10.1111/j.1365-2036.2009.03955.x
180. Mylonas A, Conrad C. Psoriasis: classical vs. paradoxical. The Yin-Yang of TNF and type I interferon. *Front Immunol.* (2018) 9:2746. doi: 10.3389/fimmu.2018.02746
181. Lindhaus C, Tittelbach J, Elsner P. Cutaneous side effects of TNF-alpha inhibitors. *J Dtsch Dermatol Ges.* (2017) 15:281–8. doi: 10.1111/ddg.13200
182. Fujimoto N, Matsuo S, Satoh T. Psoriasis vulgaris in a patient with pemphigus vulgaris on corticosteroid therapy. *J Dtsch Dermatol Ges.* (2018) 16:606–8. doi: 10.1111/ddg.13505
183. Amschler K, Meyersburg D, Kitze B, Schön MP, Mössner R. Onset of psoriasis upon interferon beta treatment in a multiple sclerosis patient. *Eur J Dermatol.* (2016) 26:211–2. doi: 10.1684/ejd.2015.2602
184. Baumgart DC, Sandborn WJ. Crohn's disease. *Lancet.* (2012) 380:1590–605. doi: 10.1016/S0140-6736(12)60026-9
185. Brand S. Crohn's disease: Th1, Th17 or both? The change of a paradigm: new immunological and genetic insights implicate Th17 cells in the pathogenesis of Crohn's disease. *Gut.* (2009) 58:1152–67. doi: 10.1136/gut.2008.163667
186. Eastaff-Leung N, Mabarrack N, Barbour A, Cummins A, Barry S. Foxp3+ regulatory T cells, Th17 effector cells, and cytokine environment in inflammatory bowel disease. *J Clin Immunol.* (2010) 30:80–9. doi: 10.1007/s10875-009-9345-1
187. Galvez J. Role of Th17 cells in the pathogenesis of human IBD. *ISRN Inflamm.* (2014) 2014:928461. doi: 10.1155/2014/928461
188. Hovhannisyan Z, Treatman J, Littman DR, Mayer L. Characterization of interleukin-17-producing regulatory T cells in inflamed intestinal mucosa from patients with inflammatory bowel diseases. *Gastroenterology.* (2011) 140:957–65. doi: 10.1053/j.gastro.2010.12.002
189. Bovenschen HJ, van de Kerkhof PC, van Erp PE, Woestenenk R, Joosten I, Koenen HJ. Foxp3+ regulatory T cells of psoriasis patients easily differentiate into IL-17A-producing cells and are found in lesional skin. *J Invest Dermatol.* (2011) 131:1853–60. doi: 10.1038/jid.2011.139
190. O'Connor WJ, Kamanaka M, Booth CJ, Town T, Nakae S, Iwakura Y, et al. A protective function for interleukin 17A in T cell-mediated intestinal inflammation. *Nat Immunol.* (2009) 10:603–9. doi: 10.1038/ni.1736
191. Hohenberger M, Cardwell LA, Oussedik E, Feldman SR. Interleukin-17 inhibition: role in psoriasis and inflammatory bowel disease. *J Dermatolog Treat.* (2018) 29:13–8. doi: 10.1080/09546634.2017.1329511
192. Goodman WA, Levine AD, Massari JV, Sugiyama H, McCormick TS, Cooper KD. IL-6 signaling in psoriasis prevents immune suppression by regulatory T cells. *J Immunol.* (2009) 183:3170–6. doi: 10.4049/jimmunol.0803721
193. Atreya R, Mudter J, Finotto S, Müllberg J, Jostock T, Wirtz S, et al. Blockade of interleukin 6 trans signaling suppresses T-cell resistance against apoptosis in chronic intestinal inflammation: evidence in crohn disease and experimental colitis *in vivo*. *Nat Med.* (2000) 6:583–8. doi: 10.1038/75068
194. Goodman WA, Young AB, McCormick TS, Cooper KD, Levine AD. Stat3 phosphorylation mediates resistance of primary human T cells to regulatory T cell suppression. *J Immunol.* (2011) 186:3336–45. doi: 10.4049/jimmunol.1001455
195. Sano S, Chan KS, DiGiovanni J. Impact of Stat3 activation upon skin biology: a dichotomy of its role between homeostasis and diseases. *J Dermatol Sci.* (2008) 50:1–14. doi: 10.1016/j.jdermsci.2007.05.016
196. Janjumratsang P, Phainupong D, Chanjanakijskul S, Roongphibulsopit P. Positive direct immunofluorescence and autoantibody profiles in psoriasis patients. *J Dermatol.* (2008) 35:508–13. doi: 10.1111/j.1346-8138.2008.00512.x
197. Dubois EL, Wierzchowiecki M, Cox MB, Weiner JM. Duration and death in systemic lupus erythematosus. An analysis of 249 cases. *JAMA.* (1979) 227:1399–402. doi: 10.1001/jama.227.12.1399
198. Tokuhiro S, Yamada R, Chang X, Suzuki A, Kochi Y, Sawada T, et al. An intronic SNP in a RUNX1 binding site of SLC22A4, encoding an organic cation transporter, is associated with rheumatoid arthritis. *Nat Genet.* (2003) 35:341–8. doi: 10.1038/ng1267
199. Prokunina L, Castillejo-López C, Oberg F, Gunnarsson I, Berg L, Magnusson V, et al. A regulatory polymorphism in PDCD1 is associated with susceptibility to systemic lupus erythematosus in humans. *Nat Genet.* (2002) 32:666–9. doi: 10.1038/ng1020
200. Perricone C, Ciccacci C, Ceccarelli F, Di Fusco D, Spinelli FR, Cipriano E, et al. TRAF3IP2 gene and systemic lupus erythematosus: association with disease susceptibility and pericarditis development. *Immunogenetics.* (2013) 65:703–9. doi: 10.1007/s00251-013-0717-6
201. Hüffmeier U, Uebe S, Ekici AB, Bowes J, Giardina E, Korendowych E, et al. Common variants at TRAF3IP2 are associated with susceptibility to psoriatic arthritis and psoriasis. *Nat Genet.* (2010) 42:996–9. doi: 10.1038/ng.688

202. Wu L, Wang C, Boisson B, Misra S, Rayman P, Finke JH, et al. The differential regulation of human ACT1 isoforms by Hsp90 in IL-17 signaling. *J Immunol.* (2014) 193:1590–9. doi: 10.4049/jimmunol.1400715
203. Chen XQ, Yu YC, Deng HH, Sun JZ, Dai Z, Wu YW, et al. Plasma IL-17A is increased in new-onset SLE patients and associated with disease activity. *J Clin Immunol.* (2010) 30:221–5. doi: 10.1007/s10875-009-9365-x
204. Wen Z, Xu L, Xu W, Yin Z, Gao X, Xiong S. Interleukin-17 expression positively correlates with disease severity of lupus nephritis by increasing anti-double-stranded DNA antibody production in a lupus model induced by activated lymphocyte derived DNA. *PLoS ONE.* (2013) 8:e58161. doi: 10.1371/journal.pone.0058161
205. Yu B, Guan M, Peng Y, Shao Y, Zhang C, Yue X, et al. Copy number variations of interleukin-17F, interleukin-21, and interleukin-22 are associated with systemic lupus erythematosus. *Arthritis Rheum.* (2011) 63:3487–92. doi: 10.1002/art.30595
206. Barreto M, Ferreira RC, Lourenço L, Moraes-Fontes MF, Santos E, Alves M, et al. Low frequency of CD4+CD25+ Treg in SLE patients: a heritabletrait associated with CTLA4 and TGFbeta gene variants. *BMC Immunol.* (2009) 10:5. doi: 10.1186/1471-2172-10-5
207. Franz B, Fritzsching B, Riehl A, Oberle N, Klemke CD, Sykora J, et al. Low number of regulatory T cells in skin lesions of patients with cutaneous lupus erythematosus. *Arthritis Rheum.* (2007) 56:1910–20. doi: 10.1002/art.22699

6

Loss of TIPE2 has Opposing Effects on the Pathogenesis of Autoimmune Diseases

Ruiling Liu[1,2†], *Xiaozhen He*[3†], *Wenwen Geng*[3], *Ting Wang*[4*] *and Qingguo Ruan*[1,4*]

[1] Center for Antibody Drug, Institute of Biomedicine and Biotechnology, Shenzhen Institutes of Advanced Technology, Chinese Academy of Sciences, Shenzhen, China, [2] University of Chinese Academy of Sciences, Beijing, China, [3] School of Medicine and Life Sciences, University of Jinan, Shandong Academy of Medical Sciences, Jinan, China, [4] State Key Laboratory Cultivation Base, Shandong Provincial Key Laboratory of Ophthalmology, Shandong Eye Institute, Shandong First Medical University & Shandong Academy of Medical Sciences, Qingdao, China

***Correspondence:**
Ting Wang
wt-ting@163.com
Qingguo Ruan
ruanqg222@hotmail.com

† These authors have contributed equally to this work

Autoimmune diseases are a physiological state wherein immune responses are directed against and damage the body's own tissues. Cytokines secreted by infiltrated inflammatory cells contribute to the pathogenesis of autoimmune diseases. TIPE2, one of the four family members of Tumor necrosis factor-α induced protein-8 (TNFAIP8), is a negative regulator of innate and adaptive immunity and plays essential roles in the maintenance of immune tolerance. However, studies on the role of TIPE2 during the development of autoimmune diseases have generated contradictory results. In the current study, we sought to determine the role of TIPE2 during the development of IMQ-induced psoriasis and Experimental Autoimmune Uveitis (EAU) in mice. Our study revealed that, while TIPE2-deficiency alleviates psoriasis, it exacerbates the development of EAU. Further studies demonstrated that, although TIPE2-deficient T cells produced more IL-17A, they do not migrate efficiently to the local inflammatory site, i.e., the skin. This in turn led to the decreased IL-17A production in the skin and consequently reduced the severity of psoriasis in TIPE2-deficient mice. However, although TIPE2-deficient T cells still produced more IL-17A in EAU model, they migrate into the inflamed eye as efficient as TIPE2-sufficient T cells, and consequently exacerbates the development of EAU in TIPE2-deficient mice. Taken together, these results indicate that TIPE2 may either promote or suppress autoimmunity depending on the specific inflammatory microenvironment in different types of autoimmune diseases.

Keywords: TIPE2, psoriasis, IL-17A, migration, EAU

INTRODUCTION

Autoimmune disease occurs when healthy body tissues were mistakenly attacked and destroyed by body's own immune system. More than 80 types of different autoimmune diseases have been reported, including psoriasis, Experimental Autoimmune Uveitis (EAU), type 1 diabetes, Experimental Autoimmune Encephalomyelitis (EAE), and Rheumatoid Arthritis (RA). Besides genetic and environmental factors, immunological factor often plays important roles during the pathogenesis of autoimmune disease which triggers the initiation of the disease as well as maintaining the disease state (1, 2). T cells, especially the IL-17A-producing Th17 cells, have been shown to play a dominant role during the pathogenesis of multiple autoimmune diseases including psoriasis and EAU (3–8). Following priming, Th17 cells migrate to local inflammatory site which was mediated by tissue selective integrins and chemokine receptors (9). While IL-17A knockout mice develop significantly less severe psoriasis and EAU (10, 11), treatment with anti-IL-17A antibody markedly reduced inflammation in both psoriatic and EAU mice (12–14).

Tumor necrosis factor-α induced protein-8-like 2 (TNFAIP8L2 or TIPE2) is one member of the TNFAIP8 family. Current study suggests that TIPE2 is a negative regulator of innate and adaptive immune responses (15). TIPE2 is preferentially expressed by immune cells and TIPE2-deficient cells are hyper-responsive to Toll-like receptor (TLR) and T cell receptor (TCR) activation. Further study revealed that TIPE2 may inhibit the activation of NF-κB in T cells and macrophages (15). Since TIPE2 is a negative regulator of immune response, it may play important roles during the pathogenesis of autoimmune disease. In fact, TIPE2 down-regulation was found in the peripheral blood mononuclear cells from patients with Systemic Lupus Erythematosus (SLE) (16). In 2016, Xu et al. reported that TIPE2 alleviates experimental SLE through the induction of M2 macrophage (17). In addition, decreased TIPE2 expression was also found to be correlated with the occurrence and development of RA (18). However, researchers have also found that TIPE2 promotes the development of colitis (19). Recently, Fayngerts et al. reported that TIPE2-deficient leukocytes were defective in polarization and chemotaxis, and consequently TIPE2-deficient mice were resistant to EAE which was mediated by leukocyte (20). Thus, the role of TIPE2 during the development of autoimmune diseases remains elusive.

In the current study, we sought to determine the role of TIPE2 during the development of IMQ-induced psoriasis and EAU in mice. Our study revealed that, although TIPE2 exacerbates the development of psoriasis through promoting the directional migration of T cells to the site of inflammation, it alleviates EAU through the suppression of IL-17A production by T cells.

MATERIALS AND METHODS

Animals

Four to six week-old wild-type and TIPE2-deficient mice in the C57BL/6 background were used in the experiments and kept under pathogen-free conditions at the animal core facility of the Shenzhen Institutes of Advanced Technology, Chinese Academy of Sciences. All efforts were made to minimize the number of mice used and to less animal distress, pain, and injury. Carbon dioxide (CO_2) was used to euthanize mice. All procedures were preapproved by the Animal Care and Use Committee of Shenzhen Institutes of Advanced Technology, Chinese Academy of Sciences.

Induction and Clinical Evaluation of Psoriasis

Commercially available IMQ cream (Aldara, Inova pharmaceuticals, USA) was smeared on the shaved back of wild-type and TIPE2-deficient mice in the C57BL/6 background at 4–6 weeks of age as previously reported (21). Alternatively, $CD3^+$ T cells were isolated from wild-type and TIPE2-deficient mice and adoptively transferred into *Rag1*$^{-/-}$ mice (10×10^6/mouse). IMQ cream was then used to induce psoriasis as mentioned above. The severity of inflammation of the back skin was evaluated according to the clinical psoriasis area and severity index (PASI) (22, 23). In order to obtain histological profiles of the back skin, skin sections were first fixed in 10% formalin, and then embedded in paraffin, sectioned, and stained with hematoxylin/eosin. Skin sections were finally examined by microscopy.

Induction and Clinical Evaluation of EAU

EAU was induced by active immunization as previously described (24). Briefly, mice were immunized with IRBP1-20 (4 mg/ml, GPTHLFQPSLVLDMAKVLLD, purchased from China Peptides) emulsified 1:1 in complete Freund's adjuvant (Chondrex, USA) with an additional 100 μl mycobacterium tuberculosis H37R (2.5 mg/ml, BD biosciences, USA) at the base of the tail and 50 μl in each thigh (400 μg peptide per mouse). An additional 200 μg bordetella pertussis toxin (Abcam, USA) was intravenously injected immediately after peptide injection. Eyes were harvested 21 days after immunization and stained with hematoxylin/eosin, and the severity of EAU was evaluated on a scale of 0–4 using previously published criteria (25).

RNA Isolation and RT-PCR

To prepare total skin cells, the back skin of the mice were collected and washed with cold washing buffer (PBS + 2% FBS), then cut into small pieces and incubated in DMEM supplemented with 0.5 mg/ml collagenase D (Sigma, USA), 0.02 mg/ml DNase (Roche, USA), and 0.1 mg/ml Dispase (Sigma, USA) for 20 min at 37°C with gentle shaking. Supernatant was collected and filtered through a 70-μm strainer (BD Biosciences, USA) to obtain single-cell suspension. Total RNA was isolated using TRIzol reagent following manufacturer's instructions (Life Technologies, USA). RNA samples were reversely transcribed using the primescript reverse transcription kit (Takara, JPN). The expression of chemokines was determined by quantitative RT-PCR using specific primers and Applied Biosystems 7500 system. When determining the relative level of gene expression, GAPDH was used as the internal control. The primers for the detection of mouse chemokines and GAPDH were synthesized as previously described (26, 27).

ELISA Assay

For cytokine assays, purified $CD4^+$ T cells from spleen and total cells from inguinal lymph node (ILN), cervical lymph node (CLN), spleen or eye were cultured at 1×10^6 cells/well in 100 μl of complete DMEM culture medium (Corning, USA) in the presence or absence of anti-CD3 (ebioscience, USA) and/or anti-CD28 (ebioscience, USA). The concentrations of anti-CD3 and anti-CD28 were indicated within the figure or figure legend. Culture supernatants were collected after 48 h; For the preparation tissue extract, total cells from the back skin of the mice were homogenized in 1% chaps (Sigma, USA) supplemented with complete protease inhibitor mixture (Roche, USA). The concentration of IL17A in the cell culture supernatant and tissue extract was determined by quantitative enzyme-linked immunosorbent assay (ELISA) per manufacturer's instructions (eBioscience, USA).

Antibodies and Flow Cytometry

Flow cytometric analyses were performed on freshly isolated cells from skin, blood, ILN, CLN, and eye. Cells were labeled with a combination of the following fluorescence-conjugated mouse mAbs: PE-anti-CD4, APC-anti-CD8, PerCP-Cy5.5-anti-CD3, APC-anti-CD183(CXCR3), APC-anti-CD184 (CXCR4), PE-anti-CD194 (CCR4), APC-anti-CD195(CCR5), PerCP/Cy5.5-anti-CD196 (CCR6), APC-anti-CD197(CCR7), and FITC-anti-CD199 (CCR9). All antibodies were purchased from BioLegend. For the intracellular staining of IL-17A, cells from the skin or eye were stimulated with PMA + ionomycin (eBioscience, USA) in the presence of GolgoStop (1:1,500 dilution, BD, USA) for 6 h. Cells were then collected and first stained with anti-CD3. After fixation and permeabilization, cells were then stained with anti-IL-17A (BioLegend, USA) per manufacturer's instructions (Invitrogen, USA). For the intracellular staining of phospho-IκBα, cells from the skin or eye were first stained with anti-CD3. After fixation and permeabilization, cells were then stained with purified anti-phospho-IκBα (Ser32/36) antibody (CST, USA), followed by staining with DyLight™ 488-conjugated goat anti-mouse IgG (BioLegend, USA) per manufacturer's instructions (Biolgend, USA). Stained cells were then examined on CytoFLEX flow cytometry system (Beckman Coulter Inc., USA).

Transwell Migration Assay

Lymphocytes were isolated from blood using mouse peripheral blood lymphocyte isolation kit (Tian Jin Hao Yang Biological Manufacture CO., LTD, China). Total T cells were isolated from blood lymphocyte and ILN using EasySep™ Mouse T Cell Isolation Kit (Stemcell, USA) and "rest" in RPMI1640 culture medium for 1 h. Migration assays were then performed using Transwells. Briefly, cells were placed on the upper layer of a cell permeable membrane of 24-well transwell plate (5 μm pore size, Corning, USA) at 5×10^4/well. IP10 (10 ng/ml, Biolegend, USA), CCL19 (10 ng/ml, Biolegend, USA), or PBS (control group) was placed below the cell permeable membrane. Following an incubation period of 3 h, the cells that have migrated through the membrane are counted by TC10 automated cell counter (Bio-Rad, USA). The chemotaxis index was calculated by dividing the number of cells that migrated in response to chemoattractant with the number of cells that migrated in the control group.

Confocal Microscopy Analysis

Total T cells were isolated from the ILN using EasySep™ Mouse T Cell Isolation Kit (Stemcell, USA). After resting in RPMI1640 culture medium for 1 h, cells were subjected to point-source stimulation with IP10 (Biologend, USA) at 1 μg/ml for 3 min at 37°C. Cells were then fixed with 4% paraformaldehyde for 15 min at room temperature, permeabilized with 0.1% TritonX-100 in PBS for 10 min and blocked with 5% normal rat serum plus 3% BSA for 1 h at room temperature. After fixation and permeabilization, cells were incubated overnight with a 1:100 dilution of Phospho-AKT (T308) antibody (Cell Signaling Technology, USA) and a 1:1,000 dilution of Phalloidin-iFluor647 (CST, USA). Cells were then washed three times and incubated for 30 min with 1:1,000 diluted DyLight™ 488 Donkey anti-rabbit IgG antibody (Biolegend, USA). Stained cells were then washed, dried and covered with ProLong Gold with DAPI (Invitrogen, USA). Images were acquired using a Leica TCS SP5 confocal microscope and analyzed using ImageJ software.

Statistical Analysis

The significance of the difference in disease severity was determined by Mann-Whitney *U*-test. The skin thickness, mean florescence intensity (MFI), level of cytokines and percentage of cells were analyzed by Student's *t*-test.

RESULTS

TIPE2-Deficiency Alleviates Psoriasis but Promotes the Development of EAU

IMQ is a ligand for TLR7/8 that when applied topically to the skin, induces psoriasis-like inflammation in susceptible mice including BABL/c and C57BL/6. The IMQ-psoriasis closely resembles human psoriasis lesions with respect to phenotypic and histological characteristics. EAU is the animal model of human uveitis that most closely resembles sympathetic ophthalmia. It is the most widely used and well-studied uveitis model. In order to determine the roles of TIPE2 in the pathogenesis of different types of autoimmune diseases, we established IMQ-induced psoriasis model and EAU model in wild-type and TIPE2-deficient mice in the C57BL/6 background. As shown in **Figure 1A**, IMQ-induced skin inflammation in TIPE2-deficient mice resulted in lower scores for erythema and scaling at the peak-stage of the disease. The difference is small but significant. Although IMQ-induced psoriasis is a T cell–dependent disease, other hematopoietic cell types may also contribute to the pathogenesis. In order to directly test the T cell–specific function of TIPE2 in psoriasis, we studied the IMQ-induced psoriasis in *Rag1*$^{-/-}$ mice that had received WT or TIPE2-deficient T cells. We found that mice received TIPE2-deficient T cells developed less severe symptoms than those reconstituted with WT T cells (**Figure 1B**). Consistent with these clinical findings, H&E-stained sections of skin from TIPE2-deficient mice demonstrated decreased epidermal thickening by **Figures 1C,D**. In contrast to the phenotype difference displayed in IMQ-induced psoriasis model, TIPE2-deficient mice exhibited more severe retinal edema and structural distortion in the EAU model (**Figure 1E**). When pathological changes in the retina were evaluated according to the scoring criteria previously reported, WT mice had a mean score of 0.8, whereas that number for TIPE2-deficient mice is 1.8 (**Figure 1F**). Similar phenotypical difference was also detected when EAU was induced in mice adoptively transferred with T cells from either WT or TIPE2-deficient mice (**Figure 1G**). Since both IMQ-induced psoriasis and EAU are T-cell mediated autoimmune disease animal model and our study has also established that TIPE2 in T cells regulates the pathogenesis of both psoriasis and EAU, in this study we focused on the roles

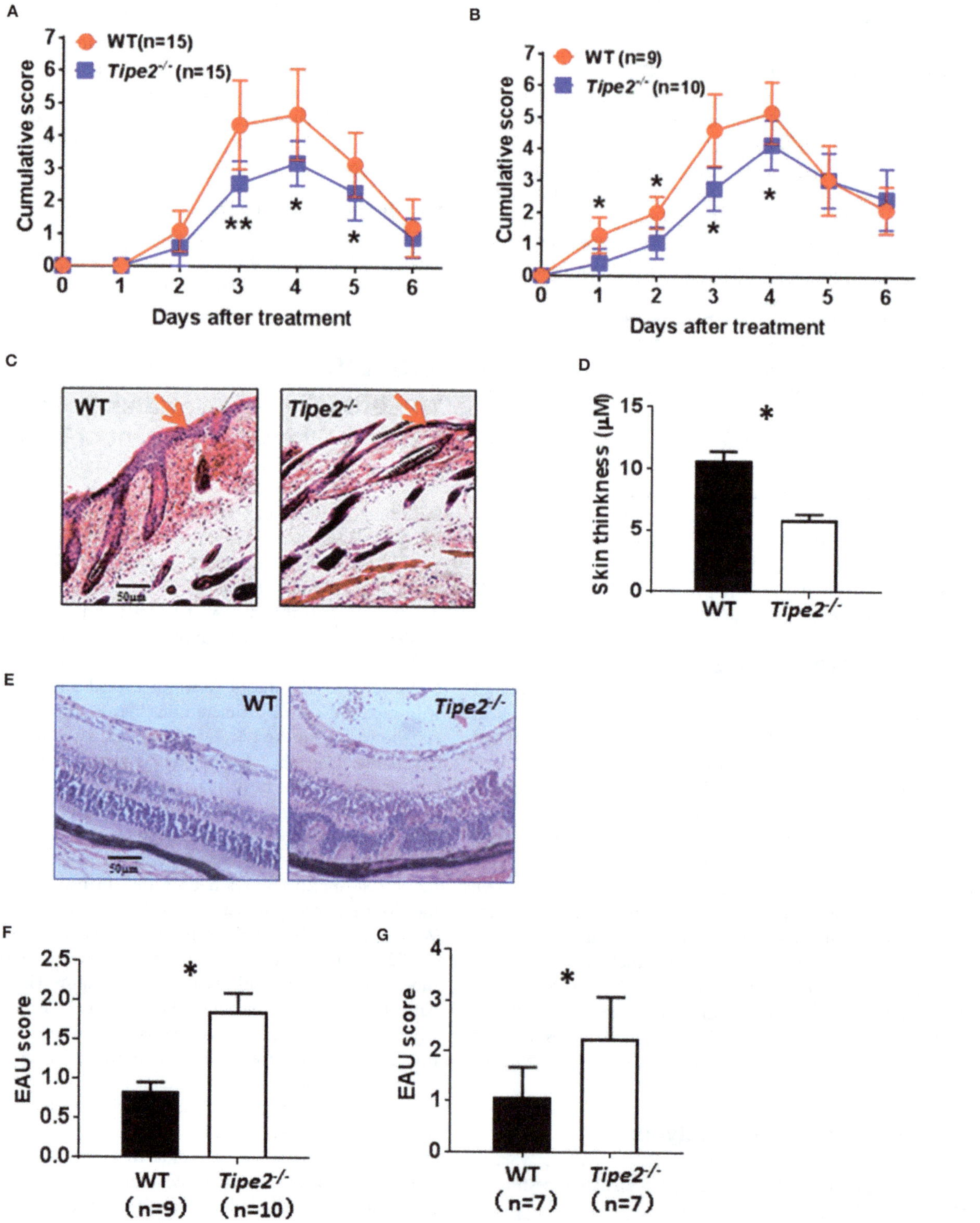

FIGURE 1 | TIPE2-deficiency alleviates psoriasis but promotes the development of EAU. **(A)** WT ($n = 15$) and TIPE2-deficient ($n = 15$) mice in the C57BL/6 background were treated with IMQ cream on the shaved back skin as mentioned in the Materials and Methods. Mice were monitored for the development of erythema and scaling on the back skin. The cumulative score (erythema plus scaling) is depicted. Data were combined from two separate experiments. **(B)** Total T cells were isolated from wild-type and TIPE2-deficient mice and adoptively transferred to *Rag1*$^{-/-}$ mice (10 × 10^6/mouse). IMQ cream was used to induce psoriasis as mentioned in the Materials and Methods. The cumulative score (erythema plus scaling) was calculated as mentioned in **(A)**. Data were

(Continued)

FIGURE 1 | combined from two separate experiments. **(C)** Mice from **(A)** were killed 6 days after the first IMQ treatment and H&E staining of the back skin of mice was performed. **(D)** Skin thickness was measured after H&E staining. **(E)** EAU was induced in WT ($n = 9$) and TIPE2-deficient ($n = 10$) mice as described in the Materials and Methods. Twenty-one days after immunization, H&E staining of the eye section was performed. Data were combined from two separate experiments. **(F)** Mice were treated as in **(E)** and EAU scores were determined on a scale of 0–4 based on the number, type, and size of lesions. **(G)** Total T cells were isolated from wild-type and TIPE2-deficient mice and adoptively transferred to *Rag1*$^{-/-}$ mice (10×10^6/mouse). EAU was induced as described in the Materials and Methods and characterized as in **(F)**. $^*P < 0.05$; $^{**}P < 0.01$.

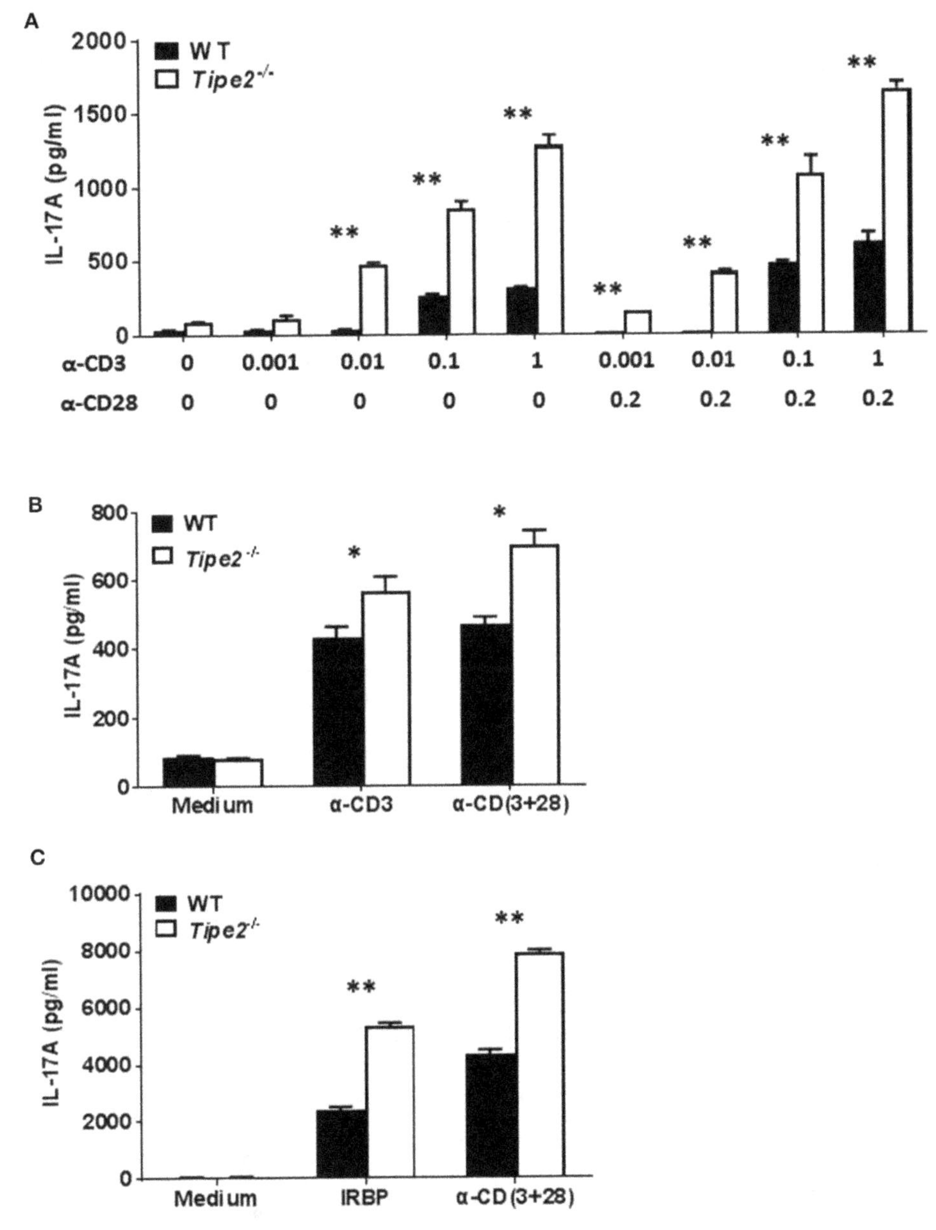

FIGURE 2 | TIPE2 suppresses IL-17A production by splenic T cells. **(A)** CD4$^+$ T cells were isolated from untreated WT ($n = 3$) and TIPE2-deficient mice ($n = 3$) and cultured with or without different concentrations (μg/ml) of plate-bound anti-CD3 plus soluble anti-CD28 as indicated. After 48 h, culture supernatants were collected and the concentration of IL-17A was determined by ELISA. Data are representative of three separate experiments. **(B)** WT ($n = 5$) and TIPE2-deficient ($n = 5$) mice were treated as in **Figure 1A** and killed 3 days after the first IMQ treatment. Total splenocytes were isolated and cultured at 1 million per well in 96-well plate with or without plate-bound anti-CD3 (0.5 μg/ml) or/and anti-CD28 (0.5 μg/ml). After 48 h, the concentration of IL-17A in the culture supernatants was determined by ELISA. Data are representative of two separate experiments. **(C)** EAU was induced in WT ($n = 4$) and TIPE2-deficient ($n = 5$) mice as in **Figure 1E** and killed 21 days following immunization. Total splenocytes were isolated and cultured at 1 million per well in 96-well plate with or without IRBP (30 μg/ml) or anti-CD3 (0.5 μg/ml) plus anti-CD28 mAb (0.5 μg/ml). After 48 h, the concentration of IL-17A in the culture supernatants was determined by ELISA. Data are representative of two separate experiments. $^*P < 0.05$; $^{**}P < 0.01$.

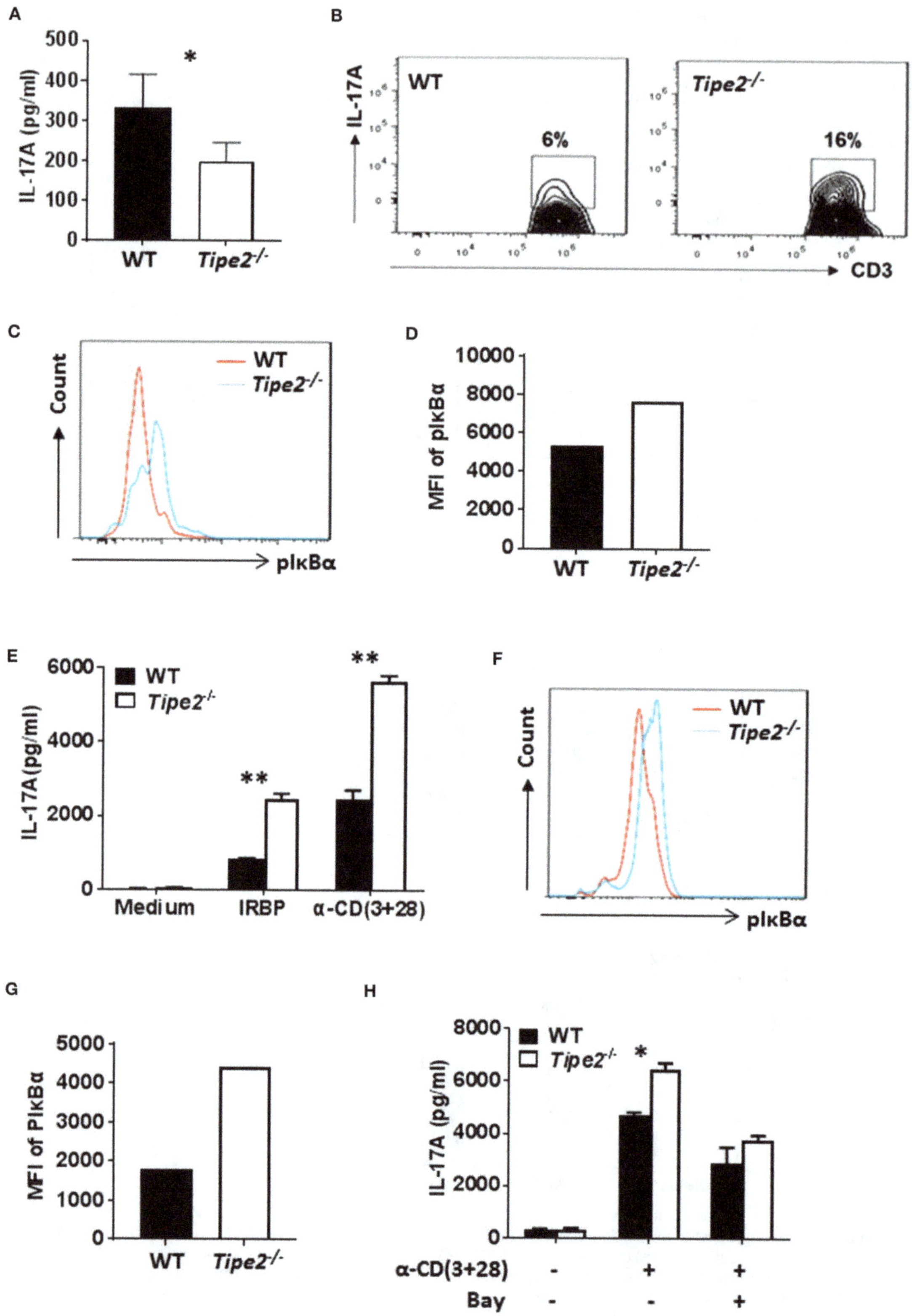

FIGURE 3 | The production of IL-17A is decreased in the skin but increased in the eye of TIPE2-deficient mice. **(A–D)** WT ($n = 5$) and TIPE2-deficient ($n = 5$) mice were treated as in **Figure 1A** and killed 3 days after the first IMQ treatment. **(A)** Tissue extracts were prepared from the back skin and the concentration of IL-17A in the tissue extract was determined by ELISA. **(B)** Total cells from the back skin were isolated and stimulated *in vitro* with PMA+ionomycin in the presence of GolgiStop

(Continued)

FIGURE 3 | for 6 h. Cells were first stained with anti-CD3, then fixed, permeabilized and stained with anti-IL-17A and examined by flow cytometry. Cells shown were gated on $CD3^+$ T cells. **(C)** Total cells from the back skin were isolated and stained with anti-CD3. After fixation and permeabilization, cells were then stained with anti-phospho-IκBα antibody, followed by staining with DyLight™ 488-conjugated goat anti-mouse IgG. Stained cells were then examined by flow cytometry. Cells shown were gated on $CD3^+$ T cells. **(D)** Relative expression level of phosphorylated IκBα was shown as the mean fluorescence intensity (MFI). **(E–H)** WT ($n = 4$) and TIPE2-deficient ($n = 5$) mice were treated as in **Figure 1E**. Mice were killed 21 days after the immunization and total cells were isolated from the eye. **(E)** Cells were cultured with or without IRBP (30 μg/ml) or anti-CD3 (0.5 μg/ml) plus anti-CD28 mAb (0.5 μg/ml). After 48 h, the concentration of IL-17A in the culture supernatants was determined by ELISA. **(F)** The level of phosphorylated IκBα was determined as in **(C)**. **(G)** Relative expression level of phosphorylated IκBα was shown as the mean fluorescence intensity (MFI). **(H)** Cells were cultured with or without plate-bound anti-CD3 (0.5 μg/ml) plus soluble anti-CD28 (0.5 μg/ml). In addition, NF-κB inhibitor BAY11-7082 (1 μM) was used to inhibit NF-κB activity as indicated. After 48 h, level of IL-17A in the supernatants was determined by ELISA. Data are representative of two separate experiments. $^*P < 0.05$; $^{**}P < 0.01$.

of TIPE2 in T cells in regular IMQ-induced psoriasis model and EAU model.

TIPE2 Suppresses the Production of IL-17A by T Cells

Both IMQ-induced psoriasis and EAU model contains a strong T cell component and the disease development is dependent on IL-17A. To determine the potential effect of TIPE2 deficiency on the production of IL-17A by T cells, we examined the expression of IL-17A produced by T cells *in vitro*. First we isolated $CD4^+$ T cells from the spleen of untreated WT and TIPE2-deficient mice and cultured them *in vitro* with or without different concentrations of plate-bound anti-CD3 and soluble anti-CD28. We found that TIPE2 deficient T cells produced significantly higher level of IL-17A (**Figure 2A**). Secondly, we isolated total splenocyte from IMQ-treated WT and TIPE2-deficient mice and cultured them *in vitro* with or without plate-bound anti-CD3 and/or soluble anti-CD28. We found that the expression of IL-17A was also significantly increased by TIPE2-deficient T cells (**Figure 2B**). Thirdly, we isolated total splenocyte from WT and TIPE2-deficient mice that have been treated to induce EAU. Cells were then cultured *in vitro* with or without IRBP or anti-CD3 plus anti-CD28. Again we found that TIPE2-deficient T cells produced significantly more IL-17A (**Figure 2C**). Taking together, these results indicate that TIPE2 is a negative regulator of IL-17A expression in T cells.

The Production of IL-17A Is Decreased in the Skin but Increased in the Eye of TIPE2-Deficient Mice

To investigate whether TIPE2 deficiency alters IL-17A production in the inflamed skin, tissue extracts were prepared from the skin of IMQ-treated WT and TIPE2-deficient mice and the production of IL-17A was measured by ELISA. We found that the production of IL-17A was significantly decreased in the skin from TIPE2-deficient mice (**Figure 3A**). This result is in consistency with the phenotype that TIPE2-deficiency alleviates IMQ-induced psoriasis. However, when flow cytometry was used to examine the percentage of IL-17-producing cells within gated $CD3^+$ T cells, we found that the percentage of IL-17A-producing cells was much higher in TIPE2-deficient mice (**Figure 3B**). In addition, we also found that the phosphorylation of Iκbα was significantly increased in TIPE2-deficient T cells (**Figures 3C,D**). Similar experiments were performed with the cells isolated from the inflamed eye of WT and TIPE2-deficient mice that have been treated to induce EAU. In consistency with the phenotype that TIPE2-deficiency promotes the development of EAU, the production of IL-17A (**Figure 3E**) and the phosphorylation of Iκbα (**Figures 3F,G**) was significantly increased by TIPE2-deficient T cells. In addition, we also found that WT and TIPE2-deficient T cells no longer displayed difference in IL-17A expression after treatment with NF-κB inhibitor BAY11-7082 (**Figure 3H**). Taking together, these results indicate that TIPE2 may suppress IL-17A production by T cells through the inhibition of NF-κB activation.

The Percentage of T Cells in TIPE2-Deficient Mice Is Decreased in the Skin but Comparable in the Eye Compared With That in WT Mice

Although TIPE2-deficient T cells produced more IL-17A, TIPE2-deficient mice produced much less IL-17A in the skin and displayed reduced severity of IMQ-induced psoriasis. To solve this paradox, we examined the percentage and absolute number of T cells in IMQ-treated WT and TIPE2-deficient mice. The results showed that, while the percentage (**Figure 4A**) and absolute number (**Figure 4B**) of $CD3^+$ T cells were significantly increased in the blood from TIPE2-deficient mice, they were significantly decreased in the skin. The percentage and absolute number of $CD3^+$ T cells were comparable in the draining lymph node (inguinal lymph node, ILN) between WT and TIPE2-deficient mice (**Figures 4A,B**). Because we have shown that TIPE2 suppresses IL-17A production by T cells during the development of IMQ-induced psoriasis (**Figure 2B**), the percentage (**Figure 4C**) and absolute number (**Figure 4D**) of $CD3^+IL\text{-}17A^+$ T cells was significantly increased in the blood and ILN as expected. However, the percentage and absolute number of $CD3^+IL\text{-}17A^+$ T cells was significantly decreased in the skin (**Figures 4C,D**). We think that this is due to the decreased percentage and number of $CD3^+$ T cells found in the skin from TIPE2-deficient mice, despite the fact that the proportion of IL-17-producing cells within gated $CD3^+$ T cells was much higher in the skin from TIPE2-deficient mice (**Figure 3B**). This may also explain why the net production of IL-17A was significantly decreased in the skin from TIPE2-deficient mice (**Figure 3A**). As for the EAU model, no significant difference was found in the inflamed eye as well as in the blood and draining lymph node (cervical lymph node, CLN) between WT and TIPE2-deficient mice in the percentage and absolute

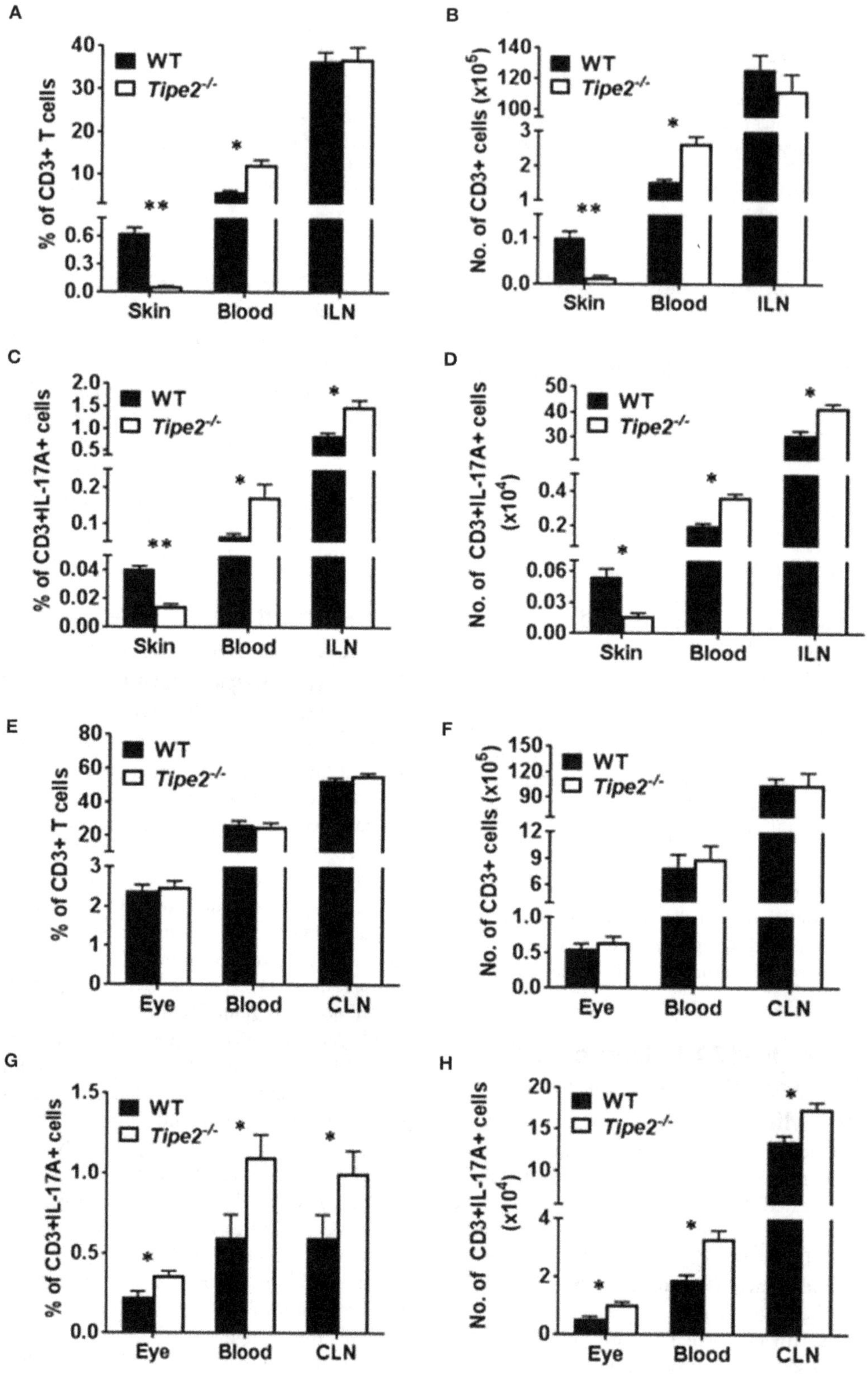

FIGURE 4 | Comparison of the percentage and absolute number of $CD3^+$ and $CD3^+IL\text{-}17A^+$ T cells in WT and TIPE2-deficient mice. **(A–D)** WT ($n = 5$) and TIPE2-deficient ($n = 5$) mice were treated as in **Figure 1A** and killed 3 days after the first IMQ treatment. The percentage **(A)** and absolute number **(B)** of $CD3^+$ T cells in the skin (0.8 cm^2), blood (0.6 ml) and ILN were determined by cell surface staining with fluorescent labeled antibody against CD3. The percentage **(C)** and number

(Continued)

FIGURE 4 | (D) of CD3$^+$IL-17A$^+$ T cells in the skin (0.8 cm^2), blood (0.6 ml) and ILN was determined by cell surface staining as described above followed by intracellular staining with fluorescent labeled antibody against IL-17A. **(E–H)** WT ($n = 6$) and TIPE2-deficient ($n = 7$) mice were treated as in **Figure 1E**. Mice were killed 21 days after the immunization and the percentage and number of CD3$^+$ **(E,F)** and CD3$^+$IL-17A$^+$ T cells **(G,H)** in the eye (one eye), blood (0.6 ml) and CLN were determined as described above. ILN, inguinal lymph node; CLN, cervical lymph node. $^*P < 0.05$; $^{**}P < 0.01$.

number of CD3$^+$ T cells (**Figures 4E,F**). However, because we have shown that TIPE2 suppresses IL-17A production by T cells during the development of EAU (**Figure 2C**), the percentage and absolute number of CD3$^+$IL-17A$^+$ T cells was significantly increased in the eye as well as in the blood and CLN from TIPE2-deficient mice (**Figures 4G,H**). Taken together, these results indicate that, although TIPE2-deficient T cells produced more IL-17A in both disease models, they are defective in migration to the skin in IMQ-induced psoriasis model but not to the eye in EAU model. Next we focused on the roles of TIPE2 in regulating T cell migration during the development of IMQ-induced psoriasis.

T Cells From IMQ-Treated TIPE2-Deficient Mice Express Normal Levels of Chemokine Receptors but Are Defective in Chemotaxis *in vitro*

During the development of psoriasis, mature activated T cells migrate through the postcapillary venules into the dermis after establishing molecular interactions mediated by tissue selective integrins and chemokine receptors (homing receptors). To determine how TIPE2 affects T cell migration during the development of psoriasis, we examined the expression of multiple chemokine receptors on the surface of CD3$^+$ T cells from the ILN and blood of IMQ-treated WT and TIPE2-deficient mice. Our results showed that the there is no significant difference in the expression of CXCR3, CXCR4, CCR4, CCR5, CCR6, CCR7, and CCR9 between IMQ-treated WT and TIPE2-deficient mice (**Figures 5A,B**). However, *in vitro* chemotaxis assay showed that TIPE2-deficient T cells from ILN were defective in migration toward IP10 and CCL19 (**Figure 5C**), which are the ligand for CCR7 and CXCR3, respectively. Similar results were found with the cells from the blood of IMQ-treated mice (**Figure 5D**). In order to exclude the possibility that decreased local chemokine production led to the defective migration of TIPE2-deficient T cells to the skin, we also examined the expression of multiple chemokines in the skin. Our results revealed that the mRNA expression of most of the chemokines was not decreased but even increased in the skin from TIPE2-deficient mice (**Figure 5E**). Because most of those chemokines were direct targets of NF-κB, it is possible that TIPE2 suppresses the production of chemokine in the skin through the inhibition of NF-κB activity.

T Cells From IMQ-Treated TIPE2-Deficient Mice Are Defective in Leading-Edge Formation During Chemotaxis

Previous studies have shown that TIPE2 promotes leading-edge formation in neutrophils through enhancing phosphoinositide-dependent signaling and cytoskeleton remodeling. Therefore, we examined the polarization of F-action and phosphor-AKT (T308) in CD3$^+$ T cells isolated from the ILN of IMQ-treated WT and TIPE2-deficient mice in response to point-source stimulation with IP10. Our results demonstrated that, although the distribution of F-actin and phosphor-AKT was aggregated on the surface of both WT and TIPE2-deficient T cells, more TIPE2-deficient T cells were not polarized (**Figures 6A,B**). Interestingly, the total amount of F-actin and phosphor-AKT were increased in TIPE2-deficient T cells (**Figure 6C**). Taking together, these results indicate that, although TIPE2 suppresses the expression of F-actin and phosphor-AKT, it promotes the leading-edge formation during chemotaxis and consequently enhances T cell directional migration.

DISCUSSION

Although it has been reported that TIPE2 is a negative immune regulator, the exact role of TIPE2 during the development of autoimmune disease remains elusive. Contradictory results have been reported when investigating the role of TIPE2 during the development of different types of autoimmune diseases. Using IMQ-induced psoriasis model and EAU model, our current study revealed that TIPE2 may either promote or suppress autoimmunity, depending on the specific inflammatory microenvironment in different types of autoimmune diseases.

Since TIPE2 functions as a negative regulator of adaptive immune response, we speculate that TIPE2-deficient mice will be more susceptible to developing psoriasis and EAU. However, our current study showed that, while TIPE2-deficient mice develop more severe EAU, they unexpectedly develop less severe IMQ-induced psoriasis. In 2017, Fayngerts et al. reported that TIPE2 functioned as a local enhancer of cytoskeleton remodeling and promoted leading-edge formation in neutrophils (20). Our previous work also showed that TIPE2 enhances the cytoskeleton remodeling and promotes the thymus egress of tTregs (28). In the current study we further confirmed that TIPE2 may promote T cell migration via the same mechanism in the psoriasis model. This would explain why TIPE2-deficient mice develop less severe IMQ-induced psoriasis. We speculate that TIPE2 may play both anti-inflammatory and pro-inflammatory roles during the development of autoimmune diseases. Although T cells produced more IL-17A in both psoriasis and EAU model, they were defective in migration to the skin but not to the inflamed eye. The final outcome depends on the balance between these two opposing effects. This theory may also explain why the IMQ-induced skin inflammation of TIPE2-deficient mice is only marginally reduced compared with that of WT mice.

However, it still remains a question why TIPE2-deficient T cells were defective in migration to the site of inflammation in one particular autoimmune disease but not in another? After priming in the draining lymph node, mature activated

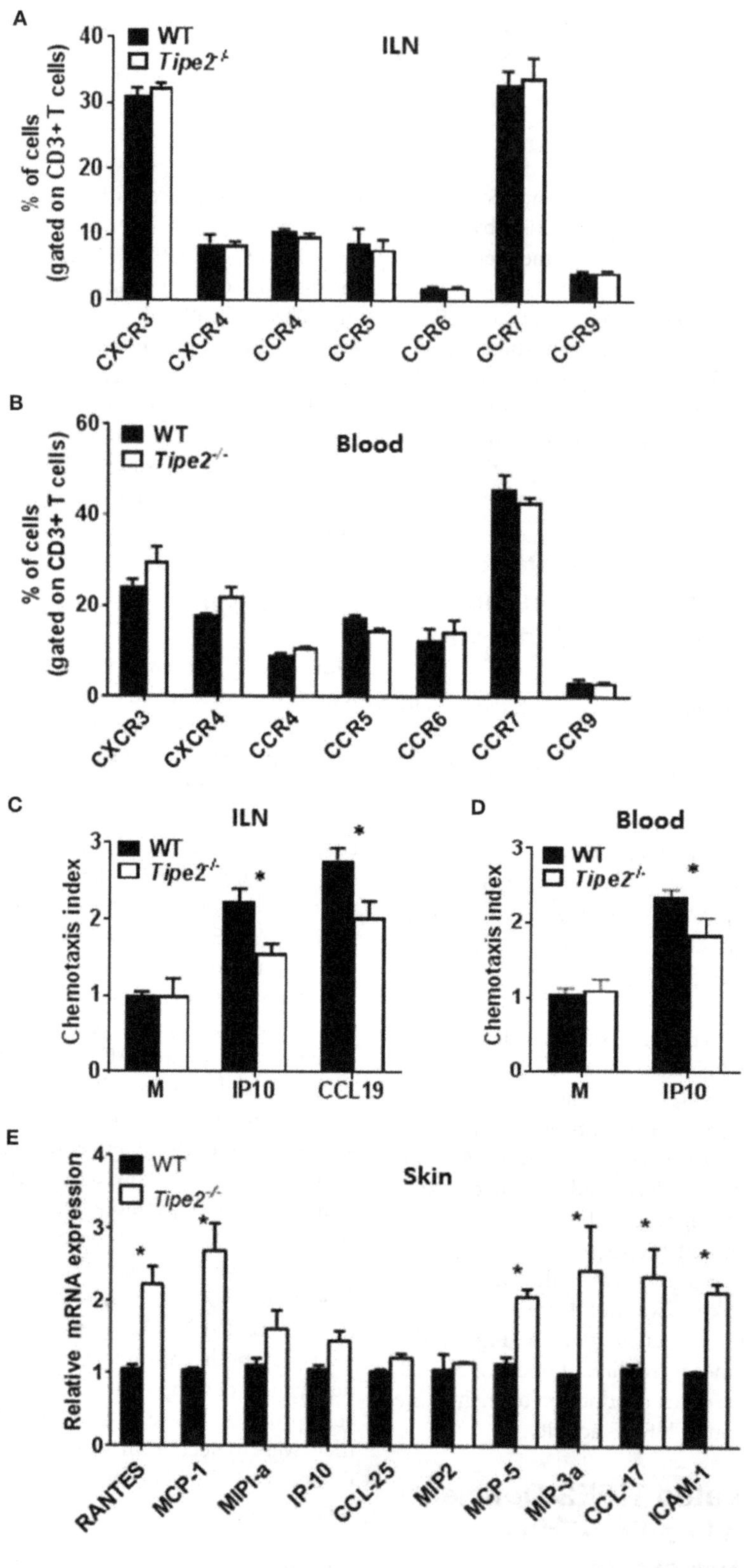

FIGURE 5 | T cells from TIPE2-deficient mice express normal levels of chemokine receptors but are defective in chemotaxis *in vitro*. WT (n = 5) and TIPE2-deficient (n = 5) mice were treated as in **Figure 1A** and killed 3 days after the first IMQ treatment. **(A)** Total cells were isolated from ILN and the expression of indicated chemokine receptors on the surface of CD3$^+$ T cells was determined by cell surface staining with florescence-labeled antibodies against CD3 and chemokine receptors. Data

(Continued)

FIGURE 5 | shown are for gated $CD3^+$ T cells. **(B)** Lymphocytes were isolated from blood and the expression of indicated chemokine receptors on the surface of $CD3^+$ T cells was determined as in **(A)**. Data shown are for gated $CD3^+$ T cells. **(C,D)** Total T cells were isolated from ILN **(C)** and blood lymphocyte **(D)**. *in vitro* transwell assay was performed to determine the migratory capacity of T cells toward IP10 and CCL19, which are the ligand for CXCR3 and CCR7, respectively. The chemotaxis index was calculated as mentioned in the Materials and Methods. **(E)** Total RNA was extracted from the back skin, and the mRNA expression of indicated chemokines was determined by quantitative RT-PCR. Data are representative of two separate experiments. ILN: inguinal lymph node. $^*P < 0.05$.

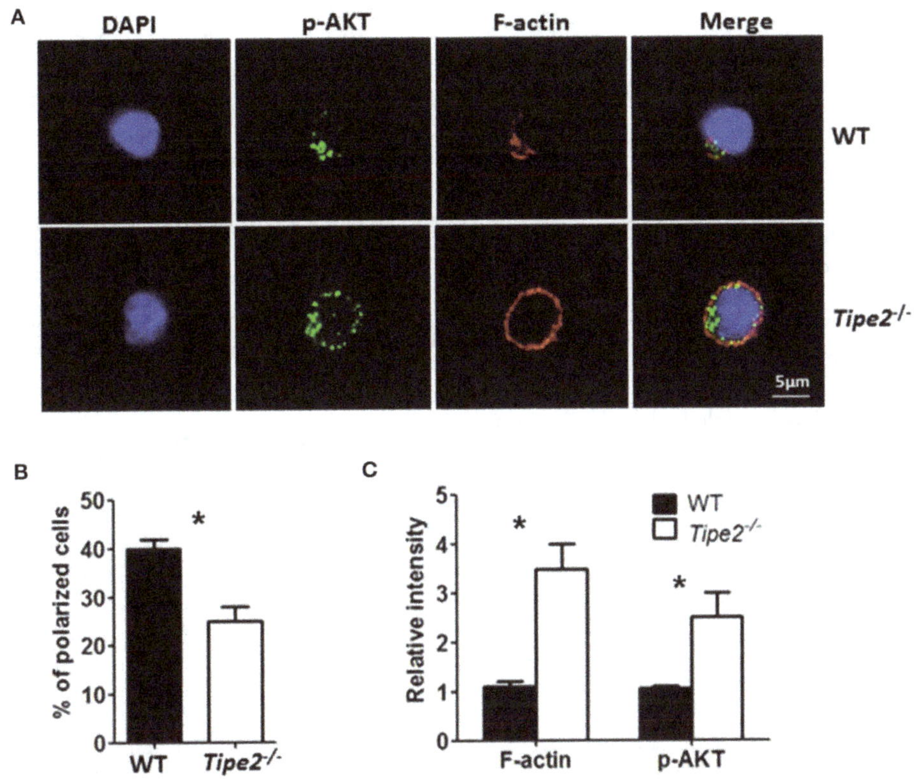

FIGURE 6 | TIPE2-deficient T cells are defective in leading-edge formation during chemotaxis. WT ($n = 5$) and TIPE2-deficient ($n = 5$) mice were treated as in **Figure 1A** and killed 3 days after the first IMQ treatment. Total T cells were isolated from inguinal lymph node and then subjected to point-source stimulation with IP10 at 1 μg/ml for 3 min at 37°C and stained with Phalloidin, anti-phospho-AKT antibody and DNA-binding dye DAPI. **(A)** The distributions of F-actin, phospho-AKT and DAPI in WT and TIPE2-deficient T cells were assessed by confocal microscopy. Data are representative of two separate experiments. **(B)** The percentages of polarized WT and TIPE2-deficient T cells were calculated. **(C)** The total intensity of F-actin and p-AKT was calculated using ImageJ. For **(B,C)**, data are pooled results from two separate experiments with more than 50 cells analyzed per genotype. $^*P < 0.05$.

Ag-specific T cells migrate through the postcapillary venules into local inflammatory site through a chemotaxis-dependent manner (29). Alternatively, primed T cells may also traffick to local inflammatory site through random migration. For example, random migration contributes to cytotoxicity of activated $CD8^+$ T-cells and may be used as a biomarker to predict the effect of immunotherapy using activated lymphocytes (30). Thus, depending on the specific inflammatory microenviroment in different types of autoimmune disease, TIPE2-deficiency may or may not affect the accumulation of T cells in the local inflammatory site. In EAU model, because pro-inflammatory leads to the breakdown of RBB (Retinal-Blood-Barrier), the majority of T cells that accumulated in the flamed eye may migrate in a chemotaxis-independent manner. The total amount of F-actin was increased in TIPE2-deficient T cells further indicates that TIPE2 in T cells may suppress non-directional cell movement.

While EAU in animals was used as a model of human uveitis, treating mice with innate TLR7/8 ligand IMQ rapidly induces dermatitis closely resembling human psoriasis. They are both T-cell mediated autoimmune diseases animal model, because only T cells can adoptively transfer those diseases (11, 14). Studies in these two disease models demonstrated that Th17 rather than Th1 cells play a critical role during their pathogenesis (10, 11). Because IL-17A is the primary Th17 cell effector cytokine, disease development was almost completely blocked in mice deficient for IL-17A or IL-17 receptor (31, 32). *In vivo* neutralization of IL-17A is able to ameliorate EAU and IMQ-induced psoriasis (12–14). While nuclear hormone receptor RORγT is a master regulator of the differentiation of IL-17-producing T cells (33), other factors such as STAT3 and NF-κB have also been shown to regulate the expression of IL-17A (34, 35). TIPE2 negatively regulates immune response through inhibiting the activity of NF-κB in T cells (36). Our results also showed that the level of phosphorylated IκBα was markedly up-regulated in TIPE2-deficient T cells derived from the inflamed eye and skin. Furthermore, we showed that WT and TIPE2-deficient T cells no longer displayed difference in IL-17A expression after treatment with NF-κB inhibitor. These results suggest that TIPE2 may inhibit the expression of IL-17A in T cells by suppressing NF-κB activity.

In addition to Th17 cells, IL-17A is also produced by a variety of cell types from the innate and adaptive immune systems (37, 38). Other types of T cells such as CD8 T cells, NKT cells and Gamma delta (γδ) T cells are also significant potential sources of IL-17A (38–40). In our current study, we didn't distinguish the T cell types in which TIPE2 inhibits the expression of IL-17A. While one group reported that Th17 cells are the major source of IL-17A in psoriatic dermis (41), others showed that the majority of IL-17A in the skin was produced by IL-23-responsive dermal γδ T cells (40, 42). Thus, future study is needed to determine the role of TIPE2 on IL-17A production in different IL-17A-producing T cells.

In summary, our study has revealed that TIPE2 can function as both a negative and positive regulator of autoimmunity. On one hand, TIPE2 could suppress inflammatory response through the inhibition of IL-17A production by T cells. On the other hand, TIPE2 could promote inflammatory response through enhancing the directional migration of T cells. The final outcome may depend on the balance of TIPE2 mediated anti-inflammatory and pro-inflammatory effects.

ETHICS STATEMENT

This study was carried out in accordance with the recommendations of the Animal Care and Use Committee of Shenzhen Institutes of Advanced Technology, Chinese Academy of Sciences. The protocol was approved by Shenzhen Institutes of Advanced Technology, Chinese Academy of Sciences.

AUTHOR CONTRIBUTIONS

QR and TW designed research and analyzed data. RL, XH, and WG performed research. QR wrote the manuscript.

ACKNOWLEDGMENTS

The authors thank Dr. Suxia Liu from Shangdong University, P. R. China for kindly providing the TIPE2 deficient mice.

REFERENCES

1. Nomura I, Gao B, Boguniewicz M, Darst MA, Travers JB, Leung DY. Distinct patterns of gene expression in the skin lesions of atopic dermatitis and psoriasis: a gene microarray analysis. *J Allergy Clin Immunol.* (2003) 112:1195–202. doi: 10.1016/j.jaci.2003.08.049
2. Harden JL, Krueger JG, Bowcock AM. The immunogenetics of psoriasis: a comprehensive review. *J Autoimmun.* (2015) 64:66–73. doi: 10.1016/j.jaut.2015.07.008
3. Ausubel FM. *Short Protocols in Molecular Biology: A Compendium of Methods From Current Protocols In Molecular Biology.* New York, NY: Greene Pub. Associates; Wiley-Interscience (1989)
4. Fierlbeck G, Rassner G. Treatment of psoriasis and psoriatic arthritis with interferon gamma. *J Invest Dermatol.* (1990) 95(6 Suppl):138s–41s. doi: 10.1111/1523-1747.ep12875040
5. Mee JB, Cork MJ, di Giovine FS, Duff GW, Groves RW. Interleukin-1: a key inflammatory mediator in psoriasis? *Cytokine.* (2006) 33:72–8. doi: 10.1016/j.cyto.2005.12.001
6. Stenderup K, Rosada C, Worsaae A, Dagnaes-Hansen F, Steiniche T, Hasselager E, et al. Interleukin-20 plays a critical role in maintenance and development of psoriasis in the human xenograft transplantation model. *Br J Dermatol.* (2009) 160:284–96. doi: 10.1111/j.1365-2133.2008.08890.x
7. Tonel G, Conrad C. Interplay between keratinocytes and immune cells–recent insights into psoriasis pathogenesis. *Int J Biochem Cell Biol.* (2009) 41:963–8. doi: 10.1016/j.biocel.2008.10.022
8. Ali FR, Warren RB. Psoriasis and susceptibility to other autoimmune diseases: an outline for the clinician. *Expert Rev Clin Immunol.* (2013) 9:99–101. doi: 10.1586/eci.12.94
9. Walsh SR, Shear NH. Psoriasis and the new biologic agents: interrupting a T-AP dance. *CMAJ.* (2004) 170:1933–41. doi: 10.1503/cmaj.1031335
10. Luger D, Silver PB, Tang J, Cua D, Chen Z, Iwakura Y, et al. Either a Th17 or a Th1 effector response can drive autoimmunity: conditions of disease induction affect dominant effector category. *J Exp Med.* (2008) 205:799–810. doi: 10.1084/jem.20071258
11. Raychaudhuri SP. Role of IL-17 in psoriasis and psoriatic arthritis. *Clin Rev Allergy Immunol.* (2013) 44:183–93. doi: 10.1007/s12016-012-8307-1
12. Zou W, Wu Z, Xiang X, Sun S, Zhang J. The expression and significance of T helper cell subsets and regulatory T cells CD(4)(+) CD(2)(5)(+) in peripheral blood of patients with human leukocyte antigen B27-positive acute anterior uveitis. *Graefes Arch Clin Exp Ophthalmol.* (2014) 252:665–72. doi: 10.1007/s00417-014-2567-9
13. Giuliari GP, Sadaka A, Hinkle DM. Biologic agents in experimental autoimmune uveitis. *Int Ophthalmol.* (2014) 34:145–56. doi: 10.1007/s10792-013-9756-0
14. Martin DA, Towne JE, Kricorian G, Klekotka P, Gudjonsson JE, Krueger JG, et al. The emerging role of IL-17 in the pathogenesis of psoriasis: preclinical and clinical findings. *J Invest Dermatol.* (2013) 133:17–26. doi: 10.1038/jid.2012.194
15. Sun H, Gong S, Carmody RJ, Hilliard A, Li L, Sun J, et al. TIPE2, a negative regulator of innate and adaptive immunity that maintains immune homeostasis. *Cell.* (2008) 133:415–26. doi: 10.1016/j.cell.2008.03.026
16. Li D, Song L, Fan Y, Li X, Li Y, Chen J, et al. Down-regulation of TIPE2 mRNA expression in peripheral blood mononuclear cells from patients with systemic lupus erythematosus. *Clin Immunol.* (2009) 133:422–7. doi: 10.1016/j.clim.2009.08.014
17. Li F, Zhu X, Yang Y, Huang L, Xu J. TIPE2 alleviates systemic lupus erythematosus through regulating macrophage polarization. *Cell Physiol Biochem.* (2016) 38:330–9. doi: 10.1159/000438633
18. Shi GS, et al. The expression of TIPE2 in patients with rheumatoid arthritis and its effect to NF-κB pathway. *China J Modern Med.* (2014) doi: 10.3969/j.issn.1005-8982.2014.04.008
19. Lou Y, Sun H, Morrissey S, Porturas T, Liu S, Hua X, et al. Critical roles of TIPE2 protein in murine experimental colitis. *J Immunol.* (2014) 193:1064–70. doi: 10.4049/jimmunol.1400415

20. Fayngerts SA, Wang Z, Zamani A, Sun H, Boggs AE, Porturas TP, et al. Direction of leukocyte polarization and migration by the phosphoinositide-transfer protein TIPE2. *Nat Immunol.* (2017) 18:ni.3866. doi: 10.1038/ni.3866
21. Fan T, Wang S, Yu L, Yi H, Liu R, Geng W, et al. Treating psoriasis by targeting its susceptibility gene Rel. *Clin Immunol.* (2016) 165:47–54. doi: 10.1016/j.clim.2016.03.009
22. van de Kerkhof PC. The Psoriasis Area and Severity Index and alternative approaches for the assessment of severity: persisting areas of confusion. *Br J Dermatol.* (1997) 137:661–2. doi: 10.1111/j.1365-2133.1997.tb03819.x
23. Bae SH, Yun SJ, Lee JB, Kim SJ, Won YH, Lee SC. Algorithm to select optimal systemic anti-psoriatic drugs in relation with patients' Psoriasis Area and Severity Index score for plaque psoriasis. *J Dermatol.* (2016) 43:643–9. doi: 10.1111/1346-8138.13195
24. Grajewski RS, Silver PB, Agarwal RK, Su SB, Chan CC, Liou GI, et al. Endogenous IRBP can be dispensable for generation of natural $CD4^+CD25^+$ regulatory T cells that protect from IRBP-induced retinal autoimmunity. *J Exp Med.* (2006) 203:851–6. doi: 10.1084/jem.20050429
25. Chan CC, Caspi RR, Ni M, Leake WC, Wiggert B, Chader GJ, et al. Pathology of experimental autoimmune uveoretinitis in mice. *J Autoimmun.* (1990) 3:247–55. doi: 10.1016/0896-8411(90)90144-H
26. Fischer FR, Santambrogio L, Luo Y, Berman MA, Hancock WW, Dorf ME. Modulation of experimental autoimmune encephalomyelitis: effect of altered peptide ligand on chemokine and chemokine receptor expression. *J Neuroimmunol.* (2000) 110:195–208. doi: 10.1016/S0165-5728(00)00351-9
27. Xiaomei L. Interleukin-17 (IL-17)-induced microRNA 873 (miR-873) contributes to the pathogenesis of experimental autoimmune encephalomyelitis by targeting A20 ubiquitin-editing enzyme. *J Biol Chem.* (2014) 289:28971–86. doi: 10.1074/jbc.M114.577429
28. Fan T, Huang X, Liu C, Liu R, Wang T, Ruan Q. Egress of murine regulatory T cells from the thymus requires TIPE2. *Biochem Biophys Res Commun.* (2018) 500:376–83. doi: 10.1016/j.bbrc.2018.04.082
29. Masopust D, Schenkel JM. The integration of T cell migration, differentiation and function. *Nat Rev Immunol.* (2013) 13:309–20. doi: 10.1038/nri3442
30. Onishi H, Kiyota A, Koya N, Tanaka H, Umebayashi M, Katano M, et al. Random migration contributes to cytotoxicity of activated $CD8^+$ T-lymphocytes but not NK cells. *Anticancer Res.* (2014) 34:3947–56.
31. Nakajima K, Kanda T, Takaishi M, Shiga T, Miyoshi K, Nakajima H, et al. Distinct roles of IL-23 and IL-17 in the development of psoriasis-like lesions in a mouse model. *J Immunol.* (2011) 186:4481–9. doi: 10.4049/jimmunol.1000148
32. van der Fits L, Mourits S, Voerman JS, Kant M, Boon L, Laman JD, et al. Imiquimod-induced psoriasis-like skin inflammation in miceis mediated via the IL-23/IL-17 axis. *J Immunol.* (2009) 182:5836–45. doi: 10.4049/jimmunol.0802999
33. Ivanov II, McKenzie BS, Zhou L, Tadokoro CE, Lepelley A, Lafaille JJ, et al. The orphan nuclear receptor RORgammat directs the differentiation program of proinflammatory $IL\text{-}17^+$ T helper cells. *Cell.* (2006) 126:1121–33. doi: 10.1016/j.cell.2006.07.035
34. Kim KW, Cho ML, Park MK, Yoon CH, Park SH, Lee SH, et al. Increased interleukin-17 production via a phosphoinositide 3-kinase/Akt and nuclear factor kappaB-dependent pathway in patients with rheumatoid arthritis. *Arthritis Res Ther.* (2005) 7:R139–48. doi: 10.1186/ar1470
35. Rubino SJ, Geddes K, Girardin SE. Innate IL-17 and IL-22 responses to enteric bacterial pathogens. *Trends Immunol.* (2012) 33:112–8. doi: 10.1016/j.it.2012.01.003
36. Shi C, Zhang S, Hong S, Pang J, Yesibulati Y, Yin P, et al. The pro-apoptotic effects of TIPE2 on AA rat fibroblast-like synoviocytes via regulation of the DR5–caspase–NF-κB pathway *in vitro*. *Oncotargets Therapy.* (2016) 9:993–1000. doi: 10.2147/OTT.S92907
37. Albanesi C, Scarponi C, Cavani A, Federici M, Nasorri F, Girolomoni G. Interleukin-17 is produced by both Th1 and Th2 lymphocytes, and modulates interferon-gamma- and interleukin-4-induced activation of human keratinocytes. *J Invest Dermatol.* (2000) 115:81–7. doi: 10.1046/j.1523-1747.2000.00041.x
38. Monteiro M, Almeida CF, Agua-Doce A, Graca L. Induced IL-17-producing invariant NKT cells require activation in presence of TGF-beta and IL-1beta. *J Immunol.* (2013) 190:805–11. doi: 10.4049/jimmunol.1201010
39. Ortega C, Fernández-AS, Carrillo JM, Romero P, Molina IJ, Moreno JC, et al. IL-17-producing $CD8^+$ T lymphocytes from psoriasis skin plaques are cytotoxic effector cells that secrete Th17-related cytokines. *J Leukoc Biol.* (2009) 86:435–43. doi: 10.1189/JLB.0109046
40. Cai Y, Shen X, Ding C, Qi C, Li K, Li X, et al. Pivotal role of dermal IL-17-producing gammadelta T cells in skin inflammation. *Immunity.* (2011) 35:596–610. doi: 10.1016/j.immuni.2011.08.001
41. Lynde CW, Poulin Y, Vender R, Bourcier M, Khalil S. Interleukin 17A: toward a new understanding of psoriasis pathogenesis. *J Am Acad Dermatol.* (2014) 71:141–50. doi: 10.1016/j.jaad.2013.12.036
42. Ramirez-Valle F, Gray EE, Cyster JG. Inflammation induces dermal Vgamma4+ gammadeltaT17 memory-like cells that travel to distant skin and accelerate secondary IL-17-driven responses. *Proc Natl Acad Sci USA.* (2015) 112:8046–51. doi: 10.1073/pnas.1508990112

7

High-Dose Intravenous Immunoglobulin in Skin Autoimmune Disease

Jochen H. O. Hoffmann and Alexander H. Enk*

Department of Dermatology, University of Heidelberg, Heidelberg, Germany

Correspondence:
Jochen H. O. Hoffmann
jochen.hoffmann@
med.uni-heidelberg.de

The immunomodulatory potential and low incidence of severe side effects of high-dose intravenous immunoglobulin (IVIg) treatment led to its successful application in a variety of dermatological autoimmune diseases over the last two decades. IVIg is usually administered at a dose of 2 g per kg body weight distributed over 2–5 days every 4 weeks. They are most commonly used as a second- or third-line treatment in dermatological autoimmune disease (pemphigus vulgaris, pemphigus foliaceus, bullous pemphigoid, mucous membrane pemphigoid, epidermolysis bullosa acquisita, dermatomyositis, systemic vasculitis, and systemic lupus erythematosus). However, first-line treatment may be warranted in special circumstances like concomitant malignancy, a foudroyant clinical course, and contraindications against alternative treatments. Furthermore, IVIg can be considered first line in scleromyxedema. Production of IVIg for medical use is strictly regulated to ensure a low risk of pathogen transmission and comparable quality of individual batches. More common side effects include nausea, headache, fatigue, and febrile infusion reactions. Serious side effects are rare and include thrombosis and embolism, pulmonary edema, renal failure, aseptic meningitis, and severe anaphylactic reactions. Regarding the mechanism of action, one can discriminate between functions of the Fcγ region and the F(ab)2 region and their effects on a cellular level. These functions are not mutually exclusive, and more than one pathway may contribute to the beneficial effects. Here, we present a historical background, details on manufacturing, hypotheses on the mechanisms of action, information on the clinical application in the abovementioned conditions, and a brief outlook on future directions of IVIg treatment in dermatology.

Keywords: scleromyxedema, vasculitis, IVIg, bullous pemhigoid, pemphigus vulgaris, epidermolysis bullosa acquisita, systemic lupus erythematosus, dermatomyositis

INTRODUCTION

The immunomodulatory potential and low incidence of severe side effects of high-dose intravenous immunoglobulin (IVIg) treatment led to its successful application in a variety of dermatological autoimmune diseases over the last two decades. From a historical perspective, the first well-documented proof-of-concept medical application of IVIg in an autoimmune disease dates back to 1981, when Imbach et al. (1) successfully treated a child with immune thrombocytopenia (ITP, formerly idiopathic thrombocytopenic purpura), a humoral and cellular autoimmune reaction

TABLE 1 | Selection of autoimmune diseases with prominent cutaneous involvement successfully treated with IVIg and common treatment regimes.

Disease entity	Common treatment regimes*
Autoimmune bullous dermatoses	
-Pemphigus vulgaris, Pemphigus foliaceus	2 g/kg bw over 2–5 days q4w
-Bullous pemphigoid	"
-Epidermolysis bullosa acquisita	"
-Mucous membrane pemphigoid	"
Collagen vascular diseases	
-Systemic lupus erythematosus	0.4–2 g/kg bw over 2–5 days q4w
Inflammatory myositides	
-Dermatomyositis	2 g/kg bw over 2–5 days q4w
Systemic vasculitides	
-ANCA-associated vasculitis	2 g/kg bw over 2–5 days q4w
-Kawasaki disease	2 g/kg bw over 12 h
Scleromyxedema	2 g/kg bw over 2–5 days q4w

*q4w, every 4 weeks; bw, body weight; IVIg, intravenous immunoglobulin. *IVIg is mostly given as an adjuvant treatment.*

against thrombocytes and megakaryocytes that results in skin purpura and organ hemorrhage. Only a few years later, Furusho et al. (2) and Newburger et al. (3) reported the successful application of IVIg in Kawasaki disease, an acute, highly febrile necrotizing systemic vasculitis that mainly affects young children, often manifests with a mucocutaneous rash and unilateral cervical lymphadenopathy, and can be complicated by potentially fatal cardiovascular involvement. Even though, to date, no randomized clinical trial exists, IVIg has since become a mainstay in the treatment of Kawasaki disease. As early as 1993, Dalakas et al. (4) reported the first randomized controlled clinical trial of IVIg in a dermatological condition demonstrating its successful application in dermatomyositis. Subsequently, IVIg has evolved as a treatment for several other dermatological autoimmune conditions, which are listed in **Table 1**. The clinical application of IVIg is, however, limited by its high cost. Therefore, to warrant a rational use of IVIg, a comprehensive clinical guideline for the use of IVIg in dermatology was first published by the European Dermatology Forum in 2009 and was recently updated in its third edition (5).

MANUFACTURING

Production of IVIg for medical use is strictly regulated to ensure a low risk of pathogen transmission and comparable quality of individual batches. Immunoglobulin concentrations in healthy human sera range from 7 to 12 g/l. Seventy-five percent of these immunoglobulins are class IgG. Modern multistep procedures allow for the purification of up to 4.5 g IgG with more than 95% purity from 1 L of plasma. Special care is taken to reduce the amount of IgA in the preparation, which can trigger severe anaphylactic reactions in patients with selective IgA deficiency. Usually, plasma from whole-blood donations or plasmapheresis of more than 10,000 donors is pooled into a single batch of IVIg. Potential pathogens are mostly inactivated during the purification process. Further steps to ensure a low risk of pathogen transmission include the epidemiological screening of donors and virological testing of donor blood and pooled plasma. Commercial IVIg preparations are usually distributed with a concentration of 50–100 g/l. Aside from IgG, the preparations usually contain sugars (sucrose, maltose, glucose), glycine, sodium chloride, and albumin. While it remains elusive whether commercial preparations differ regarding their immunomodulatory properties, the sugars contained may warrant a different approach depending on comorbidities (e.g., low glucose for diabetic patients, low sucrose for patients with renal failure, low sodium for patients with cardiovascular disease).

PRACTICAL CONSIDERATIONS AND SIDE EFFECTS

IVIg in the treatment of dermatological conditions is usually administered at a dose of 2 g per kg body weight distributed over 2–5 days every 4 weeks. For comparison, this dose is roughly four times higher than the 0.2–0.8 g per kg body weight used in the setting of substitution therapy. Given the half-life of IgG of approximately 3–4 weeks, application of 2 g/kg body weight IVIg over 2–5 days results in high peak serum concentrations. These peaks are considered by some to contribute to the beneficial treatment effects, even though no confirming data exist. At least in the treatment of immune neuropathies, an increasing body of evidence suggests that subcutaneous application of IgG with lower peak concentrations has a similar treatment effect as IVIg (6). The maximum speed of the infusion depends on the individual patient and IVIg preparation. If tolerated, it may reach 0.01 g per kg body weight per minute. Patients should drink sufficient amounts of water before and during the infusion to optimize tolerance. Adequate urine production and blood pressure should be monitored during the infusion.

More common side effects, experienced by up to 10% of patients, include nausea, headache, fatigue, and febrile infusion reactions. Oftentimes, these mild side effects can be controlled by improved hydration; modification of the infusion speed; or anti-allergic, analgesic, and antipyretic co-medication. Hemolysis and neutropenia, which are mostly mild, are thought to occur due to transferred blood-group antibodies and anti-neutrophil antibodies, respectively. Serious side effects are rare and include thrombosis and embolism, pulmonary edema, renal failure, aseptic meningitis, and severe anaphylactic reactions. These latter side effects are, in part, thought to result from impaired rheology, hypervolemia, and allergic reactions to residual IgA in the preparation. The latter reaction is mainly observed in patients with selective IgA deficiency, a rather common [prevalence of ~1:640 in industrialized western countries (7)], and except for an often mild propensity for airway infections, mostly asymptomatic defect of humoral immunity. Surprisingly, IVIg is sometimes tolerated even in this population, rendering the precise role of anti-IgA antibodies and cofactors like the route of administration in causing allergic reactions subject to further investigation (8).

MECHANISM OF ACTION AND CLINICAL USE

The mechanism of action of IVIg in the treatment of autoimmune diseases is still a matter of debate. Generally speaking, one can discriminate between functions of the Fcγ region and the $F(ab)_2$ region and their effects on a cellular level (**Figure 1**). These functions are not mutually exclusive, and given the heterogeneity of diseases IVIgs are used to treat, it is not unlikely that more than one pathway contributes to the beneficial effects. Indeed, there may be some truth to the statement that, after corticosteroids, IVIgs are the broadest immunomodulatory agent available (9).

Strong evidence for a prominent immunomodulatory function of the Fcγ fragment was reported as early as 1993, when Debre et al. (10) were able to show that transfusion of the purified Fcγ fragment is sufficient to successfully treat children with ITP. Indeed, IgG-binding Fcγ receptors were described on a variety of human cells including, among others, leucocytes and platelets. They are most effectively activated by cross-linking through binding of immune complexes. A leading hypothesis states that upregulation of the inhibitory Fcγ receptor IIB (FcγRIIB) is essential for the anti-inflammatory, immunomodulatory activity of IVIg. Supporting evidence for this hypothesis came from studies conducted by Samuelsson et al. (11), Siragam et al. (12), and Kaneko et al. (13), who could show that FcγRIIB expression is required for a response to IVIg infusion in murine models of ITP, arthritis, and nephritis, respectively. Through a series of high-impact publications, the group of Jeffrey Ravetch could subsequently demonstrate that the effects of IVIg on the Fcγ receptor repertoire were mediated not by binding of IVIg to a canonical Fcγ receptor but by a specific receptor for sialylated Fcγ fragments. Indeed, anti-inflammatory activity of IgG depends on specific sialylation of an N-linked glycan on the Fcγ region in mouse arthritis and nephritis models (14). Subsequent research demonstrated that a fully recombinant, appropriately sialylated Fcγ fragment is, in fact, sufficient to confer anti-inflammatory activity in a mouse arthritis model (15). Again using a mouse arthritis model, a specific C-type lectin, SIGN-R1, was later identified to be essential for the anti-inflammatory potential of appropriately sialylated IgG (16). Subsequently, the same group could demonstrate that humanized mice with macrophages and dendritic cells bearing the human orthologue of SIGN-R1, DC-SIGN, responded to IVIg treatment depending on DC-SIGN (17).

Another hypothesis, addressing mainly the context of ITP, states that large immune complexes are formed between IgG in IVIg and anti-D preparations and erythrocytes that inhibit macrophages competitively and via cytokine induction in the reticuloendothelial system, thereby preventing phagocytosis of platelets (18). While this hypothesis explains why anti-D IgG, sometimes given as an alternative to IVIg in ITP patients, is only effective in rhesus D-positive individuals (19), it is not easily compatible with reports that IVIg benefits in ITP were independent of the $F(ab)_2$ fragment (see previous paragraph).

On a cellular and cytokine level, IVIg was reported to induce a Th2-type immune response with production of interleukin 33 (IL33) and IL4, leading to an increased expression of FcγRIIB on splenic macrophages in a murine arthritis model (17). It should be noted, however, that previous research has suggested that IL33 and IL4 are not crucial for the beneficial effects of IVIg in murine ITP models, and patients with ITP still respond to IVIg after splenectomy (20, 21). IVIg was furthermore reported to expand regulatory T-cells in a murine experimental autoimmune encephalitis model via interaction of IVIg with DC-SIGN on dendritic cells (22); to reduce expression of stimulatory cofactors, toll-like receptors, and additional activating pathways in B-cells *ex vivo* (23, 24); and to inhibit Th17 differentiation, amplification, and function *ex vivo* (25, 26).

Very recently, two recombinant IgG1 multimers were reported that confer either several (27) or only a subset (28) of IVIg effector functions and may offer new insights into the therapeutic role of IgG subunits in IVIg formulations.

Additional hypotheses on IVIg's mechanism of action will be discussed in the following paragraphs alongside the relevant dermatological conditions.

Table 1 summarizes indications for IVIg treatment in dermatology. Due to the rarity of some of these conditions, randomized clinical trials to support the use of IVIg are not generally available.

Autoimmune Bullous Dermatoses

Autoimmune bullous dermatoses are a heterogeneous group of antibody-mediated autoimmune diseases, which manifest with bullae and erosions on the skin and mucous membranes. Prominent examples are pemphigus vulgaris and bullous pemphigoid. In pemphigus vulgaris, pathological antibodies against keratinocyte desmosomal proteins (desmoglein 3, desmoglein 1) cause intra-epidermal separation with the formation of blisters and erosions in the mouth, pharynx, and skin. Until the advent of steroid treatment, pemphigus vulgaris caused significant mortality due to malnutrition and superinfection. Even today, a subset of patients do not sufficiently respond to immunosuppressive and immunomodulatory treatment or succumb to fatal adverse effects. Bullous pemphigoid results from autoantibodies against hemidesmosomal proteins, in particular, the NC16A region of BP180. Therefore, and in contrast to pemphigus vulgaris, blister formation is sub-epidermal. The clinical course tends to be mild, and topical treatment may be sufficient. Other sub-epidermal autoimmune bullous dermatoses include epidermolysis bullosa acquisita, with anti-collagen VII autoantibodies and, consequently, the formation of deep blisters between the basal membrane and papillary dermis, and mucous membrane pemphigoid, which may result in scarring and, if affecting the eyes, loss of vision.

Treatment of recalcitrant pemphigus vulgaris and foliaceus and bullous pemphigoid with IVIg is supported by two randomized clinical trials (29, 30). **Figure 1** documents the response of a patient to IVIg treatment. Usually, IVIg is used as a third-line adjunct treatment initially flanked by high-dose systemic corticosteroids and steroid-sparing

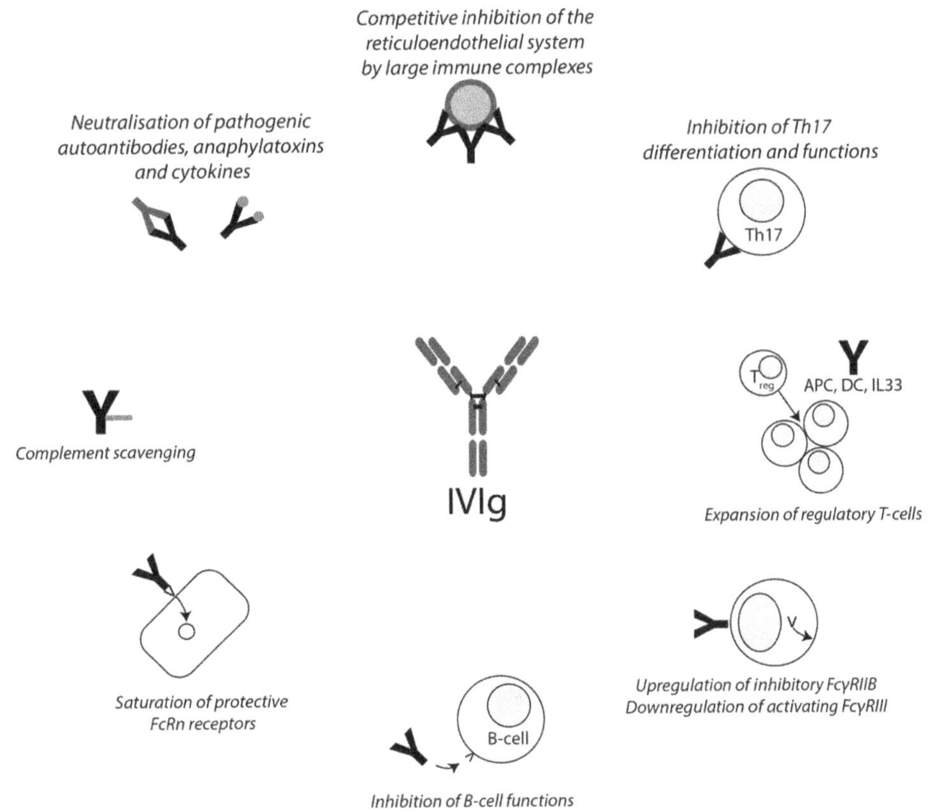

FIGURE 1 | Summary of IVIg mechanisms of action. Graphical summary of reported mechanisms of action of IVIg. IVIg effects can be mediated through the $F(ab)_2$ and Fc fragments. APC, antigen-presenting cell; DC, dendritic cell; FCγRIIB, Fcγ receptor IIB; FcRn, neonatal Fc receptor; IVIg, intravenous immunoglobulin.

immunosuppressants (5, 31). In analogy, IVIg is successfully used to treat other autoimmune bullous dermatoses including epidermolysis bullosa acquisita and mucous membrane pemphigoid (5). Once disease control is achieved, indicated by the healing of old erosions and no formation of new blisters, immunosuppressive treatment is slowly reduced and, finally, IVIg intervals may be extended to 6 weeks followed by cessation of IVIg treatment.

Regarding the mechanism of action, Li et al. (32) could demonstrate that response to IVIg treatment in murine bullous pemphigoid, pemphigus vulgaris, and pemphigus foliaceus models depended on the expression of the neonatal Fc receptor (FcRn), which regulates the half-life of serum IgG via pinocytosis and protection against lysosomal degradation. The authors put forward the hypothesis that IVIgs saturate FcRn receptors, resulting in accelerated degradation of pathogenic autoantibodies. Of note, FcRn-deficient mice developed only very mild symptoms of autoimmune bullous dermatoses, rendering the comparison with wild-type mice complex. The pathogenic relevance of FcRn in autoimmune bullous dermatoses was also demonstrated in murine experimental epidermolysis bullosa acquisita models, where FcRn deficiency protected from tissue injury [(33); for a review, see (34)]. Arguing against a prominent global role of FcRn saturation is the observation that FcRn deficiency does not preclude IVIg effects in mice with ITP (35). However, animal models of ITP usually focus on the initial phases of disease and treatment. Therefore, FcRn saturation may still contribute to the prolonged effects of IVIg treatment in autoimmune diseases. Other potential mechanisms that may contribute to IVIg's beneficial effects in autoimmune bullous dermatoses include anti-idiotypic antibodies against anti-BP180 IgG, which were demonstrated in IVIg and prevented BP180 degradation *ex vivo* (36), and a reduction of pro-inflammatory interleukin 6, which was recently demonstrated in IVIg-treated murine experimental bullous pemphigoid models (37).

Dermatomyositis

Dermatomyositis is an antibody and complement-mediated microangiopathy characteristically affecting the proximal musculature of the extremities and sun-exposed areas of the skin (38). Apart from the musculature, systemic involvement mainly affects the heart and lungs. One-third of cases are paraneoplastic. Therefore, dermatomyositis is associated with considerable mortality. In contrast to adult dermatomyositis, pediatric dermatomyositis is usually not associated with malignancy.

The treatment of dermatomyositis with IVIg is supported by a randomized clinical trial (4). A recent guideline promotes the use of IVIg as a second-line therapy after failure of systemic high-dose corticosteroids, the mainstay of dermatomyositis treatment (5). This approach is of particular use when an associated malignancy is present to reduce the need for immunosuppressive medication. Alternative second-line treatments include steroid-sparing immunosuppressants like mycophenolate mofetil, azathioprine, and methotrexate (39). The immunosuppressive medications, starting with systemic corticosteroids, are slowly reduced once disease control is achieved. Finally, IVIg intervals may be extended to 6 weeks followed by cessation of IVIg treatment.

Basta and Dalakas (40) reported that IVIg treatment prevented the formation of the complement membrane attack complex in patients with dermatomyositis. Indeed, the Fcγ fraction of IgG was shown to bind C3b, thus opsonizing it for clearance by the reticuloendothelial system (41). Additionally, Basta et al. (42) could demonstrate that the $F(ab)_2$ fraction of IgG binds and neutralizes the anaphylatoxins C3a and C5a using animal models of murine asthma and porcine C5a-induced cardiopulmonary distress. However, given the reported treatment effects of isolated Fcγ fractions, the $F(ab)_2$ fraction may not contribute equally to effects of IVIg in other diseases including ITP [see above, e.g., (10)].

Scleromyxedema

Scleromyxedema is histologically characterized by fibroblast activation, mucin deposition, and fibrosis and usually associated with paraproteinemia. The precise pathogenesis is, as of yet, unknown. Clinically, the depositions mainly affect the skin, where patients develop waxy papules and indurations that may lead to dermatogenic contractures. Systemic involvement of the peripheral and central nervous system, cardiopulmonary system, kidneys, joints, and/or muscles is observed in up to 30% of patients.

Given the unsatisfactory response and relevant associated morbidity of alternative treatments like systemic steroids, thalidomide, or melphalan, IVIg is recommended as a first-line treatment in severe scleromyxedema based on several case reports and series (5). Due to frequent relapses after cessation, long-term IVIg treatment is oftentimes necessary.

The pathogenic role of monoclonal IgG in scleromyxedema is unknown: while patient serum induced fibrosis in normal human fibroblasts, purified monoclonal patient IgG was ineffective (43). Hypotheses therefore include the blocking of an as of yet unknown circulating factor by IVIg (44). However, the mechanism of action is largely elusive and may involve various IVIg effects documented in other disease entities.

Systemic Vasculitis

Vasculitides are a heterogeneous group of diseases that result from an inflammation of the arterial blood vessels and/or post-capillary venules. They are categorized, among other criteria, by the size of the affected blood vessels and single- or multi-organ involvement according to the Chapel Hill Consensus Conference criteria (45). The symptoms largely depend on the involved organ systems. In the skin, symptoms range from papules with hemorrhage (palpable purpura) to subcutaneous nodules and necrosis depending on the size and depth of the involved blood vessels. Regarding the pathogenesis, it is possible to discriminate those types of vasculitis that involve anti-neutrophilic cytoplasmic antibodies (ANCAs), leading to neutrophil activation and degranulation, from those that result from immune complex deposition.

A randomized controlled trial indicating beneficial effects of IVIg was conducted by Jayne et al. (46) in patients with granulomatosis with polyangiitis (GPA, formerly Wegener's granulomatosis), a potentially lethal form of ANCA-associated multi-organ vasculitis. Of note, some critics of the study have later objected to the short observation period of 3 months, and a recent Cochrane review found insufficient evidence to support the use of IVIg in GPA (47). Still, the EULAR advises using IVIg as an adjuvant treatment in GPA with moderate residual disease unresponsive to high-dose systemic corticosteroids, cyclophosphamide, and rituximab (48). Based on data on IVIg in ANCA-associated vasculitis and several case reports and series documenting beneficial effects of IVIg in a variety of vasculitides, the current European guideline promotes the use of IVIg in all severe systemic vasculitides in recalcitrant cases, if other therapeutic options are contraindicated, or if the disease takes a foudroyant course (5). Alongside acetylsalicylic acid, IVIg is considered a mainstay in the treatment of Kawasaki disease, as elaborated in the introductory part of this manuscript.

In vitro data indicate that anti-idiotypic antibodies contained in IVIg can bind and neutralize ANCA (49). Whether anti-idiotypic antibodies contribute to IVIg effects in the treatment of vasculitis *in vivo* is, however, uncertain. Of note, as previously detailed in this manuscript, the $F(ab)_2$ fragment was not necessary to convey IVIg's beneficial effects in several other autoimmune diseases.

Systemic Lupus Erythematosus

Systemic lupus erythematosus (SLE) is a multi-organ collagen vascular disease, which involves characteristic anti-double-stranded DNA (anti-dsDNA) autoantibodies in the serum. Extra-cutaneous symptoms include arthritis, lupus nephritis, esophagitis, enteropathy, hepatitis, pneumonitis, interstitial lung disease, pulmonary hypertension, pericarditis, endocarditis, encephalitis, peripheral neuropathies, hematologic abnormalities, and thromboembolic disease. The skin is usually affected in a UV-dependent fashion. Individual lesions can range from erythematous macules on both cheeks (butterfly rash) to scarring erythematous, scaly plaques, and panniculitis.

The treatment of SLE depends on the involved organ systems and includes a variety of immunosuppressive agents [for a detailed review, cf. (50)]. Two randomized controlled trials reported beneficial effects of IVIg in SLE in the context of pregnancy in patients with recurrent abortions and in the treatment of lupus nephritis (51, 52). According to the European guideline, IVIg should be considered as a treatment option in all cases of severe lupus erythematosus (5). In particular, IVIg may be beneficial in the treatment of pregnant women, SLE-associated ITP, stable lupus nephritis, and neuropsychiatric disease (53).

Interestingly, affinity-purified anti-idiotypic antibodies against anti-dsDNA were effective in the treatment of an experimental murine SLE model (54). However, several of the previously detailed mechanisms can be hypothesized to contribute to the beneficial effects of IVIg in SLE [for a review, see (55)].

OUTLOOK

IVIg is successfully used to treat an expanding range of autoimmune diseases. While strong evidence points toward a prominent role of the Fcγ fragment to convey the beneficial effects of IVIg treatment, there may be more than one mechanism of action, and their precise role may vary depending on the disease in focus. It is, however, tempting to speculate that only a fraction of the components contained in IVIg formulations, e.g., specifically sialylated Fcγ fragments, are responsible for their clinical effects and that more refined preparations may make the infusions more accessible and even safer in the future.

AUTHOR CONTRIBUTIONS

JH wrote the first draft of the manuscript. JH and AE revised the work for important intellectual content. JH and AE read and approved the submitted version.

REFERENCES

1. Imbach P, Barandun S, d'Apuzzo V, Baumgartner C, Hirt A, Morell A, et al. High-dose intravenous gammaglobulin for idiopathic thrombocytopenic purpura in childhood. *Lancet.* (1981) 1:1228–31. doi: 10.1016/S0140-6736(81)92400-4
2. Furusho K, Kamiya T, Nakano H, Kiyosawa N, Shinomiya K, Hayashidera T, et al. High-dose intravenous gammaglobulin for Kawasaki disease. *Lancet.* (1984) 2:1055–8. doi: 10.1016/S0140-6736(84)91504-6
3. Newburger JW, Takahashi M, Burns JC, Beiser AS, Chung KJ, Duffy CE, et al. The treatment of Kawasaki syndrome with intravenous gamma globulin. *N Engl J Med.* (1986) 315:341–7. doi: 10.1056/NEJM198608073150601
4. Dalakas MC, Illa I, Dambrosia JM, Soueidan SA, Stein DP, Otero C, et al. A controlled trial of high-dose intravenous immune globulin infusions as treatment for dermatomyositis. *N Engl J Med.* (1993) 329:1993–2000. doi: 10.1056/NEJM199312303292704
5. Enk AH, Hadaschik EN, Eming R, Fierlbeck G, French LE, Girolomoni G, et al. European guidelines (S1) on the use of high-dose intravenous immunoglobulin in dermatology. *J Eur Acad Dermatol Venereol.* (2016) 30:1657–69. doi: 10.1111/jdv.13725
6. Leussink VI, Hartung HP, Kieseier BC, Stettner M. Subcutaneous immunoglobulins in the treatment of chronic immune-mediated neuropathies. *Ther Adv Neurol Disord.* (2016) 9:336–43. doi: 10.1177/1756285616641583
7. Hammarstrom L, Vorechovsky I, Webster D. Selective IgA deficiency (SIgAD) and common variable immunodeficiency (CVID). *Clin Exp Immunol.* (2000) 120:225–31. doi: 10.1046/j.1365-2249.2000.01131.x
8. Rachid R, Bonilla FA. The role of anti-IgA antibodies in causing adverse reactions to gamma globulin infusion in immunodeficient patients: a comprehensive review of the literature. *J Allergy Clin Immunol.* (2012) 129:628–34. doi: 10.1016/j.jaci.2011.06.047
9. Liebmann HA. Immunomodulatory drugs and monoclonal antibodies. In: *Antibody Therapy.* Switzerland: Springer (2018) p. 85–100. doi: 10.1007/978-3-319-68038-5_7
10. Debre M, Bonnet MC, Fridman WH, Carosella E, Philippe N, Reinert P, et al. Infusion of Fc gamma fragments for treatment of children with acute immune thrombocytopenic purpura. *Lancet.* (1993) 342:945–9. doi: 10.1016/0140-6736(93)92000-J
11. Samuelsson A, Towers TL, Ravetch JV. Anti-inflammatory activity of IVIG mediated through the inhibitory Fc receptor. *Science.* (2001) 291:484–6. doi: 10.1126/science.291.5503.484
12. Siragam V, Brinc D, Crow AR, Song S, Freedman J, Lazarus AH. Can antibodies with specificity for soluble antigens mimic the therapeutic effects of intravenous IgG in the treatment of autoimmune disease? *J Clin Invest.* (2005) 115:155–60. doi: 10.1172/JCI22753
13. Kaneko Y, Nimmerjahn F, Madaio MP, Ravetch JV. Pathology and protection in nephrotoxic nephritis is determined by selective engagement of specific Fc receptors. *J Exp Med.* (2006) 203:789–97. doi: 10.1084/jem.20051900
14. Kaneko Y, Nimmerjahn F, Ravetch JV. Anti-inflammatory activity of immunoglobulin G resulting from Fc sialylation. *Science.* (2006) 313:670–3. doi: 10.1126/science.1129594
15. Anthony RM, Nimmerjahn F, Ashline DJ, Reinhold VN, Paulson JC, Ravetch JV. Recapitulation of IVIG anti-inflammatory activity with a recombinant IgG Fc. *Science.* (2008) 320:373–6. doi: 10.1126/science.1154315
16. Anthony RM, Wermeling F, Karlsson MC, Ravetch JV. Identification of a receptor required for the anti-inflammatory activity of IVIG. *Proc Natl Acad Sci USA.* (2008) 105:19571–8. doi: 10.1073/pnas.0810163105
17. Anthony RM, Kobayashi T, Wermeling F, Ravetch JV. Intravenous gammaglobulin suppresses inflammation through a novel T(H)2 pathway. *Nature.* (2011) 475: U110–133. doi: 10.1038/nature10134
18. Clynes R. Immune complexes as therapy for autoimmunity. *J Clin Invest.* (2005) 115:25–7. doi: 10.1172/JCI200523994
19. Oksenhendler E, Bierling P, Brossard Y, Schenmetzler C, Girard PM, Seligmann M, et al. Anti-RH immunoglobulin therapy for human immunodeficiency virus-related immune thrombocytopenic purpura. *Blood.* (1988) 71:1499–502.
20. Cines DB, Bussel JB. How I treat idiopathic thrombocytopenic purpura (ITP). *Blood.* (2005) 106:2244–51. doi: 10.1182/blood-2004-12-4598
21. Crow AR, Song S, Semple JW, Freedman J, Lazarus AH. A role for IL-1 receptor antagonist or other cytokines in the acute therapeutic effects of IVIg? *Blood.* (2007) 109:155–8. doi: 10.1182/blood-2006-05-023796
22. Trinath J, Hegde P, Sharma M, Maddur MS, Rabin M, Vallat JM, et al. Intravenous immunoglobulin expands regulatory T cells via induction of cyclooxygenase-2-dependent prostaglandin E2 in human dendritic cells. *Blood.* (2013) 122:1419–27. doi: 10.1182/blood-2012-11-468264
23. Seite JF, Guerrier T, Cornec D, Jamin C, Youinou P, Hillion S. TLR9 responses of B cells are repressed by intravenous immunoglobulin through the recruitment of phosphatase. *J Autoimmun.* (2011) 37:190–7. doi: 10.1016/j.jaut.2011.05.014
24. Seite JF, Goutsmedt C, Youinou P, Pers JO, Hillion S. Intravenous immunoglobulin induces a functional silencing program similar to anergy in human B cells. *J Allergy Clin Immunol.* (2014) 133:181–8.e1–9. doi: 10.1016/j.jaci.2013.08.042
25. Maddur MS, Vani J, Hegde P, Lacroix-Desmazes S, Kaveri SV, Bayry J. Inhibition of differentiation, amplification, and function of human TH17 cells by intravenous immunoglobulin. *J Allergy Clin Immunol.* (2011) 127:823–30.e1–7. doi: 10.1016/j.jaci.2010.12.1102

26. Maddur MS, Sharma M, Hegde P, Lacroix-Desmazes S, Kaveri SV, Bayry J. Inhibitory effect of IVIG on IL-17 production by Th17 cells is independent of Anti-IL-17 antibodies in the immunoglobulin preparations. *J Clin Immunol.* (2013) 33:S62–S66. doi: 10.1007/s10875-012-9752-6
27. Zhang X, Owens J, Olsen HS, So E, Burch E, McCroskey MC, et al. A recombinant human IgG1 Fc multimer designed to mimic the active fraction of IVIG in autoimmunity. *JCI Insight.* (2019) 4:121905. doi: 10.1172/jci.insight.121905. [Epub ahead of print].
28. Sun H, Olsen HS, Merigeon EY, So E, Burch E, Kinsey S, et al. Recombinant human IgG1 based Fc multimers, with limited FcR binding capacity, can effectively inhibit complement-mediated disease. *J Autoimmun.* (2017) 84:97–108. doi: 10.1016/j.jaut.2017.08.004
29. Amagai M, Ikeda S, Shimizu H, Iizuka H, Hanada K, Aiba S, et al. A randomized double-blind trial of intravenous immunoglobulin for pemphigus. *J Am Acad Dermatol.* (2009) 60:595–603. doi: 10.1016/j.jaad.2008.09.052
30. Amagai M, Ikeda S, Hashimoto T, Mizuashi M, Fujisawa A, Ihn H, et al. A randomized double-blind trial of intravenous immunoglobulin for bullous pemphigoid. *J Dermatol Sci.* (2017) 85:77–84. doi: 10.1016/j.jdermsci.2016.11.003
31. Hertl M, Jedlickova H, Karpati S, Marinovic B, Uzun S, Yayli S, et al. Pemphigus. S2 guideline for diagnosis and treatment-guided by the European Dermatology Forum (EDF) in cooperation with the European Academy of Dermatology and Venereology (EADV). *J Eur Acad Dermatol Venereol.* (2015) 29:405–14. doi: 10.1111/jdv.12772
32. Li N, Zhao M, Hilario-Vargas J, Prisayanh P, Warren S, Diaz LA, et al. Complete FcRn dependence for intravenous Ig therapy in autoimmune skin blistering diseases. *J Clin Invest.* (2005) 115:3440–50. doi: 10.1172/JCI24394
33. Sesarman A, Sitaru AG, Olaru F, Zillikens D, Sitaru C. Neonatal Fc receptor deficiency protects from tissue injury in experimental epidermolysis bullosa acquisita. *J. Mol Med.* (2008) 86:951–9. doi: 10.1007/s00109-008-0366-7
34. Sesarman A, Vidarsson G, Sitaru C. The neonatal Fc receptor as therapeutic target in IgG-mediated autoimmune diseases. *Cell Mol Life Sci.* (2010) 67:2533–50. doi: 10.1007/s00018-010-0318-6
35. Crow AR, Suppa SJ, Chen X, Mott PJ, Lazarus AH. The neonatal Fc receptor (FcRn) is not required for IVIg or anti-CD44 monoclonal antibody-mediated amelioration of murine immune thrombocytopenia. *Blood.* (2011) 118:6403–6. doi: 10.1182/blood-2011-08-374223
36. Kamaguchi M, Iwata H, Mori Y, Toyonaga E, Ujiie H, Kitagawa Y, et al. Anti-idiotypic antibodies against BP-IgG prevent type XVII collagen depletion. *Front. Immunol.* (2017) 8:1669. doi: 10.3389/fimmu.2017.01669
37. Sasaoka T, Ujiie H, Nishie W, Iwata H, Ishikawa M, Higashino H, et al. Intravenous IgG reduces pathogenic autoantibodies, serum IL-6 levels, and disease severity in experimental bullous pemphigoid models. *J Invest Dermatol.* (2018) 138:1260–7. doi: 10.1016/j.jid.2018.01.005
38. Dalakas MC. Mechanisms of disease: signaling pathways and immunobiology of inflammatory myopathies. *Nat Clin Pract Rheumatol.* (2006) 2:219–27. doi: 10.1038/ncprheum0140
39. Sunderkotter C, Nast A, Worm M, Dengler R, Dorner T, Ganter H, et al. Guidelines on dermatomyositis-excerpt from the interdisciplinary S2k guidelines on myositis syndromes by the German Society of Neurology. *J Dtsch Dermatol Ges.* (2016) 14:321–38. doi: 10.1111/ddg.12909
40. Basta M, Dalakas MC. High-dose intravenous immunoglobulin exerts its beneficial effect in patients with dermatomyositis by blocking endomysial deposition of activated complement fragments. *J Clin Invest.* (1994) 94:1729–35. doi: 10.1172/JCI117520
41. Spycher M, Matozan K, Minnig K, Zehnder R, Miescher S, Hoefferer L, et al. *In vitro* comparison of the complement-scavenging capacity of different intravenous immunoglobulin preparations. *Vox. Sang.* (2009) 97:348–54. doi: 10.1111/j.1423-0410.2009.01217.x
42. Basta M, Van Goor F, Luccioli S, Billings EM, Vortmeyer AO, Baranyi L, et al. F(ab)'2-mediated neutralization of C3a and C5a anaphylatoxins: a novel effector function of immunoglobulins. *Nat Med.* (2003) 9:431–8. doi: 10.1038/nm836
43. Harper RA, Rispler J. Lichen myxedematosus serum stimulates human skin fibroblast proliferation. *Science.* (1978) 199:545–7. doi: 10.1126/science.622555
44. Rey JB, Luria RB. Treatment of scleromyxedema and the dermatoneuro syndrome with intravenous immunoglobulin. *J Am Acad Dermatol.* (2009) 60:1037–41. doi: 10.1016/j.jaad.2008.11.013
45. Jennette JC, Falk RJ, Bacon PA, Basu N, Cid MC, Ferrario F, et al. 2012 revised International Chapel Hill Consensus Conference nomenclature of vasculitides. *Arthritis Rheum.* (2013) 65:1–11. doi: 10.1002/art.37715.
46. Jayne DR, Chapel H, Adu D, Misbah S, O'Donoghue D, Scott D, et al. Intravenous immunoglobulin for ANCA-associated systemic vasculitis with persistent disease activity. *QJM.* (2000) 93:433–9. doi: 10.1093/qjmed/93.7.433
47. Fortin PM, Tejani AM, Bassett K, Musini VM. Intravenous immunoglobulin as adjuvant therapy for Wegener's granulomatosis. *Cochrane Database Syst Rev.* (2013) 1:CD007057. doi: 10.1002/14651858.CD007057.pub3
48. Yates M, Watts RA, Bajema IM, Cid MC, Crestani B, Hauser T, et al. EULAR/ERA-EDTA recommendations for the management of ANCA-associated vasculitis. *Ann Rheum Dis.* (2016) 75:1583–94. doi: 10.1136/annrheumdis-2016-209133
49. Rossi F, Dietrich G, Kazatchkine MD. Antiidiotypic suppression of autoantibodies with normal polyspecific immunoglobulins. *Res Immunol.* (1989) 140:19–31. doi: 10.1016/0923-2494(89)90004-7
50. Tunnicliffe DJ, Singh-Grewal D, Kim S, Craig JC, Tong A. Diagnosis, monitoring, and treatment of systemic lupus erythematosus: a systematic review of clinical practice guidelines. *Arthritis Care Res.* (2015) 67:1440–52. doi: 10.1002/acr.22591
51. Boletis JN, Ioannidis JP, Boki KA, Moutsopoulos HM. Intravenous immunoglobulin compared with cyclophosphamide for proliferative lupus nephritis. *Lancet.* (1999) 354:569–70. doi: 10.1016/S0140-6736(99)01575-5
52. Perricone R, De Carolis C, Kroegler B, Greco E, Giacomelli R, Cipriani P, et al. Intravenous immunoglobulin therapy in pregnant patients affected with systemic lupus erythematosus and recurrent spontaneous abortion. *Rheumatology.* (2008) 47:646–51. doi: 10.1093/rheumatology/ken046
53. Mulhearn B, Bruce IN. Indications for IVIG in rheumatic diseases. *Rheumatology.* (2015) 54:383–91. doi: 10.1093/rheumatology/keu429
54. Shoenfeld Y, Rauova L, Gilburd B, Kvapil F, Goldberg I, Kopolovic J, et al. Efficacy of IVIG affinity-purified anti-double-stranded DNA anti-idiotypic antibodies in the treatment of an experimental murine model of systemic lupus erythematosus. *Int Immunol.* (2002) 14:1303–11. doi: 10.1093/intimm/dxf099
55. Zandman-Goddard G, Blank M, Shoenfeld Y. Intravenous immunoglobulins in systemic lupus erythematosus: from the bench to the bedside. *Lupus.* (2009) 18:884–8. doi: 10.1177/0961203309106921

8

Autoantibodies in Morphea: An Update

Sangita Khatri[1], Kathryn S. Torok[2], Emily Mirizio[2], Christopher Liu[2] and Kira Astakhova[1]*

[1] *Department of Chemistry, Technical University of Denmark, Kongens Lyngby, Denmark,* [2] *Division of Rheumatology, Department of Pediatrics, Children's Hospital of Pittsburgh, University of Pittsburgh, Pittsburgh, PA, United States*

Correspondence:
Kira Astakhova
kiraas@kemi.dtu.dk

Skin autoimmune conditions belong to a larger group of connective tissue diseases and primarily affect the skin, but might also involve underlying tissues, such as fat tissue, muscle, and bone. Autoimmune antibodies (autoantibodies) play a role in autoimmune skin diseases, such as localized scleroderma also termed morphea, and systemic scleroderma, also called systemic sclerosis (SSc). The detailed studies on the biological role of autoantibodies in autoimmune skin diseases are limited. This results in a few available tools for effective diagnosis and management of autoimmune skin diseases. This review aims to provide an update on the detection and most recent research on autoantibodies in morphea. Several recent studies have indicated the association of autoantibody profiles with disease subtypes, damage extent, and relapse potential, opening up exciting new possibilities for personalized disease management. We discuss the role of existing autoantibody tests in morphea management and the most recent studies on morphea pathogenesis. We also provide an update on novel autoantibody biomarkers for the diagnosis and study of morphea.

Keywords: skin autoimmunity, morphea, autoantibody, diagnostics, personalized management

INTRODUCTION

Being a part of an abnormal immune response, autoimmune antibodies (autoantibodies) are valuable biomarkers in autoimmunity. The causality of autoantibodies in autoimmune diseases is still controversial and requires more fundamental research (1). Nevertheless, clinical assays detecting autoantibodies are commonly used to diagnose and categorize autoimmune diseases (2). Recent studies have revealed distinct autoantibody profiles among patients with autoimmune diseases, opening up new avenues for better diagnostics and personalized disease management (3).

The prototypical rheumatologic autoimmune disease of the skin, systemic sclerosis (SSc), is often defined and subcategorized by an auto-antibody profile, in addition to the extent of skin involvement (4). The presence of scleroderma-associated autoantibodies, such as autoantibodies to topoisomerase and centromeres, has enabled clinicians to better predict organ system involvement in these patients. Nevertheless, the true pathogenicity of these autoantibodies in SSc disease propagation remains to be elucidated.

A "sister" autoimmune disease to SSc in regards to its similar effect on the skin is localized scleroderma, also termed morphea. Although morphea and SSc share the same skin histopathologic changes, the distribution and pattern of skin involvement, and the associated extracutaneous and internal organ manifestations, are quite different (5). Morphea is typically distributed in patches or bands of skin inflammation and thickness either on the head, extremity, and trunk in an ipsilateral fashion (**Figure 1**). Based on the distribution patterns and depth of lesions, morphea has been divided into several clinical subtypes: circumscribed superficial morphea (plaque morphea), superficial deep morphea (deep morphea), generalized plaque morphea (multiple plaque lesions), linear scleroderma of the trunk/extremities, linear scleroderma of the head (also termed Parry–Romberg Syndrome and En coup de sabre), and pansclerotic morphea or mixed morphea (a combination of two or more of these subtypes) (6). Although morphea does not tend to have internal organ manifestations, such as interstitial lung disease or cardiac arrhythmia, the underlying and associated tissue is often affected in morphea patients, causing morbidity. The frequency of extracutaneous involvement in morphea has ranged from 20 up to 70% in the literature, depending on whether the data has been collected retrospectively or prospectively, with prospective assessment data capturing more manifestations (7–13). The most common extracutaneous manifestations (ECM) across cohorts are musculoskeletal, including arthralgia, arthritis, joint contractures, myositis, fasciitis, with associated disease-induced gait disturbance, decreased function, muscle, bone, and limb atrophy (**Figure 1**), and followed by neurologic, ophthalmologic, and dental issues occurring in ~50% of morphea patients with involvement of the head (14–16). These manifestations include seizures, headaches, hemiparesis, cranial nerve palsy, optic neuritis, uveitis, scleritis, dry eye, atrophic dental roots, dental crowding, and malocclusion. Morphea subtypes and ECM associations are different in adult vs. childhood-onset. Circumscribed superficial (plaque morphea) and generalized morphea are common in adult-onset morphea (**Figure 1A**), while linear scleroderma, both linear trunk/extremity and linear head subtypes, is more common in childhood-onset morphea (**Figure 1B**) (10, 11). To achieve personalized management schemes, these factors shall be taken into account.

In general, morphea is monitored clinically through the visualization and scoring of skin changes over time (**Figure 1**). Several clinical assessment methods have been developed to monitor morphea, such as depigmentation, induration, erythema, and the telangiectasia (DIET) score, the modified Rodnan skin score (mRSS), and the Localized Scleroderma Assessment Tool (LoSCAT) (12, 17). All of these methods assess activity and damage together, based on selected clinical parameters. The lack of a full validation of treatment response criteria of these scores limits the ability of clinicians to judge the effectiveness of these treatments. A combination of a cutaneous outcome measure in conjunction with serological biomarkers, such as autoantibodies, might be a plausible means to better classify and stratify morphea patients.

With regard to serological testing, the role of autoantibodies in morphea and their clinical application is not as clear as SSc. So far, it is recommended to use the Localized Scleroderma Assessment Tool (LoSCAT), with autoantibody tests when concurrent rheumatic and other autoimmune diseases are suspected. Suggested tests to verify this include antinuclear antibodies (ANA), antibodies to single stranded DNA (a-ssDNA), anti-histone antibodies (AHA), and anti-topoisomerase antibody type of anti-nuclear autoantibodies (anti-Scl-70).

A particular limitation of the literature in regards to autoantibody testing in morphea is that the majority of studies reporting autoantibody positivity are in context of a larger descriptive morphea cohort summary; therefore only a subset of patients have available autoantibody testing, typically guided by clinical practice instead of prospective research testing. To address this limitation, we only included cohort studies in which at least 50 morphea subjects were tested for the autoantibody of interest, in addition to prospective studies designed to test autoantibodies in morphea, to obtain more accurate frequencies and clinical correlations.

The review is organized into three parts. First, we describe the status with existing autoantibody tests (ANA, AHA, and a-ssDNA) in the context of morphea diagnosis and treatment. Here, the literature has been selected based on the number of patients with a particular autoantibody tested within each cohort (≥50 patients), and suggested associations with clinical manifestations of the disease. In the second part, we present the most recent studies on the role of autoantibodies in the pathogenesis of morphea. Here, we selected studies that included relevant controls and suggested pertinent new knowledge on morphea pathogenesis. Third, we describe emerging biomarkers in morphea research and clinical diagnostics; in this part, we select the literature based on the statistical power of the observed effects, and the appeal to potential personalized management of morphea patients.

Besides a low number of enrolled patients, a large deviation in the applied methodologies is another main problem in the field of morphea diagnostics. Therefore, we critically assessed the methodology for autoantibody testing, applied controls, and standardization methods. We also discuss the problem of the limited number of relevant animal models for morphea research, and the connection between recent studies on the potential to reveal new valuable insights into the pathogenesis of morphea, and to improve the disease management in clinics.

LABORATORY DIAGNOSTICS OF AUTOANTIBODIES IN MORPHEA

ANA Positivity in Morphea

Elevated antinuclear antibody (ANA) levels are often encountered in morphea, with larger cohort reports detecting 23–68% ANA-positive patients (see **Figure 2**; **Supplementary Table 1** and cited references). The majority of studies (>80%) describe ANA testing by Human epithelial type 2 immunofluorescence assay (Hep2 IF), with a cut-off of >1:80 in most papers, run in standardized laboratory associated with the ordering institution. Notably, both pediatric-onset and adult-onset morphea have ANA positivity in this range (**Supplementary Table 1** and cited references). One cohort study (Morphea in Adults and Children; MAC) reported a trend toward higher ANA positivity in adults (53% vs. 30% pediatrics) (10). However, in a later study with more subjects enrolled in the MAC cohort, the frequency of ANA positivity was higher in pediatric onset (27% in adults vs. 42% in pediatrics patients). The largest cohort to date with ANA testing is an international pediatric morphea cohort described by Zulian et al. in which 750 morphea patients were described, 671 in whom had ANA testing

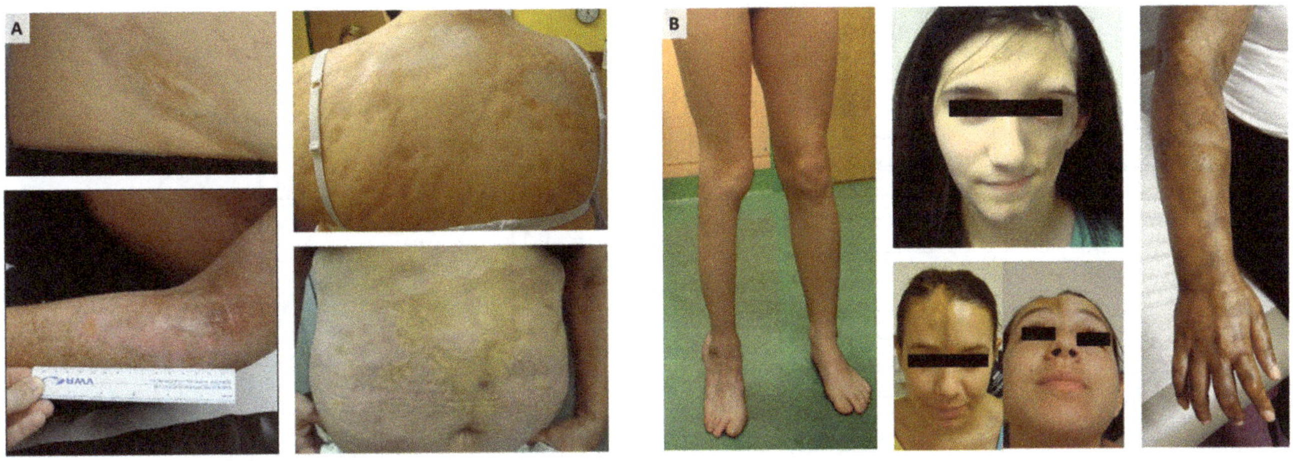

FIGURE 1 | Morphea: **(A)** Generalized morphea and plaque morphea are the most common subtypes of morphea in adult patients, while **(B)** linear scleroderma of the trunk, limbs, and head are the most common in pediatric morphea. For each photograph, written informed consent was obtained from the participant for the publication of this image.

performed (13, 18). Of these, 284 patients (42.3%) were ANA positive. ANA positivity was tested among subtypes of morphea (linear, plaque, generalized, and deep morphea) and there was no significant difference (18), with subtype ANA positivity ranging from 31 to 47%. ANA positivity has been debated to be associated with the subtype of morphea, with the initial findings of the MAC cohort supporting an association with generalized morphea and mixed morphea (generalized + linear) (10). Their later study using matched healthy case-controls compared to the morphea cohort did not find an association of ANA positivity with morphea subtype (19).

A metanalyses of ANA positivity was performed to more formally capture the average ANA positivity in morphea patients across various cohort publications. Our search strategy aimed to identify studies that described antibody testing or cohort reports in morphea (localized scleroderma). All studies that reported antibody testing were reviewed (both retrospective and prospective). Independent searches of the PubMed, Google Scholar, and Webscope databases for relevant studies was performed using the following search terms: morphea, localized scleroderma, antibody, ANA, AHA, pediatric, rheumatoid factor (RF), juvenile, morphea cohort etc. The search was limited to studies that included 50 or more patients tested for antibodies of interest. Citations were screened for duplicate studies and duplicate patient samples without blinding. Statistics software (MedCalc Software, Ostend, Belgium) was used for the statistical analysis. Outcomes were measured by calculating proportions and 95% confidence intervals (CIs) for each study, then pooled the data to derive a pooled proportion and 95% CI.

For the purpose of proportion meta-analysis, the proportions were first turned into a quantity (the Freeman-Tukey variant of the arcsine square root transformed proportion) suitable for the usual fixed and random effects summaries (20, 21). The pooled proportion was calculated as the back transform of the weighted mean of the transformed proportions, using DerSimonian weights for the random effects model (22) in the presence of significant heterogeneity. The impact of heterogeneity on the pooled estimates of the individual outcomes of the meta-analysis was assessed with the Cochran Q statistic and I^2 test, which measure the inconsistency between the study results, which was interpreted as the approximate proportion of total variation in the study estimates that was due to heterogeneity rather than sampling error (23). I^2 values of 25, 50, and 75% are considered low, moderate, and high estimates, respectively (24). As the Cochran Q test has a low sensitivity for detecting heterogeneity, a P-value of < 0.1 was considered significant for the presence of statistical heterogeneity (25). The presence of publication bias was checked with the Begg funnel plot (26), which plots the proportion (in the X axis) against the standard error of the proportion (in the Y axis). In the absence of publication bias, the proportion estimates from smaller studies are expected to be scattered above and below the summary estimate, producing a triangular or funnel shape.

The ANA positivity in primarily pediatric onset morphea patients ranged from 5.9 to 68%. The pooled ANA positivity was 29.9% (95% CI 27.3–32.5%) by the random effects model (**Figure 2**). There was significant but low heterogeneity for ANA positivity (I^2 38.3%, Cochran Q statistic 16.2, P = 0.008). Subanalyses were performed in attempt to identify patient characteristics or variables which may influence the heterogeneity, such as sex and subtype. Female sex had non-significant ($p = 0.21$) effect on the ANA+ heterogeneity. Age of patient had a significant effect on ANA+ heterogeneity ($p = 0.0001$), with the pediatric onset cohorts having more consistent ANA+ frequency compared to adult cohorts. When dichotomizing morphea subtype into linear (linear extremity/trunk and head) vs. nonlinear (generalized, plaque, deep morphea), there was also a significant impact on ANA+ which was more moderate with I^2 68%.

Although not directly related to the morphea subtype, ANA-positivity does seem to associate with disease severity in regards to the depth of the disease, association with ECMs, as well as

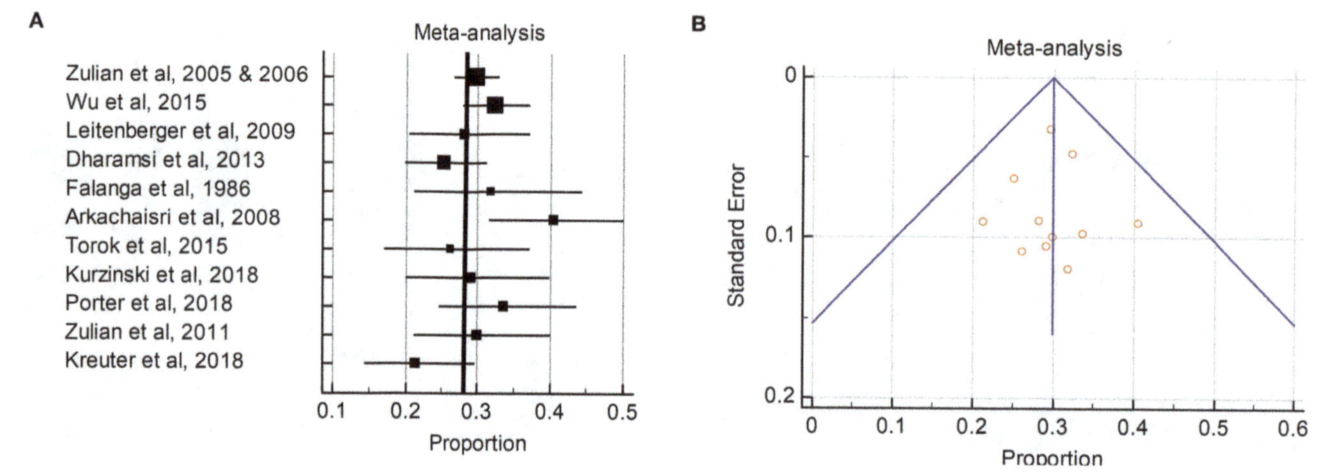

FIGURE 2 | Pooled ANA positivity in patients with morphea: **(A)** The ANA positivity (percentages) in the individual studies are represented by squares, through which the horizontal lines represent the 95% CIs. The thick vertical line represents the pooled ANA positivity from these studies; **(B)** Funnel plot of the proportion vs. the standard error of the proportion for ANA positivity. The circles represent the trials included in the meta-analysis. The line in the center indicates the summary proportion. The other lines represent the 95% CIs. Asymmetry about the pooled proportion line is consistent with the presence of minimal publication bias.

with the probability of the disease flare after remission. A study of a large pediatric international cohort ($n = 750$) reported a significant association of extracutaneous manifestations with ANA positivity (13). In this cohort, there were 168 patients (22%) with ECMs, the most common being articular (47%), followed by neurologic, vascular, ocular, and autoimmune (13). When comparing skin involvement with extracutaneous involvement subjects, the authors also noted that the erythrocyte sedimentation rate, C-reactive protein, creatinine kinase, serum IgG, and rheumatoid factor were significantly elevated in those with ECMs. Rheumatoid factor has been measured by ELISA; other clinical tests were done following standard clinical procedures utilizing pre-determined normal range for the age of the patient per test. Noteworthy, each of these laboratory tests was available for at least 350 patients, which is a limitation of several other studies. The authors argued that the positive ANA in morphea patients might be associated with either deeper tissue involvement or with a more immunogenic or true "systemic" autoimmune disease. The latter is typically associated with a myriad of positive immune activation markers (ANA, ESR, CRP, IgG, and other autoantibodies discussed next).

Data from the second largest morphea cohort published, the Childhood Arthritis and Rheumatology Research Alliance (CARRA) North American registry cohort of 381 pediatric morphea, supports the notion of ANA positivity corresponding to deeper tissue involvement (14). Using IF on Hep-2 cells, standard laboratory evaluation and cut-off, the Childhood Arthritis and Rheumatology Research Alliance (CARRA) cohort demonstrated 48% ANA positivity with a significant association of non-cutaneous disease damage with ANA, specifically for the deeper tissues of the extremity with remaining joint contractures, muscle atrophy, and extremity shortening (**Supplementary Table 1**) (14). In addition to the depth of the disease into adjacent connective tissue, ANA positivity has also been associated with cutaneous disease extent. The MAC cohort based in Texas (USA) and the National Registry of Childhood Onset Scleroderma (NRCOS) based in Pittsburgh (USA) both found that the extent of this skin disease (body surface area, number of lesions, number of areas affected, and mRSS) to be significantly associated with ANA positivity (19, 27). Similar to CARRA, the MAC cohort was tested using IF on Hep-2 cells, internal laboratory quality control, and healthy controls. Interpretation of the results has been standardized using a serum dilution series on the cells, and automated data processing to exclude the interlaboratory deviation.

In a prospective clinical cohort, the NRCOS, with full longitudinal data available from 77 morphea patients and an average follow-up of 5 years, a positive ANA at the baseline visit increased the odds of relapse (after obtaining remission) by a factor of 4.8 (95% CI [1.37–17.2]) (28). The same group more recently studied ANA positivity and more classic SSc-related autoantibodies in the NRCOS cohort (**Supplementary Table 1**). Utilizing an ANA cut-off of 1:160 via indirect immunofluorescence (IF) on Hep2 cells, 50% (35/69) pediatric morphea patients had ANA positivity, with one-third having 1:160 titer and decreasing percentages as the titer level increased, but as many as 11% had a titer of 1:1520. The most common pattern was speckled (50%), followed by homogenous, nucleolar, and centrosome (29). A panel of SSc-associated autoantibodies, including anti-topoisomerase (Scl-70), anti-centromere, U3RNP, and PM-Scl, was evaluated on all 69 subjects and were all found to be positive for 6–16% of the morphea subjects. The FIDIS™ Connective Profile SSc line immunoassay (LIA) (Euroimmun, Germany) and MagPix® (Luminex™) addressable laser bead immunoassay (ALBIA) were used to analyse morphea subject sera positivity in relation to age and sex matched healthy pediatric controls [cut-off two standard deviations (SDs) above the mean]. In general, when positive, these SSc-associated autoantibodies did not signify the diagnosis of SSc or the internal organ manifestations typically associated with SSc but correlated with morphea disease severity, such as joint contractures, musculoskeletal involvement, and skin symptoms of tingling, pain, and skin thickness (29). This supports the hypothesis that morphea (localized scleroderma) is "not just a skin disease" but that it is truly an autoimmune disease with circulating autoantibodies, associated with deeper tissue disease and more extensive connective tissue disease (28, 29).

The significant correlation of ANA and associated extrable nuclear autoantibodies with the depth of tissue involvement, extracutanous manifestations and potential for relapse in morphea, places ANA as a potential biomarker for morphea disease stratification and management, either individually or as a composite indictor with clinical variables, such as the mLoSSI, and other immune markers, such as cytokines of interest in the field, CXCL9 and CXCL10 (30, 31). CARRA investigators support ANA positivity in the prediction of muscle involvement, as is was associated with muscle atrophy, joint contracture and/or limb shortening, along with elevated muscle enzymes, CPK and aldolase, in a large North American cohort (32). A positive ANA at the baseline clinical visit for a morphea patient should prompt the clinician to closely monitor (1) the depth of the lesion, which may include further evaluation with MRI of the fascia, muscle, tendon and joint, especially the linear and generalized plaque morphea subtypes (33, 34), and (2) clinical signs of disease relapse, both during quiescent disease while on treatment and after systemic treatment course is completed (28, 35). The design of clinical trials for morphea are currently under discussion, with inclusion of ANA and other autoantibodies as exploratory biomarkers.

Anti-histone and ss-DNA Antibodies in Morphea

In an original report of a Japanese cohort studied in the 1990s (36), anti-histone antibodies (AHAs) were positive in 47% (23/49) of the cohort. This was studied by immunoblotting and ELISA, using manual data processing, internal quality control, and a titration curve from certified tests for quantification purposes. AHA titers correlated positively with the number of lesions, larger distribution of lesions, and muscle involvement. More recent large cohort analyses in North America and Europe have also studied AHA positivity in morphea and have found similar associations (**Figure 3; Supplementary Table 2**). A North American nested case-control study, including both pediatric and adult morphea subjects ($n = 187$) and age, sex, and race-matched controls ($n = 149$) who were all tested for AHA via ELISA, found a significant difference in AHA positivity between morphea subjects and controls (12 vs. 2%, $p < 0.001$) (19). AHA positivity was more frequently present in the linear morphea subtype compared to the generalized plaque morphea (18 vs. 7%, $p = 0.04$) (19). The AHA may indeed associate with the linear morphea subtype, as the other large North American cohort, the NRCOS, consisting of 60% patients with linear disease subtype, reports a relatively high AHA positivity (32–39%) in a longitudinal study of subjects (30, 38). Consistent with original findings in Japan (36), in this North American cohort, AHA correlated with general disease burden, such as number of lesions and number of sites with skin involvement, especially if $\geq$ two cutaneous sites (as dictated by the LoSCAT score) were affected. AHA levels also correlated with the depth of the lesion, reflected by the presence of joint contractures (27, 30, 38). Although the AHA seemed to predict severity, it was not found to be a predictor of disease relapse prospectively in the NRCOS cohort (28).

Interestingly, in NRCOS, the AHA levels did have some immunological correlation to T-helper (T_H) cell-associated cytokines evaluated by Luminex, including T_H1-associated cytokines (IL-12p70, IFN- γ, IL-2), T_H2-associated cytokines (Il-4, IL-13), and T_H17 associated cytokines (IL-17a, IL-17e, IL-17f, IL-d22, IL-23) (37). The Luminex assay has been standardized using age-matched healthy controls and internal laboratory quality control. Sensitivity down to a couple of molecules/uL samples is a great advantage of a Luminex detection methodology; in addition, all data have been processed automatically. Immune activation, reflected by cutaneous disease activity, was noted in this cohort's earlier reports, with a subset of patients having longitudinal changes in their AHA levels corresponding to changes in the disease activity status (38).

Around the same time the AHA was being described in morphea, the research group in Pittsburgh identified an antibody to DNA in morphea. Originally it was thought to be directed to double-stranded (ds) DNA, but an investigation with the *Crithidia lucillae* IF assay determined negative antibodies to double-stranded DNA (a-dsDNA), but a positive anti-single stranded DNA (a-ssDNA) antibodies (27). Herein, internal laboratory control and a non-matched healthy cohorts were applied, and the data was processed automatically. Further, the study of 39 patients in this cohort found that 51% of the morphea subjects had positive anti-ssDNA, with a positive correlation between anti-ssDNA antibody and joint contracture or active disease with a duration of longer than 2 years (27) (**Supplementary Table 2**). These general findings were validated in a Japanese cohort, led by Takehara and Sato, who found 50% morphea subjects with a positive anti-ssDNA, which correlated with deeper involvement of the muscle and fascia (39). Anti-ssDNA levels also correlated positively with the disease activity in a subgroup of patients (39). Later studies in the childhood-onset Pittsburgh cohort, NRCOS, continued to find anti-ssDNA positivity in ~30–44% of their morphea subjects, associated with more extensive skin involvement, active disease, and inflammatory cytokines IFN-α2 and IL-33, signifying immunologically active disease (30, 38). Noteworthy, anti-ssDNA positivity did not predict relapse in this cohort followed longitudinally (28).

Double positivity for AHA and anti-ssDNA was associated with a more severe morphea phenotype with deep tissue involvement and joint contracture, especially in childhood-onset, but also adult onset (38). In contrast, the other North American cohort, MAC, found a much lower positivity of anti-ssDNA, finding 6–8% positivity among combined adult and pediatric-onset morphea, which was not significantly different from their control cohort (7%) (19, 40). It is unclear why there is a degree of difference, potentially due to the different testing methods (41),

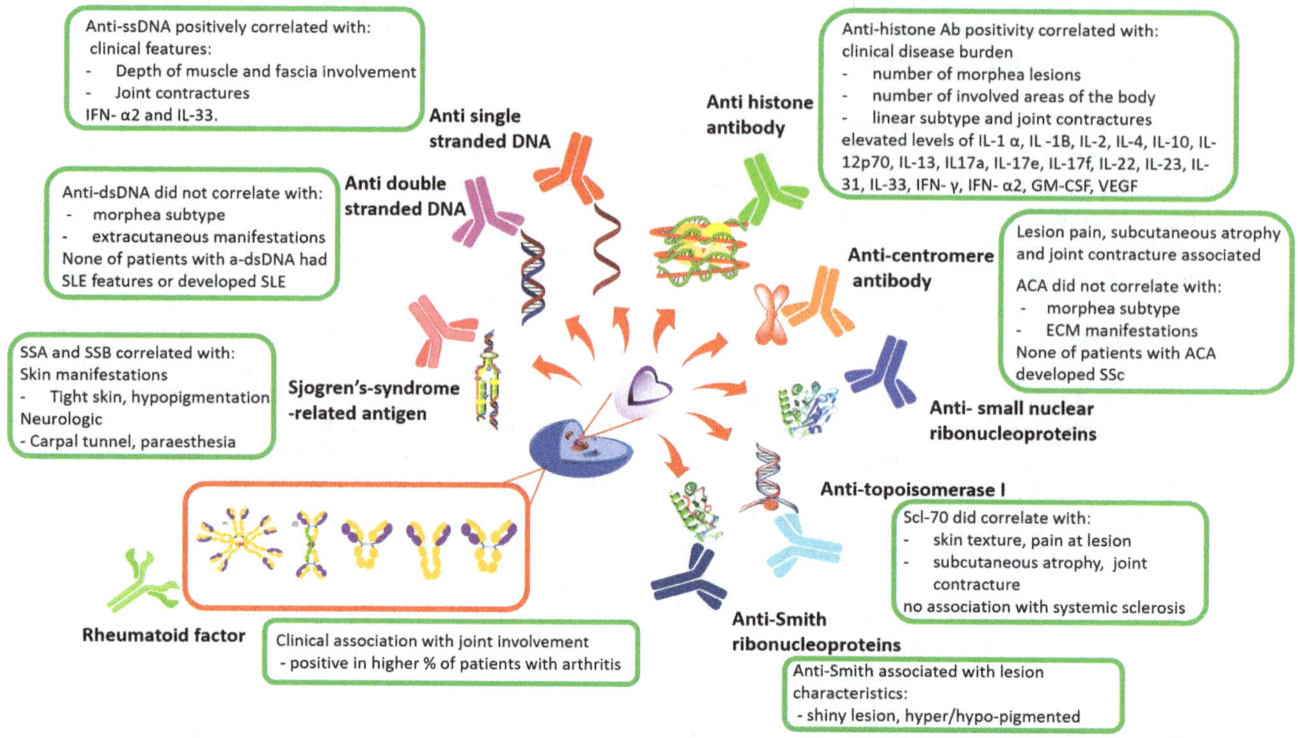

FIGURE 3 | General overview of morphea autoantibodies in relation to clinical features. Anti-ssDNA, Anti-single stranded DNA; IFNx, Interferon; ILx, Interleukin; SSA, Sjogren's-syndrome-related antigen A; SSB, Sjogren's-syndrome-related antigen B; Scl-70, Topoisomerase I; ACA, Anti-centromere antibody; ECM, Extracutaneous manifestations; SSc, Systemic Sclerosis; SLE, Systemic lupus erythematosus; GM-CSF, Granulocyte-macrophage colony-stimulating factor; VEGF, Vascular endothelial growth factor; Ab, Antibody (9, 10, 13, 18, 19, 27–30, 37, 38).

ELISA compared to IF. IF is believed to be more accurate. IF also has an automated data processing vs. the often manually performed ELISA.

In the dermatology-based United States cohort, the MAC cohort, patients with a double positivity for ss-DNA and AHA or ANA, indicated more severe morphea including functional limitations in linear disease (anti-ssDNA, $p = 0.005$; and AHA, $p = 0.006$), extensive body surface area involvement (anti-ssDNA, $p = 0.01$; and ANA, $p = 0.005$), and higher skin damage (ANA, $p = 0.004$) (19).

In concert with the ANA's ability to reflect deeper disease, such as fascia, muscle, and joint involvement, with resultant joint contractures, AHA and ss-DNA positivity share this relationship and could guide the clinician's management. This would include a more complete examination of the underlying connective tissue with a thorough joint examination and the use of available adjunct measures to monitor the depth and activity status of morphea in deeper tissues, such as MRI and Ultrasound (33, 34). A combination of positive antibodies between ANA, AHA, and ss-DNA should signify to the clinician a more severe immunophenotype with potential progression to joint contracture, which may influence decisions to initiate systemic medications and the length of treatment. Unlike ANA positivity at the baseline assessment, AHA and anti-ssDNA antibodies do not appear to influence disease relapse to assist in assessment of recurrence.

Systemic Sclerosis and Systemic Lupus Erythematosus Autoantibodies in Morphea

Antibodies against the traditional extractable nuclear antigens (ENAs), such as anti-dsDNA, SSA/B, Smith/RNP, anti-Scl-70, and anti-centromere Abs, are seldom in morphea, with general percentages of positivity ranging from 1 to 15% internationally in both pediatric and adult onset morphea [**Supplementary Table 3**; (9, 10, 13, 18, 29)]. These serum autoantibodies were obtained clinically, and abnormal values were referenced to the normal range of laboratory parameters of each of the participating centers. It is important to note that clinical development of the connective tissue diseases typically associated with these ENAs, such as SLE, Sjogrens' or SSc, was not documented in any of these cohort studies (**Supplementary Table 3**). Only a few studies investigated clinical associations of morphea patients with these ENAs. The international pediatric cohort compared morphea subtype and presence of extracutaneous manifestation with the presence of ds-DNA, Scl-70, and centromere antibodies and did not find any associations (13, 18). However, in the prospectively collected NRCOS cohort, when comparing detailed clinical variables of morphea, such as lesion characteristics of thickness, subcutaneous atrophy, and patient symptoms, such as pain at site of the lesion, more correlations were detected with these ENAs (**Supplementary Table 3**) (29).

Rheumatoid Factor

Rheumatoid factor (RF), which is typically associated with adult rheumatoid arthritis, was positive in 3–16% of morphea patients in the reported cohorts internationally (**Supplementary Table 3**). These serum RF values were obtained clinically, and abnormal values were referenced to the normal range of laboratory parameters of each of the participating centers. The largest cohort tested were childhood-onset patients ($n = 464$). Of this cohort, 16% of subjects were RF positive which correlated positively with arthritis and musculoskeletal manifestations (18), providing evidence for increased clinical monitoring of the joints of positive RF patients (42–44).

ROLE OF AUTOANTIBODIES IN THE PATHOGENESIS OF MORPHEA

There are several recent studies aimed at an improved understanding of the basic biology of morphea. A better understanding of the underlying mechanisms in morphea, especially during the active inflammatory phase, would lead to more direct and efficient therapies (45). According to Jacobe et al. specific HLA class I and class II alleles are associated with generalized and linear subtypes of morphea (40). Notably, the morphea-associated alleles are different from those found in SSc, suggesting that morphea is immunogenetically distinct. Risk alleles in morphea are also associated with conditions such as rheumatoid arthritis (RA) and other autoimmune conditions (40). The role of HLA products in regulating interactions of immune cells is well-known (46), and therefore, the specific HLA profile of morphea could lead to B cells producing certain cytokines and autoantibodies contributing to disease progression (40, 47).

Cytokine and autoantibody profiles and their relationship to clinical features in morphea have been described. It is believed that the imbalance between Th1/Th2/Th17 cell subsets drives inflammation in the early stages of disease (Th1 and Th17 predominant) and fibrosis in the later stages of morphea (Th2 predominant) (47). As in SSc, T-helper (Th) cells and their associated cytokines have been suggested to contribute significantly to the pathophysiology of the disease. This was confirmed by the presence of cytokines from Th cells in the sera and tissues of patients (**Figure 4**) (37).

Kurzinski and Torok analyzed the available experimental data on cytokines in morphea and compared them to available clinical disease severity and activity features (37). They confirmed that cytokines of Th1, Th2, and Th17 cell responses likely contribute to the pathogenesis of both SSc and morphea. Prior studies support the theory of Th1/Th2 imbalance in SSc propagating disease in a Th2 manner, leading to skin fibrosis and damage. Early presence of the pro-inflammatory cytokines IL-2 and IL-6 inducing Th17 in morphea patients suggests that an early increase of Th1 cytokines mediates the active, inflammatory phase of the disease (which was further supported by their later work) (30), and the subsequent inflammation and transition to the fibrotic damage phase is achieved via Th17. This is further supported by the elevated Th17 effector cytokines 2–4 years after the initial onset of disease. In turn, Th2 effector cytokines shown to be present at elevated levels in morphea promote the development of tissue damage and fibrosis later in the course of the disease (37).

Badea et al. reviewed step-wise development of morphea (**Figure 4**) (48). In early inflammatory stages, environmental stimuli and genetic factors activate mononuclear cells that in turn induce perivascular infiltration of the skin. At this stage, ANA, cytokines, and other soluble cell-adhesion molecules are elevated, confirming on-going immune activation. At stage 2, functional and structural changes occurred to the microvascular system, and adhesion molecules including ICAM-1 and VCAM-1, were upregulated in response to various cytokines and cell mediators (IFN-γ, IL-1, TNFs). The third stage is the least understood, and it is believed to involve a large release of cytokines by the lymphocytes. IL-4, IL-6, and IL-8 are among those overproduced cytokines. Stage four involves hardening of the skin from excessive cellular proliferation and deposition of collagen and other extracellular matrix components. This stage of LS progression has the most deleterious effects and is believed to be driven by excess IL-4 and TGF-β (48). This general pathogenesis model has been confirmed by *in vitro* studies in cohorts of morphea patients at different disease stages, and by knock-out mouse models (Tsk). Using novel antigens *in vivo* could bring new insights into pathogenesis. Moreover, detailed studies of T and B cell populations in morphea vs. controls, e.g., SSc and psoriasis, are lacking (49).

Osmola-Mankowska et al. added new knowledge to the existing picture of morphea pathogenesis, by proposing the underseen role of dendritic cells (DCs) in it (**Figure 4**) (50). In brief, an unknown natural ligand activates DC to produce IFN-α and IFN-β that in turn activate myeloid DCs (mDCs). mDCs activate autoreactive B and T cells via MHC molecules, which then leads to skin autoimmunity and morphea in particular. The hypothesis has been confirmed by both *in vitro* and *in vivo* studies and is an exciting new knowledge with potential therapeutic outcomes (50). T-cell subtyping has been successfully used to identify *in vivo* the regulatory pathways associated with morphea, specifically, confirming that apoptotic bodies bearing CD8, activate CD205 of DCs. This knowledge allows the application of already existing therapies to morphea, such as pDC regulating SLE drug candidates (Anti-BDCA-2 Abs and nanobodies).

Verification of the role of autoantibodies in morphea is complicated by only a few available animal models. Marangoni et al. reviewed available models of scleroderma (51) and provided details on nine key mouse models available today, created by exogenous administration of fibrosis-inducing agents (bleomycin, Ad-TGFβ1$^{223/225}$), and by genetic manipulation (e.g., Tsk-2 and Fbn-1 mutants). The high diversity of skin disease symptoms complicates creating a reliable model for morphea. The authors suggest using genome-wide expression analysis to match the animal models to the appropriate subtypes of human clinical disease. Additionally, there is a high deviation in methodology for inducing scleroderma pathogenesis with bleomycin and Ad-TGFβ1$^{223/225}$ that remains unresolved. In spite of this, mouse models of cutaneous fibrosis are proven to

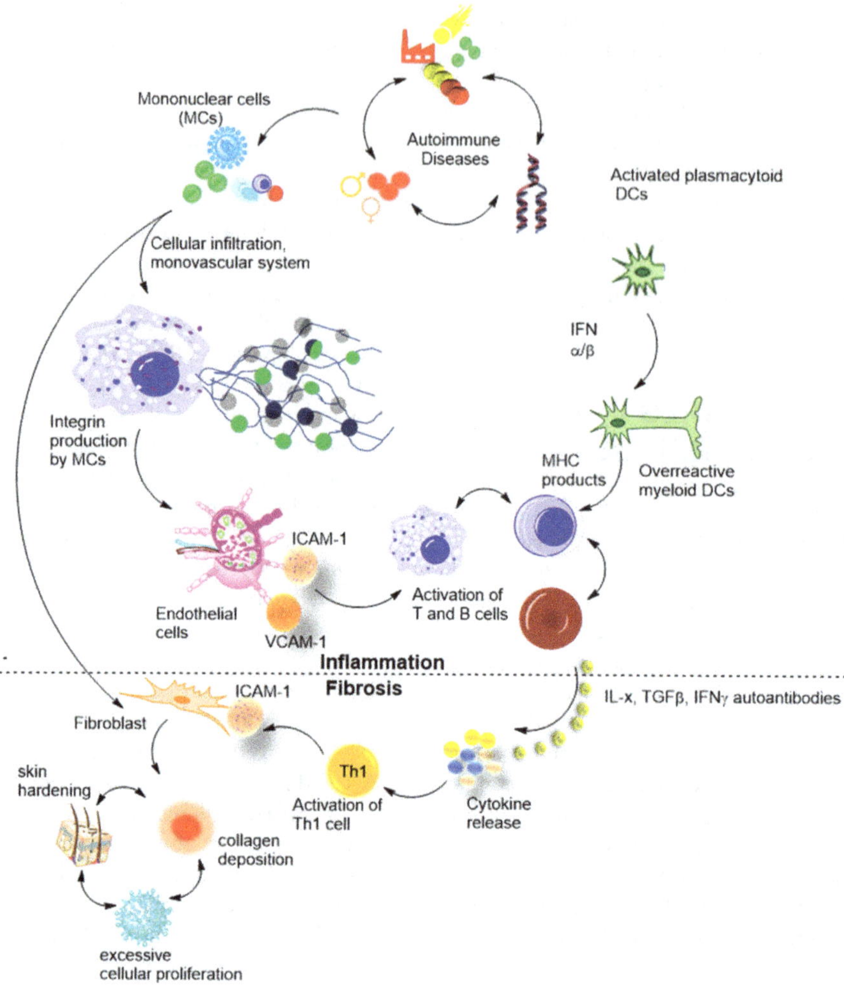

FIGURE 4 | Biological mechanisms involved in morphea, and suggested roles of cytokines and autoantibodies.

be useful to study underlying mechanisms of the disease and its linkage to other conditions (51).

Several other mouse models of skin fibrosis were reported as useful to study the onset of the disease (52). Tsk1 and Tsk2 models are developed through mutations in fibrillin gene *FBN1* leading to fibrinogenesis. It is known that fibrillin-1 is a component of connective tissue microfibrils and is important in correcting elastic fiber assembly. Second, fibrillin-1 can partially control TGF-β availability via confirmed interactions with TGF-β binding proteins 1 and 4. Genetic analysis of 6-week-old Tsk mutant mice indicated morphea related effects: upregulated collagen synthesis, increased bone morphogenic protein, and connective tissue growth factor. Additionally, Wnt signaling proteins that interfere with TGF-β are overproduced. With regard to serology, 88% of Tsk mutant models are ANA positive, and also contain AHA, anti-Scl-70, and anti-RNApol II antibodies (52). This makes Tsk models potent tools for studying autoantibodies in morphea. A limitation is the fact that Tsk model lacks inflammation histologically, therefore it reflects SSc skin condition more than morphea skin. Bleomycin-induced mouse is an alternative to Tsk for studies of morphea which develops a skin inflammation and a set of autoantibodies (51, 52).

EMERGING AUTOANTIBODY BIOMARKERS IN MORPHEA

Autoantibodies to the dense fine speckled 70 kDa antigen (anti-DFS70) is a hot topic in autoimmune research and diagnostics at the moment. Anti-DFS70 are reported to be more common in individuals who do not have an antinuclear antibody (ANA)-associated rheumatic disease (AARD) than in patients with AARD. So far, the frequency of anti-DFS70 antibodies has been thoroughly studied in adults but not in pediatric populations. The primary objective of a recent observational study was to determine the frequency of anti-DFS70 in pediatric AARD including morphea, and reference cohorts (53). Sera from 743 children with AARD and related conditions and 345 samples from controls [healthy children and suspected for AARD] were tested for anti-DFS70 antibodies. Using a novel

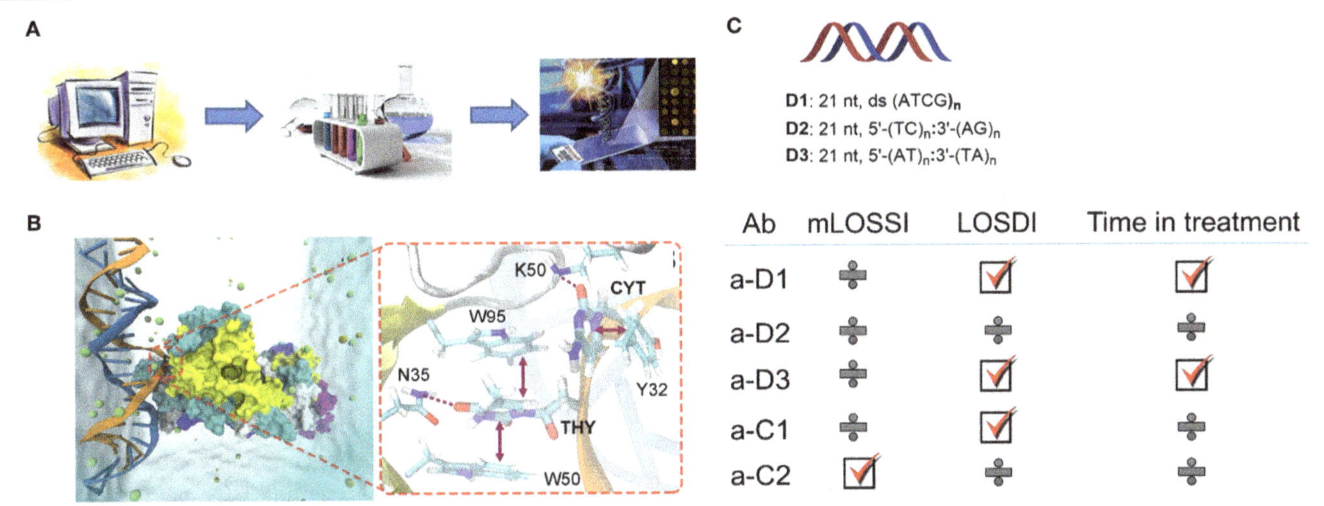

FIGURE 5 | Synthetic DNA, RNA, and LNA antigens in morphea (56). **(A)** A general approach to the design including computation, library screening, and ELISA; **(B)** representative molecular dynamics result for dsDNA antigen and autoantibody showing key interactions contributing to the binding; **(C)** Representative antigens selected for the study of the pediatric morphea cohort, and correlations of ELISA results with modified localized scleroderma skin severity index (mLOSSI), index of disease damage (LOSDI), and time in treatment. C1 and C2 were commercial controls used in the study, calf thymus DNA, and G-quadruplex human DNA.

chemiluminescence assay, anti-DFS70 antibodies were elevated in 2.1% of healthy children and 4.5% of sera from ANA positive pediatric samples. Information on standardization procedure was missing for anti-DFS70 that might lead to deviation from other cohorts. Notably, in line with previous studies which suggest an overlap of morphea with other diseases, the frequency of anti-DFS70 was highest in juvenile morphea (13.8%), along with juvenile dermatomyositis (18.2%), childhood SLE (5.7%), and juvenile idiopathic arthritis (2.5%) (53).

In our recent study, we developed a series of synthetic oligonucleotides (54, 55) that allowed us to investigate the details on the antigen recognition by autoimmune antibodies in pediatric morphea (**Figure 5**) (56). In this work, we hypothesized that having a sequence-controlled rationally designed DNA, RNA, and locked nucleic acid (LNA) antigen might provide new insights into sequence-specific binding of anti-ssDNA and anti-dsDNA. Typically used in nucleic acid diagnostics and gene therapy (57, 58) synthetic oligo- and poly-nucleotides are poorly explored in immunology. However, these molecules have major advantages of high purity, controlled chemical content and a possibility to incorporate functional tags (54, 55). To design new antigens which were 21–63 nucleotide long oligo- and polymers, we successfully combined computation and library screening (56, 59). The study has been benchmarked to SLE ($n = 30$) and healthy controls ($n = 80$); standardization has been done using internal laboratory control and external calibrators provided by Odense University Hospital, Denmark, and Stanford University Hospital, CA, USA. Besides dramatically improving the analytical specificity of the assay, our data suggest a potential link between antibodies to DNA and the disease state in morphea. Moreover, introducing chemical modification (LNA) into antigens completely changed the binding of corresponding antibodies and their clinical relevance. The strongest observed effect was seen for the localized scleroderma skin damage index (LoSDI) on the IgG antibodies to TC dinucleotide-rich dsDNA ($p < 0.001$) (56). Synthetic DNA and analogs are therefore a new promising class of antigens that could bring light into sequence specificity of anti-DNA antibodies in morphea and related diseases. Lack of confirmation for antigen-antibody reactivity in a relevant morphea animal model is a limitation of this work.

Looking for gene association of autoimmune diseases including morphea is a rapidly developing research field with high potential to provide new insights into pathogenesis and new biomarkers. Earlier, Torok et al. reported an up-regulated IFN-related gene CXCL10 in pediatric morphea subjects (30). Simultaneously, O'Brien et al. investigated transcriptional and cytokine profiles in 87 adult morphea subjects and 26 healthy controls (31). This study identified a disease severity association for CXCL9, which was present at increased levels in active morphea subjects (37%) along with Th1 cell cytokines (57%). Related gene CXCL10 was upregulated in 44% morphea subjects but did not correlate with disease severity (31). CXCL9/10 studies also led to a new hypothesis on the onset of morphea. As a result of cutaneous overproduction of IFN-γ by cutaneous macrophages, Th1 imbalance in the skin could be a contributing factor to disease progression. Thus, local skin autoimmunity could be the driver of the disease in contrast to the systemic dysregulation in SSc (31). In (31), a higher number of healthy controls and additional disease controls could be included to support this study.

CONCLUSIONS

As this review summarizes, morphea (localized scleroderma) is a complex disease with a diverse profile of clinical manifestations and still unresolved issues with serological diagnosis, clear knowledge on pathogenesis, and missing of effective management routes. In this scoping review, we selected studies based on the number of enrolled patients with autoantibody testing (≥50 patients), relevance to studies of morphea pathogenesis, and reported emerging animal models and biomarkers that could lead to improved personalized morphea management. Up to 50% of patients in cohorts described herein have elevated levels of three main autoantibodies: ANA, AHA, and anti-ssDNA, whereas other autoantibodies are observed at frequencies below 10%.

These autoantibodies associate with more severe disease, including lesion depth and spread, associating with more severe morphea subtypes and extracutaneous manifestations. The presence of two or more of these autoantibodies appears to have a cumulative effect on correlation to disease affecting the deep muscle, fasica and tendons, resulting in joint contracture and limited mobility. Rheumatoid factor also appears to be a strong indicator of deeper tissue disease with arthritis association. Taken together, patients with ANA, AHA, ss-DNA, or RF positivity in isolation, or more importantly in combination, are at higher risk for muscle and joint morbidity. Extra care should be taken to ensure these patients have a detailed musculoskeletal examination (in addition to a thorough cutaneous assessment), and if possible, consider imaging deeper tissue to monitor the depth of moprhea involvement and the disease activity status (i.e.,–edema of the fascia on MRI).

Furthermore, morphea patients with multiple autoantibody positivity might have a more robust B cell activation, promoting such antibodies, and may benefit from anti-CD20 therapy, such as Rituximab, currently available for rheumatoid arthritis and other connective tissue disease indications (60). Only a few case reports are available evaluating Rituximab in morphea, but do show successful response (including improvement of deeper tissue via MRI evaluation) in previous recalcitrant disease (61, 62). Another potential therapeutic target in morphea is between the T cell and antigen presenting cell (DC or B-cell) communication, via abatacept, a fusion protein that inhibits CD80/86 interaction with CD28. This can dampen B cell:T-cell interactions and T-cell functional activation, which in turn would lead to less inflammatory driven fibrosis and potentially less auto-antibody production. A few cases reports have described successful treatment of morphea with abatacept, especially widespread disease or deeper disease (monitored by MRI in some) (63–65). Further clinical studies in trial format are warranted to further understand the utility of these biologic agents in treating morphea.

Pathogenesis of morphea remains being a black box, although there are several recent works that bring new knowledge to the field. The reported association with HLA I and HLA II alleles defined by Jacobe et al., could be a breakthrough in the genotype based diagnosis, subtyping and research on morphea (40). Genomic association with CXCL9 is another exciting direction toward these goals (31). Recently, a role of DCs in the critical step of morphea development has been recently confirmed (50). Tsk animal models show high levels of autoantibodies and similar fibrotic skin features to human morphea, making Tsk mouse a valuable model for further studies, although the inflammatory state is somewhat limited in the Tsk mouse (51, 52). As more information is gained about the underlying mechanisms of morphea, diagnosis and treatments can become more accurate and better personalized. Importantly, improving scleroderma patients' early diagnosis before extracutaneous manifestations occur should improve patients long term recovery (45, 66).

Furthermore, beneficial autoantibodies having protective effects against the development of immune-mediated diseases and conventional antibodies depend on the activation of T and B lymphocytes by antigen presenting DCs and share common ontogeny (67, 68). Thus, it is suspected that the disturbance in the homeostasis of autoantibodies can trigger autoimmune diseases. Cabral-Marques reported that dysregulation of autoantibody-targeting G protein-coupled receptors (GPCRs) can trigger the development of rheumatic diseases including rheumatoid arthritis and SSc. Sera from 84 patients with SSc and 491 healthy controls were tested for anti- GPCRs antibodies. Using commercial solid-phase sandwich ELISA, anti-GPCRs concentration were either elevated or decreased in sera of SSc and rheumatoid arthritis in contrast to healthy samples. Hence, the discovery of anti-GPCR autoantibodies in pathogenesis of rheumatic diseases opens up opportunities for new investigations in autoimmune diseases including morphea and SSc (68).

The potential impact of synthetic biology and computational chemistry in improving the efficacy and specificity of existing antigens might present an exciting new approach in the management of morphea. For example, a combined computation and library screening provided with a new TC rich dsDNA antigen that allows for detecting autoantibodies associated with skin damage index.

Increased evidence shows that environmental factors and other diseases may have an impact on morphea. Emerging biomarkers including anti-DFS70 and anti-LNA/DNA, aim at detecting these associations, which opens up new pathways for managing difficult and rare cases of morphea (69, 70).

AUTHOR CONTRIBUTIONS

SK and KA: prepared initial draft. All authors collected and analyzed data and research papers, prepared graphics, proof read the paper, and prepared the final version.

REFERENCES

1. Cotton CV, Spencer LG, New RP, Cooper RG. The utility of comprehensive autoantibody testing to differentiate connective tissue disease associated and idiopathic interstitial lung disease subgroup cases. *Rheumatology.* (2017) 56:1264–71. doi: 10.1093/rheumatology/kew320
2. Kontny E, Lewandowska-Poluch A, Chmielinska M, Olesinska M. Subgroups of Sjögren's syndrome patients categorised by serological profiles: clinical and immunological characteristics. *Reumatologia.* (2018) 56:346–53. doi: 10.5114/reum.2018.80711
3. Navallas M, Inarejos Clemente EJ, Iglesias E, Rebollo-Polo M, Antón J, Navarro OM. Connective tissue disorders in childhood: are they all the same? *Radiographics.* (2019) 39:229–50. doi: 10.1148/rg.2019180078
4. Steen VD, Medsger TA. Improvement in skin thickening in systemic sclerosis associated with improved survival. *Arthritis Rheum.* (2001) 44:2828–35. doi: 10.1002/1529-0131(200112)44:12<2828::AID-ART470>3.0.CO;2-U
5. Bernatsky S, Joseph L, Pineau CA, Belisle P, Hudson M, Clarke AE. Scleroderma prevalence: demographic variations in a population-based sample. *Arthritis Rheum.* (2009) 61:400–4. doi: 10.1002/art.24339
6. Laxer RM, Zulian F. Localized scleroderma. *Curr Opin Rheumatol.* (2006) 18:606–13. doi: 10.1097/01.bor.0000245727.40630.c3
7. Ardalan K, Zigler CK, Torok KS. Predictors of longitudinal quality of life in juvenile localized scleroderma. *Arthritis Care Res.* (2017) 69:1082–7. doi: 10.1002/acr.23101
8. Condie D, Grabell D, Jacobe H. Comparison of outcomes in adults with pediatric-onset morphea and those with adult-onset morphea: a cross-sectional study from the morphea in adults and children cohort. *Arthritis Rheumatol.* (2014) 66:3496–504. doi: 10.1002/art.38853
9. Kreuter A, Wischnewski J, Terras S, Altmeyer P, Stücker M, Gambichler T. Coexistence of lichen sclerosus and morphea: a retrospective analysis of 472 patients with localized scleroderma from a German tertiary referral center. *J Am Acad Dermatol.* (2012) 67:1157–62. doi: 10.1016/j.jaad.2012.04.003
10. Leitenberger JJ, Cayce RL, Haley RW, Adams-Huet B, Bergstresser PR, Jacobe HT. Distinct autoimmune syndromes in morphea: a review of 245 adult and pediatric cases. *Arch Dermatol.* (2009) 145:545–50. doi: 10.1001/archdermatol.2009.79
11. Li SC. Scleroderma in children and adolescents: localized scleroderma and systemic sclerosis. *Pediatr Clin North Am.* (2018) 65:757–81. doi: 10.1016/j.pcl.2018.04.002
12. Li SC, Li X, Pope E, Stewart K, Higgins GC, Rabinovich CE, et al. New features for measuring disease activity in pediatric localized scleroderma. *J Rheumatol.* (2018) 45:1680–8. doi: 10.3899/jrheum.171381
13. Zulian F, Vallongo C, Woo P, Russo R, Ruperto N, Harper J, et al. Localized scleroderma in childhood is not just a skin disease. *Arthritis Rheum.* (2005) 52:2873–81. doi: 10.1002/art.21264
14. *Description of the Juvenile Localized Scleroderma Subgroup of the Childhood Arthritis and Rheumatology Research Alliance (CARRA) Registry—ACR Meeting Abstracts.* Available online at: https://acrabstracts.org/abstract/description-of-the-juvenile-localized-scleroderma-subgroup-of-the-childhood-arthritis-and-rheumatology-research-alliance-carra-registry/ (accessed May 25, 2019).
15. Kister I, Inglese M, Laxer RM, Herbert J. Neurologic manifestations of localized scleroderma: a case report and literature review. *Neurology.* (2008) 71:1538–45. doi: 10.1212/01.wnl.0000334474.88923.e3
16. Moko SB, Mistry Y, Blandin de Chalain TM. Parry-Romberg syndrome: intracranial MRI appearances. *J Craniomaxillofac Surg.* (2003) 31:321–4. doi: 10.1016/S1010-5182(03)00028-3
17. Arkachaisri T, Vilaiyuk S, Torok KS, Medsger TA. Development and initial validation of the localized scleroderma skin damage index and physician global assessment of disease damage: a proof-of-concept study. *Rheumatology.* (2010) 49:373–81. doi: 10.1093/rheumatology/kep361
18. Zulian F, Athreya BH, Laxer R, Nelson AM, Feitosa de Oliveira SK, Punaro MG, et al. Juvenile localized scleroderma: clinical and epidemiological features in 750 children. An international study. *Rheumatology.* (2006) 45:614–20. doi: 10.1093/rheumatology/kei251
19. Dharamsi JW, Victor S, Aguwa N, Ahn C, Arnett F, Mayes MD, et al. Morphea in adults and children cohort III: nested case-control study–the clinical significance of autoantibodies in morphea. *JAMA Dermatol.* (2013) 149:1159–65. doi: 10.1001/jamadermatol.2013.4207
20. Freeman MF, Tukey JW. Transformations related to the angular and the square root. *Ann Math Statist.* (1950) 21:607–11. doi: 10.1214/aoms/1177729756
21. Miller JJ. The inverse of the Freeman – Tukey double arcsine transformation. *Am Stat.* (1978) 32:138. doi: 10.1080/00031305.1978.10479283
22. DerSimonian R, Laird N. Meta-analysis in clinical trials. *Control Clin Trials.* (1986) 7:177–88. doi: 10.1016/0197-2456(86)90046-2
23. www.iecs.org.ar/cochrane/guias/Handbook_4-2-2.pdf
24. Higgins JPT, Thompson SG. Quantifying heterogeneity in a meta-analysis. *Stat Med.* (2002) 21:1539–58. doi: 10.1002/sim.1186
25. Lau J, Ioannidis JP, Schmid CH. Quantitative synthesis in systematic reviews. *Ann Intern Med.* (1997) 127:820–6. doi: 10.7326/0003-4819-127-9-199711010-00008
26. Dear KBG, Begg CB. An approach for assessing publication bias prior to performing a meta-analysis. *Stat Sci.* (1992) 7:237–45. doi: 10.1214/ss/1177011363
27. Falanga V, Medsger TA, Reichlin M, Rodnan GP. Linear scleroderma. Clinical spectrum, prognosis, and laboratory abnormalities. *Ann Intern Med.* (1986) 104:849–57. doi: 10.7326/0003-4819-104-6-849
28. Kurzinski KL, Zigler CK, Torok KS. Prediction of disease relapse in a cohort of paediatric patients with localized scleroderma. *Br J Dermatol.* (2019) 180:1183–9. doi: 10.1111/bjd.17312
29. *Autoantibody Testing in Pediatric Localized Scleroderma (LS) - ACR Meeting Abstracts.* Available online at: https://acrabstracts.org/abstract/autoantibody-testing-in-pediatric-localized-scleroderma-ls/ (accessed March 27, 2019)
30. Torok KS, Kurzinski K, Kelsey C, Yabes J, Magee K, Vallejo AN, et al. Peripheral blood cytokine and chemokine profiles in juvenile localized scleroderma: T-helper cell-associated cytokine profiles. *Semin Arthritis Rheum.* (2015) 45:284–93. doi: 10.1016/j.semarthrit.2015.06.006
31. O'Brien JC, Rainwater YB, Malviya N, Cyrus N, Auer-Hackenberg L, Hynan LS, et al. Transcriptional and cytokine profiles identify CXCL9 as a biomarker of disease activity in morphea. *J Invest Dermatol.* (2017) 137:1663–70. doi: 10.1016/j.jid.2017.04.008
32. Wu EY, Li SC, Torok KS, Virkud YV, Fuhlbrigge RC, Rabinovich CE, et al. Baseline description of the juvenile localized scleroderma subgroup from the childhood arthritis and rheumatology research alliance legacy registry. *ACR Open Rheumatol.* (2019) 1:119–24. doi: 10.1002/acr2.1019
33. Eutsler EP, Horton DB, Epelman M, Finkel T, Averill LW. Musculoskeletal MRI findings of juvenile localized scleroderma. *Pediatr Radiol.* (2017) 47:442–9. doi: 10.1007/s00247-016-3765-x
34. Schanz S, Henes J, Ulmer A, Kötter I, Fierlbeck G, Claussen CD, et al. Response evaluation of musculoskeletal involvement in patients with deep morphea treated with methotrexate and prednisolone: a combined MRI and clinical approach. *Am J Roentgenol.* (2013) 200:W376–82. doi: 10.2214/AJR.12.9335
35. Mirsky L, Chakkittakandiyil A, Laxer RM, O'Brien C, Pope E. Relapse after systemic treatment in pediatric morphoea. *Br J Dermatol.* (2012) 166:443–5. doi: 10.1111/j.1365-2133.2011.10535.x
36. Sato S, Ihn H, Soma Y, Igarashi A, Tamaki T, Kikuchi K, et al. Antihistone antibodies in patients with localized scleroderma. *Arthritis Rheum.* (1993) 36:1137–41. doi: 10.1002/art.1780360815
37. Kurzinski K, Torok KS. Cytokine profiles in localized scleroderma and relationship to clinical features. *Cytokine.* (2011) 55:157–64. doi: 10.1016/j.cyto.2011.04.001
38. Arkachaisri T, Fertig N, Pino S, Medsger TA. Serum autoantibodies and their clinical associations in patients with childhood- and adult-onset linear scleroderma. A single-center study. *J Rheumatol.* (2008) 35:2439–44. doi: 10.3899/jrheum.080098
39. Takehara K, Sato S. Localized scleroderma is an autoimmune disorder. *Rheumatology.* (2005) 44:274–9. doi: 10.1093/rheumatology/keh487
40. Jacobe H, Ahn C, Arnett FC, Reveille JD. Major histocompatibility complex class I and class II alleles may confer susceptibility to or protection against morphea: findings from the Morphea in Adults and Children cohort. *Arthritis Rheumatol.* (2014) 66:3170–7. doi: 10.1002/art.38814
41. Takehara K, Moroi Y, Nakabayashi Y, Ishibashi Y. Antinuclear antibodies in localized scleroderma. *Arthritis Rheum.* (1983) 26:612–6. doi: 10.1002/art.1780260506

42. Zulian F, Vallongo C, Patrizi A, Belloni-Fortina A, Cutrone M, Alessio M, et al. A long-term follow-up study of methotrexate in juvenile localized scleroderma (morphea). *J Am Acad Dermatol.* (2012) 67:1151–6. doi: 10.1016/j.jaad.2012.03.036
43. Knobler R, Moinzadeh P, Hunzelmann N, Kreuter A, Cozzio A, Mouthon L, et al. European dermatology forum S1-guideline on the diagnosis and treatment of sclerosing diseases of the skin, Part 1: localized scleroderma, systemic sclerosis and overlap syndromes. *J Eur Acad Dermatol Venereol.* (2017) 31:1401–24. doi: 10.1111/jdv.14458
44. Mimura Y, Ihn H, Jinnin M, Asano Y, Yamane K, Tamaki K. Rheumatoid factor isotypes in localized scleroderma. *Clin Exp Dermatol.* (2005) 30:405–8. doi: 10.1111/j.1365-2230.2005.01776.x
45. Brady SM, Shapiro L, Mousa SA. Current and future direction in the management of scleroderma. *Arch Dermatol Res.* (2016) 308:461–71. doi: 10.1007/s00403-016-1647-6
46. Gough SCL, Simmonds MJ. The HLA region and autoimmune disease: associations and mechanisms of action. *Curr Genom.* (2007) 8:453–65. doi: 10.2174/138920207783591690
47. Hasegawa M, Fujimoto M, Kikuchi K, Takehara K. Elevated serum levels of interleukin 4 (IL-4), IL-10, and IL-13 in patients with systemic sclerosis. *J Rheumatol.* (1997) 24:328–32. doi: 10.1016/0923-1811(96)89424-2
48. Badea I, Taylor M, Rosenberg A, Foldvari M. Pathogenesis and therapeutic approaches for improved topical treatment in localized scleroderma and systemic sclerosis. *Rheumatology.* (2009) 48:213–21. doi: 10.1093/rheumatology/ken405
49. Caielli S, Veiga DT, Balasubramanian P, Athale S, Domic B, Murat E, et al. A CD4+ T cell population expanded in lupus blood provides B cell help through interleukin-10 and succinate. *Nat Med.* (2019) 25:75–81. doi: 10.1038/s41591-018-0254-9
50. Osmola-Mankowska A, Teresiak-Mikołajczak E, Danczak-Pazdrowska A, Kowalczyk M, Zaba R, Adamski Z. The role of dendritic cells and regulatory T cells in the pathogenesis of morphea. *Cent Eur J Immunol.* (2015) 40:103–8. doi: 10.5114/ceji.2015.50841
51. Marangoni RG, Varga J, Tourtellotte WG. Animal models of scleroderma: recent progress. *Curr Opin Rheumatol.* (2016) 28:561–70. doi: 10.1097/BOR.0000000000000331
52. Smith GP, Chan ESL. Molecular pathogenesis of skin fibrosis: insight from animal models. *Curr Rheumatol Rep.* (2010) 12:26–33. doi: 10.1007/s11926-009-0080-7
53. Schmeling H, Mahler M, Levy DM, Moore K, Stevens AM, Wick J, et al. Autoantibodies to dense fine speckles in pediatric diseases and controls. *J Rheumatol.* (2015) 42:2419–26. doi: 10.3899/jrheum.150567
54. Astakhova IK, Kumar TS, Campbell MA, Ustinov AV, Korshun VA, Wengel J. Branched DNA nanostructures efficiently stabilised and monitored by novel pyrene-perylene 2'-α-L-amino-LNA FRET pairs. *Chem Commun.* (2013) 49:511–3. doi: 10.1039/C2CC37547H
55. Astakhova IK, Pasternak K, Campbell MA, Gupta P, Wengel J. A locked nucleic acid-based nanocrawler: designed and reversible movement detected by multicolor fluorescence. *J Am Chem Soc.* (2013) 135:2423–6. doi: 10.1021/ja311250w
56. Samuelsen S, Jørgensen CD, Mellins ED, Torok KS, Astakhova K. Detection of autoimmune antibodies in localized scleroderma by synthetic oligonucleotide antigens. *PLoS ONE.* (2018) 13:e0195381. doi: 10.1371/journal.pone.0195381
57. Astakhova K. Toward non-enzymatic ultrasensitive identification of single nucleotide polymorphisms by optical methods. *Chemosensors.* (2014) 2:193–206. doi: 10.3390/chemosensors2030193
58. Taskova M, Madsen CS, Jensen KJ, Hansen LH, Vester B, Astakhova K. Antisense oligonucleotides internally labeled with peptides show improved target recognition and stability to enzymatic degradation. *Bioconjug Chem.* (2017) 28:768–74. doi: 10.1021/acs.bioconjchem.6b00567
59. Klecka M, Thybo C, Macaubas C, Solov'yov I, Simard J, Balboni IM, et al. Autoantibody profiling in lupus patients using synthetic nucleic acids. *Sci Rep.* (2018) 8:5554. doi: 10.1038/s41598-018-23910-5
60. Lafyatis R, Kissin E, York M, Farina G, Viger K, Fritzler MJ, et al. B cell depletion with rituximab in patients with diffuse cutaneous systemic sclerosis. *Arthritis Rheum.* (2009) 60:578–83. doi: 10.1002/art.24249
61. Traboulsi D, Kaminska EA, Barr SG, Hunter C, Mydlarski PR. Morphea associated with primary biliary cirrhosis and Waldenstrom macroglobulinemia: response to rituximab. *JAAD Case Rep.* (2018) 4:784–7. doi: 10.1016/j.jdcr.2018.04.016
62. Chimenti MS, Teoli M, Di Stefani A, Giunta A, Esposito M, Perricone R. Resolution with rituximab of localized scleroderma occurring during etanercept treatment in a patient with rheumatoid arthritis. *Eur J Dermatol.* (2013) 23:273–4. doi: 10.1684/ejd.2013.1929
63. Stausbøl-Grøn B, Olesen AB, Deleuran B, Deleuran MS. Abatacept is a promising treatment for patients with disseminated morphea profunda: presentation of two cases. *Acta Derm Venereol.* (2011) 91:686–8. doi: 10.2340/00015555-1136
64. Adeeb F, Anjum S, Hodnett P, Kashif A, Brady M, Morrissey S, et al. Early- and late-stage morphea subtypes with deep tissue involvement is treatable with Abatacept (Orencia). *Semin Arthritis Rheum.* (2017) 46:775–81. doi: 10.1016/j.semarthrit.2016.08.018
65. Fage SW, Arvesen KB, Olesen AB. Abatacept improves skin-score and reduces lesions in patients with localized scleroderma: a case series. *Acta Derm Venereol.* (2018) 98:465–6. doi: 10.2340/00015555-2878
66. Saracino AM, Denton CP, Orteu CH. The molecular pathogenesis of morphoea: from genetics to future treatment targets. *Br J Dermatol.* (2017) 177:34–46. doi: 10.1111/bjd.15001
67. Ludwig RJ, Vanhoorelbeke K, Leypoldt F, Kaya Z, Bieber K, McLachlan SM, et al. Mechanisms of autoantibody-induced pathology. *Front Immunol.* (2017) 8:603. doi: 10.3389/fimmu.2017.00603
68. Cabral-Marques O, Marques A, Giil LM, De Vito R, Rademacher J, Günther J, et al. GPCR-specific autoantibody signatures are associated with physiological and pathological immune homeostasis. *Nat Commun.* (2018) 9:5224. doi: 10.1038/s41467-018-07598-9
69. Cho JH, Gregersen PK. Genomics and the multifactorial nature of human autoimmune disease. *N Engl J Med.* (2011) 365:1612–23. doi: 10.1056/NEJMra1100030
70. Denton CP, Ong VH. Targeted therapies for systemic sclerosis. *Nat Rev Rheumatol.* (2013) 9:451–64. doi: 10.1038/nrrheum.2013.46

9

Tyrosine Kinases in Autoimmune and Inflammatory Skin Diseases

Kata P. Szilveszter, Tamás Németh and Attila Mócsai**

Department of Physiology, Semmelweis University School of Medicine, Budapest, Hungary

***Correspondence:**
Kata P. Szilveszter
szilveszter.kata@med.semmelweis-univ.hu
Attila Mócsai
mocsai.attila@med.semmelweis-univ.hu

Tyrosine kinases relay signals from diverse leukocyte antigen receptors, innate immune receptors, and cytokine receptors, and therefore mediate the recruitment and activation of various leukocyte populations. Non-receptor tyrosine kinases of the Jak, Src, Syk, and Btk families play major roles in various immune-mediated disorders, and small-molecule tyrosine kinase inhibitors are emerging novel therapeutics in a number of those diseases. Autoimmune and inflammatory skin diseases represent a broad spectrum of immune-mediated diseases. Genetic and pharmacological studies in humans and mice support the role of tyrosine kinases in several inflammatory skin diseases. Atopic dermatitis and psoriasis are characterized by an inflammatory microenvironment which activates cytokine receptors coupled to the Jak-Stat signaling pathway. Jak kinases are also implicated in alopecia areata and vitiligo, skin disorders mediated by cytotoxic T lymphocytes. Genetic studies indicate a critical role for Src-family kinases and Syk in animal models of autoantibody-mediated blistering skin diseases. Here, we review the various tyrosine kinase signaling pathways and their role in various autoimmune and inflammatory skin diseases. Special emphasis will be placed on identification of potential therapeutic targets, as well as on ongoing preclinical and clinical studies for the treatment of inflammatory skin diseases by small-molecule tyrosine kinase inhibitors.

Keywords: tyrosine kinases, signaling, Syk, Jak, Src-family, dermatitis, psoriasis, autoimmune blistering diseases

INTRODUCTION

Tyrosine kinases are intracellular enzymes mediating tyrosine phosphorylation of downstream molecules. They play a critical role in signal transduction by various cell surface receptors including, among others, growth factor receptors, adhesion receptors, immunoreceptors, and cytokine receptors. Given their role in multiple signaling processes and disease pathogenesis, tyrosine kinases have emerged as excellent therapeutic targets for the targeted therapy of various diseases. Indeed, small molecule tyrosine kinase inhibitors became important contributors to the pharmacological control of a diverse array of diseases including various malignant processes and immune-mediated diseases such as autoimmune and inflammatory conditions (1).

Inflammatory joint diseases such as rheumatoid arthritis have been in the focus of the development of tyrosine kinase inhibitors for therapeutic purposes within the area of immune mediated diseases (2). This has culminated in the regulatory approval of Jak inhibitors for the treatment of rheumatoid arthritis and certain related disease states (3). Besides inflammatory arthritis, inflammatory skin diseases are another major group of diseases with a major pathogenetic component of various immune cells and immunological pathways. Several lines of evidence indicate the contribution of various tyrosine kinases to the development and progression of diverse inflammatory skin diseases. Those issues suggest that tyrosine kinase inhibitors may provide therapeutic benefit in inflammatory skin diseases.

In this review article, we summarize our current knowledge and understanding of the role of tyrosine kinases in autoimmune and inflammatory skin diseases. We first provide an overview of the various receptor and non-receptor tyrosine kinases and their role in immunological and inflammatory processes. We then summarize the role of the various tyrosine kinases in specific autoimmune or inflammatory skin diseases. Special emphasis is placed on genetic studies in mice and humans indicating a role for tyrosine kinase pathways in inflammatory skin diseases, as well as the preclinical and clinical development of tyrosine kinases inhibitors for the targeted pharmacological therapy of those diseases.

SIGNAL TRANSDUCTION BY TYROSINE KINASES

Non-receptor Tyrosine Kinases

Non-receptor tyrosine kinases are intracellular tyrosine kinases without a direct role in sensing extracellular cues. Nevertheless, these tyrosine kinases are often coupled to various cell surface receptors and are intimately involved in the transmission of extracellular signals to downstream intracellular signaling pathways and cellular effector functions.

There are a total of 10 different non-receptor tyrosine kinase families. Of those, we will discuss Janus kinases (also known as Jak-family kinases), Src-family kinases, and the Syk tyrosine kinase, as well as members of the Btk kinase family.

Janus Kinase Family

The Janus kinase family consists of four members: Jak1, Jak2, Jak3, and Tyk2. While Jak1, Jak2, and Tyk2 are ubiquitously expressed, the expression of Jak3 is limited to the hematopoietic compartment.

These kinases are primarily involved in the signal transduction of various cytokine receptors which are grouped into type I (extracellular WSXWS sequence present; e.g., IL-2, IL-6, GH, EPO, G-CSF, and GM-CSF receptors) and type II (no extracellular WSXWS sequence; e.g., IFN-α, IFN-β, and IL-10 receptors) cytokine receptors. Since Jak-coupled cytokine receptors act as dimers, Jak family kinase activity is also mediated by involving two Jak-family kinases. In most cases, the two cooperating kinases are different ("heterodimers," although they do not form a firm dimer), although Jak2 can also cooperate with another Jak2 molecule ("homodimer"). Upon ligand binding, the conformational changes of the receptor and/or ligand-induced dimerization promotes Jak activation, which leads to autophosphorylation of tyrosine residues of the kinase itself, further augmenting its kinase activity. Jaks then phosphorylate the receptor chains, allowing the recruitment of various signal transducer and activator of transcription (Stat) transcription factors. Stat molecules are then also phosphorylated by Jak kinases, leading to dimerization and translocation to the nucleus where they activate or repress gene expression and influence epigenetic alterations (**Figure 1**). These basic signaling principles are conserved across the diverse array of different biological functions of the Jak-Stat signaling pathway.

Despite the complex and promiscuous nature of receptor association of the different Jak family kinases, human inherited traits and mouse genetic studies have revealed several critical functions of the different Jak kinases. Jak1 is essential for the signaling through type II cytokine receptors (such as IFN receptors), as well as through receptors that utilize the common γ-chain (γc) or the shared gp130 subunit. Jak1 deficiency in mice leads to defective lymphoid development and neurological defects resulting in perinatal lethality without disturbing other hemopoietic lineages (4). Signaling downstream of type II IFNs and receptors with shared gp130 subunit also require Jak2 (besides Jak1), whereas, Jak2 mediated signaling is not required for lymphoid development. IL-3 receptor and several hormone-like receptors (EPO, TPO, GH, PRL) signal through Jak2 alone. Deletion of Jak2 leads to embryonic lethality due to failure of definitive erythropoiesis in mice, likely due to the role of Jak2 in signaling by cytokine receptors involved in the regulation of hematopoiesis and, especially, erythropoiesis (5, 6). Jak3 expression is essentially limited to hematopoietic cells and it is known that it constitutively and exclusively binds to γc-containing receptors including IL-2 and IL-4 receptors. Jak3 mutation in humans leads to severe combined immunodeficiency (7, 8) and studies using *Jak3*$^{-/-}$ mice further confirmed the critical role of Jak3 in lymphoid development (9, 10). Tyk2 is important in IL-12 and IL-23-mediated T cell responses and IFN signaling (11, 12). *Tyk2*$^{-/-}$ mice are viable but susceptible to infections, and macrophages fail to respond to LPS both *in vitro* and *in vivo* (13, 14).

Given their central role in cytokine signaling it is not surprising that Jaks have a role in several immune mediated diseases involving autoimmunity, transplant rejection, and malignancies. Therefore, pharmacological targeting of Jaks was plausible and Jak inhibitors have been extensively studied in several clinical studies. A critical aspect of Jak inhibitors is their selectivity profile for the different Jak family kinases which determines the spectrum of their biological effects. **Table 1** provides a list and the selectivity profile of currently available Jak inhibitors based on cell-free assays. The mechanism of action of those drugs is competitive binding to the ATP binding site of the kinase domain therefore inhibiting phosphorylation and activation of Jaks, except for the case of PF6615600 and BMS986165 (15). PF6615600 mediates a covalent, irreversible Jak3 inhibition through a non-conserved Cys residue in the ATP binding pocket, whereas BMS986165 binds to the pseudokinase domain of Tyk2 (15). First generation Jak inhibitors (tofacitinib, ruxolitinib, baricitinib, and oclacitinib) tend to be less selective among the Jak family kinases due to structural similarities in the ATP binding site of different Jaks, whereas more selective inhibitors were developed during later stages of drug development. Discrepancies between biochemical and cellular potencies of Jak inhibitors have been reported, potentially due to the dominant role of one Jak over another in certain cytokine signaling pathways (16).

The most studied Jak inhibitor is tofacitinib, which ameliorated autoimmune arthritides in various animal models

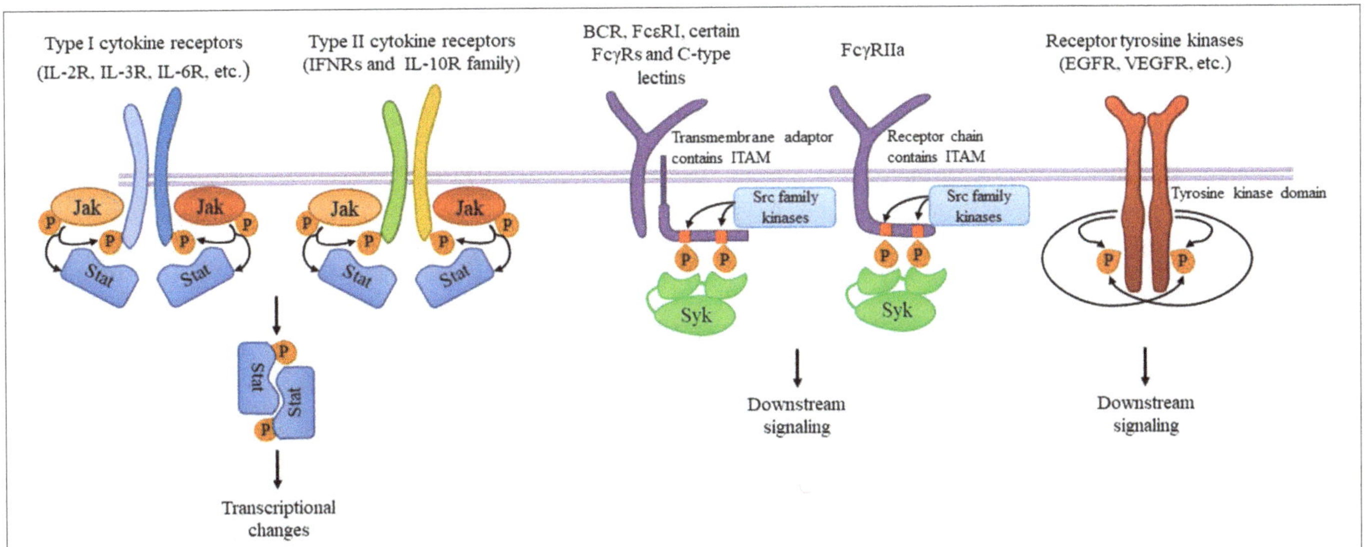

FIGURE 1 | Tyrosine kinases and their signaling pathways. Type I and type II cytokine receptors utilize Janus kinases for the initiation of downstream signaling. Type I cytokine receptor superfamily shares a common amino acid motif WSXWS. Within this family receptors containing the common γ chain (γc) recognize IL-2, IL-4, and IL-13 among others utilizing Jak1 and Jak3. Cytokines including IL-3 and IL-6 are also recognized by type I cytokine receptors acting through Jak1/Jak2 heterodimers or Jak2 homodimers, respectively. The type II cytokine receptor family includes receptors activated by interferons (IFNs) and the IL-10 family utilizing heterodimers of Jak1 along with Jak2 or Tyk2. Ligand binding leads to Jak activation resulting in phosphorylation of the receptor and downstream signal transducers and activators known as Stats mediating transcriptional changes (more information in the text). Src-family kinases and Syk are involved in several immune cell signaling pathways like immunoreceptor, integrin and C-type lectin signaling. Upon ligand binding, activation of Src-family kinases leads to the phosphorylation of tyrosine residues in immunoreceptor tyrosine-based activation motifs (ITAMs), that can be part of a transmembrane adaptor molecule like in case of B cell receptor (BCR), FcεRI, and certain FcγRs and C-type lectins, or of the receptor chain itself like in FcγRIIa in humans. Syk is recruited to the dually phosphorylated ITAMs and becomes activated resulting in the recruitment and activation of various further adapter proteins promoting downstream signaling. Receptor tyrosine kinases, for example EGFR and VEGFR have intrinsic tyrosine kinase activity leading to auto-and transphosphorylation of the receptor chains upon ligand binding. Recruitment of several adaptors and effector molecules through SH2 and phosphotyrosine binding domains mediate downstream signaling.

(17–20) and proved to be effective in several phase II and III studies in the treatment of rheumatoid arthritis, leading to regulatory approval by both the FDA and EMA (2, 21). Jak inhibitors are also currently under investigation in other immune mediated diseases like inflammatory bowel disease, transplant rejection, and multiple dermatological disorders. Excellent reviews about the current state of Jak inhibitors and ongoing clinical trials have been published recently (3, 15, 22).

Src-Family Kinases and the Syk Tyrosine Kinase

The Src kinase family includes nine members (including Hck, Fgr, Lyn, and Lck) which are involved in many signaling pathways in immune cells including immunoreceptor as well as integrin signaling. Src-family kinase activity is regulated by tyrosine phosphorylation and Src homology 2 and 3 (SH2 and SH3) mediated protein-protein interactions with partner proteins containing phosphotyrosine or proline-rich motifs, respectively. Src-family kinases are ubiquitously expressed, although different cells express different family members. Within the immune system, T cells express Lck and Fyn, B cells express Fyn, Lyn, and Blk, and myeloid cells express Hck, Fgr, and Lyn (23). Spleen tyrosine kinase (Syk) is a tandem SH2 domain-containing enzyme acting mostly downstream of Src-family kinases. Syk is expressed in most hematopoietic lineage cells except for T-cells (and, partially, NK-cells) where a closely related kinase, ZAP-70 is expressed and performs a similar function (24).

Immunoreceptors such as B cell receptors (BCR), T cell receptors (TCR), and various activating Fc receptors of innate immune cells are physically associated with transmembrane adapter proteins carrying immunoreceptor tyrosine-based activation motifs (ITAMs). Ligand-receptor interaction results in the enzymatic activation of Src-family kinases phosphorylating the ITAM motifs in the receptor subunits (24). Dually phosphorylated ITAMs are recognized by the tandem SH2 domains of Syk (or ZAP-70 in T cells and NK cells), leading to the recruitment and activation of various further adapter proteins and the activation of several downstream signaling pathways leading to cellular responses (**Figure 1**). Leukocyte integrin "outside-in" signaling also requires Src family kinases and Syk, resulting in adhesion-induced activation of immune cells (24–28). Some inhibitory receptors containing immunoreceptor tyrosine-based inhibitory motifs (ITIMs) also act through Src-family kinases (mostly Lyn), resulting in phosphatase activation and downmodulating of activating signals.

T cell development requires TCR-based signaling and Src-family kinases, particularly Lck. In case of B lymphocytes, Lyn kinase has primary role in BCR signaling. Paradoxically, B cell-specific deletion of Lyn not only results in the expected defects in B cell development, but also leads to autoimmunity (29). Myeloid cells primarily express Hck, Fgr, and Lyn which have a critical but overlapping role in the activation of neutrophils and macrophages through Fcγ receptors, as well as through

TABLE 1 | Jak inhibitors and their selectivity profile.

Compound	Primary target(s)	IC_{50} in cell free assay (nM)			
		Jak1	Jak2	Jak3	Tyk2
Tofacitinib	Jak3, Jak2, and Jak1	112	20	1	34
Ruxolitinib	Jak1 and Jak2	3.3	2.8	428	19
Baricitinib	Jak1 and Jak2	5.9	5.7	560	53
Delgocitinib	Jak1, Jak2	2.8	2.6	13	58
Momelotinib	Jak1, Jak2	11	18	155	n.a
Filgotinib	Jak1 > Jak2	10	28	810	116
Solcitinib	Jak1	8–9	108	539	225
Upadacitinib	Jak1	47	120	2,300	4,700
Itacitinib	Jak1	2	63	>2,000	795
Abrocitinib	Jak1	29	803	>10,000	1,253
PF-06651600	Jak3	>10,000	>10,000	33,1	>10,000
PF-06700841	Tyk2 > Jak1	n.a	n.a	n.a	n.a
BMS986165	Tyk2	n.a	n.a	n.a	2–14
SAR-20347	Tyk2	23	26	41	0.6

Obtained from MedChemExpress and Selleckchem. n.a, not available.

β_1 and β_2 integrins. A prominent feature of Src-family kinases is a significant functional overlap between individual family members. Therefore, in contrast to Jak kinases, individual Src-family kinases are not essential for a given response and complete inhibition of a signaling pathway often requires combinational deletion of multiple kinases in myeloid cells. FcγR mediated phagocytosis is slowed in macrophages lacking Hck, Fgr, and Lyn (30). Adhesion-induced activation is also abrogated in neutrophils lacking Hck, Fgr, and Lyn including oxidative burst, degranulation, and cell spreading (28). Their role has also been shown in chemokine and cytokine responses (31). Moreover, $Hck^{-/-}Lyn^{-/-}Fgr^{-/-}$ triple knockout but not single or double knockout animals were completely protected from autoantibody induced arthritis due to the defective generation of inflammatory environment without affecting the intrinsic migratory capacity of myeloid cells (32).

Currently available Src-family inhibitors have limited selectivity, also inhibiting various other tyrosine kinases such as c-Kit, EGFR, or Abl (summarized in **Table 2**). Those inhibitors are often used in cancer therapy based on their effects on kinases other than Src-family kinases. As an example, dasatinib and bosutinib are potent multi-target inhibitors of Abl, Kit, and several members of the Src kinase family. Beside their therapeutic use in hematological malignancies, they have been found to be relevant in inflammatory conditions as well both *in vitro* and *in vivo* in immune-mediated experimental models (48–51).

Syk and ZAP-70 are also essential for the development of mature B and T cells, respectively (24, 52, 53). Syk deficiency leads to perinatal lethality due to defective separation of lymphoid and blood vessels (54). In the myeloid compartment, Syk is a key protein mediating Fc receptor and integrin mediated signaling and also mediates downstream signaling of C-type lectins like Dectin-1 recognizing fungal antigens (55, 56). Deficiency of the Syk kinase produces profound defects in neutrophil/macrophage

TABLE 2 | Inhibitors of the Src-family and Syk.

Compound	Primary target(s) (IC_{50} in cell free assay)	Other targets (IC_{50} in cell free assay)	Clinical relevance
Dasatinib	Src (0.8 nM), Abl (<1 nM)	c-Kit (79 nM)	Approved in chronic myeloid leukemia and acute lymphoblastic leukemia (33)
Bosutinib (34)	Src (1.2 nM), Abl (1 nM)	n.a	Approved in chronic myeloid leukemia (35)
PP1 (36)	Lck (5 nM), Fyn (6 nM)	Hck (20 nM), Src (170 nM), Bcr-Abl (1 μM), Kit (75 nM), EGFR (250 nM)	–
PP2 (36)	Lck (4 nM), Fyn (5 nM), Hck (5 nM)	EGFR (480 nM), other 56 kinases at 10 μM (37)	–
Fostamatinib (38)	Syk (41 nM), Flt3	79 kinases <100 nM (39)	Approved in immune thrombocytopenia (40)
Entospletinib (41)	Syk (7.7 nM)	TNK1 (<100 nM) (39)	Investigated in hematological malignancies (42)
P505-15 (43)	Syk (1–2 nM)	Fgr (81 nM), Yes (123 nM), MLK1 (88 nM)	–
RO9021 (44)	Syk (5.6 nM)	n.a	–
PRT318 (45)	Syk (4 nM)	n.a	–
TAK-659 (46)	Syk (3.2 nM)	Flt3 (4.6 nM), ZAP-70 (75 nM), Jak3 (114 nM), VEGFR2 (135 nM)	Investigated in hematological malignancies and solid tumors (47)

Obtained from MedChemExpress and Selleckchem. n.a, not available.

integrin signaling and responses to immune complexes, resulting in significantly reduced stimulation of respiratory burst, degranulation and cell spreading (57–59). Syk-deficient bone marrow chimeras proved to be completely protected from autoantibody-induced arthritis that is due to enzymes specifically expressed in neutrophils (60–62). The partially selective Syk inhibitor fostamatinib showed clinical benefit in rheumatoid arthritis patients (63) and has been also investigated in other autoimmune and allergic diseases but considerable adverse events possibly due to its poor selectivity profile led to the suspension of further investigations in RA. New and more specific Syk inhibitors have been developed in the past few years (summarized in **Table 2**) that show promising results in this regard according to *in vitro* results, animal models of autoimmune arthritis and phase I clinical trials (41, 43, 44, 64).

Cerdulatinib and gusacitinib represent dual inhibitors of Syk and Jak kinases and cerdulatinib demonstrated efficacy in experimental arthritis (65). The concept that dual inhibition may result in a stronger therapeutic response is favorable, however it can also represent a limitation by the increased risk of toxicity.

Bruton's Tyrosine Kinase

Bruton's tyrosine kinase (Btk) is involved in the development and activation of B cells through BCR and Toll-like receptor (TLR) signaling (66). Patients with loss-of-function mutations in the Btk gene suffer from immunodeficiency due to the absence of mature B cells and immunoglobulins (67, 68). Similarly, deficiency of Btk in mice results in an impaired differentiation of B cells (69). In addition, transgenic mice that overexpress human Btk display systemic autoimmune response with spontaneous germinal center formation, increased cytokine production (IFNγ and IL-6) and anti-nuclear autoantibodies (ANAs) (70). Btk and other members of the Btk family like Tec kinase are also expressed in myeloid cells regulating maturation and effector function (71). Btk inhibitors interacting with the ATP binding site have been developed and proved to be effective in several systemic autoimmune mouse models like arthritis and lupus models (72, 73).

Receptor Tyrosine Kinases

Receptor tyrosine kinases represent a large family of receptors recognizing various hormones, cytokines, and growth factors (74). They form dimeric combinations upon ligand binding resulting in auto- and transphosphorylation and the recruitment and activation of effectors containing SH2 and phosphotyrosine binding domains, leading to multiple downstream signaling (**Figure 1**).

EGFR and its related receptors, PDGFRs, VEGF receptors and their intact signaling are essential for normal embryonic development and adult tissue homeostasis including cell survival, proliferation, adhesion and migration. Their deregulation has been associated with many human diseases, including immune-mediated disorders and cancer. Targeted therapy by receptor tyrosine kinase inhibitors revolutionized cancer therapy (75). VEGF receptors mediate angiogenesis and lymphangiogenesis during the inflammation process regulating immune cell recruitment and resolution of inflammation.

TYROSINE KINASES IN INFLAMMATORY SKIN DISEASES

Atopic Dermatitis

Atopic dermatitis (AD) is the most common inflammatory skin disease. A T_H2 dominated immune response is essential in the pathogenesis causing eczematous dermatitis with intense pruritus accompanied by elevated serum concentrations of IgE. AD is commonly associated with other T_H2 mediated allergic diseases called the "atopic-allergic march" (76).

Pathogenesis—Pivotal Role of Barrier Disruption and Subsequent TSLP Production

The fundamental lesion is currently thought to be an impaired barrier function that can be due to disrupted expression of essential barrier proteins like filaggrin (77, 78). Subsequent increased penetration of cutaneous and environmental antigens leads to the production of keratinocyte-derived cytokines including thymic stromal lymphopoietin (TSLP). TSLP is thought to be a critical factor driving the pathogenesis of atopic diseases. TSLP receptor is widely expressed in cells that contribute to AD (dendritic cells, T cells, B cells, mast cells, eosinophils, epithelial cells, and sensory neurons) utilizing the Jak-Stat pathway in humans. However, interestingly, it seems that murine TSLP receptor activates Stats by the Btk-family kinase Tec without the involvement of Janus kinases (79). Tamoxifen-induced keratinocyte-specific TSLP-deficient mice displayed drastically reduced allergic skin inflammation in a tape-stripping- and ovalbumin-induced AD model accompanied by the impairment of T_H2 response and allergen-induced sensitization (80). In contrast, overexpression of TSLP in keratinocytes triggered massive itching behavior together with the development of AD-like dermatitis (81). Therefore, intradermal TSLP injection is often used to induce AD-like dermatitis in mice. Wilson et al. showed that it triggers itch sensation within minutes independently from the presence of adaptive immunity or mast cells (82). They also showed that TSLP receptors are present in sensory neurons innervating the skin and TSLP-evoked neuronal activation was responsible for itch sensation.

T_H2 Mediated Allergic Responses—Key Role of T_H2 Cytokines in AD

The importance of the T_H2 pathway is further supported by the observation that transgenic mice overexpressing the T_H2 cytokines IL-4 or IL-13 spontaneously develop skin inflammation that is frequently used as an animal model for AD (83). IL-4 and IL-13 are recognized by the type I cytokine receptor (IL-4 receptor) containing the γc subunit that signals through Jak1 and Jak3. Besides regulating IgE production in B cells and promoting the differentiation of T_H2 lymphocytes, the IL4 receptor is also constitutively expressed by keratinocytes. Stimulation of IL-4 receptors leads to cytokine and chemokine production and downregulation of genes involved in keratinocyte differentiation (such as filaggrin) *in vitro*. This suggests that IL-4 receptor signaling in keratinocytes can further contribute to barrier impairment and inflammation in AD (84–87). Moreover, type 2 cytokines are also capable of activating sensory neurons directly depending on IL-4 receptor and Jak signaling, thus contributing to the development of chronic itch in AD (88). Dupilumab, a monoclonal antibody against the α subunit of the IL-4 receptors that blocks signaling from both IL-4 and IL-13 was effective in phase III studies (89, 90) and it was the first biologic agent approved by the FDA and EMA in the treatment of adults with moderate-to-severe atopic dermatitis (91).

Contribution of IgE-Mediated Signaling to the Allergic Response in AD

Elevated IgE levels and IgE autoreactivity were also suggested to contribute to the development and severity of AD. Beside mast cells and basophils, significant FcεRI expression has been shown in professional antigen presenting cells in atopic skin lesions. FcεRIs crosslinked with IgE are expected to use ITAM-dependent pathways including Src-family kinases and Syk to facilitate degranulation, internalization of allergens and antigen presentation promoting T_H2 immunity (92).

Chronic Phase—Transition Into T_H1-Type Inflammation

T_H1 and IFNγ-mediated responses are thought to dominate the chronic phase of the disease (83). Animal models of hapten-, or allergen-induced contact dermatitis resemble pathogenetic features of both acute and chronic AD involving the disruption of the barrier as a primary event followed by sensitization, inflammation, increased epidermal proliferation, and changes in keratinocyte-differentiation (83).

The Jak-Stat Pathway in Preclinical Studies

The above mentioned pathogenetic features strongly suggest the role of the Jak-Stat pathway in AD (**Figure 2**). Accordingly, Yasuda et al. showed that gain of function mutation in Jak1 resulted in a spontaneous dermatitis phenotype (93). Generation of bone marrow chimeras revealed that Jak1 expression in non-hematopoietic cells was responsible for the development of dermatitis, but Jak1 acting in immune cells exacerbated the dermatitis symptoms and disease severity. They claimed that a possible molecular mechanism behind these findings was that hyperactivation of Jak1 pathway in epidermal keratinocytes resulted in a skin barrier defect due to the overexpression of serine proteases (93). The Jak3 inhibitor tofacitinib reduced ear-swelling and scratching behavior in an allergen-induced dermatitis model, especially upon topical application (94). Inhibition of Jak1 and Jak2 by topically applied ruxolitinib or momelotinib successfully decreased inflammation in a hapten-induced hypersensitivity model as well as in TSLP-induced dermatitis in mice together with the down-regulation of mRNA expression of IL-4, IL-5, IFNγ, and TSLP in the skin (95, 96). Oral administration of delgocitinib (JTE-052) efficiently reduced inflammation in a murine model of hapten-induced hypersensitivity. Moreover, delgocitinib inhibited proliferation and activation of T cells, but did not affect the number of DCs migrated to the draining lymph node during the sensitization phase (97). Delgocitinib was even found to be superior to conventional therapeutic agents like cyclosporine or tacrolimus ointment in hapten- and in TSLP-induced murine dermatitis models with respect to ear thickness, microscopic phenotype, inflammatory cytokine production, and serum IgE level (98). Another study suggested that delgocitinib might directly enhance keratinocyte differentiation *in vitro* (87). Delgocitinib treatment increased the expression of filaggrin and loricrin, genes that are known to be involved in keratinocyte differentiation, in primary human keratinocytes. In addition, IL-4 receptor-mediated downregulation of these genes was reversed upon delgocitinib treatment. Transepidermal water loss was also reduced upon delgocitinib treatment *in vivo* in a murine dry skin model which does not induce immune cell infiltration, indicating that Jak inhibition can improve skin barrier function independently of affecting immune cell activation (87). Taken together, the Jak-Stat pathway seems to be a central component of AD development, mediating multiple aspects of the pathogenesis such as type II cytokine signaling and TSLP-mediated inflammation, itching, keratinocyte disruption, and barrier impairment together with IFNγ-driven responses in the chronic phase. These findings strongly suggest a therapeutic utility of Jak inhibitors in human AD.

Jak Inhibitors in Clinical Trials

Given the substantial interest toward Jak inhibitors, a large amount of data is available from case reports, retrospective studies and open-label studies in the field of treatment of inflammatory skin diseases. In this review we are focusing on randomized, placebo-controlled phase II-III clinical trials that meet the standards of accepted evidence-based medicine (**Table 3**).

Both topical tofacitinib and ruxolitinib treatment significantly improved skin inflammation and pruritus in AD patients in phase II studies (99, 100). In addition, the TRuE-AD phase III clinical trial has just started with the aim of assessing the efficacy of topical ruxolitinib treatment with long-term safety extension period in a larger cohort (101). Studies evaluating efficacy and safety of novel, more selective Jak inhibitors have also shown promising results. Patients treated with baricitinib in combination with topical corticosteroids achieved greater reduction in disease severity than corticosteroids alone (102). In another phase III trial, baricitinib as a monotherapy met its primary endpoint in AD patients (103). Per os abrocitinib and upadacitinib also significantly improved the Eczema Area and Severity Index and reduced pruritus compared to placebo [NCT02780167, (104), respectively]. Emerging number of studies are currently recruiting patients to evaluate efficacy and long-term safety up to 2 years in AD patients (**Table 3**).

Psoriasis

IL-23 Is Crucial to Activate IL-17-Mediated Effector Responses

Psoriasis is a common chronic inflammatory skin disease characterized by epidermal hyperplasia and parakeratosis together with the accumulation of inflammatory cells in the dermis, clinically causing red scaly papules and plaques. Activation of the IL-23/IL-17 axis plays a pivotal role in the pathogenesis of the disease (**Figure 3**). Resident immune cells such as dendritic cells and macrophages are considered to be initially activated through Toll like receptors that lead to the production of cytokines including IL-23 and TNFα that are known to be critical for IL-17 production in human psoriatic skin (105, 106). In fact, intradermal injection of IL-23 alone results in a skin pathology that strongly mimics human disease and is therefore commonly used as an animal model of psoriasis (107). IL-23 is known to induce the differentiation of T_H17 cells that are considered as a major source of IL-17 in humans (106). However, activated dermal γδ T cells were also implicated as major IL-17-producing cells upon IL-23 stimulation in mouse models of psoriasis (108). IL-17 and IL-22 (another T_H17 cytokine) then act as effectors inducing keratinocyte proliferation and hyperkeratosis. They also enhance the production of inflammatory cytokines and chemokines (including IL-1β, CCL20, and IL-8) by keratinocytes, leading to recruitment of other effector cells like neutrophils, further contributing to tissue damage and establishing the inflammatory milieu (109).

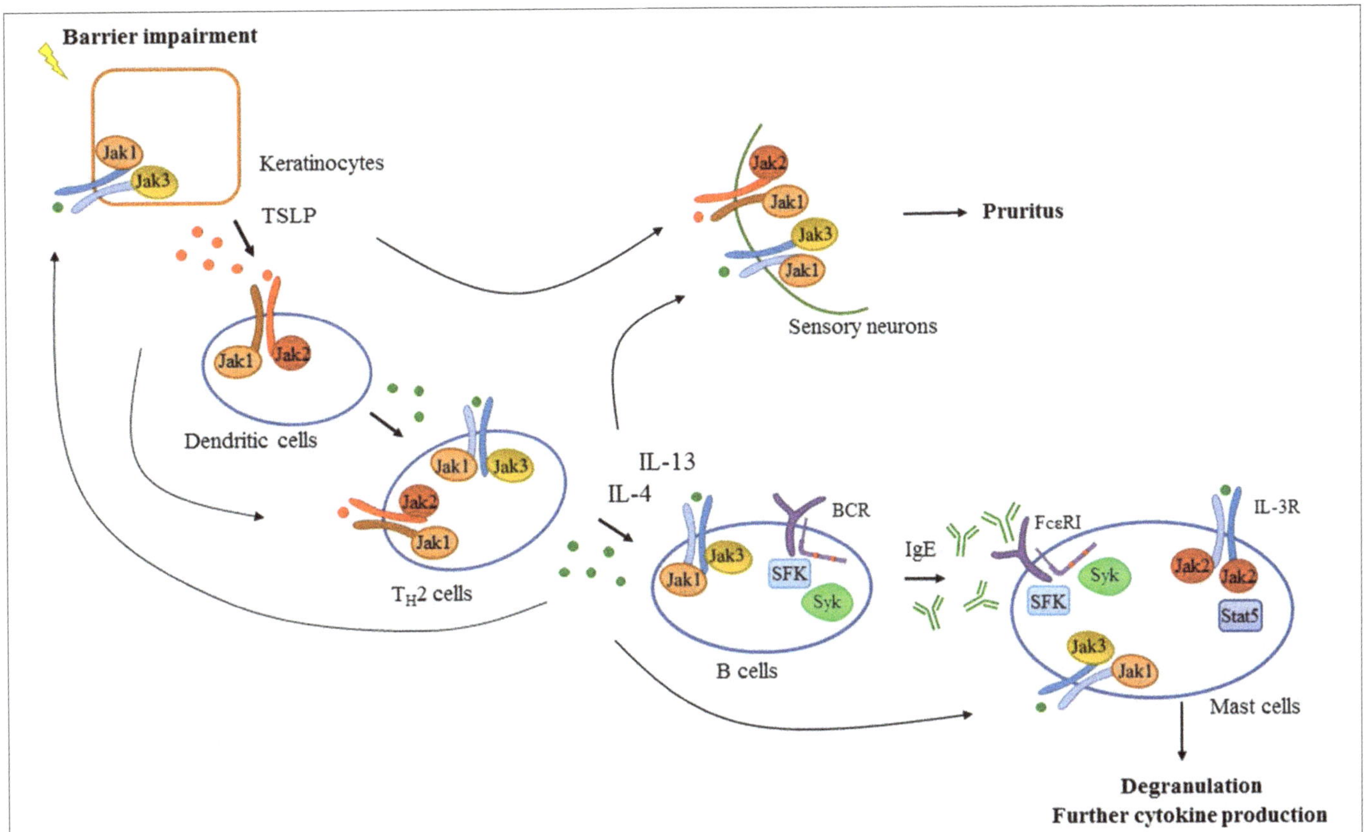

FIGURE 2 | Tyrosine kinases in the development of atopic dermatitis. Barrier impairment is one of the initial steps in the pathogenesis of atopic dermatitis which leads to the production of TSLP by keratinocytes that activates dendritic cells in a Jak1/Jak2 dependent manner in the skin. Proinflammatory mediators produced by dendritic cells and keratinocytes drive the activation and differentiation of $CD4^+$ T cells toward the T_H2 phenotype. Activated T_H2 cells produce several cytokines including IL-4 and IL-13 which promote isotype switch and IgE production in B cells acting through receptors with the common γ chain (γc) utilizing the Jak1/Jak3 heterodimer. Additionally, intact B cell receptor (BCR) signaling involving Src-family kinases (SFK) and Syk is essential for normal B cell development. Downstream effector cells like mast cells recognize IgE through FcεRI in a Src-family and Syk dependent manner leading to degranulation and the production of proinflammatory mediators contributing to the development of atopic dermatitis. There are several feedback loops and shortcuts in this pathway facilitating inflammation utilizing tyrosine kinases. T_H2 cytokines also promote the activation of keratinocytes and effector immune cells like mast cells requiring intact Jak signaling. Activation of mast cells through IL-3R/Jak2/Stat5 pathway was also found to be important in allergen-induced dermatitis in mice. Furthermore, TSLP and T_H2 cytokines acting through a Jak dependent manner in sensory neurons were found to mediate pruritus in atopic dermatitis in addition to mast cell-derived compounds such as histamine.

Jak-Stat Signaling in Psoriasis

A number of novel biological therapies (including monoclonal antibodies against IL-23, IL-17, and IL-17R) have been approved for the treatment of psoriasis in the last few years (110). IL-23 receptors rely on Jak2/Tyk2 heterodimer-mediated signaling, implicating their role in the pathogenesis of the disease. Several genes of Jak-Stat signaling pathway have also shown to be associated with psoriasis (111). This was further supported by a genetic approach showing that Tyk2-deficient mice had significantly reduced ear swelling and epidermal hyperplasia upon injection with IL-23. In addition, infiltration of various leukocytes (including different T cell subsets, neutrophils, and macrophages) and the production of the pro-inflammatory cytokines IL-17 and IL-22 were also impaired in the absence of Tyk2 (112). Downstream signaling components like Stat3, a key factor in T_H17 differentiation, was also found to be upregulated in human psoriatic lesions (113). Sano et al. showed that constitutive expression of Stat3 in keratinocytes resulted in a dermatitis phenotype closely resembling psoriasis (113). Epidermal hyperplasia, parakeratosis and dermal infiltration of immune cells occurred upon tape stripping or wounding of the skin, and in some mice, it occurred even spontaneously. The development of psoriatic lesions in these mice required both hyperactive Stat3 in keratinocytes and activated T cells in the dermis. Furthermore, inhibition of Stat3 with decoy oligonucleotides successfully inhibited disease development and even reversed disease severity showing that Stat3 may be an important regulator of genes in keratinocytes in the development of psoriasis cooperating with T cells (113).

Jak Inhibitors in the Treatment of Psoriasis

Pharmacological inhibition of the Jak-Stat pathway showed promising results in murine models of psoriasis reducing disease pathology, keratinocyte-activation, and proinflammatory cytokine levels (95, 98, 114). In addition, a number of clinical trials investigate the effect of different Jak inhibitors in

TABLE 3 | Phase II and III clinical trials studying Jak inhibitors in atopic dermatitis.

Drug name	Identifier	Status	Phase, administration	Enrollment	Duration
Tofacitinib	NCT02001181	Completed (99)	IIa, topical	69	4-week
Ruxolitinib	NCT03011892	Completed (100)	IIb, topical	307	8-week dose-ranging and additional 4-week optional open-label treatment
	NCT03745638; NCT03745651	Underway (101)	III, topical	1,200	8-week and long-term safety extension period
Delgocitinib	NCT03725722	Recruiting	IIb, topical	250	8-week dose-ranging
Baricitinib	NCT02576938	Completed (102)	II, per os	124	16-week in combination with TCS
	NCT03334396; NCT03334422	Met primary endpoint (103)	III, per os	1,350	16-week
	NCT03334435	Recruiting	III, per os	1,500	52-week to evaluate long-term safety
	NCT03428100	Recruiting	III, per os	500	16-week in those who cannot have cyclosporin
	NCT03435081	Recruiting	III, per os	450	16-week dose-ranging study
	NCT03559270	Recruiting	III, per os	300	2-year in those who have completed NCT03435081
	NCT03733301	Recruiting	III, per os	300	16-week in combination with TCS
Abrocitinib	NCT02780167	Completed, results online	IIb, per os	269	12-week dose-range study
	NCT03796676	Recruiting	III, per os	225, adolescents	12-week with other topical therapy
	NCT03575871; NCT03349060	Recruiting	III, per os	375	12-week
	NCT03422822	Recruiting	III, per os	2,300	Approximately 2 years who have completed a qualifying phase III study
	NCT03627767	Recruiting	III, per os	1,370	Over 40 weeks in those who responded well to an initial 12-week treatment
	NCT03720470	Recruiting	III, per os	700	12-week, efficacy compared to dupilumab at 2 weeks
Upadacitinib	NCT02925117	Completed (104)	III, per os	166	16-week
	NCT03738397	Recruiting	III, per os	650	24-week treatment, 12-week follow-up
	NCT03661138	Recruiting	III, per os	264	Up to 141 weeks, evaluating safety
	NCT03568318	Recruiting	III, per os	810	16-week combined with TCS
	NCT03607422; NCT03569293	Recruiting	III, per os	810	16-week

psoriasis (**Table 4**). Short-term oral tofacitinib therapy resulted in significant clinical improvement in patients with moderate-to-severe plaque psoriasis (116) along with reducing epidermal thickness, DC and T cell numbers and the expression of psoriasis-related genes in the lesional skin (115). Several additional phase III studies were completed evaluating the long-term safety and efficacy of the treatment. Oral administration of tofacitinib was non-inferior to parenteral etanercept indicating that tofacitinib may provide a more convenient therapeutic option (117). Tofacitinib also demonstrated sustained efficacy in patients with psoriasis through up to 52 months and was well-tolerated with an acceptable safety profile detailed later (118, 121, 122, 130). In a 56-week withdrawal and retreatment study, patients who received continuous treatment maintained a response more effectively, however, 60% of patients who relapsed upon tofacitinib withdrawal recaptured a response with tofacitinib (119).

Topical treatment provides an excellent opportunity to overcome possible systemic adverse effects. Tofacitinib ointment also showed greater efficacy compared to vehicle at week 8, but failed to be superior to placebo at week 12 in a phase IIb study (123). Topical ruxolitinib was found to be well-tolerated, safe, and efficacious in short-term treatment in a smaller cohort of patients (124).

Oral treatment of novel, more selective inhibitors also improved symptoms and were well-tolerated in patients with psoriasis in phase II trials (125–127, 129). Since IL-12/IL-23-mediated signaling relies on Jak2/Tyk2 heterodimers, specific inhibition of these kinases may provide further improvement in psoriasis patients. Due to the critical role of Jak2 in hemopoietic development, inhibition of Tyk2 seem to be plausible in the treatment of psoriatic patients. Indeed, BMS986165 showed promising results in a 12-week phase II trial enrolling 267 patients (128) and a phase III study is currently recruiting patients to compare oral BMS986165 treatment to placebo and currently available treatment apremilast (NCT03624127 and NCT03611751).

Syk Tyrosine Kinase in IL-17-Mediated Inflammation

Little is known about the role of Syk in psoriasis. The pattern recognition receptor Dectin-1 was implicated in the disease process, suggesting that recognition of fungal antigens in a

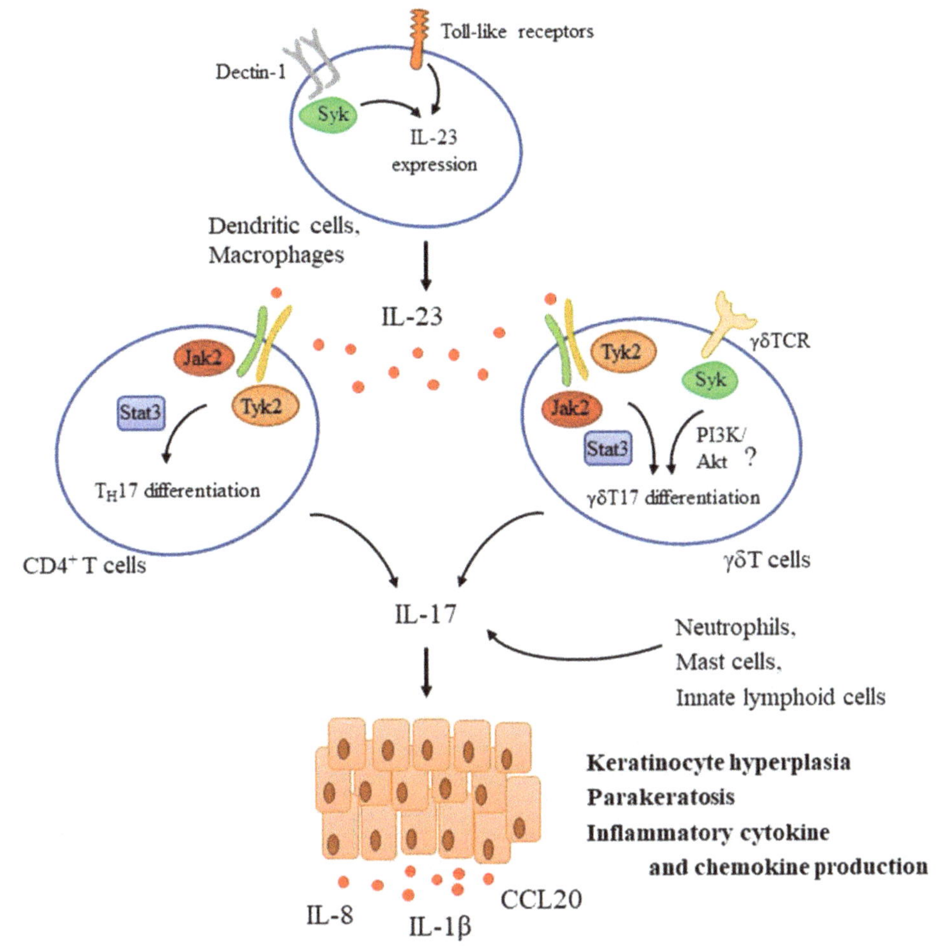

FIGURE 3 | Tyrosine kinases in the IL-23/IL-17 axis during psoriasis pathogenesis. IL-23 is a key mediator driving psoriasis pathogenesis. It is expressed by dendritic cells upon their activation through Toll-like receptors (TLR) and Dectin-1, the latter one utilizing Syk. IL-23 promotes the differentiation of $CD4^+$ T cells and γδT cells as well toward T_H17 and γδT17, respectively via a Jak2/Tyk2-Stat3-mediated pathway and also induces the expression of IL-17. TCR activation in γδ T cells was also proposed to be important for mediating IL-17 production and psoriatic skin lesions, utilizing Syk and probably the PI3K/Akt pathway. In addition to T_H17 and γδT17 cells, other sources of IL-17 include neutrophils, mast cells, and innate lymphoid cells. IL-17 then acts as an effector acting mainly on keratinocytes mediating hyperproliferation, parakeratosis, and production of several inflammatory chemokines and cytokines like IL-1β, IL-8, and CCL20.

Syk and CARD9 dependent manner promotes the maturation of DCs and their ability to induce IL-17 production by T_H17 cells (55). In addition, another source of IL-17 is γδ T cells, which utilize Syk as a dominant proximal kinase of the γδ TCR signaling pathway. Furthermore, skin inflammation was ameliorated in mice lacking the adaptor molecule RhoH that recruits Syk to the TCR in imiquimod-induced psoriasis model (131). These findings suggest that Syk may contribute to IL-17 production, but its actual relevance in case of psoriasis needs further investigation.

Role of Growth Factor Receptors in AD and Psoriasis

EGF receptor family members in keratinocytes facilitate epidermal differentiation and plays a crucial role in wound healing as well as in carcinogenesis. Though epidermal hyperplasia is a hallmark of both AD and psoriasis, the contribution of EGF receptor signaling to inflammatory skin disorders is poorly understood. Psoriatic lesions are known to overexpress EGFR and ligands like amphiregulin. Transgenic overexpression of amphiregulin in either basal or suprabasal epidermis causes severe psoriasis-like hyperplasia and skin inflammation in mice (132, 133). In line with that, neutralizing antibodies against amphiregulin reduce epidermal thickness of human psoriatic lesions transplanted onto mice with severe combined immunodeficiency (134). However, mice lacking another EGFR ligand epiregulin develop severe chronic dermatitis showing complicated modulating role of EGFR signaling pathways in the epidermis (135). Mice lacking epidermal EGFR spontaneously develop skin inflammation, decreased host defense and deficient skin barrier function (136). Proinflammatory cytokines such as IFNγ was also suggested to transactivate EGFR leading to the downregulation of the expression of chemokines like CCL2, CCL5, and CXCL10. In line with that, EGFR inhibition resulted in the aggravation of allergic

TABLE 4 | Phase II and III clinical trials studying Jak inhibitors in psoriasis.

Drug name	Identifier	Status	Phase, administration	Enrollment	Duration
Tofacitinib	NCT01710046	Completed (115)	IIa, per os	12	12-week
	NCT00678210	Completed (116)	IIb, per os	197	12-week
	NCT01241591	Completed (117)	III, per os	1,101	12-week non-inferiority trial compared to etanercept
	NCT01519089	Completed (118)	III, per os	95	52-week evaluating long-term safety
	NCT01186744	Completed (119)	III, per os	666	56-week withdrawal and retreatment study
	NCT01276639 and NCT01309737	Completed (120)	III, per os	901 and 960	52-week
	NCT01815424	Completed (121)	III, per os	266	52-week
	NCT01163253	Terminated as it met its objectives (122)	III, per os	2,867	median duration 35.6 months open-label extension study who completed qualifying phase II/III studies
	NCT01831466	Completed (123)	IIb, topical	430	12-week
Ruxolitinib	NCT00820950	Completed (124)	II, topical	29	28-day
	NCT00778700	Completed, no results available	II, topical	199	12-week
Baricitinib	NCT01490632	Completed (125)	IIb, per os	271	12-week
Abrocitinib	NCT02201524	Terminated (126)	II, per os	59	4-week terminated due to changes in sponsors development priorities
PF-06700841	NCT02969018	Completed	IIa, per os	212	12-week, results online
	NCT03850483	Not yet recruiting	IIb, topical	240	12-week
Itacitinib	NCT01634087	Completed (127)	II, per os	50	28-day
BMS986165	NCT02931838	Completed (128)	II, per os	267	12-week
	NCT03624127 and NCT03611751	Recruiting	III, per os	600 and 1,000	Non-inferiority study compared to apremilast
Solcitinib	NCT01782664	Completed (129)	IIa, per os	68	12-week

contact dermatitis in mice by enhanced chemokine production of keratinocytes, promoting subsequent leukocyte recruitment (137). In contrast, IL-8 gene expression is actively induced by the EGFR ligands in keratinocytes (135, 137). In turn, IL-8 could contribute to activating the metalloprotease-dependent release of EGFR ligands by acting on its specific receptor in cancer cells (138), indicating the possibility of a positive feedback loop both for epidermal hyperplasia and neutrophil accumulation.

It is also well-known that EGFR inhibitor therapy in malignancies often causes inflammatory or toxic effects on the skin, and such side effects even act as strong predictors of good response to treatment (139).

Psoriasis and atopic dermatitis are both characterized by altered angiogenesis and lymphangiogenesis (140). Hyperplastic hyperpermeable dermal blood vessels can be detected in psoriatic skin lesions and transgenic delivery of VEGF to the skin results in a profound inflammatory skin condition resembling psoriasis (141) while topical application of VEGFR inhibitor successfully prevented disease development in the mouse model of psoriasis (142). Interestingly, stimulation of lymphangiogenesis by VEGFR-3 or via administration of its ligand VEGF-C inhibited inflammatory cell infiltration by oxazolone-induced skin inflammation (143, 144). This indicates that blood vessels contribute to the development of inflammatory environment by helping inflammatory cell infiltration while lymphatic vessels may limit skin inflammation by helping their elimination. Thus, selectivity can be especially important upon targeting VEGFRs in malignancies.

Alopecia Areata and Vitiligo

Both alopecia areata and vitiligo are characterized by IFNγ producing autoreactive cytotoxic T lymphocytes that attack hair follicles and melanocytes, respectively.

Alopecia areata (AA) is the main cause of non-scarring hair loss most commonly occurring in the scalp. The upregulation of several Jak-Stat pathway components downstream of γ-chain containing cytokines (which are known to promote the activity and survival of IFNγ-producing cytotoxic T cells) was detected in AA skin both from humans and mice. In a mouse model of AA, systemic administration of Jak inhibitors successfully prevented the development of disease. Moreover, both systemic and topical administration was able to reverse established disease and even promoted hair regrowth (145). Gene expression and immunofluorescent studies from mouse skin showed that expression and activity of the Jak-Stat pathway is dynamically changing during the hair follicle cycle. Moreover, Jak inhibition promoted the entry into the hair cycle and subsequent hair regrowth by activating hair follicle stem cells in healthy mice and also in lymphocyte-deficient mouse strains (146). This dual effect further justifies the investigation of Jak inhibitors in the treatment of AA. Some open label phase II clinical studies showed that Jak inhibitor treatment resulted in significant hair regrowth and improvement of AA in patients with better response if administered orally instead of topical formulations. Hair loss typically reoccurred after discontinuation of therapy within months (147–149). There are several active randomized, double-blind, placebo-controlled phase II clinical trials on the efficacy and safety of topical and oral Jak inhibitors in AA (**Table 5**), promising further insight into these issues in the near future.

In case of vitiligo cytotoxic T cell-mediated melanocyte destruction causes depigmentation leading to the occurrence of white spots throughout the body surface of patients. IFNγ produced by activated melanocyte-specific cytotoxic T lymphocytes is strongly implicated in the disease pathogenesis by promoting further T cell accumulation in the skin through IFNγ-dependent chemokines like CXCL10 (150). In addition, IFNγ was found to directly induce melanocyte senescence and apoptosis of primary human melanocytes which could be attenuated by siRNA against Jak2 and Stat1, but not Jak1. IFNγ treatment also resulted in the accumulation of reactive oxygen species and the production of proinflammatory cytokines like IL-6 which are considered as important contributing factors facilitating a vitiligo-prone environment in the skin (151).

Given the multiple role of IFNγ in vitiligo, inhibition of the Jak-Stat pathway may represent a promising therapeutic strategy. Beside some case reports and retrospective studies showing benefits of Jak inhibitors treating vitiligo patients (152, 153), so far only one open label phase II proof of concept pilot trial has been completed. This showed that topical ruxolitinib treatment provided significant repigmentation in facial vitiligo in a small cohort of patients (154). A randomized double-blind, dose-ranging, placebo-controlled phase II trial is now ongoing for evaluating the efficacy of ruxolitinib cream in vitiligo (NCT03099304). Another randomized controlled phase IIb trial is currently recruiting patients for evaluating per os treatment with novel selective Jak inhibitors (NCT03715829, also see in **Table 5**).

An additional important aspect of AA and vitiligo is that these diseases mostly cause cosmetic concern with emotional problems. Therefore, analyzing the safety and benefit profile of potential treatments is extremely important and Jak inhibitors should be very carefully tested in this regard.

Pemphigus

Pemphigus vulgaris and foliaceus are severe autoimmune blistering skin diseases with autoantibodies that are directed against the desmosomal cadherins, mainly desmoglein 3 (Dsg3) and Dsg1. These are required for the proper intercellular adhesion of keratinocytes and autoantibody deposition results in flaccid blister formation within the epidermis affecting mucous membranes and skin. Pemphigus vulgaris (PV) can be life threatening causing significant loss of the physical barrier. Application of artificial barriers like ointments can improve barrier function but there is an unmet need for definitive treatment.

Given the central role of Btk and Syk in B cell development and activation, these kinases may promote pathogenic antibody production in pemphigus. An inhibitor of Btk is under current evaluation in an open-label phase II clinical trial in pemphigus (NCT02704429) moreover, a randomized, double-blind placebo-controlled phase III study is already recruiting patients (NCT03762265).

IgG4 is the major subclass of autoantibodies in pemphigus and it is known to have limited ability to activate complement. Accordingly, acantholysis in pemphigus has been demonstrated to be independent from complement and Fc receptors (155, 156). Anti-Dsg3 IgG was able to directly induce the destruction of desmosomes by steric hindrance, promoting the internalization of Dsg3 (157, 158) and interfering with desmosome turnover (159). Recently it has been shown that Dsg3 transcription is negatively regulated by Stat3 in keratinocytes and corticosteroid treatment upregulates Dsg3 expression by inhibiting Stat3 through a yet unknown mechanism possibly involving Jaks (160). Those results suggest that specific inhibition of the Jak-Stat3 pathway may also be beneficial without the known adverse effects of steroids. T_H2 cytokines like IL-4, IL-9, and IL-21, that utilize Jak-family kinases are known to contribute to the induction and regulation of autoantibody production in pemphigus (161, 162) therefore Jak inhibitors also serve as a potential treatment, but preclinical or clinical studies are yet to be done (163).

Binding of pathogenic IgG can also trigger outside-in signaling in keratinocytes eliciting acantholysis and apoptosis. Moreover, autoantibody binding also promoted secretion of inflammatory cytokines from keratinocytes, which may augment the pathogenic autoimmune response (164). However, the precise molecular mechanism is at present unclear. Several downstream mediators were implicated involving activation of EGFR-mediated signaling and focal adhesion kinase in keratinocytes (165–169). In a recent report, Src family kinases were implicated in autoantibody-mediated desmosome disassembly (170). Src phosphorylation was induced in keratinocytes upon *in vitro* antibody treatment obtained from PV patients. Loss of cell cohesion caused by anti-Dsg3 antibody was abolished upon Src inhibition by PP2 both *in vitro* and *in vivo* in a neonatal mouse model. However, inhibition of Src was not protective in some cases against PV-Ig-induced loss-of-keratinocyte-cohesion in keratinocyte monolayer, nor in intact human skin (170). These results underlie the need for further investigations of keratinocyte signaling in pemphigus pathogenesis.

Pemphigoid Diseases

Pemphigoid diseases are characterized by autoantibody production against distinct components of the dermal-epidermal junction leading to dermal-epidermal separation and tense blister formation (171).

Bullous pemphigoid (BP) is the most prevalent autoimmune bullous disease. Antibody formation directed against key hemidesmosomal components BP180 (also called type XVII collagen), and/or BP230 results in subepidermal blistering phenotype. Urticarial plaques and pruritus are also present in most of the cases which is a unique symptom among the pemphigoid group. Epidermolysis bullosa acquisita (EBA) is a very rare disease characterized by autoantibodies directed against

TABLE 5 | Phase II and III clinical trials studying Jak inhibitors in alopecia areata and vitiligo.

Disease	Drug name	Identifier	Status	Phase, administration	Enrollment	Duration
Alopecia areata	Baricitinib	NCT03570749	Ongoing	II/III, per os	725	36-week
	PF-06651600 and PF-06700841	NCT02974868	Ongoing	IIa, per os	142	24-week with extension period up to 2 years
	Delgocitinib	NCT02561585	Results submitted	II, topical	31	12-week
Vitiligo	Ruxolitinib	NCT03099304	Ongoing	II, topical	157	1-year with 1 year open-label extension
	PF-06651600 and PF06700841	NCT03715829	Recruiting	IIb, per os	330	60-week with 24 weeks dose ranging and 24 week extension period

type VII collagen (C7), the key anchoring fibril in the upper dermis, also causing subepidermal blister formation (172).

Essential Role of Antibody-Deposition in Pemphigoid Diseases

Antibody deposition to the basement membrane is the key feature in the pathogenesis, demonstrated by the fact that passive transfer of either anti-BP180 or anti-C7 antibodies isolated either from human patients or generated against human or murine antigens result in a severe blistering phenotype in mice (173–176). These approaches became useful experimental models to investigate the effector phase of autoantibody-mediated pemphigoid diseases. Several studies showed that deposition of antibodies are followed by the activation of the complement system and the recruitment of neutrophils mediating tissue damage and blister formation (177–181). Eosinophils and mast cells are also considered as contributors of blister formation by producing mediators facilitating further neutrophil recruitment and tissue damage (182–184). However, there are controversies in the literature especially regarding the role of mast cells (185). It has been proposed that autoantibodies can also directly affect epidermal cell—extracellular matrix integrity (186–188) and can trigger morphological and functional changes in keratinocytes (189) including IL-6 and IL-8 production (190) which can promote the recruitment of neutrophils (**Figure 4**).

Pathways Mediating Immune-Complex Recognition and Leukocyte Migration

Signaling through complement receptors and recognition of deposited immune complexes by neutrophils through activating Fcγ receptors was essential for blister formation both *in vitro* using human cryosections and in *in vivo* mouse models (191–193). FcεRI signaling in mast cells, eosinophils and basophils have also been implicated in immune complex recognition because IgE isotypes of autoantibodies can also be detected in many patients in addition to IgG (194, 195). Actual pathogenetic relevance of IgE and FcεRI was further supported by the fact that omalizumab treatment was able to reduce the number of blisters and itching in BP patients (196). However, the role of other potential participants, namely β_2 integrins, which are known to be involved in the migration of neutrophils to the inflamed area, is not entirely clear. Mac-1-deficient neonatal mice developed impaired neutrophil infiltration and were resistant to blister formation after 24 h of a single anti-BP180 treatment (197). In contrast, another study in the experimental model of EBA induced by repeated anti-C7 injections found that the absence of Mac-1 led to an even exacerbated disease phenotype (198). Therefore, further experiments are needed to reveal the role of β_2 integrins in pemphigoid diseases.

Src-Family Kinases and Syk in Pemphigoid Diseases

Fc receptor-mediated signaling is strongly dependent of intracellular tyrosine kinases like Src-family kinases and Syk (24, 25). Given the central role of immune complex recognition by Fc receptors of resident and recruited innate immune cells, Src-family kinases and Syk may have an important role in the development of pemphigoid diseases. Indeed, triple knockout mice lacking Hck, Fgr, and Lyn, three Src-family kinases expressed in the myeloid compartment, were completely protected in an autoantibody induced model of EBA (32). Neutrophils lacking Hck, Fgr, and Lyn also failed to produce superoxide in response to C7-containing immune complexes (199), which has been shown to be important in mediating tissue damage in the skin (200). The Syk tyrosine kinase, which is recruited to ITAM sequences phosphorylated by Src-family kinases, was also found indispensable for the effector phase of the disease (199, 201). Analysis of Syk-deficient bone marrow chimeras revealed that Syk deficiency completely protected mice from anti-C7 antibody-induced skin disease and abrogated the accumulation of key cytokines and chemokines, as well as the infiltration of leukocytes, at the site of inflammation (199). Moreover, Syk deficient neutrophils failed to release CXCL2 or leukotriene B_4 upon activation by immobilized C7-anti-C7 immune complexes *in vitro*. Integrin signaling also acts through Src kinases and Syk, however, *in vivo* migratory capacity either of Syk deficient or Src-family triple knockout neutrophils remained unaffected (199). Furthermore, neutrophil-specific expression of the CARD9 adaptor protein was also found to contribute to the development of the disease, as complete or neutrophil-specific CARD9 deletion partially protected mice from anti-C7 antibody-induced skin inflammation, likely due to CARD9-dependent regulation of neutrophil gene expression changes (202).

Taken together, Fc receptors and β_2 integrins signal through Src-family kinases and Syk which are indispensable for immune-complex and adhesion-induced activation of effector cells

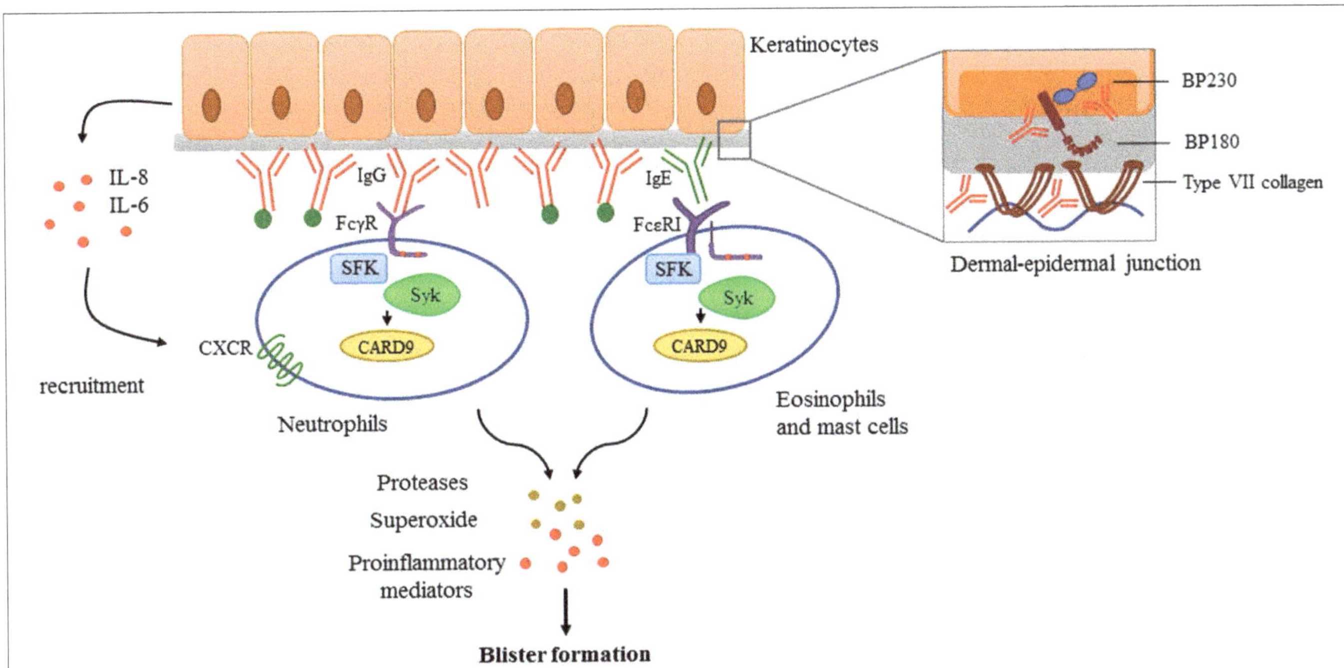

FIGURE 4 | Antibody-mediated signaling in pemphigoid diseases. Pemphigoid diseases are characterized by autoantibody production against components of the dermal-epidermal junction (DEJ) like BP180 and BP230 in case of bullous pemphigoid, or against type VII collagen in patients with epidermolysis bullosa acquisita (Structure of the DEJ with special attention to the above-mentioned autoantigens is shown on the upper right panel). Autoantibody deposition along the DEJ results in the activation of the complement system (indicated with green dots) and initiation of keratinocyte-responses involving IL-6 and IL-8 production. This leads to recruitment of innate effector cells like neutrophils, eosinophils, and mast cells. Recognition of deposited immune complexes through Fc receptors utilizing Src-family kinases (SFK), Syk, and CARD9 is critical for the development of pemphigoid diseases, as shown by genetic studies using transgenic animals (see more detail in the text). Immune complex-mediated activation of effectors leads to the release of reactive oxygen species, proteases, and the production of proinflammatory mediators culminating into blister formation.

(neutrophils, macrophages and, possibly, eosinophils and mast cells) without affecting their intrinsic migratory capacity. Src and Syk kinases are also responsible for the amplification of the inflammation process through the release of mediators that recruit neutrophils and/or directly damage dermal-epidermal junction in experimental pemphigoid models like proteases and superoxide. Therefore, these non-receptor tyrosine kinases may be good candidates for therapeutic intervention in the future, even though the development of specific inhibitors has yet to be solved.

Presence of Jaks in Pemphigoid Diseases

Several proinflammatory cytokine levels are elevated in blister fluid of BP patients such as IL-1β, IL-4, IL-6, IL-8, and TSLP (172, 203–205), and many of them act through the Jak-Stat pathway. In line with that, the expression of Jak-Stat proteins was found to be also elevated in skin lesions of BP patients (206). A meeting abstract discussed that pharmacological inhibition of Jak2 impaired the induction of EBA by antibody transfer and had therapeutic effects too in immunization-induced EBA model (207). However, there are no clinical studies using Jak inhibitors in pemphigoid diseases. A case report has been published about successfully treating a BP patient with anti-IL-4 antibody (208). The low number of clinical studies in general with novel therapeutic options is possibly due to the fact that BP usually affects elderly patients, therefore one should very carefully balance risk-benefit ratio in case of novel systemic treatments with special attention to inflammation and carcinogenesis.

Systemic Lupus Erythematosus

Almost all patients with systemic lupus erythematosus (SLE) develop lupus-specific cutaneous symptoms at some point in the disease course. There are also patients with cutaneous lupus that do not meet other diagnostic criteria for SLE. SLE is characterized by autoreactive B cells and autoantibody formation which proposes the role for Syk and Btk, non-receptor tyrosine kinases mediating BCR signaling, in disease development. The partially selective Syk inhibitor fostamatinib prevented the development of skin disease and significantly reduced established skin disease in lupus-prone mice (209). In addition, Btk inhibiton significantly attenuated the lupus-associated cutaneous disease phenotypes in mice (210). Systemic inflammatory conditions mediated by secretion of proinflammatory cytokines that act through Jaks is also important in SLE cutaneous manifestations (211–215). Indeed, Jak inhibition by ruxolitinib prevented the development of cutaneous lupus lesions in lupus-prone mice (216). However, baricitinib failed to improve skin manifestations in systemic lupus patients in a phase II trial, despite the fact that the overall systemic symptoms were effectively reduced by the drug (217).

Neutrophilic Dermatoses

Neutrophilic dermatoses represent a group of disorders characterized by massive neutrophil infiltration in the skin without evidence of infection. Signs of systemic inflammation often accompanies skin pathology and they are often associated with malignancies and autoimmune diseases like RA and inflammatory bowel diseases. Interestingly, autoinflammatory diseases share various common features with neutrophilic dermatoses suggesting some similarities in the pathogenesis (218). Since an excellent review has been currently published about mechanisms of inflammation in neutrophil dermatoses (219), here we are focusing on evidence about the importance of tyrosine kinases.

Abnormalities in neutrophil function is obviously implicated in the pathogenesis. The SH2 domain-containing tyrosine phosphatase SHP-1 is essential for inhibiting proinflammatory signal transduction and loss-of-function mutation of SHP-1 in mice causes severe cutaneous inflammation resembling human neutrophilic dermatoses. Kanneganti and her group showed that IL-1α signaling through IL-1R and adaptor protein Myd88 drives inflammation in this model where tyrosine phosphorylation of Myd88 is counterregulated by SHP-1 and Syk (220). Dysfunction of SHP-1 leads to the release of Syk from inhibition resulting in excessive expression of proinflammatory mediators and other effector molecules. Downstream of Syk, the CARD9 adaptor protein was also found to be a key mediator in cutaneous inflammation in the aforementioned model (221).

Cytokine dysregulation are considered as contributing factors to the development of the disease. Elevation of serum G-CSF was detected in patients with active disease of unknown origin (222), moreover, G-CSF is a common cause of drug-induced neutrophilic dermatosis (223). G-CSFR signals through Jak2 suggesting a possible role of Jak2 creating cytokine dysregulation. In addition, increased expression of IFNγ was also described in patients and rare genetic autoinflammatory diseases characterized by high IFNγ production also represent neutrophilic dermatosis where Jak inhibitor therapy significantly improved symptoms in some cases (224).

ADVERSE EVENTS DURING JAK INHIBITOR TREATMENT IN INFLAMMATORY DISEASES

Safety information from long-term studies of Jak inhibitor treatment are limited due to the novelty of these drugs. Most data are available from RA patients (225), but there is slowly emerging information from patients with skin inflammation and several long-term safety-assessing trials are currently recruiting patients (**Tables 3–5**).

Safety profile is considered generally acceptable, infections and laboratory abnormalities can be observed as major adverse events (226). The increased risk of infections was similar to that observed by the use of biologics, with the exception of higher risk for varicella zoster infection which should be taken into consideration. Cytopenias, mostly anemia and neutropenia relatively often occur likely due to Jak2 inhibition but rarely severe. Elevated serum cholesterol level has been also mentioned in patients treated with Jak inhibitors (227). It was usually sustained after the first few months and was controllable by statin therapy. Among less frequent adverse events thromboembolism was documented, however most patients already suffer from increased risk due to chronic systemic inflammation which further complicates the picture (228). One of the most serious concerns is the possibility of the development of malignancies upon long-term Jak inhibitor treatment. Current studies have not shown higher risk (225), but longer follow-up is needed to properly address this matter.

Taken together, Jak inhibitor treatment has not higher risk than biologics overall. However, skin diseases often present as less severe but chronic symptoms where risk/benefit ratio should be carefully considered upon choosing appropriate treatment. Nevertheless, the possibility of topical application represents an excellent opportunity which deserve further elaboration.

CONCLUSION AND FUTURE DIRECTIONS

The highly effective treatment of various malignancies by tyrosine kinase inhibitors and the regulatory approval of Jak inhibitors for the targeted therapy of rheumatoid arthritis has generated major interest in the therapeutic targeting of other diseases, including inflammatory skin diseases, by tyrosine kinase inhibitors. Besides the most extensively studied Jak inhibitors, compounds targeting other kinases such as Syk, Src-family kinases, or Btk are also expected to emerge as new therapeutics for inflammatory dermatitis. The more and more detailed understanding of individual kinase family members and the development of novel inhibitors with more specifically tailored specificities toward individual kinases are expected to lead to more refined therapies driving the field toward personalized targeted therapeutic approaches. Skin diseases also provide unique opportunities for the development of novel small molecule therapeutics, mostly through the opportunity of topical application without systemic side effects. On the other hand, the cosmetic aspects of skin diseases and the role of skin and mucous membranes as critical barriers between the internal and external environment also present substantial challenges during the development of novel therapeutics. Taken together, the scientific community may expect exciting major advances in the field of understanding and targeting tyrosine kinases in inflammatory skin diseases in the coming years.

AUTHOR CONTRIBUTIONS

KS and AM wrote the manuscript. TN provided intellectual advice.

ACKNOWLEDGMENTS

We thank members of our research group for inspiring discussions. We dedicate this work to the memory of Tibor Vántus who played a fundamental role in promoting the development of tyrosine kinase inhibitors to target inflammatory processes and inflammatory disease pathogenesis in our group.

REFERENCES

1. Gadina M. Advances in kinase inhibition: treating rheumatic diseases and beyond. *Curr Opin Rheumatol.* (2014) 26:237–43. doi: 10.1097/BOR.0000000000000023
2. Mocsai A, Kovacs L, Gergely P. What is the future of targeted therapy in rheumatology: biologics or small molecules? *BMC Med.* (2014) 12:43. doi: 10.1186/1741-7015-12-43
3. Schwartz DM, Kanno Y, Villarino A, Ward M, Gadina M, O'Shea JJ. JAK inhibition as a therapeutic strategy for immune and inflammatory diseases. *Nat Rev Drug Discov.* (2017) 16:843–62. doi: 10.1038/nrd.2017.201
4. Rodig SJ, Meraz MA, White JM, Lampe PA, Riley JK, Arthur CD, et al. Disruption of the Jak1 gene demonstrates obligatory and nonredundant roles of the Jaks in cytokine-induced biologic responses. *Cell.* (1998) 93:373–83. doi: 10.1016/S0092-8674(00)81166-6
5. Parganas E, Wang D, Stravopodis D, Topham DJ, Marine JC, Teglund S, et al. Jak2 is essential for signaling through a variety of cytokine receptors. *Cell.* (1998) 93:385–95. doi: 10.1016/S0092-8674(00)81167-8
6. Neubauer H, Cumano A, Muller M, Wu H, Huffstadt U, Pfeffer K. Jak2 deficiency defines an essential developmental checkpoint in definitive hematopoiesis. *Cell.* (1998) 93:397–409. doi: 10.1016/S0092-8674(00)81168-X
7. Macchi P, Villa A, Giliani S, Sacco MG, Frattini A, Porta F, et al. Mutations of Jak-3 gene in patients with autosomal severe combined immune deficiency (SCID). *Nature.* (1995) 377:65–8. doi: 10.1038/377065a0
8. Russell SM, Tayebi N, Nakajima H, Riedy MC, Roberts JL, Aman MJ, et al. Mutation of Jak3 in a patient with SCID: essential role of Jak3 in lymphoid development. *Science.* (1995) 270:797–800. doi: 10.1126/science.270.5237.797
9. Nosaka T, van Deursen JM, Tripp RA, Thierfelder WE, Witthuhn BA, McMickle AP, et al. Defective lymphoid development in mice lacking Jak3. *Science.* (1995) 270:800–2. doi: 10.1126/science.270.5237.800
10. Park SY, Saijo K, Takahashi T, Osawa M, Arase H, Hirayama N, et al. Developmental defects of lymphoid cells in Jak3 kinase-deficient mice. *Immunity.* (1995) 3:771–82. doi: 10.1016/1074-7613(95)90066-7
11. Shimoda K, Kato K, Aoki K, Matsuda T, Miyamoto A, Shibamori M, et al. Tyk2 plays a restricted role in IFN alpha signaling, although it is required for IL-12-mediated T cell function. *Immunity.* (2000) 13:561–71. doi: 10.1016/S1074-7613(00)00055-8
12. Karaghiosoff M, Neubauer H, Lassnig C, Kovarik P, Schindler H, Pircher H, et al. Partial impairment of cytokine responses in Tyk2-deficient mice. *Immunity.* (2000) 13:549–60. doi: 10.1016/S1074-7613(00)00054-6
13. Karaghiosoff M, Steinborn R, Kovarik P, Kriegshauser G, Baccarini M, Donabauer B, et al. Central role for type I interferons and Tyk2 in lipopolysaccharide-induced endotoxin shock. *Nat Immunol.* (2003) 4:471–7. doi: 10.1038/ni910
14. Shaw MH, Boyartchuk V, Wong S, Karaghiosoff M, Ragimbeau J, Pellegrini S, et al. A natural mutation in the Tyk2 pseudokinase domain underlies altered susceptibility of B10.Q/J mice to infection and autoimmunity. *Proc Natl Acad Sci USA.* (2003) 100:11594–9. doi: 10.1073/pnas.1930781100
15. Virtanen A, Haikarainen T, Raivola J, Silvennoinen O. Selective JAKinibs: prospects in inflammatory and autoimmune diseases. *BioDrugs.* (2019) 33:15–32. doi: 10.1007/s40259-019-00333-w
16. Yu V, Pistillo J, Archibeque I, Han Lee J, Sun B-C, Schenkel LB, et al. Differential selectivity of JAK2 inhibitors in enzymatic and cellular settings. *Exp Hematol.* (2013) 41:491–500. doi: 10.1016/j.exphem.2013.01.005
17. Yarilina A, Xu K, Chan C, Ivashkiv LB. Regulation of inflammatory responses in tumor necrosis factor-activated and rheumatoid arthritis synovial macrophages by JAK inhibitors. *Arthritis Rheum.* (2012) 64:3856–66. doi: 10.1002/art.37691
18. LaBranche TP, Jesson MI, Radi ZA, Storer CE, Guzova JA, Bonar SL, et al. JAK inhibition with tofacitinib suppresses arthritic joint structural damage through decreased RANKL production. *Arthritis Rheum.* (2012) 64:3531–42. doi: 10.1002/art.34649
19. Ghoreschi K, Jesson MI, Li X, Lee JL, Ghosh S, Alsup JW, et al. Modulation of innate and adaptive immune responses by tofacitinib (CP-690,550). *J Immunol.* (2011) 186:4234–43. doi: 10.4049/jimmunol.1003668
20. Milici AJ, Kudlacz EM, Audoly L, Zwillich S, Changelian P. Cartilage preservation by inhibition of Janus kinase 3 in two rodent models of rheumatoid arthritis. *Arthritis Res Ther.* (2008) 10:R14. doi: 10.1186/ar2365
21. Gomez-Puerta JA, Mocsai A. Tyrosine kinase inhibitors for the treatment of rheumatoid arthritis. *Curr Top Med Chem.* (2013) 13:760–73. doi: 10.2174/15680266113139990094
22. Gadina M, Johnson C, Schwartz D, Bonelli M, Hasni S, Kanno Y, et al. Translational and clinical advances in JAK-STAT biology: the present and future of jakinibs. *J Leukoc Biol.* (2018) 104:499–514. doi: 10.1002/JLB.5RI0218-084R
23. Lowell CA. Src-family kinases: rheostats of immune cell signaling. *Mol Immunol.* (2004) 41:631–43. doi: 10.1016/j.molimm.2004.04.010
24. Mocsai A, Ruland J, Tybulewicz VL. The SYK tyrosine kinase: a crucial player in diverse biological functions. *Nat Rev Immunol.* (2010) 10:387–402. doi: 10.1038/nri2765
25. Berton G, Mocsai A, Lowell CA. Src and Syk kinases: key regulators of phagocytic cell activation. *Trends Immunol.* (2005) 26:208–14. doi: 10.1016/j.it.2005.02.002
26. Futosi K, Mocsai A. Tyrosine kinase signaling pathways in neutrophils. *Immunol Rev.* (2016) 273:121–39. doi: 10.1111/imr.12455
27. Jakus Z, Fodor S, Abram CL, Lowell CA, Mocsai A. Immunoreceptor-like signaling by β2 and β3 integrins. *Trends Cell Biol.* (2007) 17:493–501. doi: 10.1016/j.tcb.2007.09.001
28. Mocsai A, Ligeti E, Lowell CA, Berton G. Adhesion-dependent degranulation of neutrophils requires the Src family kinases Fgr and Hck. *J Immunol.* (1999) 162:1120–6.
29. Lamagna C, Hu Y, DeFranco AL, Lowell CA. B cell-specific loss of Lyn kinase leads to autoimmunity. *J Immunol.* (2014) 192:919–28. doi: 10.4049/jimmunol.1301979
30. Fitzer-Attas CJ, Lowry M, Crowley MT, Finn AJ, Meng F, DeFranco AL, et al. Fcγ receptor-mediated phagocytosis in macrophages lacking the Src family tyrosine kinases Hck, Fgr, and Lyn. *J Exp Med.* (2000) 191:669–82. doi: 10.1084/jem.191.4.669
31. Mocsai A, Jakus Z, Vantus T, Berton G, Lowell CA, Ligeti E. Kinase pathways in chemoattractant-induced degranulation of neutrophils: the role of p38 mitogen-activated protein kinase activated by Src family kinases. *J Immunol.* (2000) 164:4321–31. doi: 10.4049/jimmunol.164.8.4321
32. Kovacs M, Nemeth T, Jakus Z, Sitaru C, Simon E, Futosi K, et al. The Src family kinases Hck, Fgr, and Lyn are critical for the generation of the *in vivo* inflammatory environment without a direct role in leukocyte recruitment. *J Exp Med.* (2014) 211:1993–2011. doi: 10.1084/jem.20132496
33. Lindauer M, Hochhaus A. Dasatinib. *Recent Results Cancer Res.* (2018) 212:29–68. doi: 10.1007/978-3-319-91439-8_2
34. Puttini M, Coluccia AM, Boschelli F, Cleris L, Marchesi E, Donella-Deana A, et al. *In vitro* and *in vivo* activity of SKI-606, a novel Src-Abl inhibitor,

against imatinib-resistant Bcr-Abl+ neoplastic cells. *Cancer Res.* (2006) 66:11314–22. doi: 10.1158/0008-5472.CAN-06-1199

35. Amsberg GK, Schafhausen P. Bosutinib in the management of chronic myelogenous leukemia. *Biologics.* (2013) 7:115–22. doi: 10.2147/BTT.S30182
36. Hanke JH, Gardner JP, Dow RL, Changelian PS, Brissette WH, Weringer EJ, et al. Discovery of a novel, potent, and Src family-selective tyrosine kinase inhibitor. Study of Lck- and FynT-dependent T cell activation. *J Biol Chem.* (1996) 271:695–701. doi: 10.1074/jbc.271.2.695
37. Brandvold KR, Steffey ME, Fox CC, Soellner MB. Development of a highly selective c-Src kinase inhibitor. *ACS Chem Biol.* (2012) 7:1393–8. doi: 10.1021/cb300172e
38. Braselmann S, Taylor V, Zhao H, Wang S, Sylvain C, Baluom M, et al. R406, an orally available spleen tyrosine kinase inhibitor blocks fc receptor signaling and reduces immune complex-mediated inflammation. *J Pharmacol Exp Ther.* (2006) 319:998–1008. doi: 10.1124/jpet.106.109058
39. Sharman J, Hawkins M, Kolibaba K, Boxer M, Klein L, Wu M, et al. An open-label phase 2 trial of entospletinib (GS-9973), a selective spleen tyrosine kinase inhibitor, in chronic lymphocytic leukemia. *Blood.* (2015) 125:2336–43. doi: 10.1182/blood-2014-08-595934
40. Connell NT, Berliner N. Fostamatinib for the treatment of chronic immune thrombocytopenia. *Blood.* (2019) 133:2027–30. doi: 10.1182/blood-2018-11-852491
41. Currie KS, Kropf JE, Lee T, Blomgren P, Xu J, Zhao Z, et al. Discovery of GS-9973, a selective and orally efficacious inhibitor of spleen tyrosine kinase. *J Med Chem.* (2014) 57:3856–73. doi: 10.1021/jm500228a
42. Liu D, Mamorska-Dyga A. Syk inhibitors in clinical development for hematological malignancies. *J Hematol Oncol.* (2017) 10:145. doi: 10.1186/s13045-017-0512-1
43. Coffey G, DeGuzman F, Inagaki M, Pak Y, Delaney SM, Ives D, et al. Specific inhibition of spleen tyrosine kinase suppresses leukocyte immune function and inflammation in animal models of rheumatoid arthritis. *J Pharmacol Exp Ther.* (2012) 340:350–9. doi: 10.1124/jpet.111.188441
44. Liao C, Hsu J, Kim Y, Hu DQ, Xu D, Zhang J, et al. Selective inhibition of spleen tyrosine kinase (SYK) with a novel orally bioavailable small molecule inhibitor, RO9021, impinges on various innate and adaptive immune responses: implications for SYK inhibitors in autoimmune disease therapy. *Arthritis Res Ther.* (2013) 15:R146. doi: 10.1186/ar4329
45. Reilly MP, Sinha U, Andre P, Taylor SM, Pak Y, Deguzman FR, et al. PRT-060318, a novel Syk inhibitor, prevents heparin-induced thrombocytopenia and thrombosis in a transgenic mouse model. *Blood.* (2011) 117:2241–6. doi: 10.1182/blood-2010-03-274969
46. Lam B, Arikawa Y, Cramlett J, Dong Q, de Jong R, Feher V, et al. Discovery of TAK-659 an orally available investigational inhibitor of Spleen Tyrosine Kinase (SYK). *Bioorg Med Chem Lett.* (2016) 26:5947–50. doi: 10.1016/j.bmcl.2016.10.087
47. Kaplan JB, Gordon LI, Infante JR, Popat R, Rambaldi A, Madan S, et al. Updated results from a phase 1 study of TAK-659, an investigational and reversible SYK inhibitor, in Patients (Pts) with advanced solid tumor or lymphoma malignancies. *Blood.* (2016) 128:624.
48. Futosi K, Nemeth T, Pick R, Vantus T, Walzog B, Mocsai A. Dasatinib inhibits proinflammatory functions of mature human neutrophils. *Blood.* (2012) 119:4981–91. doi: 10.1182/blood-2011-07-369041
49. Azizi G, Goudarzvand M, Afraei S, Sedaghat R, Mirshafiey A. Therapeutic effects of dasatinib in mouse model of multiple sclerosis. *Immunopharmacol Immunotoxicol.* (2015) 37:287–94. doi: 10.3109/08923973.2015.1028074
50. da Silva AL, Magalhaes RF, Branco VC, Silva JD, Cruz FF, Marques PS, et al. The tyrosine kinase inhibitor dasatinib reduces lung inflammation and remodelling in experimental allergic asthma. *Br J Pharmacol.* (2016) 173:1236–47. doi: 10.1111/bph.13430
51. Guo K, Bu X, Yang C, Cao X, Bian H, Zhu Q, et al. Treatment effects of the second-generation tyrosine kinase inhibitor dasatinib on autoimmune arthritis. *Front Immunol.* (2018) 9:3133. doi: 10.3389/fimmu.2018.03133
52. Turner M, Mee PJ, Costello PS, Williams O, Price AA, Duddy LP, et al. Perinatal lethality and blocked B-cell development in mice lacking the tyrosine kinase Syk. *Nature.* (1995) 378:298–302. doi: 10.1038/378298a0
53. Cheng AM, Rowley B, Pao W, Hayday A, Bolen JB, Pawson T. Syk tyrosine kinase required for mouse viability and B-cell development. *Nature.* (1995) 378:303–6. doi: 10.1038/378303a0
54. Abtahian F, Guerriero A, Sebzda E, Lu MM, Zhou R, Mocsai A, et al. Regulation of blood and lymphatic vascular separation by signaling proteins SLP-76 and Syk. *Science.* (2003) 299:247–51. doi: 10.1126/science.1079477
55. LeibundGut-Landmann S, Gross O, Robinson MJ, Osorio F, Slack EC, Tsoni SV, et al. Syk- and CARD9-dependent coupling of innate immunity to the induction of T helper cells that produce interleukin 17. *Nat Immunol.* (2007) 8:630–8. doi: 10.1038/ni1460
56. Gross O, Poeck H, Bscheider M, Dostert C, Hannesschlager N, Endres S, et al. Syk kinase signalling couples to the Nlrp3 inflammasome for anti-fungal host defence. *Nature.* (2009) 459:433–6. doi: 10.1038/nature07965
57. Mocsai A, Zhou M, Meng F, Tybulewicz VL, Lowell CA. Syk is required for integrin signaling in neutrophils. *Immunity.* (2002) 16:547–58. doi: 10.1016/S1074-7613(02)00303-5
58. Mocsai A, Abram CL, Jakus Z, Hu Y, Lanier LL, Lowell CA. Integrin signaling in neutrophils and macrophages uses adaptors containing immunoreceptor tyrosine-based activation motifs. *Nat Immunol.* (2006) 7:1326–33. doi: 10.1038/ni1407
59. Crowley MT, Costello PS, Fitzer-Attas CJ, Turner M, Meng F, Lowell C, et al. A critical role for Syk in signal transduction and phagocytosis mediated by Fcgamma receptors on macrophages. *J Exp Med.* (1997) 186:1027–39. doi: 10.1084/jem.186.7.1027
60. Jakus Z, Simon E, Balazs B, Mocsai A. Genetic deficiency of Syk protects mice from autoantibody-induced arthritis. *Arthritis Rheum.* (2010) 62:1899–910. doi: 10.1002/art.27438
61. Nemeth T, Futosi K, Szilveszter K, Vilinovszki O, Kiss-Papai L, Mocsai A. Lineage-specific analysis of Syk function in autoantibody-induced arthritis. *Front Immunol.* (2018) 9:555. doi: 10.3389/fimmu.2018.00555
62. Elliott ER, Van Ziffle JA, Scapini P, Sullivan BM, Locksley RM, Lowell CA. Deletion of Syk in neutrophils prevents immune complex arthritis. *J Immunol.* (2011) 187:4319–30. doi: 10.4049/jimmunol.1100341
63. Weinblatt ME, Kavanaugh A, Burgos-Vargas R, Dikranian AH, Medrano-Ramirez G, Morales-Torres JL, et al. Treatment of rheumatoid arthritis with a Syk kinase inhibitor: a twelve-week, randomized, placebo-controlled trial. *Arthritis Rheum.* (2008) 58:3309–18. doi: 10.1002/art.23992
64. Coffey G, Rani A, Betz A, Pak Y, Haberstock-Debic H, Pandey A, et al. PRT062607 achieves complete inhibition of the spleen tyrosine kinase at tolerated exposures following oral dosing in healthy volunteers. *J Clin Pharmacol.* (2017) 57:194–210. doi: 10.1002/jcph.794
65. Coffey G, Betz A, DeGuzman F, Pak Y, Inagaki M, Baker DC, et al. The novel kinase inhibitor PRT062070 (Cerdulatinib) demonstrates efficacy in models of autoimmunity and B-cell cancer. *J Pharmacol Exp Ther.* (2014) 351:538–48. doi: 10.1124/jpet.114.218164
66. Rip J, de Bruijn MJW, Appelman MK, Pal Singh S, Hendriks RW, Corneth OBJ. Toll-like receptor signaling drives Btk-mediated autoimmune disease. *Front Immunol.* (2019) 10:95. doi: 10.3389/fimmu.2019.00095
67. Tsukada S, Saffran DC, Rawlings DJ, Parolini O, Allen RC, Klisak I, et al. Deficient expression of a B cell cytoplasmic tyrosine kinase in human X-linked agammaglobulinemia. *Cell.* (1993) 72:279–90. doi: 10.1016/0092-8674(93)90667-F
68. Vetrie D, Vorechovsky I, Sideras, Holland J, Davies A, Flinter F, et al. The gene involved in X-linked agammaglobulinaemia is a member of the src family of protein-tyrosine kinases. *Nature.* (1993) 361:226–33. doi: 10.1038/364362a0
69. Middendorp S, Dingjan GM, Hendriks RW. Impaired precursor B cell differentiation in Bruton's tyrosine kinase-deficient mice. *J Immunol.* (2002) 168:2695–703. doi: 10.4049/jimmunol.168.6.2695
70. Kil LP, de Bruijn MJ, van Nimwegen M, Corneth OB, van Hamburg JP, Dingjan GM, et al. Btk levels set the threshold for B-cell activation and negative selection of autoreactive B cells in mice. *Blood.* (2012) 119:3744–56. doi: 10.1182/blood-2011-12-397919
71. Fiedler K, Sindrilaru A, Terszowski G, Kokai E, Feyerabend TB, Bullinger L, et al. Neutrophil development and function critically depend on Bruton tyrosine kinase in a mouse model of X-linked agammaglobulinemia. *Blood.* (2011) 117:1329–39. doi: 10.1182/blood-2010-04-281170
72. Corneth OBJ, Klein Wolterink RGJ, Hendriks RW. BTK Signaling in B cell differentiation and autoimmunity. *Curr Top Microbiol Immunol.* (2016) 393:67–105. doi: 10.1007/82_2015_478

73. Horwood NJ, Urbaniak AM, Danks L. Tec family kinases in inflammation and disease. *Int Rev Immunol.* (2012) 31:87–103. doi: 10.3109/08830185.2012.670334
74. Lemmon MA, Schlessinger J. Cell signaling by receptor tyrosine kinases. *Cell.* (2010) 141:1117–34. doi: 10.1016/j.cell.2010.06.011
75. Roskoski R Jr. The ErbB/HER family of protein-tyrosine kinases and cancer. *Pharmacol Res.* (2014) 79:34–74. doi: 10.1016/j.phrs.2013.11.002
76. Weidinger S, Beck LA, Bieber T, Kabashima K, Irvine AD. Atopic dermatitis. *Nat Rev Dis Primers.* (2018) 4:1. doi: 10.1038/s41572-018-0001-z
77. Palmer CN, Irvine AD, Terron-Kwiatkowski A, Zhao Y, Liao H, Lee SP, et al. Common loss-of-function variants of the epidermal barrier protein filaggrin are a major predisposing factor for atopic dermatitis. *Nat Genet.* (2006) 38:441–6. doi: 10.1038/ng1767
78. Sandilands A, O'Regan GM, Liao H, Zhao Y, Terron-Kwiatkowski A, Watson RM, et al. Prevalent and rare mutations in the gene encoding filaggrin cause ichthyosis vulgaris and predispose individuals to atopic dermatitis. *J Invest Dermatol.* (2006) 126:1770–5. doi: 10.1038/sj.jid.5700459
79. Wohlmann A, Sebastian K, Borowski A, Krause S, Friedrich K. Signal transduction by the atopy-associated human thymic stromal lymphopoietin (TSLP) receptor depends on Janus kinase function. *Biol Chem.* (2010) 391:181–6. doi: 10.1515/bc.2010.029
80. Leyva-Castillo JM, Hener, Jiang H, Li M. TSLP produced by keratinocytes promotes allergen sensitization through skin and thereby triggers atopic march in mice. *J Invest Dermatol.* (2013) 133:154–63. doi: 10.1038/jid.2012.239
81. Yoo J, Omori M, Gyarmati D, Zhou B, Aye T, Brewer A, et al. Spontaneous atopic dermatitis in mice expressing an inducible thymic stromal lymphopoietin transgene specifically in the skin. *J Exp Med.* (2005) 202:541–9. doi: 10.1084/jem.20041503
82. Wilson SR, The L, Batia LM, Beattie K, Katibah GE, McClain SP, et al. The epithelial cell-derived atopic dermatitis cytokine TSLP activates neurons to induce itch. *Cell.* (2013) 155:285–95. doi: 10.1016/j.cell.2013.08.057
83. Jin H, He R, Oyoshi M, Geha RS. Animal models of atopic dermatitis. *J Invest Dermatol.* (2009) 129:31–40. doi: 10.1038/jid.2008.106
84. Howell MD, Kim BE, Gao P, Grant AV, Boguniewicz M, Debenedetto A, et al. Cytokine modulation of atopic dermatitis filaggrin skin expression. *J Allergy Clin Immunol.* (2007) 120:150–5. doi: 10.1016/j.jaci.2007.04.031
85. Bao L, Shi VY, Chan LS. IL-4 regulates chemokine CCL26 in keratinocytes through the Jak1, 2/Stat6 signal transduction pathway: implication for atopic dermatitis. *Mol Immunol.* (2012) 50:91–7. doi: 10.1016/j.molimm.2011.12.008
86. Bao L, Shi VY, Chan LS. IL-4 up-regulates epidermal chemotactic, angiogenic, and pro-inflammatory genes and down-regulates antimicrobial genes *in vivo* and *in vitro*: relevant in the pathogenesis of atopic dermatitis. *Cytokine.* (2013) 61:419–25. doi: 10.1016/j.cyto.2012.10.031
87. Amano W, Nakajima S, Kunugi H, Numata Y, Kitoh A, Egawa G, et al. The Janus kinase inhibitor JTE-052 improves skin barrier function through suppressing signal transducer and activator of transcription 3 signaling. *J Allergy Clin Immunol.* (2015) 136:667–77.e7. doi: 10.1016/j.jaci.2015.03.051
88. Oetjen LK, Mack MR, Feng J, Whelan TM, Niu H, Guo CJ, et al. Sensory neurons co-opt classical immune signaling pathways to mediate chronic itch. *Cell.* (2017) 171:217–28.e13. doi: 10.1016/j.cell.2017.08.006
89. Beck LA, Thaci D, Hamilton JD, Graham NM, Bieber T, Rocklin R, et al. Dupilumab treatment in adults with moderate-to-severe atopic dermatitis. *N Engl J Med.* (2014) 371:130–9. doi: 10.1056/NEJMoa1314768
90. Blauvelt A, de Bruin-Weller M, Gooderham M, Cather JC, Weisman J, Pariser D, et al. Long-term management of moderate-to-severe atopic dermatitis with dupilumab and concomitant topical corticosteroids (LIBERTY AD CHRONOS): a 1-year, randomised, double-blinded, placebo-controlled, phase 3 trial. *Lancet.* (2017) 389:2287–303. doi: 10.1111/imj.67_13578
91. Shirley M. Dupilumab: first global approval. *Drugs.* (2017) 77:1115–21. doi: 10.1007/s40265-017-0768-3
92. Novak N, Tepel C, Koch S, Brix K, Bieber T, Kraft S. Evidence for a differential expression of the FcepsilonRIgamma chain in dendritic cells of atopic and nonatopic donors. *J Clin Invest.* (2003) 111:1047–56. doi: 10.1172/JCI200315932
93. Yasuda T, Fukada T, Nishida K, Nakayama M, Matsuda M, Miura I, et al. Hyperactivation of JAK1 tyrosine kinase induces stepwise, progressive pruritic dermatitis. *J Clin Invest.* (2016) 126:2064–76. doi: 10.1172/JCI82887
94. Fukuyama T, Ehling S, Cook E, Baumer W. Topically administered Janus-Kinase inhibitors tofacitinib and oclacitinib display impressive antipruritic and anti-inflammatory responses in a model of allergic dermatitis. *J Pharmacol Exp Ther.* (2015) 354:394–405. doi: 10.1124/jpet.115.223784
95. Fridman JS, Scherle PA, Collins R, Burn T, Neilan CL, Hertel D, et al. Preclinical evaluation of local JAK1 and JAK2 inhibition in cutaneous inflammation. *J Invest Dermatol.* (2011) 131:1838–44. doi: 10.1038/jid.2011.140
96. Jin W, Huang W, Chen L, Jin M, Wang Q, Gao Z, et al. Topical application of JAK1/JAK2 inhibitor momelotinib exhibits significant anti-inflammatory responses in DNCB-induced atopic dermatitis model mice. *Int J Mol Sci.* (2018) 19:E3973. doi: 10.3390/ijms19123973
97. Amano W, Nakajima S, Yamamoto Y, Tanimoto A, Matsushita M, Miyachi Y, et al. JAK inhibitor JTE-052 regulates contact hypersensitivity by downmodulating T cell activation and differentiation. *J Dermatol Sci.* (2016) 84:258–65. doi: 10.1016/j.jdermsci.2016.09.007
98. Tanimoto A, Shinozaki Y, Yamamoto Y, Katsuda Y, Taniai-Riya E, Toyoda K, et al. A novel JAK inhibitor JTE-052 reduces skin inflammation and ameliorates chronic dermatitis in rodent models: comparison with conventional therapeutic agents. *Exp Dermatol.* (2018) 27:22–29. doi: 10.1111/exd.13370
99. Bissonnette R, Papp KA, Poulin Y, Gooderham M, Raman M, Mallbris L, et al. Topical tofacitinib for atopic dermatitis: a phase IIa randomized trial. *Br J Dermatol.* (2016) 175:902–11. doi: 10.1111/bjd.14871
100. Incyte Corporation. *Incyte Announces Positive Data from Phase 2b Trial of Ruxolitinib Cream in Patients with Atopic Dermatitis* (2018). Available online at: https://www.businesswire.com/news/home/20180913005058/en/Incyte-Announces-Positive-Data-Phase-2b-Trial
101. Incyte Corporation. *Incyte Announces First Patient Treated in Phase 3 Clinical Trial Program for Ruxolitinib Cream in Atopic Dermatitis* (2018). Available online at: https://www.businesswire.com/news/home/20181220005644/en/
102. Incyte Corporation. *Baricitinib Meets Primary Endpoint in Phase 2 Study of Patients with Moderate-to-Severe Atopic Dermatitis* (2017). Available onlilne at: https://www.prnewswire.com/news-releases/baricitinib-meets-primary-endpoint-in-phase-2-study-of-patients-with-moderate-to-severe-atopic-dermatitis-300518896.html
103. *Lilly Announces Top-Line Phase 3 Results for Baricitinib in Patients with Moderate to Severe Atopic Dermatitis.* Eli Lilly & Company (2019). Available online at: https://www.prnewswire.com/news-releases/lilly-announces-top-line-phase-3-results-for-baricitinib-in-patients-with-moderate-to-severe-atopic-dermatitis-300788783.html
104. AbbVie. *AbbVie's Upadacitinib (ABT-494) Meets Primary Endpoint in Phase 2b Study in Atopic Dermatitis* (2017). Available online at: https://news.abbvie.com/news/abbvies-upadacitinib-abt-494-meets-primary-endpoint-in-phase-2b-study-in-atopic-dermatitis.htm
105. Greb JE, Goldminz AM, Elder JT, Lebwohl MG, Gladman DD, Wu JJ, et al. Psoriasis. *Nat Rev Dis Primers.* (2016) 2:16082. doi: 10.1038/nrdp.2016.82
106. Di Cesare A, Di Meglio P, Nestle FO. The IL-23/Th17 axis in the immunopathogenesis of psoriasis. *J Invest Dermatol.* (2009) 129:1339–50. doi: 10.1038/jid.2009.59
107. Singh TP, Zhang HH, Hwang ST, Farber JM. IL-23- and imiquimod-induced models of experimental psoriasis in mice. *Curr Protoc Immunol.* (2019) 125:e71. doi: 10.1002/cpim.71
108. Cai YH, Shen XY, Ding CL, Qi CJ, Li KJ, Li X, et al. Pivotal role of dermal IL-17-producing γδ T cells in skin inflammation. *Immunity.* (2011) 35:596–610. doi: 10.1016/j.immuni.2011.10.006
109. Dainichi T, Kitoh A, Otsuka A, Nakajima S, Nomura T, Kaplan DH, et al. The epithelial immune microenvironment (EIME) in atopic dermatitis and psoriasis. *Nat Immunol.* (2018) 19:1286–98. doi: 10.1038/s41590-018-0256-2
110. Rendon A, Schakel K. Psoriasis pathogenesis and treatment. *Int J Mol Sci.* (2019) 20:E1475. doi: 10.3390/ijms20061475
111. Singh S, Pradhan D, Puri P, Ramesh V, Aggarwal S, Nayek A, et al. Genomic alterations driving psoriasis pathogenesis. *Gene.* (2019) 683:61–71. doi: 10.1016/j.gene.2018.09.042

112. Ishizaki M, Muromoto R, Akimoto T, Sekine Y, Kon S, Diwan M, et al. Tyk2 is a therapeutic target for psoriasis-like skin inflammation. *Int Immunol.* (2014) 26:257–67. doi: 10.1093/intimm/dxt062
113. Sano S, Chan KS, Carbajal S, Clifford J, Peavey M, Kiguchi K, et al. Stat3 links activated keratinocytes and immunocytes required for development of psoriasis in a novel transgenic mouse model. *Nat Med.* (2005) 11:43–9. doi: 10.1038/nm1162
114. Works MG, Yin F, Yin CC, Yiu Y, Shew K, Tran TT, et al. Inhibition of TYK2 and JAK1 ameliorates imiquimod-induced psoriasis-like dermatitis by inhibiting IL-22 and the IL-23/IL-17 axis. *J Immunol.* (2014) 193:3278–87. doi: 10.4049/jimmunol.1400205
115. Krueger J, Clark JD, Suarez-Farinas M, Fuentes-Duculan J, Cueto I, Wang CQ, et al. Tofacitinib attenuates pathologic immune pathways in patients with psoriasis: a randomized phase 2 study. *J Allergy Clin Immunol.* (2016) 137:1079–90. doi: 10.1016/j.jaci.2015.12.1318
116. Papp KA, Menter A, Strober B, Langley RG, Buonanno M, Wolk R, et al. Efficacy and safety of tofacitinib, an oral Janus kinase inhibitor, in the treatment of psoriasis: a Phase 2b randomized placebo-controlled dose-ranging study. *Br J Dermatol.* (2012) 167:668–77. doi: 10.1111/j.1365-2133.2012.11168.x
117. Bachelez H, van de Kerkhof PC, Strohal R, Kubanov A, Valenzuela F, Lee JH, et al. Tofacitinib versus etanercept or placebo in moderate-to-severe chronic plaque psoriasis: a phase 3 randomised non-inferiority trial. *Lancet.* (2015) 386:552–61. doi: 10.1016/S0140-6736(14)62113-9
118. Asahina A, Etoh T, Igarashi A, Imafuku S, Saeki H, Shibasaki Y, et al. Oral tofacitinib efficacy, safety and tolerability in Japanese patients with moderate to severe plaque psoriasis and psoriatic arthritis: a randomized, double-blind, phase 3 study. *J Dermatol.* (2016) 43:869–80. doi: 10.1111/1346-8138.13258
119. Bissonnette R, Iversen L, Sofen H, Griffiths CE, Foley P, Romiti R, et al. Tofacitinib withdrawal and retreatment in moderate-to-severe chronic plaque psoriasis: a randomized controlled trial. *Br J Dermatol.* (2015) 172:1395–406. doi: 10.1111/bjd.13551
120. Papp KA, Menter MA, Abe M, Elewski B, Feldman SR, Gottlieb AB, et al. Tofacitinib, an oral Janus kinase inhibitor, for the treatment of chronic plaque psoriasis: results from two randomized, placebo-controlled, phase III trials. *Br J Dermatol.* (2015) 173:949–61. doi: 10.1111/bjd.14018
121. Zhang J, Tsai TF, Lee MG, Zheng M, Wang G, Jin H, et al. The efficacy and safety of tofacitinib in Asian patients with moderate to severe chronic plaque psoriasis: a Phase 3, randomized, double-blind, placebo-controlled study. *J Dermatol Sci.* (2017) 88:36–45. doi: 10.1016/j.jdermsci.2017.05.004
122. Valenzuela F, Korman NJ, Bissonnette R, Bakos N, Tsai TF, Harper MK, et al. Tofacitinib in patients with moderate-to-severe chronic plaque psoriasis: long-term safety and efficacy in an open-label extension study. *Br J Dermatol.* (2018) 179:853–62. doi: 10.1111/bjd.16798
123. Papp KA, Bissonnette R, Gooderham M, Feldman SR, Iversen L, Soung J, et al. Treatment of plaque psoriasis with an ointment formulation of the Janus kinase inhibitor, tofacitinib: a Phase 2b randomized clinical trial. *BMC Dermatol.* (2016) 16:15. doi: 10.1186/s12895-016-0051-4
124. Punwani N, Scherle P, Flores R, Shi J, Liang J, Yeleswaram S, et al. Preliminary clinical activity of a topical JAK1/2 inhibitor in the treatment of psoriasis. *J Am Acad Dermatol.* (2012) 67:658–64. doi: 10.1016/j.jaad.2011.12.018
125. Papp KA, Menter MA, Raman M, Disch D, Schlichting DE, Gaich C, et al. A randomized phase 2b trial of baricitinib, an oral Janus kinase (JAK) 1/JAK2 inhibitor, in patients with moderate-to-severe psoriasis. *Br J Dermatol.* (2016) 174:1266–76. doi: 10.1111/bjd.14403
126. Schmieder GJ, Draelos ZD, Pariser DM, Banfield C, Cox L, Hodge M, et al. Efficacy and safety of the Janus kinase 1 inhibitor PF-04965842 in patients with moderate-to-severe psoriasis: phase II, randomized, double-blind, placebo-controlled study. *Br J Dermatol.* (2018) 179:54–62. doi: 10.1111/bjd.16004
127. Bissonnette R, Luchi M, Fidelus-Gort R, Jackson S, Zhang H, Flores R, et al. A randomized, double-blind, placebo-controlled, dose-escalation study of the safety and efficacy of INCB039110, an oral janus kinase 1 inhibitor, in patients with stable, chronic plaque psoriasis. *J Dermatolog Treat.* (2016) 27:332–8. doi: 10.3109/09546634.2015.1115819
128. Papp K, Gordon K, Thaci D, Morita A, Gooderham M, Foley P, et al. Phase 2 trial of selective tyrosine kinase 2 inhibition in psoriasis. *N Engl J Med.* (2018) 379:1313–21. doi: 10.1056/NEJMoa1806382
129. Ludbrook VJ, Hicks KJ, Hanrott KE, Patel JS, Binks MH, Wyres MR, et al. Investigation of selective JAK1 inhibitor GSK2586184 for the treatment of psoriasis in a randomized placebo-controlled phase IIa study. *Br J Dermatol.* (2016) 174:985–95. doi: 10.1111/bjd.14399
130. Papp KA, Krueger JG, Feldman SR, Langley RG, Thaci D, Torii H, et al. Tofacitinib, an oral Janus kinase inhibitor, for the treatment of chronic plaque psoriasis: long-term efficacy and safety results from 2 randomized phase-III studies and 1 open-label long-term extension study. *J Am Acad Dermatol.* (2016) 74:841–50. doi: 10.1016/j.jaad.2016.01.013
131. Muro R, Nitta T, Nakano K, Okamura T, Takayanagi H, Suzuki H. γδ TCR recruits the Syk/PI3K axis to drive proinflammatory differentiation program. *J Clin Invest.* (2018) 128:415–26. doi: 10.1172/JCI95837
132. Cook PW, Piepkorn M, Clegg CH, Plowman GD, DeMay JM, Brown JR, et al. Transgenic expression of the human amphiregulin gene induces a psoriasis-like phenotype. *J Clin Invest.* (1997) 100:2286–94. doi: 10.1172/JCI119766
133. Cook PW, Brown JR, Cornell KA, Pittelkow MR. Suprabasal expression of human amphiregulin in the epidermis of transgenic mice induces a severe, early-onset, psoriasis-like skin pathology: expression of amphiregulin in the basal epidermis is also associated with synovitis. *Exp Dermatol.* (2004) 13:347–56. doi: 10.1111/j.0906-6705.2004.00183.x
134. Bhagavathula N, Nerusu KC, Fisher GJ, Liu G, Thakur AB, Gemmell L, et al. Amphiregulin and epidermal hyperplasia: amphiregulin is required to maintain the psoriatic phenotype of human skin grafts on severe combined immunodeficient mice. *Am J Pathol.* (2005) 166:1009–16. doi: 10.1016/S0002-9440(10)62322-X
135. Pastore S, Mascia F, Mariotti F, Dattilo C, Mariani V, Girolomoni G. ERK1/2 regulates epidermal chemokine expression and skin inflammation. *J Immunol.* (2005) 174:5047–56. doi: 10.4049/jimmunol.174.8.5047
136. Lichtenberger BM, Gerber PA, Holcmann M, Buhren BA, Amberg N, Smolle V, et al. Epidermal EGFR controls cutaneous host defense and prevents inflammation. *Sci Transl Med.* (2013) 5:199ra111. doi: 10.1126/scitranslmed.3005886
137. Mascia F, Mariani V, Girolomoni G, Pastore S. Blockade of the EGF receptor induces a deranged chemokine expression in keratinocytes leading to enhanced skin inflammation. *Am J Pathol.* (2003) 163:303–12. doi: 10.1016/S0002-9440(10)63654-1
138. Tanida S, Joh T, Itoh K, Kataoka H, Sasaki M, Ohara H, et al. The mechanism of cleavage of EGFR ligands induced by inflammatory cytokines in gastric cancer cells. *Gastroenterology.* (2004) 127:559–69. doi: 10.1053/j.gastro.2004.05.017
139. Lacouture ME. Mechanisms of cutaneous toxicities to EGFR inhibitors. *Nat Rev Cancer.* (2006) 6:803–12. doi: 10.1038/nrc1970
140. Varricchi G, Granata F, Loffredo S, Genovese A, Marone G. Angiogenesis and lymphangiogenesis in inflammatory skin disorders. *J Am Acad Dermatol.* (2015) 73:144–53. doi: 10.1016/j.jaad.2015.03.041
141. Xia YP, Li B, Hylton D, Detmar M, Yancopoulos GD, Rudge JS. Transgenic delivery of VEGF to mouse skin leads to an inflammatory condition resembling human psoriasis. *Blood.* (2003) 102:161–8. doi: 10.1182/blood-2002-12-3793
142. Halin C, Fahrngruber H, Meingassner JG, Bold G, Littlewood-Evans A, Stuetz A, et al. Inhibition of chronic and acute skin inflammation by treatment with a vascular endothelial growth factor receptor tyrosine kinase inhibitor. *Am J Pathol.* (2008) 173:265–77. doi: 10.2353/ajpath.2008.071074
143. Huggenberger R, Siddiqui SS, Brander D, Ullmann S, Zimmermann K, Antsiferova M, et al. An important role of lymphatic vessel activation in limiting acute inflammation. *Blood.* (2011) 117:4667–78. doi: 10.1182/blood-2010-10-316356
144. Huggenberger R, Ullmann S, Proulx ST, Pytowski B, Alitalo K, Detmar M. Stimulation of lymphangiogenesis via VEGFR-3 inhibits chronic skin inflammation. *J Exp Med.* (2010) 207:2255–69. doi: 10.1084/jem.20100559
145. Xing L, Dai Z, Jabbari A, Cerise JE, Higgins CA, Gong W, et al. Alopecia areata is driven by cytotoxic T lymphocytes and is reversed by JAK inhibition. *Nat Med.* (2014) 20:1043–9. doi: 10.1038/nm.3645

146. Harel S, Higgins CA, Cerise JE, Dai Z, Chen JC, Clynes R, et al. Pharmacologic inhibition of JAK-STAT signaling promotes hair growth. *Sci Adv.* (2015) 1:e1500973. doi: 10.1126/sciadv.1500973
147. Kennedy Crispin M, Ko JM, Craiglow BG, Li S, Shankar G, Urban JR, et al. Safety and efficacy of the JAK inhibitor tofacitinib citrate in patients with alopecia areata. *JCI Insight.* (2016) 1:e89776. doi: 10.1172/jci.insight.89776
148. Mackay-Wiggan J, Jabbari A, Nguyen N, Cerise JE, Clark C, Ulerio G, et al. Oral ruxolitinib induces hair regrowth in patients with moderate-to-severe alopecia areata. *JCI Insight.* (2016) 1:e89790. doi: 10.1172/jci.insight.89790
149. Liu LY, Craiglow BG, King BA. Tofacitinib 2% ointment, a topical Janus kinase inhibitor, for the treatment of alopecia areata: a pilot study of 10 patients. *J Am Acad Dermatol.* (2018) 78:403–4.e1. doi: 10.1016/j.jaad.2017.10.043
150. Rashighi M, Agarwal P, Richmond JM, Harris TH, Dresser K, Su MW, et al. CXCL10 is critical for the progression and maintenance of depigmentation in a mouse model of vitiligo. *Sci Transl Med.* (2014) 6:223ra23. doi: 10.1126/scitranslmed.3007811
151. Wang S, Zhou M, Lin F, Liu D, Hong W, Lu L, et al. Interferon-γ induces senescence in normal human melanocytes. *PLoS ONE.* (2014) 9:e93232. doi: 10.1371/journal.pone.0093232
152. Craiglow BG, King BA. Tofacitinib Citrate for the treatment of vitiligo: a pathogenesis-directed therapy. *JAMA Dermatol.* (2015) 151:1110–2. doi: 10.1001/jamadermatol.2015.1520
153. Liu LY, Strassner JP, Refat MA, Harris JE, King BA. Repigmentation in vitiligo using the Janus kinase inhibitor tofacitinib may require concomitant light exposure. *J Am Acad Dermatol.* (2017) 77:675–82.e1. doi: 10.1016/j.jaad.2017.05.043
154. Rothstein B, Joshipura D, Saraiya A, Abdat R, Ashkar H, Turkowski Y, et al. Treatment of vitiligo with the topical Janus kinase inhibitor ruxolitinib. *J Am Acad Dermatol.* (2017) 76:1054–60.e1. doi: 10.1016/j.jaad.2017.02.049
155. Rock B, Labib RS, Diaz LA. Monovalent Fab' immunoglobulin fragments from endemic pemphigus foliaceus autoantibodies reproduce the human disease in neonatal Balb/c mice. *J Clin Invest.* (1990) 85:296–9. doi: 10.1172/JCI114426
156. Anhalt GJ, Till GO, Diaz LA, Labib RS, Patel HP, Eaglstein NF. Defining the role of complement in experimental pemphigus vulgaris in mice. *J Immunol.* (1986) 137:2835–40.
157. Calkins CC, Setzer SV, Jennings JM, Summers S, Tsunoda K, Amagai M, et al. Desmoglein endocytosis and desmosome disassembly are coordinated responses to pemphigus autoantibodies. *J Biol Chem.* (2006) 281:7623–34. doi: 10.1074/jbc.M512447200
158. Mao X, Choi EJ, Payne AS. Disruption of desmosome assembly by monovalent human pemphigus vulgaris monoclonal antibodies. *J Invest Dermatol.* (2009) 129:908–18. doi: 10.1038/jid.2008.339
159. Spindler V, Waschke J. Pemphigus-A disease of desmosome dysfunction caused by multiple mechanisms. *Front Immunol.* (2018) 9:136. doi: 10.3389/fimmu.2018.00136
160. Mao X, Cho MJT, Ellebrecht CT, Mukherjee EM, Payne AS. Stat3 regulates desmoglein 3 transcription in epithelial keratinocytes. *JCI Insight.* (2017) 2:92253. doi: 10.1172/jci.insight.92253
161. Satyam A, Khandpur S, Sharma VK, Sharma A. Involvement of T(H)1/T(H)2 cytokines in the pathogenesis of autoimmune skin disease-Pemphigus vulgaris. *Immunol Invest.* (2009) 38:498–509. doi: 10.1080/08820130902943097
162. Tavakolpour S, Tavakolpour V. Interleukin 4 inhibition as a potential therapeutic in pemphigus. *Cytokine.* (2016) 77:189–95. doi: 10.1016/j.cyto.2015.09.017
163. Tavakolpour S. Tofacitinib as the potent treatment for refractory pemphigus: a possible alternative treatment for pemphigus. *Dermatol Ther.* (2018) 31:e12696. doi: 10.1111/dth.12696
164. Vodo D, Sarig O, Geller S, Ben-Asher E, Olender T, Bochner R, et al. Identification of a functional risk variant for pemphigus vulgaris in the ST18 gene. *PLoS Genet.* (2016) 12:e1006008. doi: 10.1371/journal.pgen.1006008
165. Gil MP, Modol T, Espana A, Lopez-Zabalza MJ. Inhibition of FAK prevents blister formation in the neonatal mouse model of pemphigus vulgaris. *Exp Dermatol.* (2012) 21:254–9. doi: 10.1111/j.1600-0625.2012.01441.x
166. Frusic-Zlotkin M, Raichenberg D, Wang X, David M, Michel B, Milner Y. Apoptotic mechanism in pemphigus autoimmunoglobulins-induced acantholysis-possible involvement of the EGF receptor. *Autoimmunity.* (2006) 39:563–75. doi: 10.1080/08916930600971836
167. Chernyavsky AI, Arredondo J, Kitajima Y, Sato-Nagai M, Grando SA. Desmoglein versus non-desmoglein signaling in pemphigus acantholysis: characterization of novel signaling pathways downstream of pemphigus vulgaris antigens. *J Biol Chem.* (2007) 282:13804–12. doi: 10.1074/jbc.M611365200
168. Rubenstein DS, Diaz LA. Pemphigus antibody induced phosphorylation of keratinocyte proteins. *Autoimmunity.* (2006) 39:577–86. doi: 10.1080/08916930600971885
169. Sanchez-Carpintero I, Espana A, Pelacho B, Lopez Moratalla N, Rubenstein DS, Diaz LA, et al. *In vivo* blockade of pemphigus vulgaris acantholysis by inhibition of intracellular signal transduction cascades. *Br J Dermatol.* (2004) 151:565–70. doi: 10.1111/j.1365-2133.2004.06147.x
170. Kugelmann D, Rotzer V, Walter E, Egu DT, Fuchs MT, Vielmuth F, et al. Role of Src and cortactin in pemphigus skin blistering. *Front Immunol.* (2019) 10:626. doi: 10.3389/fimmu.2019.00626
171. Schmidt E, Zillikens D. Pemphigoid diseases. *Lancet.* (2013) 381:320–32. doi: 10.1016/S0140-6736(12)61140-4
172. Bagci IS, Horvath ON, Ruzicka T, Sardy M. Bullous pemphigoid. *Autoimmun Rev.* (2017) 16:445–55. doi: 10.1016/j.autrev.2017.03.010
173. Liu Z, Sui W, Zhao M, Li Z, Li N, Thresher R, et al. Subepidermal blistering induced by human autoantibodies to BP180 requires innate immune players in a humanized bullous pemphigoid mouse model. *J Autoimmun.* (2008) 31:331–8. doi: 10.1016/j.jaut.2008.08.009
174. Liu Z, Diaz LA, Troy JL, Taylor AF, Emery DJ, Fairley JA, et al. A passive transfer model of the organ-specific autoimmune disease, bullous pemphigoid, using antibodies generated against the hemidesmosomal antigen, BP180. *J Clin Invest.* (1993) 92:2480–8. doi: 10.1172/JCI1 16856
175. Woodley DT, Ram R, Doostan A, Bandyopadhyay P, Huang Y, Remington J, et al. Induction of epidermolysis bullosa acquisita in mice by passive transfer of autoantibodies from patients. *J Invest Dermatol.* (2006) 126:1323–30. doi: 10.1038/sj.jid.5700254
176. Sitaru C, Mihai S, Otto C, Chiriac MT, Hausser I, Dotterweich B, et al. Induction of dermal-epidermal separation in mice by passive transfer of antibodies specific to type VII collagen. *J Clin Invest.* (2005) 115:870–8. doi: 10.1172/JCI200521386
177. Liu Z, Giudice GJ, Swartz SJ, Fairley JA, Till GO, Troy JL, et al. The role of complement in experimental bullous pemphigoid. *J Clin Invest.* (1995) 95:1539–44. doi: 10.1172/JCI117826
178. Liu Z, Giudice GJ, Zhou X, Swartz SJ, Troy JL, Fairley JA, et al. A major role for neutrophils in experimental bullous pemphigoid. *J Clin Invest.* (1997) 100:1256–63. doi: 10.1172/JCI119639
179. Li Q, Ujiie H, Shibaki A, Wang G, Moriuchi R, Qiao HJ, et al. Human IgG1 monoclonal antibody against human collagen 17 noncollagenous 16A domain induces blisters via complement activation in experimental bullous pemphigoid model. *J Immunol.* (2010) 185:7746–55. doi: 10.4049/jimmunol.1000667
180. Sitaru C, Chiriac MT, Mihai S, Buning J, Gebert A, Ishiko A, et al. Induction of complement-fixing autoantibodies against type VII collagen results in subepidermal blistering in mice. *J Immunol.* (2006) 177:3461–8. doi: 10.4049/jimmunol.177.5.3461
181. Mihai S, Chiriac MT, Takahashi K, Thurman JM, Holers VM, Zillikens D, et al. The alternative pathway of complement activation is critical for blister induction in experimental epidermolysis bullosa acquisita. *J Immunol.* (2007) 178:6514–21. doi: 10.4049/jimmunol.178.10.6514
182. Amber KT, Valdebran M, Kridin K, Grando SA. The role of eosinophils in bullous pemphigoid: a developing model of eosinophil pathogenicity in mucocutaneous disease. *Front Med.* (2018) 5:201. doi: 10.3389/fmed.2018.00201
183. Chen R, Ning G, Zhao ML, Fleming MG, Diaz LA, Werb Z, et al. Mast cells play a key role in neutrophil recruitment in experimental bullous pemphigoid. *J Clin Invest.* (2001) 108:1151–8. doi: 10.1172/JCI11494
184. Heimbach L, Li Z, Berkowitz P, Zhao M, Li N, Rubenstein DS, et al. The C5a receptor on mast cells is critical for the autoimmune skin-blistering disease bullous pemphigoid. *J Biol Chem.* (2011) 286:15003–9. doi: 10.1074/jbc.M111.221036

185. Kasprick A, Yu X, Scholten J, Hartmann K, Pas HH, Zillikens D, et al. Conditional depletion of mast cells has no impact on the severity of experimental epidermolysis bullosa acquisita. *Eur J Immunol.* (2015) 45:1462–70. doi: 10.1002/eji.201444769

186. Hiroyasu S, Ozawa T, Kobayashi H, Ishii M, Aoyama Y, Kitajima Y, et al. Bullous pemphigoid IgG induces BP180 internalization via a macropinocytic pathway. *Am J Pathol.* (2013) 182:828–40. doi: 10.1016/j.ajpath.2012.11.029

187. Ujiie H, Sasaoka T, Izumi K, Nishie W, Shinkuma S, Natsuga K, et al. Bullous pemphigoid autoantibodies directly induce blister formation without complement activation. *J Immunol.* (2014) 193:4415–28. doi: 10.4049/jimmunol.1400095

188. Iwata H, Kamio N, Aoyama Y, Yamamoto Y, Hirako Y, Owaribe K, et al. IgG from patients with bullous pemphigoid depletes cultured keratinocytes of the 180-kDa bullous pemphigoid antigen (type XVII collagen) and weakens cell attachment. *J Invest Dermatol.* (2009) 129:919–26. doi: 10.1038/jid.2008.305

189. Tie D, Da X, Natsuga K, Yamada N, Yamamoto O, Morita E. Bullous pemphigoid IgG induces cell dysfunction and enhances the motility of epidermal keratinocytes via Rac1/proteasome activation. *Front Immunol.* (2019) 10:200. doi: 10.3389/fimmu.2019.00200

190. Schmidt E, Reimer S, Kruse N, Jainta S, Brocker EB, Marinkovich MP, et al. Autoantibodies to BP180 associated with bullous pemphigoid release interleukin-6 and interleukin-8 from cultured human keratinocytes. *J Invest Dermatol.* (2000) 115:842–8. doi: 10.1046/j.1523-1747.2000.00141.x

191. Zhao ML, Trimbeger ME, Li N, Diaz LA, Shapiro SD, Liu Z. Role of FcRs in animal model of autoimmune bullous pemphigoid. *J Immunol.* (2006) 177:3398–405. doi: 10.4049/jimmunol.177.5.3398

192. Schulze FS, Beckmann T, Nimmerjahn F, Ishiko A, Collin M, Kohl J, et al. Fcγ receptors III and IV mediate tissue destruction in a novel adult mouse model of bullous pemphigoid. *Am J Pathol.* (2014) 184:2185–96. doi: 10.1016/j.ajpath.2014.05.007

193. Sitaru C, Kromminga A, Hashimoto T, Brocker EB, Zillikens D. Autoantibodies to type VII collagen mediate Fcgamma-dependent neutrophil activation and induce dermal-epidermal separation in cryosections of human skin. *Am J Pathol.* (2002) 161:301–11. doi: 10.1016/S0002-9440(10)64182-X

194. Dimson OG, Giudice GJ, Fu CL, Van den Bergh F, Warren SJ, Janson MM, et al. Identification of a potential effector function for IgE autoantibodies in the organ-specific autoimmune disease bullous pemphigoid. *J Invest Dermatol.* (2003) 120:784–8. doi: 10.1046/j.1523-1747.2003.12146.x

195. Freire PC, Munoz CH, Stingl G. IgE autoreactivity in bullous pemphigoid: eosinophils and mast cells as major targets of pathogenic immune reactants. *Br J Dermatol.* (2017) 177:1644–53. doi: 10.1111/bjd.15924

196. Yu KK, Crew AB, Messingham KA, Fairley JA, Woodley DT. Omalizumab therapy for bullous pemphigoid. *J Am Acad Dermatol.* (2014) 71:468–74. doi: 10.1016/j.jaad.2014.04.053

197. Liu Z, Zhao M, Li N, Diaz LA, Mayadas TN. Differential roles for beta2 integrins in experimental autoimmune bullous pemphigoid. *Blood.* (2006) 107:1063–9. doi: 10.1182/blood-2005-08-3123

198. Deng FY, Chen Y, Zheng JF, Huang QNA, Cao XT, Zillikens D, et al. CD11b-deficient mice exhibit an increased severity in the late phase of antibody transfer-induced experimental epidermolysis bullosa acquisita. *Exp Dermatol.* (2017) 26:1175–8. doi: 10.1111/exd.13434

199. Nemeth T, Virtic O, Sitaru C, Mocsai A. The Syk tyrosine kinase is required for skin inflammation in an *in vivo* mouse model of epidermolysis bullosa acquisita. *J Invest Dermatol.* (2017) 137:2131–9. doi: 10.1016/j.jid.2017.05.017

200. Chiriac MT, Roesler J, Sindrilaru A, Scharffetter-Kochanek K, Zillikens D, Sitaru C. NADPH oxidase is required for neutrophil-dependent autoantibody-induced tissue damage. *J Pathol.* (2007) 212:56–65. doi: 10.1002/path.2157

201. Samavedam UK, Mitschker N, Kasprick A, Bieber K, Schmidt E, Laskay T, et al. Whole-genome expression profiling in skin reveals sYK as a key regulator of inflammation in experimental epidermolysis Bullosa acquisita. *Front Immunol.* (2018) 9:249. doi: 10.3389/fimmu.2018.00249

202. Nemeth T, Futosi K, Sitaru C, Ruland J, Mocsai A. Neutrophil-specific deletion of the CARD9 gene expression regulator suppresses autoantibody-induced inflammation *in vivo*. *Nat Commun.* (2016) 7:11004. doi: 10.1038/ncomms11004

203. Schmidt E, Bastian B, Dummer R, Tony HP, Brocker EB, Zillikens D. Detection of elevated levels of IL-4, IL-6, and IL-10 in blister fluid of bullous pemphigoid. *Arch Dermatol Res.* (1996) 288:353–7. doi: 10.1007/BF02507102

204. Schmidt E, Mittnacht A, Schomig H, Dummer R, Brocker EB, Zillikens D. Detection of IL-1 alpha, IL-1 beta and IL-1 receptor antagonist in blister fluid of bullous pemphigoid. *J Dermatol Sci.* (1996) 11:142–7. doi: 10.1016/0923-1811(95)00435-1

205. Schmidt E, Ambach A, Bastian B, Brocker EB, Zillikens D. Elevated levels of interleukin-8 in blister fluid of bullous pemphigoid compared with suction blisters of healthy control subjects. *J Am Acad Dermatol.* (1996) 3:310–2. doi: 10.1016/S0190-9622(96)80146-0

206. Juczynska K, Wozniacka A, Waszczykowska E, Danilewicz M, Wagrowska-Danilewicz M, Wieczfinska J, et al. Expression of the JAK/STAT signaling pathway in bullous pemphigoid and dermatitis herpetiformis. *Mediators Inflamm.* (2017) 2017:6716419. doi: 10.1155/2017/6716419

207. Samavedam U, Scheuber J, Seavey M, Koga H, Witte M, Schulze F, et al. Therapeutic efficacy of a novel selective JAK2 inhibitor (CEP-33779) in organ-specific, autoantibody-induced tissue injury. *J Invest Dermatol.* (2014) 134:S16.

208. Kaye A, Gordon SC, Deverapalli SC, Her MJ, Rosmarin D. Dupilumab for the treatment of recalcitrant bullous pemphigoid. *JAMA Dermatol.* (2018) 154:1225–6. doi: 10.1001/jamadermatol.2018.2526

209. Deng GM, Liu L, Bahjat FR, Pine PR, Tsokos GC. Suppression of skin and kidney disease by inhibition of spleen tyrosine kinase in lupus-prone mice. *Arthritis Rheum.* (2010) 62:2086–92. doi: 10.1002/art.27452

210. Chalmers SA, Wen J, Doerner J, Stock A, Cuda CM, Makinde HM, et al. Highly selective inhibition of Bruton's tyrosine kinase attenuates skin and brain disease in murine lupus. *Arthritis Res Ther.* (2018) 20:10. doi: 10.1186/s13075-017-1500-0

211. Yu C, Chang C, Zhang J. Immunologic and genetic considerations of cutaneous lupus erythematosus: a comprehensive review. *J Autoimmun.* (2013) 41:34–45. doi: 10.1016/j.jaut.2013.01.007

212. Deng GM, Tsokos GC. Pathogenesis and targeted treatment of skin injury in SLE. *Nat Rev Rheumatol.* (2015) 11:663–9. doi: 10.1038/nrrheum.2015.106

213. Robinson ES, Werth VP. The role of cytokines in the pathogenesis of cutaneous lupus erythematosus. *Cytokine.* (2015) 73:326–34. doi: 10.1016/j.cyto.2015.01.031

214. Chasset F, Arnaud L. Targeting interferons and their pathways in systemic lupus erythematosus. *Autoimmun Rev.* (2018) 17:44–52. doi: 10.1016/j.autrev.2017.11.009

215. Deng GM. Pathogenesis of skin injury of systemic lupus erythematosus. *Curr Rheumatol Rep.* (2018) 20:5. doi: 10.1007/s11926-018-0713-9

216. Chan ES, Herlitz LC, Jabbari A. Ruxolitinib attenuates cutaneous lupus development in a mouse lupus model. *J Invest Dermatol.* (2015) 135:1912–5. doi: 10.1038/jid.2015.107

217. Wallace DJ, Furie RA, Tanaka Y, Kalunian KC, Mosca M, Petri MA, et al. Baricitinib for systemic lupus erythematosus: a double-blind, randomised, placebo-controlled, phase 2 trial. *Lancet.* (2018) 392:222–31. doi: 10.1016/S0140-6736(18)31363-1

218. Satoh TK, Mellett M, Contassot E, French LE. Are neutrophilic dermatoses autoinflammatory disorders? *Br J Dermatol.* (2018) 178:603–13. doi: 10.1111/bjd.15105

219. Marzano AV, Ortega-Loayza AG, Heath M, Morse D, Genovese G, Cugno M. Mechanisms of inflammation in neutrophil-mediated skin diseases. *Front Immunol.* (2019) 10:1059. doi: 10.3389/fimmu.2019.01059

220. Gurung P, Fan G, Lukens JR, Vogel P, Tonks NK, Kanneganti TD. Tyrosine kinase SYK licenses MyD88 adaptor protein to instigate IL-1α-mediated inflammatory disease. *Immunity.* (2017) 46:635–48. doi: 10.1016/j.immuni.2017.03.014

221. Tartey S, Gurung P, Samir P, Burton A, Kanneganti TD. Cutting edge: dysregulated CARD9 signaling in neutrophils drives inflammation in a mouse model of neutrophilic dermatoses. *J Immunol.* (2018) 201:1639–44. doi: 10.4049/jimmunol.1800760

222. Kawakami T, Ohashi S, Kawa Y, Takahama H, Ito M, Soma Y, et al. Elevated serum granulocyte colony-stimulating factor levels in patients with active phase of sweet syndrome and patients with active behcet disease: implication in neutrophil apoptosis dysfunction. *Arch Dermatol.* (2004) 140:570–4. doi: 10.1001/archderm.140.5.570
223. White JM, Mufti GJ, Salisbury JR, du Vivier AW. Cutaneous manifestations of granulocyte colony-stimulating factor. *Clin Exp Dermatol.* (2006) 31:206–7. doi: 10.1111/j.1365-2230.2005.01996.x
224. Boyadzhiev M, Marinov L, Boyadzhiev V, Iotova V, Aksentijevich I, Hambleton S. Disease course and treatment effects of a JAK inhibitor in a patient with CANDLE syndrome. *Pediatr Rheumatol Online J.* (2019) 17:19. doi: 10.1186/s12969-019-0322-9
225. Yamaoka K. Janus kinase inhibitors for rheumatoid arthritis. *Curr Opin Chem Biol.* (2016) 32:29–33. doi: 10.1016/j.cbpa.2016.03.006
226. Strober BE, Gottlieb AB, van de Kerkhof PCM, Puig L, Bachelez H, Chouela E, et al. Benefit-risk profile of tofacitinib in patients with moderate-to-severe chronic plaque psoriasis: pooled analysis across six clinical trials. *Br J Dermatol.* (2019) 180:67–75. doi: 10.1111/bjd.17149
227. Wolk R, Armstrong EJ, Hansen PR, Thiers B, Lan S, Tallman AM, et al. Effect of tofacitinib on lipid levels and lipid-related parameters in patients with moderate to severe psoriasis. *J Clin Lipidol.* (2017) 11:1243–56. doi: 10.1016/j.jacl.2017.06.012
228. Scott IC, Hider SL, Scott DL. Thromboembolism with Janus Kinase (JAK) inhibitors for rheumatoid arthritis: how real is the risk? *Drug Saf.* (2018) 41:645–53. doi: 10.1007/s40264-018-0651-5

10

Characteristic Pattern of IL-17RA, IL-17RB and IL-17RC in Monocytes/ Macrophages and Mast Cells from Patients with Bullous Pemphigoid

Stéphane Nesmond[1], Céline Muller[1], Richard Le Naour[1,2], Manuelle Viguier[3], Philippe Bernard[1,3†], Frank Antonicelli[1,4†] and Sébastien Le Jan[1*†]

[1] Laboratory of Dermatology, EA7509 IRMAIC, University of Reims-Champagne-Ardenne, Reims, France, [2] Department of Biological Sciences, UFR Pharmacy, University of Reims Champagne-Ardenne, Reims, France, [3] Department of Dermatology, University Hospital, University of Reims-Champagne-Ardenne, Reims, France, [4] Department of Biological Sciences, Immunology, UFR Odontology, University of Reims-Champagne-Ardenne, Reims, France

Correspondence:
Sébastien Le Jan
sebastien.le-jan@univ-reims.fr

† These authors have contributed equally to this work

Inflammation is largely implicated in bullous pemphigoid (BP), the most frequent skin auto-immune blistering disease. IL-17, essentially IL-17A/F, has been involved in blister formation through regulation of protease production, and its specific serum profile within BP was related to disease outcome. However, relationships between IL-17 family ligands and receptors are quite complex with six different IL-17 isoforms, and five different receptors. We here aimed at clarifying the contribution of the IL-17 axis in BP by characterizing not only the expression of IL-17 receptor (IL-17R) members within immune cells isolated from BP patients (PMNs, $n = 9$; T-lymphocytes, $n = 10$; and monocytes, $n = 10$) but also the expression of IL-17 isoforms in sera ($n = 83$), and blister fluid ($n = 31$) of BP patients. We showed that at diagnosis, IL-17RA and IL-17RC expression were significantly increased in monocytes isolated from BP patients as compared to those from control subjects ($p = 0.006$ and $p = 0.016$, respectively). Notably, both IL-17RA and IL-17RC mRNA expression remained elevated in BP monocytes at time of relapse. We further demonstrated a significant increase of all IL-17 isoforms tested in BP blister fluid compared with BP serum (IL-17A, $p < 0.0001$; IL-17A/F, $p < 0.0001$; IL-17B, $p = 0.0023$; IL-17C, $p = 0.0022$; IL-17E, $p < 0.0001$). Among all, IL-17B was the only cytokine for which a significant decreased concentration within blister fluid was observed in BP patients with severe disease compared to patients with moderate disease ($p = 0.012$). We further evidenced a significant negative correlation between IL-17B levels and blister/erosion BPDAI subscore ($r = -0.52$, $p = 0.003$). We finally identified mast cells as a potential target of IL-17B in lesional skin of BP patients. In conclusion, we showed here that IL-17RA and IL-17RC expression in monocyte was associated with disease activity and evidenced *in situ* a negative correlation between BP disease activity and IL-17B, whose effects could be mediated by IL-17RB expressed by mast cell in BP lesional skin.

Keywords: autoimmunity, inflammation, bullous pemphigoid, IL-17 receptors, IL-17 isoforms

INTRODUCTION

Bullous pemphigoid (BP) is the most frequent blistering skin disease of autoimmune origin and affects mainly the elderly (1–6). Clinical features of BP are intense pruritus associated with tense bullae, inflammatory erythematous plaques, and itching (1, 2, 6, 7). BP is characterized by the production of autoantibodies against two proteins of the hemidesmosome structure, BP180, and BP230 (8–13). The binding of BP autoantibodies onto their target induces blister formation by activating complement pathway, which triggered subsequent recruitment of inflammatory cells at the dermal–epidermal junction. Secretion of inflammatory key mediators by inflammatory cells leads up to an overexpression of proteases, such as the matrix metalloproteinase-9 (MMP-9) and the neutrophil elastase, which are involved in dermal–epidermal splitting (14–23). However, autoantibody level does not explain all clinical features of BP (24), suggesting that other regulatory mechanisms are involved in the inflammatory response associated with BP. In this line, we previously showed that IL-17 within the blister fluid (BF) of BP patients was related to MMP-9 production (25), and that specific patterns of IL-17 within the serum of BP patients were related to BP outcome (26). Moreover, anti-IL-17 therapy was revealed quite promising by using experimental murine and human-derived models of BP (27). However, these studies mostly concerned IL-17A and IL-17A/F isoforms, and to our knowledge, no study has evaluated the expression of the receptors of those cytokines yet, or the type of cells expressing those receptors in patients with BP.

IL-17 receptor family is composed of five members from IL-17RA to IL-17RE. The subunit IL-17RA is ubiquitous (28–31) and is a common co-receptor subunit for other members of the IL-17 family. IL-17RA pairs with IL-17RC to bind either IL-17A or IL-17F as covalent homodimers, but also IL-17A/IL-17F as heterodimers (32, 33). However, the association of IL-17RA with other members of the IL-17 receptor family shifts the affinity toward other members of the IL-17 family (34). Indeed, combination of IL-17RA with IL-17RB binds IL-17E as covalent homodimers (35–37). Besides, IL-17RA can also associate with IL-17RE to bind IL-17C as homodimers (38). However, the involvement of IL-17RA is not compulsory, as IL-17RB forms homodimers to target IL-17B as covalent homodimers (39). Up to now, no ligand for IL-17RD has been discovered yet. Also, the receptor of IL-17D remains unknown. In BP, IL-17A production has been mainly attributed to neutrophils, $CD3^{+}$ T-lymphocytes, and mast cells (25, 27). Besides, IL-17RC expression was found increased in the skin of BP patients, whereas IL-17RA expression was unchanged (27). However, to better understand the role of IL-17 axis in BP, the pattern of IL-17 receptor isoform expression, and the cell types expressing those receptors both in the skin of BP patients and in the circulating immune blood cells need to be further investigated.

In this prospective study, we investigated the IL-17R isoform expression in immune blood cells of BP patients. We also analyzed the expression of IL-17 isoforms in the sera and in the BF of BP patients. To investigate the clinical involvement of the different IL-17 members in BP, we performed correlation studies between IL-17 concentration within the BF and the BPDAI (bullous pemphigoid disease activity index). Finally, to further delineate the role of IL-17 members in the inflammatory response within the BF associated with clinical activity of BP, we evaluated the expression of the respective IL-17 receptors at the surface of immune cells in lesional skin of patients.

MATERIALS AND METHODS

Patients and Study Design

This prospective, single-center study was conducted between September 2013 and July 2017 in the Department of Dermatology at Reims University Hospital (French Referral Center for Autoimmune Bullous Diseases), under the approval of the Ethic Committee of the University Hospital of Reims (CNIL authorization DR-2013-320). In accordance with the Helsinki Declaration, all subjects gave their informed and written consent before their inclusion in the study. Patients that were included presented blistering skin dermatosis fulfilling at least three of four clinical criteria for BP according to Vaillant et al. (40), and in lesional skin, a basal lamina continuous deposit of IgG and/or C3 is revealed by direct immunofluorescence (IF) microscopy. Exclusion criteria were administration of a specific treatment for more than 2 days, pregnancy, and expected survival shorter than 3 months. Sera and blood cells were collected at different time points: at diagnosis (D0), 360 days after the diagnosis (D360), and at the time of a relapse (if it occurred). When possible, BF was collected at diagnosis (D0). Control samples were obtained from age- and sex-matched patients admitted to the department of traumatology, and orthopedic surgery of the same hospital. Controls that were included in the study did not have any autoimmune diseases and any clinical or biological signs of inflammation.

Clinical Characteristics of BP Patients

Clinical data recorded at baseline were gender, age, and clinical activity of the disease evaluated by the Bullous Pemphigoid Disease Area Index (BPDAI) score (7). The BPDAI measures separate scores for mucous membrane and skin activities, the latter evaluating separately both cutaneous urticaria/erythema (non-bullous phase), and cutaneous blisters/erosions (blistering phase). As previously reported (41), a global BPDAI score ≥ 56 at baseline defined a severe disease while a global BPDAI score <56 defined a moderate disease.

Cell Isolation

Peripheral blood mononuclear cells (PBMCs) and polymorphonuclear cells (PMNs) were isolated by density-gradient centrifugation from EDTA-treated whole blood (Granulosep, Eurobio-Abcys, France). Monocytes were then purified from PBMCs by means of positive selection with CD14 immunomagnetic beads (MACS; Miltenyi Biotec, Germany), according to the manufacturer's instructions. Then, flow through was used to isolate T lymphocytes by means of negative selection with the pan T-cell Isolation Kit from Miltenyi Biotec (MACS).

IL-17R Gene Expression Analysis

Total RNA was extracted from isolated cells (3M, 5M, 7M, and 4M for monocytes, lymphocytes, PMNs, and PBMCs, respectively) using TRI-Reagent (Euromedex, Bas-Rhin, France) according to the manufacturer's protocol. cDNAs were synthetized and amplified using the Maxima First Strand cDNA kit with dsDNAse (Life Technologies), according to the manufacturer's instructions. The expression of IL-17RA, IL-17RB, IL-17RC, IL-17RD, IL-17RE, and β2-microglobulin (β_2M) was analyzed by real-time quantitative PCR using the Power SYBR Green PCR Master Mix (Applied Biosystems) on the Stratagene Mx3005P (Agilent Technologies). Relative quantification was performed with β_2M as a reference gene. Results were analyzed by using the MxPro QPCR software, and the fold regulation was calculated by using the $2^{-\Delta\Delta CT}$ method. Primer sequences (Eurofins) used to detect IL-17RA, IL-17RB, IL-17RC, IL-17RD, IL-17RE, and β_2M are detailed in **Table 1**.

Cytokine Measurement in Biological Fluids From BP Patients

IL-17A, IL-17A/F, IL-17B, IL-17C, and IL-17E were measured in control sera ($n = 46$), BP sera ($n = 83$), and BP BF ($n = 31$) using a U-PLEX assay (MesoScale Diagnostics; Rockville; USA). U-PLEX technology allows multiplex measurement of up to 10 cytokines within a single well in a volume of 50 μL. This technique is based on electro-chemiluminescence detection. Briefly biotinylated capture antibodies were coupled to U-PLEX linkers. The U-PLEX linkers then self-assembled onto unique spots on the U-PLEX plate. After binding to the capture antibodies, detection antibodies conjugated with electro-chemiluminescent labels (MSD GOLD SULFO-TAG) bound to the analytes to complete the sandwich immunoassay. The plate was then placed into an MSD instrument (SECTOR S6000 plate reader) to acquire data. Data analysis was performed by using MSD Workbench software. Limits of detection (LLOD) were 1.6 pg/ml for IL-17A, 3.0 pg/ml for IL-17A/F, 1.0 pg/ml for IL-17B, 3.0 pg/ml for IL-17C, and 0.76 pg/ml for IL-17E.

IL-17R Detection in Isolated Monocytes From BP Patients

IL-17RA and IL-17RC expression was analyzed in monocytes isolated from BP patients and control subjects by immunocytochemistry (ICC). Isolated monocytes were cytospun and fixed with paraformaldehyde 4% (VWR). The primary antibodies rabbit anti-human IL-17RA (Bioss Antibodies, bs-2606R), and rabbit anti-human IL-17RC (Bioss Antibodies, bs-2607R) were applied to the cells and incubated overnight at 4°C. Chicken anti-rabbit IgG Alexa Fluor 594 (Life technologies, A21442) was used as secondary antibodies. Nuclei were stained with Hoechst 33342 (Thermofisher, Waltham, MA).

IL-17R Detection in BP Skin Biopsy Specimen

Double IF staining were performed to analyze IL-17RA, IL-17RB, and IL-17RC expression on paraformaldehyde-fixed and paraffin-embedded lesional skin biopsy specimens from three BP patients before introduction of any treatment. All biopsies were obtained from the Pathology Department of Reims University Hospital. Briefly, after heat-induced antigen retrieval in Tris 10 mM EDTA buffer pH 9 and blocking in PBS 1×/BSA 3%, the primary antibodies rabbit anti-human IL-17RA (Bioss Antibodies, bs-2606R), rabbit anti-human IL-17RB (Gene Tex, GTX81729), rabbit anti-IL-17RC (Bioss Antibodies, bs-2607R), mouse anti-human mast cell tryptase clone AA1 (Dako,

TABLE 1 | Primer sequences used for amplification of IL-17R member and β2M genes by real-time quantitative PCR.

Oligonucleotide	Forward sequence	Reverse sequence
IL-17RA	TGCCCCTGTGGGTGTACTGGT	GCAGGCAGGCCATCGGTGTA
IL-17RB	TACCCCGAGAGCCGACCGTT	GGCATCTGCCCCGGAGTACCCA
IL-17RC	CTGCCCTTGTGCAGTTTGG	CAGATTCGTACCTCACTCCCTA
IL-17RD	AGGCCTGGGTGAGGAGGAACC	GGGGAATCAGAGGGAGGCAGCA
IL-17RE	CCACCTTCAGGCCATGCAGCC	CTGTCATCCGTGTGGGAGGCC
β_2M	ACCCCCACTGAAAAAGATGA	ATCTTCAAACCTCCATGATG

TABLE 2 | Baseline clinical characteristics of patients with BP.

(A) In the whole BP population included ($n = 83$)

Number of daily new blisters*	21 ± 36
BPDAI total score*	40 ± 27
BPDAI skin activity score*	38 ± 26
- Blisters/erosions score*	25 ± 17
- Erythema/urticaria score*	14 ± 14
Patients with severe disease[a], *n* (%)	22 (26)
Patients with relapse[b], *n* (%)	12 (14)

(B) In the subgroups of BP patients with ($n = 12$) and without relapse ($n = 71$)

	BP without relapse	BP with relapse	*p*-value
Number of daily new blisters*	21 ± 36	22 ± 32	0.2
BPDAI total score*	38 ± 27	49 ± 25	0.1
BPDAI skin activity score*	37 ± 27	47 ± 25	0.2
- Blisters/erosions score*	24 ± 17	32 ± 21	0.2
- Erythema/urticaria score*	14 ± 15	15 ± 12	0.5

(C) In the subsets of BP patients with moderate ($n = 61$) and with severe disease ($n = 22$)

	Moderate BP	Severe BP	*p*-value
Number of daily new blisters*	9 ± 13	57 ± 52	0.0001
BPDAI total score*	26 ± 15	77 ± 17	0.0001
BPDAI skin activity score*	25 ± 15	75 ± 15	0.0001
- Blisters/erosions score*	17 ± 11	47 ± 13	0.0001
- Erythema/urticaria score*	9 ± 10	28 ± 16	0.0001

[a] *Severe disease was defined by BPDAI ≥ 56 (41).*
[b] *Relapse was defined as the reappearance of at least three daily new blisters along with pruriginous, erythematous, or urticarial plaques.*
Mann–Whitney's test was used for statistical analysis.
* *Mean ± SD.*

M7052), mouse anti-human CD163 (Novusbio, NB110-59935), and mouse anti-myeloperoxidase FITC (Abcam, ab11729) were applied and incubated overnight 4°C. Goat anti-mouse IgG Alexa Fluor 488 (Life technologies, A11029) and chicken anti-rabbit IgG Alexa Fluor 594 (Life Technologies, A21442) were used as secondary antibodies. Nuclei were stained with Hoechst 33342 (Thermofisher, Waltham, MA).

ICC and IF staining were visualized on an AxioObserver Z1 microscope (ZEISS) spinning disk ILAS 2 (Roper scientific). Image analysis was performed by using Metamorph software (Roper Scientific).

Statistical Analysis

Statistical significance was inferred when necessary. GraphPad Prism 5 software (GraphPad, La Jolla, CA) was used for statistical analysis. Results are presented as mean ± SEM (standard error of the mean). Normality test was performed to evaluate Gaussian's distribution of the different population tested. We used non-parametric Mann–Whitney's test to compare two independent groups and non-parametric Wilcoxon's test to compare paired groups of population; chi-square test was used to evaluate qualitative variables. Pearson's correlation test was performed to explore the relationship between continuous variables. Results were considered significant when $p < 0.05$.

RESULTS

Characteristics of the Studied Population

A total of 83 patients with BP were included in the study. The mean age at diagnosis was 81 years old and the sex ratio F/M was 1.9. A population of control subjects ($n = 46$) was used with no significant difference regarding these factors. At diagnosis, the total BPDAI score in the whole BP population was 40 ± 27 (**Table 2**). BP patients received superpotent topical corticosteroids as treatment, in association or not with systemic immunomodulators. Among the 83 patients included, 61 patients had a moderate BP, 22 patients a severe BP, 12 (14%) relapsed, 19 patients (24%) died, and 6 (7%) were lost during the year of follow-up. Baseline clinical characteristics of BP patient subgroups according to outcome are displayed in **Table 2**.

IL-17 Receptor Family Members in Immune Circulating Cells in BP

We first investigated the expression of each IL-17 receptor family member in circulating immune cells of patients with BP. At the time of diagnosis, circulating immune cells issued from BP patients or control subjects showed differential expression profile of each IL-17 receptor member. Indeed, whereas PMN cells mainly expressed IL-17RA mRNA (**Figure 1A**), lymphocytes expressed all IL-17 receptor members, except IL-17RD (data not shown), both in patients with BP and in control subjects (**Figure 1B**). In addition, in both lymphocytes and PMNs, no statistical differences could be observed at diagnosis between cells originated from BP patients and cells issued from control subjects. In contrast, a significant increase of IL-17RA, and IL-17RC mRNA expression ($p = 0.006$ and $p = 0.016$, respectively) was evidenced in monocytes from BP patients ($n = 10$) as compared with control subjects ($n = 6$) (**Figure 1C**). The overexpression of both receptors in monocytes from BP patients was also demonstrated at the protein level by IF staining (**Figure 1D**). Evaluation of the longitudinal variation of these receptors was realized on BP patients with an ongoing remission ($n = 7$), and in BP patients with relapse ($n = 5$) for whom blood samples were available. Baseline clinical characteristics in these subgroups of BP patient with and without relapse were similar to those displayed in **Table 2** (data not shown). Both IL-17RA and IL-17RC mRNA increased expressions were significantly abolished after 1 year of treatment (D360) as compared to the level detected at the time of diagnosis (D0) ($p = 0.016$ and $p = 0.016$, respectively) in monocytes from patients with ongoing remission (**Figure 2A**). In contrast, in patients with relapse, both IL-17RA, and IL-17RC mRNA expression remained elevated at time of relapse ($D_{Relapse}$). Indeed, no significant decrease of both IL-17RA and IL-17RC was demonstrated at time of relapse compared with diagnosis (**Figure 2B**).

IL-17 Isoforms in Serum and BF of Patients With BP

We next examined the expression of the IL-17 ligands including IL-17A, IL-17A/F, IL-17B, IL-17C, and IL-17E in biological fluids that could bind to the above-described IL-17R members expressed by circulating immune cells originated from BP patients. At the time of diagnosis, all tested IL-17 isoforms were detected in sera of control subjects ($n = 46$), and in sera ($n = 83$), and BF ($n = 31$) of patients with BP (**Figure 3**). Whatever the IL-17 isoforms analyzed, no significant differences were evidenced between sera from BP patients and sera from control subjects. In contrast, in BF of BP patients, the mean levels of each IL-17 isoform were all significantly increased as compared to BP sera concentrations (IL-17A, $p < 0.0001$; IL-17A/F, $p < 0.0001$; IL-17B, $p < 0.01$; IL-17C, $p < 0.01$; IL-17E, $p < 0.0001$) (**Figure 3**).

IL-17 Isoforms and Disease Activity

Investigation of whether the IL-17 isoform levels within the BF varied according to disease activity at diagnosis was performed on 16 BP patients with "mild to moderate" disease and on 15 BP patients with "severe" disease (**Figure 4A**). These subgroups were characterized by an increase of the total BPDAI score and skin subscores in BP patients with severe disease (BPDAI total score: 72 ± 14 vs. 39 ± 13, $p = 0.0001$; BPDAI skin activity subscore: 71 ± 14 vs. 38 ± 13, $p = 0.0001$; blisters/erosions subscore: 43 ± 11 vs. 26 ± 9, $p = 0.0003$; erythema/urticaria subscore: 29 ± 16 vs. 12 ± 10, $p = 0.003$ for severe and moderate BP patients, respectively). **Figure 4A** showed that IL-17B level was significantly higher (~3-fold, $p = 0.01$) in BF of BP patients with a mild to moderate disease as compared with levels measured in BF of BP patients with a severe disease. None of the other IL-17 isoforms showed significant variations according to disease extent. Deeper investigation revealed a significant and negative correlation between IL-17B and total BPDAI score ($n = 31$, $r = -0.51$, $p = 0.004$). Further analysis with respect to BPDAI subscores showed that IL-17B concentrations in BF were negatively correlated with the total skin BPDAI subscore ($n = 31$, $r = -0.51$, $p = 0.003$), and the skin blisters/erosions

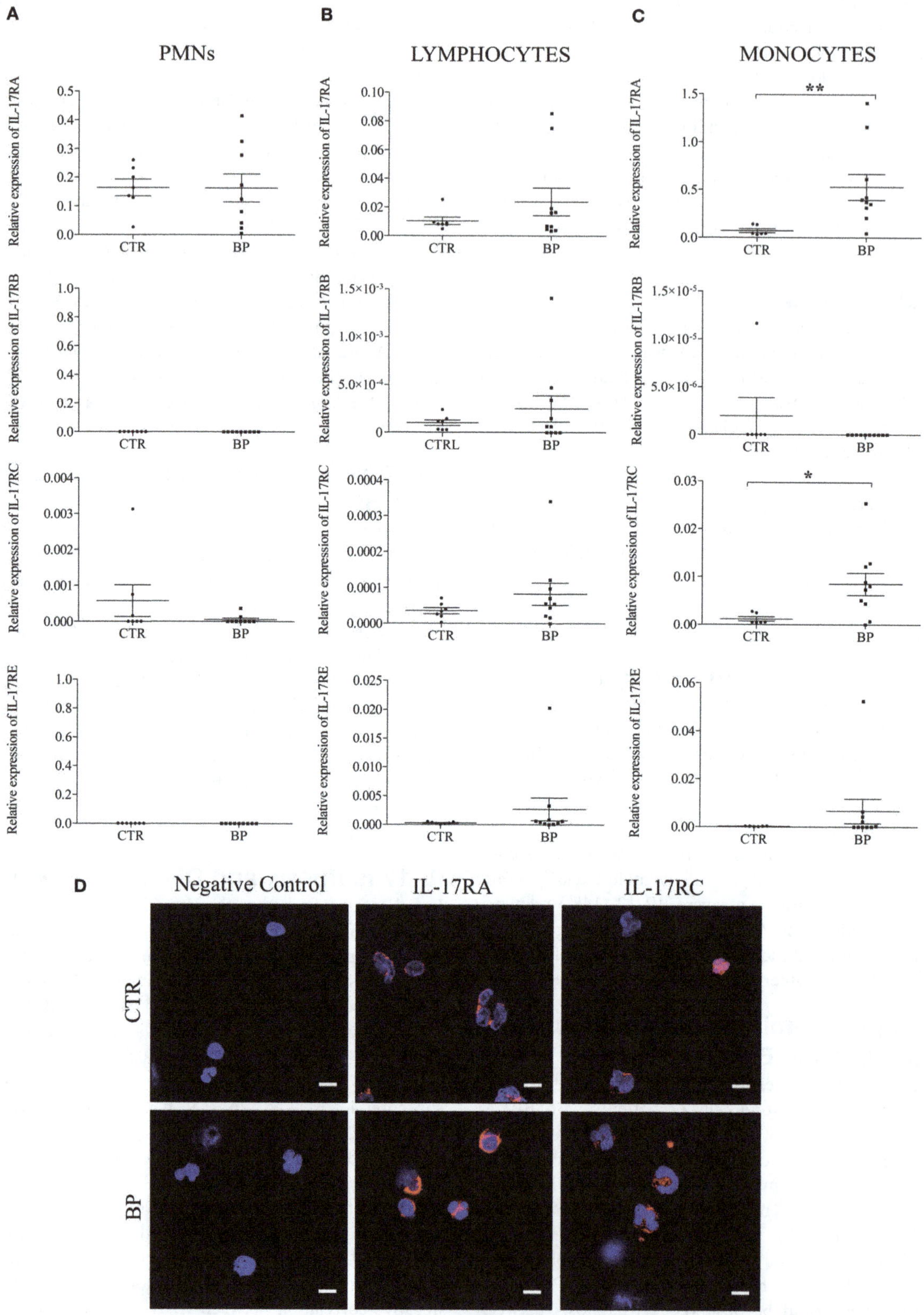

FIGURE 1 | IL-17RA and IL-17RC mRNA expressions were increased in monocytes isolated from blood of patients with BP. The mRNA expression of IL-17RA, IL-17RB, IL-17RC, and IL-17RE were analyzed by real-time quantitative PCR in polymorphonuclear cells (PMNs) **(A)**, in lymphocytes **(B)**, and in monocytes

(Continued)

FIGURE 1 | (C) isolated from blood of control subjects (CTR), and of patients with BP at diagnosis (BP). Lines represent the mean, and non-parametric Mann–Whitney's test was used for statistical analysis (*$p < 0.05$; **$p < 0.01$). **(D)** Monocytes from BP patients and control subjects were stained for IL-17RA or IL-17RC. Negative control: primary antibodies were not added. Nuclei were counterstained with Hoechst (blue). Scale bar = 10 μm.

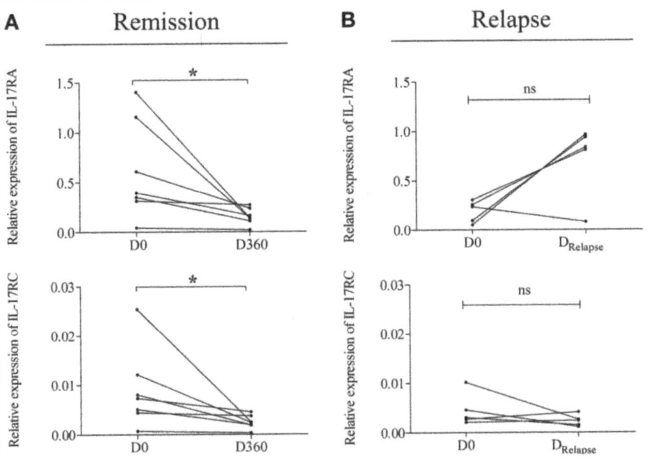

FIGURE 2 | Analysis of IL-17RA and IL-17RC expression in monocytes issued from patients with BP according to disease outcome. IL-17RA and IL-17RC mRNA expressions were analyzed in monocytes of BP patients with ongoing remission **(A)** and of BP patients who relapsed **(B)**, at diagnosis (D_0), and at day 360 (D_{360}), or at the time of relapse ($D_{Relapse}$), respectively. Non-parametric paired Wilcoxon's test was used for statistical analysis (*$p < 0.05$; ns = non-significant).

BPDAI subscore ($n = 31$, $r = -0.52$, $p = 0.003$) but not with the erythema/urticaria BPDAI subscore ($n = 31$, $r = -0.27$, $p = 0.14$) (**Figure 4B**).

IL-17 Receptor Expression in Lesional Skin of BP Patients

Finally, we wondered which cells within the blister cavity could be targeted by IL-17B. Double staining for IL-17RB and either mast cell (tryptase), macrophage (CD163), or neutrophil (myeloperoxidase, MPO) markers was performed in biopsies of BP patients ($n = 3$). Double staining revealed co-localization between IL-17RB and mast cell marker. Conversely, IL-17RB was not expressed by macrophages or neutrophils in blister cavity. In contrast, IL-17RA, and IL-17RC were expressed by both $CD163^+$ macrophages and MPO^+ neutrophils in blister cavity (**Figure 5**).

DISCUSSION

In this study, we demonstrated that IL-17 R expression displayed a peculiar pattern, with IL-17RA, and IL-17RC increased expression in monocyte and macrophages, whereas IL-17 RB was detected in mast cells. Noteworthy, IL-17RA and IL-17RC expression remained elevated in BP patients who relapsed under corticosteroid treatment. Furthermore, we also found that IL-17 A, B C, E, and F isoforms were all increased in the BF of BP patients. Although such IL-17 production suggested a broad involvement of the IL-17 axis in BP with active skin lesions before starting treatment, we only evidenced a negative correlation between BP disease activity and IL-17B, which could be mediated by IL-17RB expressed by mast cell in BP lesional skin.

We also showed that at the active phase of the disease and before treatment, IL-17RA and IL-17RC expressions were increased in monocyte, but neither in lymphocytes nor in neutrophils. Furthermore, no variation was observed in PBMCs (data not shown), suggesting that the overexpression is mainly restricted to monocytes. Actually, the critical role of monocytes in BP was already illustrated in a previous study showing that monocytes but not lymphocytes from BP patients responded to CXCL10 by increasing MMP-9 secretion (42). Thus, although all IL-17 receptors were detected in circulating blood cells, the overexpression of IL-17RA and IL-17RC in monocytes suggests that those receptors could play a critical role in BP. Actually, IL-17RA, and IL-17RC overexpression in monocytes could participate in BP relapse mechanisms as we observed that their expression was downregulated in BP patients whose disease was controlled by treatment, but remained overexpressed in BP patients who relapsed. Such results are in line with the IL-17 overexpression in the serum of BP patients with relapse under treatment (26) and with the capacity of those sera to increase NETosis in BP (43). This is also in setting with the fact that IL-17RC expression was found increased in the skin of BP patients (27), although in this study the authors found that IL-17RA expression remained unchanged. Indeed, in relation with the variations in monocytes, we also observed that IL-17RA and IL-17RC were markedly expressed by macrophages in the lesional skin of BP patients. Noteworthy, such IL-17RA, and IL-17RC expression in blister cavity was also demonstrated on neutrophils, further advocating on the role of both macrophages, and neutrophils in the dermal–epidermal cleavage upon IL-17 stimulation (25–27, 42, 43). Therefore, altogether, our results showed that investigation of both IL-17 isoforms and IL-17RA/RC may represent adequate tools to predict BP activity and outcome.

Here, we evidenced for the first time the expression of the different isoforms of IL-17 in the serum and in the BF of patients with BP. Furthermore, all of the IL-17 isoforms were produced at a higher level in the BF as compared to the serum of BP patients, suggesting a local production of these cytokines within the bullous area. However, the different IL-17 isoforms were produced at different levels. This is of importance as we also demonstrated that the expression of IL-17 receptors varied according to the immune cell types analyzed. Thus, this suggests that in BP, all combination of IL-17/IL-17R could be formed depending on the receptor types expressed at the surface of the cells, and on the affinity between these couples. IL-17A expression has already been mainly attributed to neutrophils, $CD3^+$ T-lymphocytes, and mast cells (25, 27). The expression

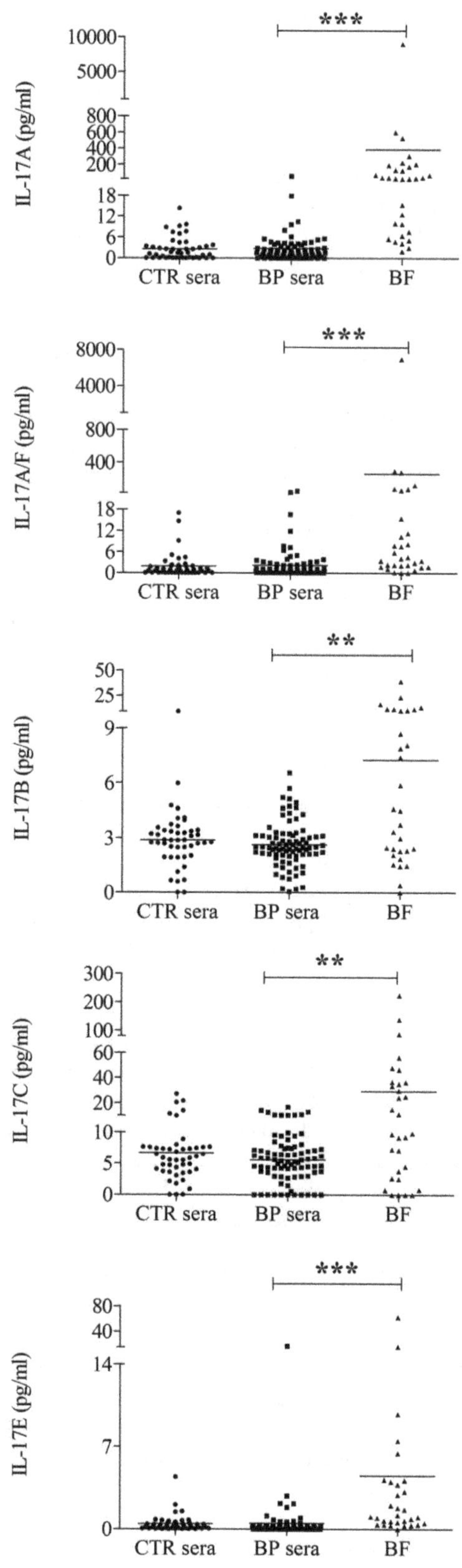

FIGURE 3 | The expression of each IL-17 isoform tested was increased in blister fluid of BP patients. The concentrations of IL-17A, IL-17A/F, IL-17B, *(Continued)*

FIGURE 3 | IL-17C, and IL-17E were measured at the time of diagnosis in serum (BP sera), and blister fluid (BF) of BP patients, and in serum of control subjects (CTR sera) using U-PLEX cytokine multiplex assay. Lines represent the mean, and non-parametric Mann–Whitney's test was used for statistical analysis (**$p < 0.01$; ***$p < 0.001$).

of other isoforms of IL-17 is much less defined. The expression of IL-17B and IL-17C has been attributed to T-cells (44). The expression of IL-17E has also been found to be produced by immune cells such as macrophage, lymphocyte, or mast cell (37, 45). Although the origin of the different IL-17 isoforms and of their receptors still needs to be further documented, the expression of all of those molecules of the IL-17 axis might conduct to a very intricate network in BP.

At baseline, only IL-17B expression was correlated with the BPDAI scores. Thus, we evidenced here, for the first time in BP, an IL-17 cytokine isoform capable of discriminating BP patients according to disease activity with the particularity that a negative correlation was observed between IL-17B and BP activity. Although further studies are required to demonstrate whether IL-17B expression is only a marker of disease activity or if this cytokine has a specific role in the regulation of the inflammatory response in BP, previous observation supports the idea that IL-17B could have a protective role in the process of inflammation (46). In BP, BPDAI subscore analysis showed that IL-17B was negatively correlated with the skin blisters/erosions lesions but not with the erythema/urticaria lesions. Therefore, IL-17B might not be involved in the pre-bullous phase of the disease. In contrast, the negative correlation between IL-17B and blisters and erosions lesions suggests that a BP patient with high IL-17B level would not form many blisters and erosions, and *vice versa*. IL-17B could interfere on BP pathogenesis by several mechanisms. On one hand, IL-17B could bind to IL-17RB, and scavenger at least in part IL-17RA to form the heterodimer IL-17RA/IL-17RB. This would reduce the pool of IL-17RA to enable to transduce the pathogenic effects of IL-17A and IL-17F either as homodimers or as heterodimers. In this way, this could limit the effects of IL-17E (IL-25) that bind to the IL-17RA/RB homodimer (46). On the other hand, binding of IL-17B onto its receptor could also transduce an anti-inflammatory response. Indeed, it has been shown that IL-17B is an anti-inflammatory cytokine (46). Given that IL-17RB is expressed by mucosal epithelial cells, such effects could be involved in the regulation of mucosal inflammation that occurs in certain patients with BP (47). However, why a patient would express a higher IL-17B than another patient is still unknown, and whether this level varies according to disease extent for a specific patient still needs to be investigated.

Besides, IL-17B concentrations within the BF were correlated neither with the anti-BP180NC16A nor with the anti-BP230 autoantibody titers (data not shown), suggesting that, in BP, IL-17B production was disconnected from the autoimmune process, which initiates blister formation. Also, no correlation was observed between serum and BF concentrations (data not shown), suggesting that IL-17B is mainly produced at the skin lesional site. Although we mentioned the pathogenic role of IL-17A or IL-17A/F above, we did not find any correlation with

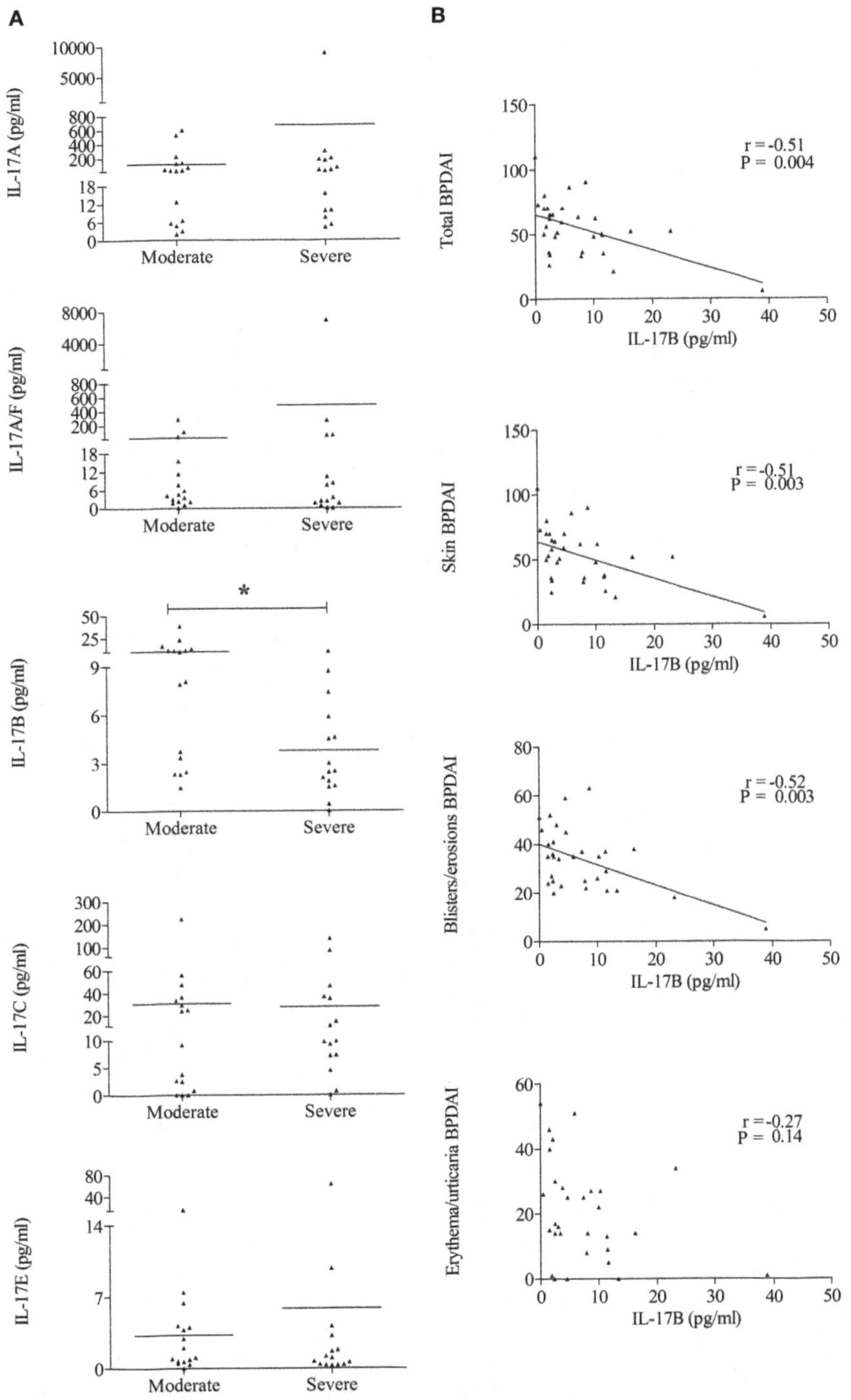

FIGURE 4 | IL-17B levels were decreased in BP patients with severe disease extent and negatively correlated with blisters/erosions BPDAI subscore. **(A)** IL-17A, IL-17A/F, IL-17B, IL-17C, and IL-17E concentrations measured at the time of diagnosis in BF were analyzed according to the disease extent. "Moderate" stands for BP patients with a BPDAI <56 and "Severe" for BP patients with a BPDAI ≥56. Non-parametric Mann–Whitney's test was used for statistical analysis (* $p < 0.05$). **(B)** Correlations between total, skin, blisters/erosions, or erythema/urticaria BPDAI scores, and IL-17B levels in BF were analyzed using the Pearson's correlation test.

IL-17A or IL-17A/F with the BPDAI score and subscores. A potential explanation could be that the binding of an IL-17 isoform onto an IL-17 receptor may modulate the affinity and specificity of other IL-17 isoform receptor-binding event. This is of interest as this suggests that besides the IL-17RA pathways, other IL-17/IL-17R signaling cascades may be involved in the pathophysiology of BP. Noteworthy, IL-17RB also associates with IL-17RA to transduce the effects of IL-17E. In our study, we

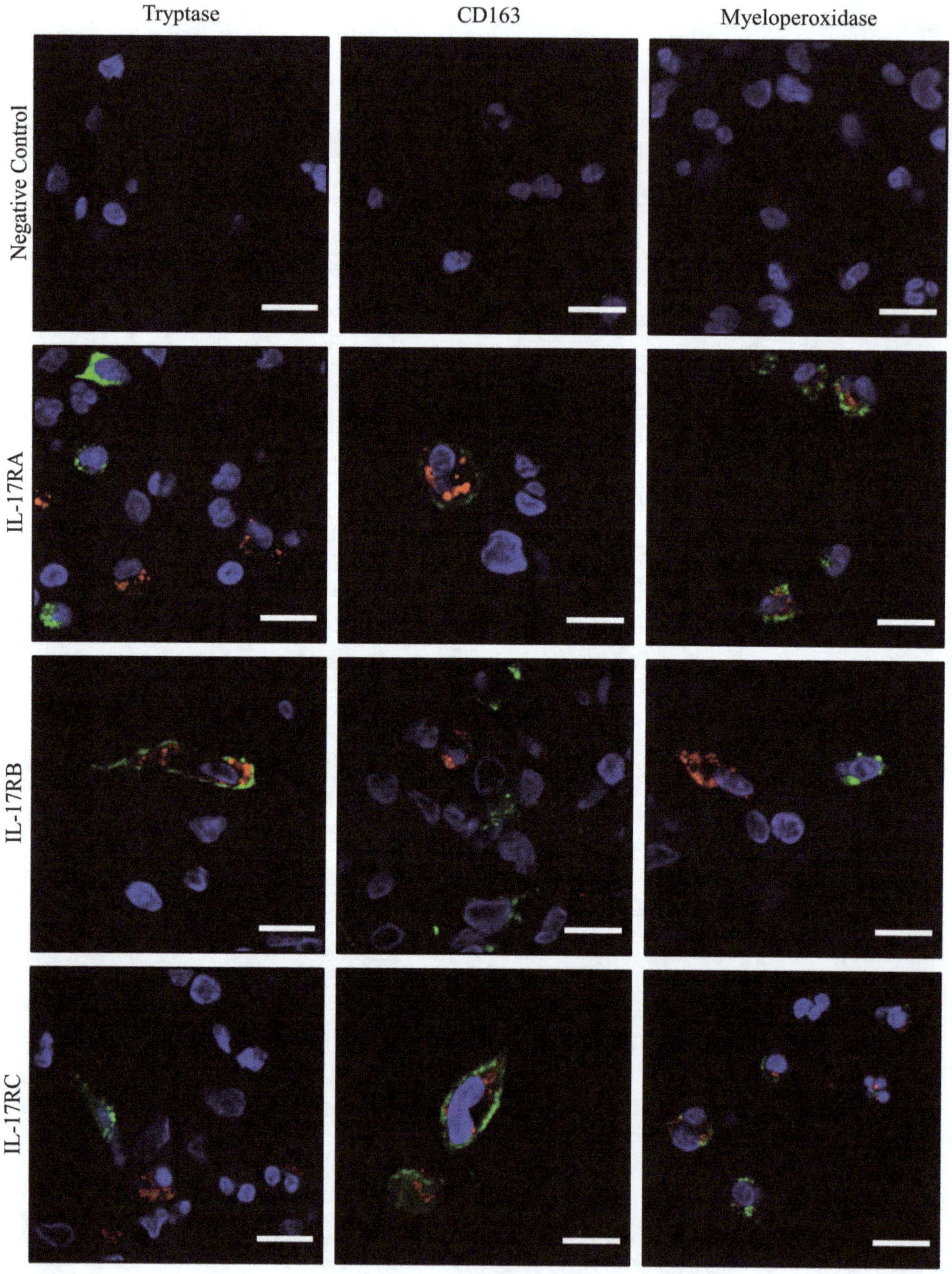

FIGURE 5 | IL-17RA, IL-17RB, and IL-17RC showed differential pattern of expression in immune cells associated to lesional skin of patients with BP. Paraffin-embedded skin biopsy specimen of blistering skin from BP patients ($n = 3$) were subjected to double immunofluorescence staining for IL-17RA, IL-17RB, and IL-17RC (in red), and either Tryptase, CD163, or myeloperoxidase (MPO) (in green) with Hoechst counterstain. Negative control: primary antibodies were not added. Scale bar = 10 μm.

evidenced that the *in situ* expression of IL-17RB was attributed to mast cell within the blister cavity. This is in line with a previous study showing that mast cells expressed and responded to IL-17E, which also has IL-17RB as receptor (37). Thus, altogether, our results suggest that antagonist mechanisms may be involved in the formation of different IL-17 cytokine, and receptor complexes. However, further studies are required to better understand how the IL-17 network is related with clinical disease activity in BP.

Regarding the IL-17 cytokine family, up to now, the main focus was given to IL-17A and IL-17A/F in BP. In this study, our results promote the investigation of IL-17 RA and IL-17 RC as new relevant predicting factors in BP. Furthermore, we previously showed that IL-17A/F was a relevant marker of BP outcome (26), and a recent publication showed promising results in the use of anti-IL-17A by using both animal model of BP and a human-derived model of BP (27). Nevertheless, the therapeutic approach targeting the IL-17 axis should be seen from a broader angle. Actually, the IL-17RA isoform is ubiquitous and can combine with most of the other IL-17 receptor isoforms to conduct the message delivered by the different IL-17 isoforms. Indeed, we showed an increase of IL-17RA and IL-17RC at time of diagnosis of patients with BP. Thus, blocking the IL-17RA isoform would limit the effects of IL-17A and IL-17F. Although this still needs to be demonstrated, this could also limit the effects of other IL-17 isoforms that require the IL-17RA to transduce their effects such as the IL-17E, whose concentration is increased in the BF of BP patients. In contrast, this could favor the anti-inflammatory effects of IL-17B, which is independent of IL-17RA. Therefore, in BP like in other dermatologic diseases such as psoriasis, inhibiting IL-17RA may represent a good therapeutic option (48–50).

Taken together, the results of our study provide a better understanding of the pattern of IL-17 and IL-17 receptor isoforms in BP. In particular, this is the first study investigating the expression of IL-17 receptors by immune cells from patients with BP. We showed that, in BP, the expression of IL-17RA and IL-17RC in monocyte and macrophages are related to disease outcome, whereas IL-17B was negatively correlated to disease activity. Although further studies are required to demonstrate the role of the IL-17B/IL-17RB axis in the pathophysiology of this disease, our study highlighted an intricate IL-17 network with potential antagonist effects of these members of the IL-17 family.

ETHICS STATEMENT

The studies involving human participants were reviewed and approved by Ethic Committee of the University Hospital of Reims (CNIL authorization DR-2013-320). The patients/participants provided their written informed consent to participate in this study.

AUTHOR CONTRIBUTIONS

PB, FA, and SL designed the study. SN, CM, and SL performed experiments. SN, CM, RL, PB, FA, and SL analyzed clinical and biological data. SN and SL performed the statistical analyses. CM, MV, and PB contributed to the clinical data collection. SN, RL, PB, FA, and SL wrote the manuscript. All authors critically evaluated the data and approved the final version for publication.

ACKNOWLEDGMENTS

We thank Dr. Christine Terryn from the PICT platform of the University of Reims Champagne-Ardenne for providing microscopy equipment and for technical assistance. We also thank Dr. Anne Durlach from the laboratory of Pol Bouin for providing all of the histological samples.

REFERENCES

1. Joly P, Baricault S, Sparsa A, Bernard P, Bédane C, Duvert-Lehembre S, et al. Incidence and mortality of bullous pemphigoid in France. *J Investig Dermatol.* (2012) 132:1998–2004. doi: 10.1038/jid.2012.35
2. Bernard P, Vaillant L, Labeille B, Bedane C, Arbeille B, Denoeux J-P, et al. Incidence and distribution of subepidermal autoimmune bullous skin diseases in three French regions. *Arch Dermatol.* (1995) 131:48–52. doi: 10.1001/archderm.131.1.48
3. Bernard P, Antonicelli F. Bullous pemphigoid: a review of its diagnosis, associations and treatment. *Am J Clin Dermatol.* (2017) 18:513–28. doi: 10.1007/s40257-017-0264-2
4. Witte M, Zillikens D, Schmidt E. Diagnosis of autoimmune blistering diseases. *Front Med.* (2018) 5:296. doi: 10.3389/fmed.2018.00296
5. Kridin K, Ludwig RJ. The growing incidence of bullous pemphigoid: overview and potential explanations. *Front Med.* (2018) 5:220. doi: 10.3389/fmed.2018.00220
6. Genovese G, Di Zenzo G, Cozzani E, Berti E, Cugno M, Marzano AV. New insights into the pathogenesis of bullous pemphigoid: 2019 Update. *Front Immunol.* (2019) 10:1506. doi: 10.3389/fimmu.2019.01506
7. Murrell DF, Daniel BS, Joly P, Borradori L, Amagai M, Hashimoto T, et al. Definitions and outcome measures for bullous pemphigoid: recommendations by an international panel of experts. *J Am Acad Dermatol.* (2012) 66:479–85. doi: 10.1016/j.jaad.2011.06.032
8. Stanley JR, Tanaka T, Mueller S, Klaus-Kovtun V, Roop D. Isolation of complementary DNA for bullous pemphigoid antigen by use of patients' autoantibodies. *J Clin Invest.* (1988) 82:1864–70. doi: 10.1172/JCI113803
9. Giudice GJ, Emery DJ, Diaz LA. Cloning and primary structural analysis of the bullous pemphigoid autoantigen BP180. *J Investig Dermatol.* (1992) 99:243–50. doi: 10.1111/1523-1747.ep12616580
10. Zillikens D, Rose PA, Balding SD, Liu Z, Olague-Marchan M, Diaz LA, et al. Tight clustering of extracellular BP180 epitopes recognized by bullous pemphigoid autoantibodies. *J Investig Dermatol.* (1997) 109:573–9. doi: 10.1111/1523-1747.ep12337492
11. Thoma-Uszynski S, Uter W, Schwietzke S, Schuler G, Borradori L, Hertl M.

Autoreactive T and B cells from bullous pemphigoid (BP) patients recognize epitopes clustered in distinct regions of BP180 and BP230. *J Immunol.* (2006) 176:2015–23. doi: 10.4049/jimmunol.176.3.2015

12. Di Zenzo G, Thoma-Uszynski S, Fontao L, Calabresi V, Hofmann SC, Hellmark T, et al. Multicenter prospective study of the humoral autoimmune response in bullous pemphigoid. *Clin Immunol.* (2008) 128:415–26. doi: 10.1016/j.clim.2008.04.012
13. Koga H, Teye K, Ishii N, Ohata C, Nakama T. High index values of enzyme-linked immunosorbent assay for BP180 at baseline predict relapse in patients with bullous pemphigoid. *Front Med.* (2018) 5:139. doi: 10.3389/fmed.2018.00139
14. Niimi Y, Pawankar R, Kawana S. Increased expression of matrix metalloproteinase-2, matrix metalloproteinase-9 and matrix metalloproteinase-13 in lesional skin of bullous pemphigoid. *Int Arch Allergy Immunol.* (2006) 139:104–13. doi: 10.1159/0000 90385
15. Verraes S, Hornebeck W, Bernard P, Polette M, Borradori L. Respective contribution of neutrophil elastase and matrix metalloproteinase 9 in the degradation of BP180 (type XVII collagen) in Human Bullous Pemphigoid. *J Investig Dermatol.* (2001) 117:1091–6. doi: 10.1046/j.0022-202x.2001. 01521.x
16. Hertl M. T cell control in autoimmune bullous skin disorders. *J Clin Investig.* (2006) 116:1159–66. doi: 10.1172/JCI28547
17. Fairley JA, Burnett CT, Fu C-L, Larson DL, Fleming MG, Giudice GJ. A Pathogenic role for IgE in autoimmunity: bullous pemphigoid IgE reproduces the early phase of lesion development in human skin grafted to nu/nu mice. *J Investig Dermatol.* (2007) 127:2605–11. doi: 10.1038/sj.jid.57 00958
18. Liu Z, Diaz LA, Troy JL, Taylor AF, Emery DJ, Fairley JA, et al. A passive transfer model of the organ-specific autoimmune disease, bullous pemphigoid, using antibodies generated against the hemidesmosomal antigen, BP180. *J Clin Invest.* (1993) 92:2480–8. doi: 10.1172/JCI1 16856
19. Nishie W, Sawamura D, Goto M, Ito K, Shibaki A, McMillan JR, et al. Humanization of autoantigen. *Nat Med.* (2007) 13:378–83. doi: 10.1038/nm1496
20. Schulze FS, Beckmann T, Nimmerjahn F, Ishiko A, Collin M, Köhl J, et al. Fcγ receptors III and IV mediate tissue destruction in a novel adult mouse model of bullous pemphigoid. *Am J Pathol.* (2014) 184:2185–96. doi: 10.1016/j.ajpath.2014.05.007
21. Hirose M, Recke A, Beckmann T, Shimizu A, Ishiko A, Bieber K, et al. Repetitive immunization breaks tolerance to type XVII collagen and leads to bullous pemphigoid in mice. *J Immunol.* (2011) 187:1176–83. doi: 10.4049/jimmunol.1100596
22. Liu Z, Giudice GJ, Swartz SJ, Fairley JA, Till GO, Troy JL, et al. The role of complement in experimental bullous pemphigoid. *J Clin Invest.* (1995) 95:1539–44. doi: 10.1172/JCI117826
23. Natsuga K, Nishie W, Shinkuma S, Ujiie H, Nishimura M, Sawamura D, et al. Antibodies to pathogenic epitopes on type XVII collagen cause skin fragility in a complement-dependent and -independent manner. *J Immunol.* (2012) 188:5792–9. doi: 10.4049/jimmunol.1003402
24. Fichel F, Barbe C, Joly P, Bedane C, Vabres P, Truchetet F, et al. Clinical and immunologic factors associated with bullous pemphigoid relapse during the first year of treatment: a multicenter, prospective study. *JAMA Dermatol.* (2014) 150:25–33. doi: 10.1001/jamadermatol.2013.5757
25. Le Jan S, Plée J, Vallerand D, Dupont A, Delanez E, Durlach A, et al. Innate immune cell-produced IL-17 sustains inflammation in bullous pemphigoid. *J Invest Dermatol.* (2014) 134:2908–17. doi: 10.1038/jid.2014.263
26. Plée J, Le Jan S, Giustiniani J, Barbe C, Joly P, Bedane C, et al. Integrating longitudinal serum IL-17 and IL-23 follow-up, along with autoantibodies variation, contributes to predict bullous pemphigoid outcome. *Sci Rep.* (2015) 5:18001. doi: 10.1038/srep18001
27. Chakievska L, Holtsche MM, Künstner A, Goletz S, Petersen B-S, Thaci D, et al. IL-17A is functionally relevant and a potential therapeutic target in bullous pemphigoid. *J Autoimmun.* (2019) 96:104–12. doi: 10.1016/j.jaut.2018.09.003
28. Ramirez-Carrozzi V, Sambandam A, Luis E, Lin Z, Jeet S, Lesch J, et al. IL-17C regulates the innate immune function of epithelial cells in an autocrine manner. *Nat Immunol.* (2011) 12:1159–66. doi: 10.1038/ni.2156
29. Moseley TA, Haudenschild DR, Rose L, Reddi AH. Interleukin-17 family and IL-17 receptors. *Cytokine Growth Factor Rev.* (2003) 14:155–74. doi: 10.1016/S1359-6101(03)00002-9
30. Silva WA, Covas DT, Panepucci RA, Proto-Siqueira R, Siufi JLC, Zanette DL, et al. The profile of gene expression of human marrow mesenchymal stem cells. *Stem Cells.* (2003) 21:661–9. doi: 10.1634/stemcells.21-6-661
31. Kuestner RE, Taft DW, Haran A, Brandt CS, Brender T, Lum K, et al. Identification of the IL-17 receptor related molecule IL-17RC as the receptor for IL-17F. *J Immunol.* (2007) 179:5462–73. doi: 10.4049/jimmunol.179.8.5462
32. Wright JF, Guo Y, Quazi A, Luxenberg DP, Bennett F, Ross JF, et al. Identification of an interleukin 17F/17A heterodimer in activated human CD4+ T cells. *J Biol Chem.* (2007) 282:13447–55. doi: 10.1074/jbc.M700499200
33. Wright JF, Bennett F, Li B, Brooks J, Luxenberg DP, Whitters MJ, et al. The human IL-17F/IL-17A heterodimeric cytokine signals through the IL-17RA/IL-17RC receptor complex. *J Immunol.* (2008) 181:2799–805. doi: 10.4049/jimmunol.181.4.2799
34. Gaffen SL. Structure and signalling in the IL-17 receptor superfamily. *Nat Rev Immunol.* (2009) 9:556. doi: 10.1038/nri2586
35. Lee J, Ho W-H, Maruoka M, Corpuz RT, Baldwin DT, Foster JS, et al. IL-17E, a novel proinflammatory ligand for the IL-17 receptor homolog IL-17Rh1. *J Biol Chem.* (2001) 276:1660–4. doi: 10.1074/jbc.M0082 89200
36. Maezawa Y, Nakajima H, Suzuki K, Tamachi T, Ikeda K, Inoue J-I, et al. Involvement of TNF receptor-associated factor 6 in IL-25 receptor signaling. *J Immunol.* (2006) 176:1013–8. doi: 10.4049/jimmunol.176. 2.1013
37. Fallon PG, Ballantyne SJ, Mangan NE, Barlow JL, Dasvarma A, Hewett DR, et al. Identification of an interleukin (IL)-25–dependent cell population that provides IL-4, IL-5, and IL-13 at the onset of helminth expulsion. *J Exp Med.* (2006) 203:1105–16. doi: 10.1084/jem.20051615
38. Chang SH, Reynolds JM, Pappu BP, Chen G, Martinez GJ, Dong C. Interleukin-17C promotes Th17 cell responses and autoimmune disease *via* interleukin-17 receptor E. *Immunity.* (2011) 35:611–21. doi: 10.1016/j.immuni.2011.09.010
39. Shi Y, Ullrich SJ, Zhang J, Connolly K, Grzegorzewski KJ, Barber MC, et al. A novel cytokine receptor–ligand pair: identification, molecular characterization, and *in vivo* immunomodulatory activity. *J Biol Chem.* (2000) 275:19167–76. doi: 10.1074/jbc.M910228199
40. Vaillant L. Evaluation of clinical criteria for diagnosis of bullous pemphigoid. *Arch Dermatol.* (1998) 134:1075. doi: 10.1001/archderm.134.9.1075
41. Lévy-Sitbon C, Barbe C, Plee J, Goeldel A-L, Antonicelli F, Reguiaï Z, et al. Assessment of bullous pemphigoid disease area index during treatment: a prospective study of 30 patients. *Dermatology.* (2014) 229:116–22. doi: 10.1159/000362717
42. Riani M, Le Jan S, Plée J, Durlach A, Le Naour R, Haegeman G, et al. Bullous pemphigoid outcome is associated with CXCL10-induced matrix metalloproteinase 9 secretion from monocytes and neutrophils but not lymphocytes. *J Allergy Clin Immunol.* (2017) 139:863–72.e3. doi: 10.1016/j.jaci.2016.08.012
43. Giusti D, Bini E, Terryn C, Didier K, Le Jan S, Gatouillat G, et al. NET formation in bullous pemphigoid patients with relapse is modulated by IL-17 and IL-23 interplay. *Front Immunol.* (2019) 10:701. doi: 10.3389/fimmu.2019.00701
44. Yamaguchi Y, Fujio K, Shoda H, Okamoto A, Tsuno NH, Takahashi K, et al. IL-17B and IL-17C are associated with TNF-production and contribute to the exacerbation of inflammatory arthritis. *J Immunol.* (2007) 179:7128–36. doi: 10.4049/jimmunol.179.10.7128
45. Dong C. Regulation and pro-inflammatory function of interleukin-17 family cytokines. *Immunol Rev.* (2008) 226:80–6. doi: 10.1111/j.1600-065X.2008.00709.x
46. Reynolds JM, Lee Y-H, Shi Y, Wang X, Angkasekwinai P, Nallaparaju KC, et al. Interleukin-17B antagonizes interleukin-25-mediated mucosal

inflammation. *Immunity.* (2015) 42:692–703. doi: 10.1016/j.immuni.2015.03.008

47. Clapé A, Muller C, Gatouillat G, Le Jan S, Barbe C, Pham B-N, et al. Mucosal involvement in bullous pemphigoid is mostly associated with disease severity and to absence of anti-BP230 autoantibody. *Front Immunol.* (2018) 9:479. doi: 10.3389/fimmu.2018.00479
48. Leonardi C, Matheson R, Zachariae C, Cameron G, Li L, Edson-Heredia E, et al. Anti-interleukin-17 monoclonal antibody ixekizumab in chronic plaque psoriasis. *N Engl J Med.* (2012) 366:1190–9. doi: 10.1056/NEJMoa1109997
49. Griffiths CEM, Reich K, Lebwohl M, van de Kerkhof P, Paul C, Menter A, et al. Comparison of ixekizumab with etanercept or placebo in moderate-to-severe psoriasis (UNCOVER-2 and UNCOVER-3): results from two phase 3 randomised trials. *Lancet.* (2015) 386:541–51. doi: 10.1016/S0140-6736(15)60125-8
50. Papp KA, Leonardi C, Menter A, Ortonne J-P, Krueger JG, Kricorian G, et al. Brodalumab, an anti-interleukin-17-receptor antibody for psoriasis. (2012) 366:1181–9. doi: 10.1056/NEJMoa1109017

11

Skin and Systemic Inflammation in Schnitzler's Syndrome are Associated with Neutrophil Extracellular Trap Formation

Hanna Bonnekoh [1,2], *Jörg Scheffel* [1,2], *Jim Wu* [1], *Sheila Hoffmann* [3], *Marcus Maurer* [1,2] and *Karoline Krause* [1,2*]

[1] *Department of Dermatology and Allergy, Allergie-Centrum-Charité, Berlin Institute of Health, Charité – Universitätsmedizin Berlin, Freie Universität Berlin, Humboldt-Universität zu Berlin, Berlin, Germany,* [2] *Autoinflammation Reference Center Charité (ARC2), Berlin Institute of Health, Charité – Universitätsmedizin Berlin, Freie Universität Berlin, Humboldt-Universität zu Berlin, Berlin, Germany,* [3] *German Center for Neurodegenerative Diseases, Berlin, Germany*

Correspondence:
Karoline Krause
karoline.krause@charite.de

Schnitzler's syndrome is a rare autoinflammatory disorder characterized by interleukin-1ß-mediated and neutrophil-dominated inflammation. Neutrophil extracellular traps (NETs) are web-like structures of decondensed chromatin, histones, and antimicrobial peptides released by neutrophils. NETs were initially described in the context of pathogen defense but are also involved in autoimmune-mediated skin diseases. Here, we assessed the role of neutrophil extracellular trap formation (NETosis) in Schnitzler's syndrome. Immunofluorescence co-staining of myeloperoxidase and subnucleosomal complex was performed on lesional skin samples from patients with Schnitzler's syndrome, other neutrophilic dermatoses (cryopyrin-associated periodic syndrome, Sweet syndrome, and pyoderma gangrenosum), urticarial vasculitis and chronic spontaneous urticaria as well as healthy control skin. Blood neutrophils from patients with Schnitzler's syndrome and controls were isolated, and NETosis was induced by phorbol 12-myristate 13-acetate (PMA). Also, NETosis of control neutrophils induced by symptomatic Schnitzler's syndrome sera, cytokines and sub-threshold PMA doses was studied. Immunofluorescence co-staining revealed widespread and substantial NET formation in lesional skin of Schnitzler's syndrome patients but absence of NETs in chronic spontaneous urticaria and control skin. Neutrophils undergoing NETosis were observed in the skin of other neutrophilic diseases too. Correspondingly, blood neutrophils from Schnitzler's syndrome patients showed significantly elevated NETosis rates compared to control neutrophils following stimulation with PMA. Increased NETosis correlated well with high levels of C-reactive protein (CRP). SchS patients with the lowest NETosis rates had persistent joint and bone pain despite IL-1 blockade. Stimulation of control neutrophils and sub-threshold PMA with sera of symptomatic Schnitzler's syndrome patients disclosed enhanced NETosis as compared to control sera. Our results suggest that the induction of NET formation by neutrophils contributes to skin and systemic inflammation and may support the resolution of local inflammation in Schnitzler's syndrome.

Keywords: Schnitzler's syndrome, neutrophil extracellular traps, neutrophils, autoinflammation, autoimmunity, neutrophilic dermatosis

INTRODUCTION

Schnitzler's syndrome (SchS) is a rare acquired autoinflammatory disease defined by recurrent urticarial rash, monoclonal gammopathy, and systemic inflammation that presents with fever episodes, muscle, bone, and joint pain (1). Until now, little is known about the exact pathophysiology of SchS. As in other autoinflammatory diseases, interleukin-1ß (IL-1β) functions as a key mediator of inflammation (2). In the skin of SchS patients, IL-1ß, and related cytokines are upregulated and produced by dermal mast cells and neutrophils (3, 4). The urticarial rash in SchS corresponds to neutrophil-rich dermal infiltrates classified as neutrophilic dermatosis. This term comprises a heterogeneous group of non-infectious inflammatory skin diseases characterized by the predominance of neutrophils in lesional skin (5). The specific role of neutrophils in SchS, however, is still ill-defined.

Neutrophils are part of the innate immune system and are responsible for the first line defense against pathogens by degranulating and secreting granule-stored antibacterial proteins as well as phagocytosis. Moreover, neutrophils are known to release neutrophil extracellular traps (NETs), which are web-like structures of decondensed chromatin, histones, and antimicrobial peptides that were initially described in the context of pathogen defense (6). NETs are also involved in various immune-mediated disorders as well as autoimmune diseases, and they contribute to the cutaneous inflammation in systemic lupus erythematosus (SLE) and psoriasis (7, 8). Recently, NETs were shown to regulate IL-1ß-mediated systemic inflammation in the autoinflammatory disease familial Mediterranean fever (FMF) (9) and were linked to arthritic inflammation in patients with gout (10).

In this study, we assessed NET formation in the lesional skin and peripheral blood of patients with SchS.

MATERIALS AND METHODS

Patients and Patient Samples

Lesional skin biopsies (ø 3–4 mm) were obtained from symptomatic patients with SchS (based on the Straßbourg diagnostic criteria (1)) or chronic spontaneous urticaria (CSU) who were treated at the Department of Dermatology, Charité - Universitätsmedizin Berlin. At the time of the skin biopsy, patients did not receive anti-IL-1-therapy or other immunomodulatory therapies. In addition, lesional skin samples from patients with Cryopyrin-associated periodic syndrome (CAPS), urticarial vasculitis (UV), and other neutrophilic dermatoses (Sweet syndrome [SwS] and pyoderma gangrenosum [PG]) as well as skin samples from healthy control subjects who underwent bariatric, plastic or breast reduction surgery, were obtained from the Department of Surgery, Charité—Universitätsmedizin Berlin. Also, blood samples from SchS patients (canakinumab-treated within the last 8 weeks and untreated patients) and healthy donors were taken. Blood samples were derived from SchS patients who underwent skin biopsy and from additional SchS patients. The mean disease duration in SchS patients was 10.45 years when tests were performed. Skin and blood specimens from individual patients were obtained at different time points. The study was approved by the local ethics committee (EA4/005/15, EA1/007/17), and patients provided written and oral informed consent.

Immunofluorescence Staining of Skin Samples

Paraffin sections (5 μm) of lesional skin (SchS $n = 8$, CSU $n = 5$, CAPS $n = 3$, UV $n = 5$, SwS $n = 4$, PG $n = 4$) and healthy control skin ($n = 10$) were prepared and processed for immunofluorescence staining. We stained hematoxylin eosin, myeloperoxidase (MPO) as well as subnucleosomal complex as a marker for NET formation and used DAPI (4',6-Diamidino-2-phenylindole dihydrochloride 10236276001, Roche Diagnostics Deutschland GmbH, Mannheim) for counterstaining of nuclei. MPO (1:400 392105 MAB3174 R&D Systems, Inc., Minneapolis, USA) was incubated with the secondary antibody (1:600 30 min room temperature, Alexa Fluor® 488-conjugated AffiniPure goat-anti-mouse IgG, 115-545-146; Jackson Immuno Research, West Grove, USA) and mouse normal serum 4% was added (1 h room temperature). The Alexa 488-labeled MPO antibody (overnight 4°C) was followed by incubation with Alexa 594 (1:200 30 min room temperature, Alexa Fluor® 594-conjugated Fab AffiniPure goat-anti-mouse IgG, 115-585-062; Jackson Immuno Research, West Grove, USA) labeled monoclonal mouse-anti-human-subnucleosomal complex (Histone 2A, 2B, chromatin) antibody (1:1,500 1 h room temperature). Samples of tonsil tissue served as positive controls for staining MPO and were derived from routine tissue sampling of the Department of Pathology, Charité – Universitätsmedizin Berlin. Sections omitting the primary antibody served as negative controls.

Isolation and Stimulation of Neutrophils

Peripheral blood neutrophils from SchS patients ($n = 12$; canakinumab-treated patients $n = 9$, untreated patients $n = 3$; **Table S1**) and healthy controls ($n = 12$) were isolated by using a neutrophil isolation kit (MACSxpress® neutrophil isolation kit human, MACS Miltenyi Biotec GmbH, Bergisch-Gladbach, Germany, no. 130-104-434). Neutrophils were assessed for spontaneous NET formation (incubation with RPMI medium with 2% fetal calf serum for 130 min) and for NET formation after stimulation with 20 nM phorbol 12-myristate 13-acetate (PMA) for 80, 100, and 130 min as previously described (11). Neutrophils were isolated and processed in pairs of one patient and one healthy control at a time.

Abbreviations: CAPS, Cryopyrin-associated periodic syndrome; CRP, C-reactive protein; CSU, Chronic spontaneous urticaria; DAPI, 4',6-Diamidino-2-phenylindole dihydrochloride; FMF, Familial Mediterranean fever; IL, Interleukin; IL-1RA, Interleukin-1-receptor antagonist; MPO, Myeloperoxidase; NETs, Neutrophil extracellular traps; NLRP, Nucleotide binding domain like receptor protein; PG, Pyoderma gangrenosum; PGA, Physician global assessment; PMA, Phorbol 12-myristate 13-acetate; SAA, Serum amyloid A; SchS, Schnitzler's syndrome; SLE, Systemic lupus erythematosus; SwS, Sweet syndrome; UV, Urticarial vasculitis.

In addition, NET formation of healthy control neutrophils by SchS sera (10% serum concentration) from symptomatic patients ($n = 12$), combined with RPMI medium with 2% fetal calf serum as well as sub-threshold (0.05 nM) PMA doses for 130 min, was assessed. Sera from healthy individuals ($n = 14$) served as controls. Also, NET formation of control neutrophils and neutrophils from SchS patients was assessed after stimulation with IL-1β (10–50 ng/ml), IL-6 (10–100 ng/ml), IL-17 (20–100 ng/ml), or IL-8 (20–100 ng/ml) as well as with a combination of proinflammatory cytokines (IL-1β, IL-6, IL-17, IL-8) and subthreshold PMA.

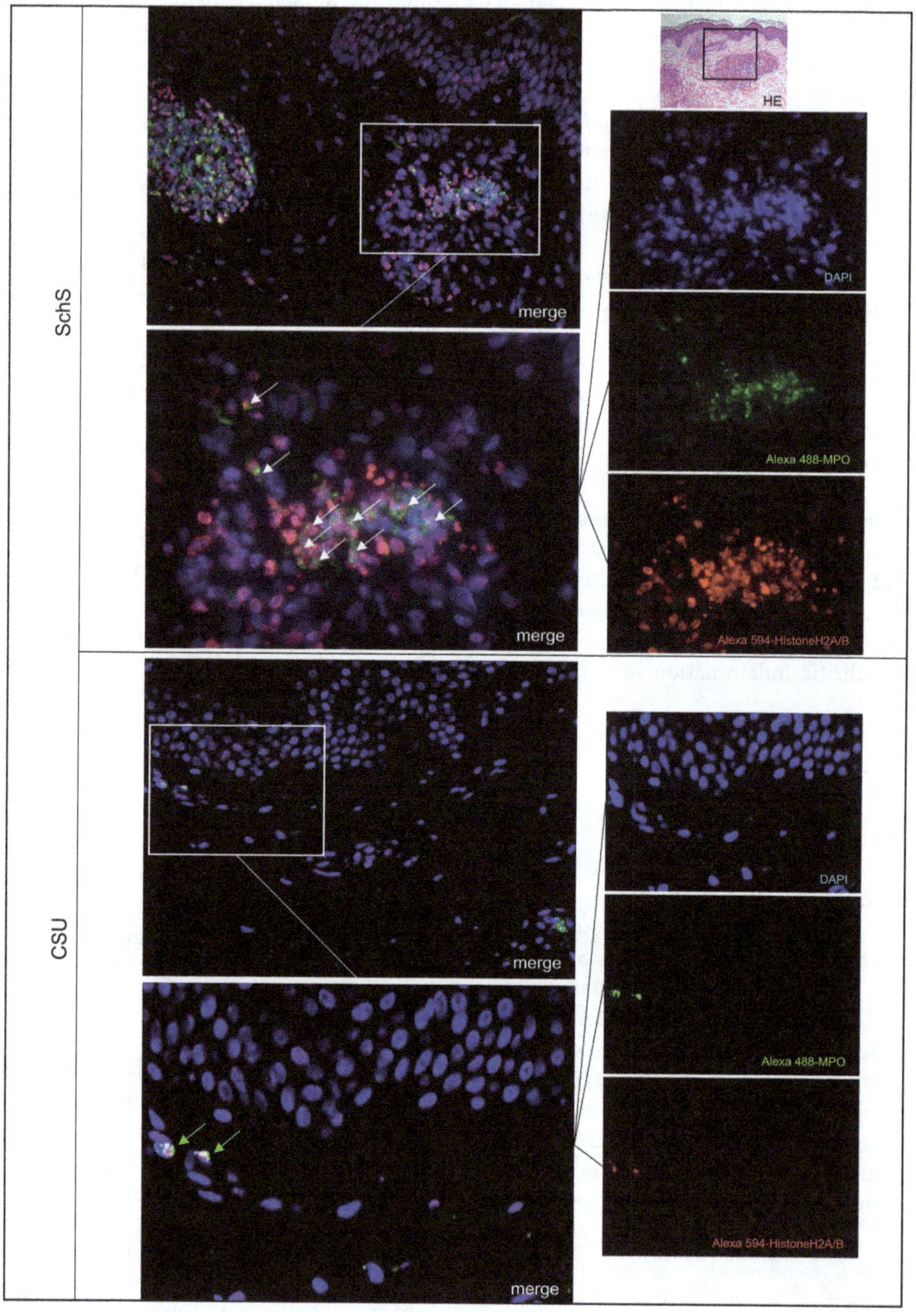

FIGURE 1 | Marked NET formation in lesional skin of Schnitzler's syndrome (SchS) patient vs. absence of NET formation in chronic spontaneous urticaria (CSU) patient. Exemplified fluorescence images showing marked and aggregated NET formation characterized by nuclear expansion and extracellular web-like DNA-fibers (white arrows) in the lesional dermis of a SchS patient vs. absence of NETosis of neutrophils (green arrows) in lesional dermis of a CSU patient. Neutrophils (Alexa 488-MPO–green) undergoing NETosis (subnucleosomal complex Histone H2A, H2B, chromatin Alexa 594–red). Nuclei are counterstained with DAPI (blue) (original magnification 200x). Overview: Hematoxylin-Eosin staining of infiltrate in lesional skin of SchS patient (original magnification 200x).

NET Detection by Immunofluorescence Staining and Quantification of NET Formation of Peripheral Blood and Skin Neutrophils

Samples were stained (immunofluorescence co-staining of DAPI and subnucleosomal complex), and microscopic images of peripheral blood neutrophils were analyzed by ImageJ as previously described (12). In brief, 5 microscopic images of each coverslip were randomly taken per experiment (100x magnification). Image files were loaded in the ImageJ software and for total cell number, the DAPI fluorescence image stack was analyzed (automatic particle analysis, 20 pixels minimum size). For neutrophils undergoing NETosis, the anti-subnucleosomal complex fluorescence image stack was counted automatically. To clearly distinguish between non-NETting and NETting cells, exposure times were calibrated to show no fluorescence signal in non-stimulated neutrophils (negative control) and full fluorescence signal of anti-subnucleosomal antibody in the PMA 130 min.-stimulated samples (positive control). We kept this threshold value of exposure time constant for each experiment. Relative NETosis rates were calculated by using the highest NETosis rate per experiment as 100%. NETosis in the skin was assessed by percentages of neutrophils undergoing NETosis per high power field. Stainings were analyzed by one blinded researcher who counted all neutrophils undergoing NETosis in five exemplified high power fields per skin sample (400x magnification). Cases of dense neutrophilic infiltration with wide-spread NETosis covering the HPF, were assessed as 100%. Exemplified stainings of NETosis were analyzed by confocal microscopy.

Assessment of Serum Inflammation Markers and Physician Global Assessment

Sera of canakinumab-treated SchS patients ($n = 8$) were analyzed for C-reactive protein (CRP, Ref. <5.0 mg/l), serum amyloid A (SAA, Ref. <6.4 mg/l), and total blood neutrophil count (Ref. 1.5–7.7/nl) at the time of neutrophil stimulation. For analysis of S100A8/9 (Ref. <2.94 μg/ml) and interleukin-1-receptor antagonist (IL-1RA, Ref. <500 pg/ml), sera of $n = 5$ canakinumab treated patients were available. We also assessed quantitative immunoglobulins (IgM, Ref. < 2.3 g/l; IgG, Ref. 7–16 g/l). In addition, physician global assessment (PGA, categories: urticarial rash, fatigue, fever, myalgia/bone pain and arthralgia, score 0–4; maximum score: 20) was performed.

Statistical Analysis

Statistical analysis was performed for non-parametric data by using the Mann Whitney *U*-Test. Correlation analyses for inflammation marker concentrations as well as PGA and NETosis rates were performed by Spearman's rank coefficient. For all analyses, SPSS version 22.0 and Graph Pad Prism version 6.0 were used. Statistical significance was considered by $p \leq 0.05$.

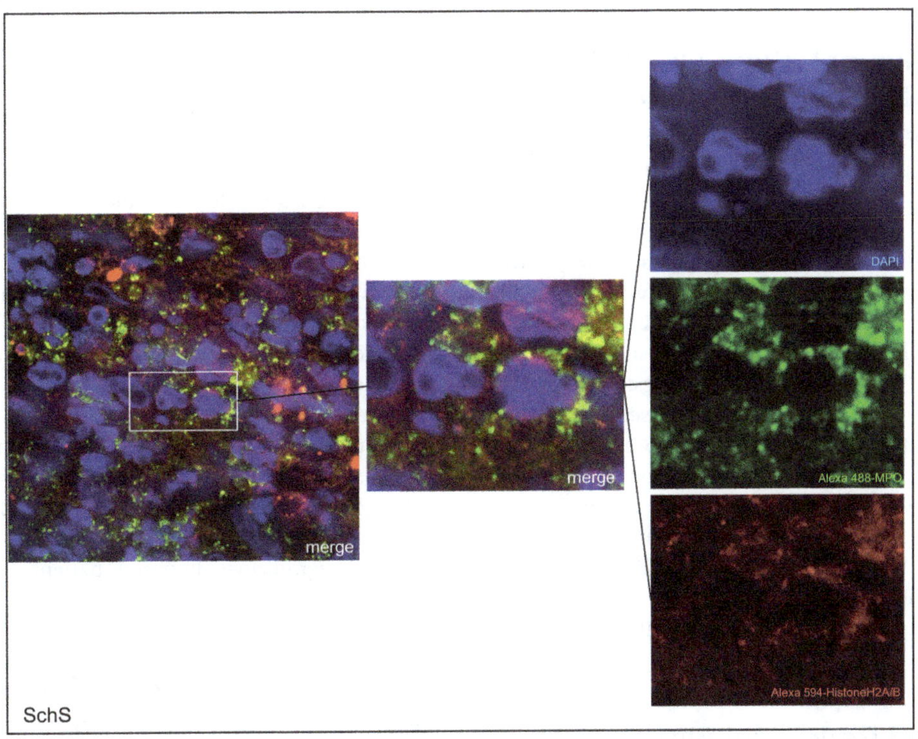

FIGURE 2 | Confocal microscopic images of Schnitzler's syndrome (SchS) skin tissue. Neutrophils (Alexa 488-MPO–green) undergoing NETosis (subnucleosomal complex Histone H2A, H2B, chromatin Alexa 594–red) are demonstrated by extracelluar co-localization of subnucleosomal complex and MPO. Nuclei are counterstained with DAPI (blue) (original magnification 1,000x).

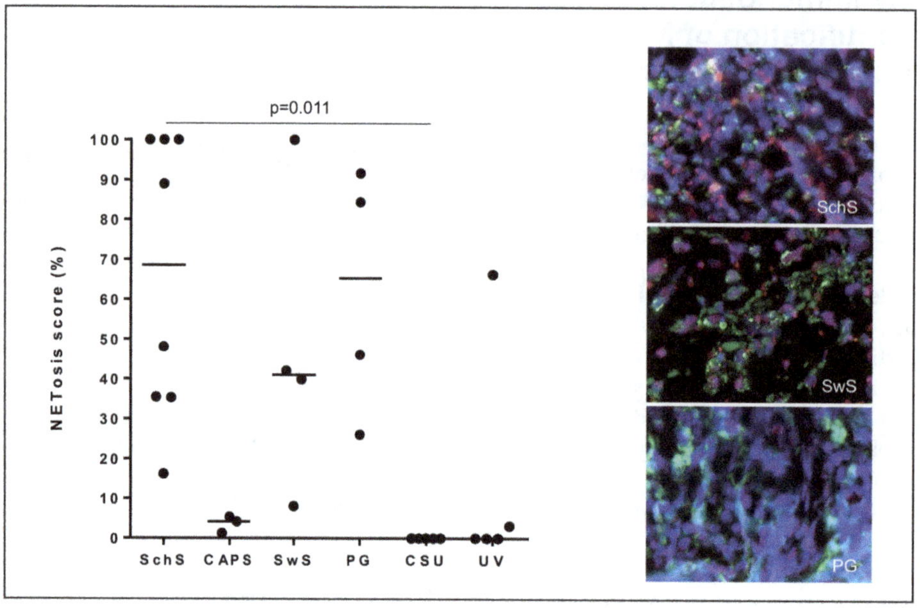

FIGURE 3 | NETosis - immunoreactivity score in %: High NETosis rates in lesional dermis of Schnitzler's syndrome (SchS) patients as well as Sweet syndrome (SwS) patients and pyoderma gangrenosum (PG) patients. In lesional skin of Cryopyrin-associated periodic syndrome (CAPS) patients, only single neutrophils underwent NETosis. In $n = 2/5$ patients with urticarial vasculitis patients (UV) NETting neutrophils (single cells or aggregated NETs) were detected. Absence of NETosis rates in lesional dermis of CSU patients. Bars indicate median values. Exemplified fluorescence images showing dense neutrophilic infiltration with marked and aggregated NET formation characterized by nuclear expansion and extracellular web-like DNA-fibers in the lesional dermis of a SchS patient (top), SwS patient (middle) and PG patient (bottom). Neutrophils (Alexa 488-MPO - green) undergoing NETosis (subnucleosomal complex Histone H2A, H2B, chromatin Alexa 594 – red). Nuclei are counterstained with DAPI (blue) (original magnification 400x).

RESULTS

The Lesional Skin of Patients With SchS Is Characterized by Abundant Infiltrates of Neutrophils That Undergo NETosis

Lesional skin of SchS patients showed stronger neutrophilic cell infiltrates as compared to CSU (**Figure S1**). Immunofluorescence co-staining revealed marked and aggregated NET formation in lesional skin of all untreated SchS patients ($n = 8$) with highest median NETosis scores (68.54%) (**Figures 1, 3**). This could be confirmed by confocal microscopy (**Figure 2**) which demonstrated extracellular co-localization of subnucleosomal complex and MPO in SchS lesional skin. Interestingly, marked and aggregated NET formation was also present in lesional dermal skin of patients with SwS, (median score 40.99%) and PG (median score 65.28%) (**Figure 3**). Only single neutrophils undergoing NETosis were observed in CAPS patients (median score 4.17%), whereas $n = 2/5$ UV patients presented with single or marked aggregated NETs (median score 0%) (**Figure 3**). There was an absence of NETs in the skin of CSU patients ($n = 5$) (**Figures 1, 3**; SchS vs. CSU $p = 0.011$) and healthy controls ($n = 10$) (data not shown).

PMA-Stimulated Peripheral Blood Neutrophils of SchS Patients Show Higher NETosis Rates Than Healthy Controls

Blood neutrophils from the majority of canakinumab-treated patients ($n = 6/9$ for 80 min and 100 min, $n = 9/9$ for 130 min) and all untreated SchS patients showed higher NETosis rates of PMA-stimulated (20 nM) blood neutrophils. NETosis rates of PMA-stimulated blood neutrophils from SchS patients increased over time compared to healthy control neutrophils with significant difference after 100 min ($p = 0.045$) and 130 min ($p = 0.007$) of PMA-stimulation (**Figures 4A,B**). However, considerable variability was observed in both groups and between experiments. Incubation of neutrophils with RPMI medium alone resulted in near absent NETosis rates in both SchS patients and healthy controls. Patients on IL-1 blockade (canakinumab; $n = 6$) showed similar results compared to untreated patients ($n = 3$) without significant differences between both patient groups (**Figure 4B,** # marked as untreated patients).

Stimulation with individual or combined proinflammatory cytokines IL-1β, IL-6, IL-8, IL-17 in different concentrations and together with PMA showed higher NETosis rates of blood neutrophils in single SchS patients, but there was no overall statistical significance between patients and healthy controls (data not shown).

SchS Sera Induce High Rates of NETosis in Healthy Donor Neutrophils

Stimulation of healthy control neutrophils with serum of untreated symptomatic SchS patients showed near absence of NETosis rates, which is comparable to stimulation with healthy control sera as well as to stimulation with RPMI medium. Co-stimulation of healthy control neutrophils with

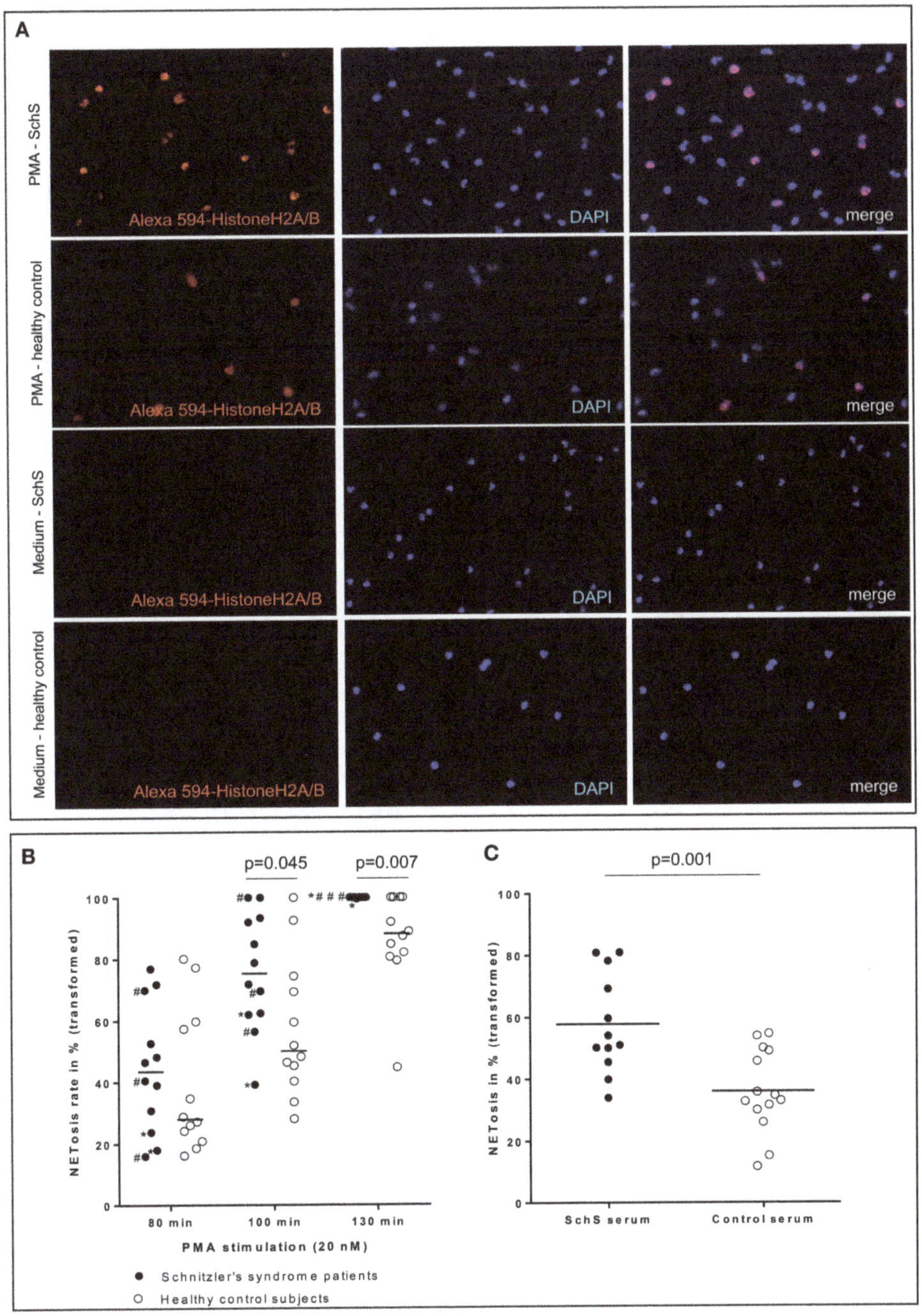

FIGURE 4 | (A) Higher NETosis rates of blood neutrophils in Schnitzler's syndrome (SchS) patient vs. healthy control after 130 min of PMA stimulation: Fluorescence images of peripheral blood neutrophils of a patient with SchS compared to healthy control: NET formation of isolated neutrophils (subnucleosomal complexe Histone H2A, H2B, chromatin Alexa 594 – red). Nuclei are counterstained with DAPI (blue) (original magnification 100x) **(B)** Higher NETosis rates of neutrophils in SchS vs. healthy controls: NETosis rates in % of blood neutrophils in IL-1-inhibitor treated and untreated SchS patients (# marked untreated patients) vs. healthy controls after 80, 100, and 130 min following 20 nM PMA stimulation. *patients with persistent joint/bone inflammation despite IL-1 blockade. **(C)** Higher NETosis rates after SchS serum stimulated control neutrophils compared to control serum stimulation: NETosis rates in % of control blood neutrophils after stimulation with 0.05 nM PMA and 10% serum of symptomatic SchS patients and healthy controls. Bars indicate median values.

serum of untreated symptomatic SchS patients and sub-threshold PMA (0.05 nM) disclosed significantly higher NETosis rates as compared to control sera and sub-threshold PMA ($p = 0.001$) (**Figure 4C**).

High NETosis Rates Significantly Correlate With Increased Inflammation Markers

Due to the continuous anti-IL-1 blockade in the majority of patients, inflammation markers were barely elevated. Still, a

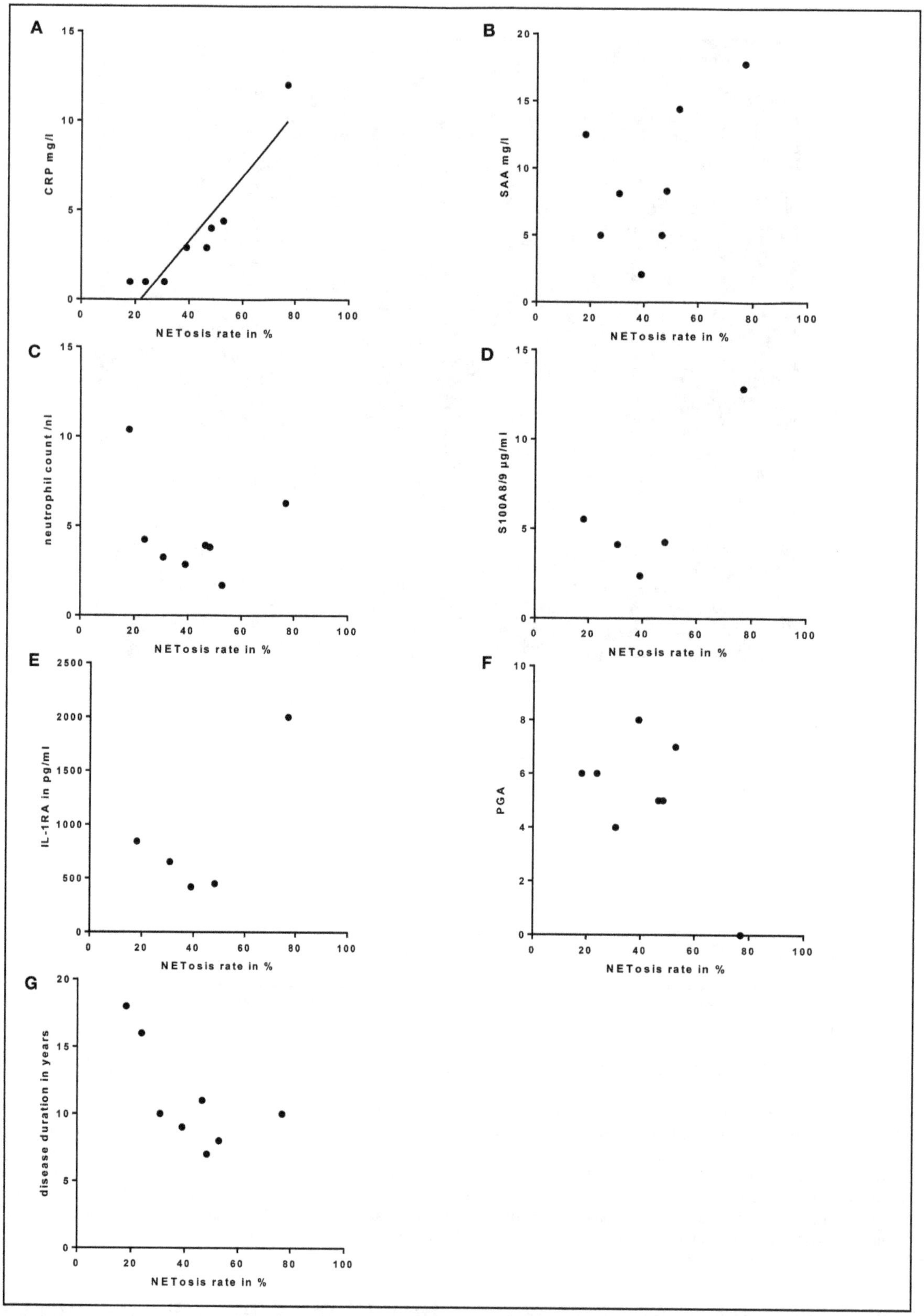

FIGURE 5 | Correlation between serum markers, physician global assessment (PGA), disease duration and NETosis rates: **(A)** Correlation between high NETosis rates and high C-reactive protein (CRP) levels for 80 min PMA stimulation in Schnitzler's syndrome patients ($p = 0.000$; $r = 0.970$). No significant correlation between

(Continued)

FIGURE 5 | NETosis rates and serum levels of **(B)** serum amyloid A (SAA), **(C)** total blood neutrophil count, **(D)** S100A8/9, **(E)** interleukin-1-receptor antagonist (IL-1RA), **(F)** PGA or **(G)** disease duration was observed in Schnitzler's syndrome patients. The dotted lines indicate normal values (CRP, SAA, neutrophil count, S100A8/9, IL-1RA) and minimal disease activity (PGA).

strong correlation between high NETosis rates and high CRP levels (for 80 min PMA stimulation $p = 0.000$; $r = 0.970$) was identified (**Figure 5A**). In contrast, no significant correlation between NETosis rates and markers of subclinical inflammation (SAA, S100A8/9, IL-1RA), neutrophil count, disease duration or clinical disease activity assessed by PGA was observed (**Figure 5**). Also, we could not detect a significant correlation between NETosis rates of symptomatic SchS patients and immunoglobulin levels. The two SchS patients with the lowest NETosis rates had persistent joint and bone pain despite IL-1 blockade (**Figure 4B, *** marked patients with persistent joint and bone pain). Vice versa, 2 out of 3 patients with high NETosis rates had only mild bone pain/arthralgia.

DISCUSSION

Our results demonstrate increased amounts of neutrophils undergoing NETosis in lesional skin and peripheral blood of SchS patients as compared to CSU and/or healthy controls. To the best of our knowledge, this is the first study which reports NETosis in SchS. Furthermore, it supports the significance of NET formation in autoinflammatory diseases as previously described for FMF and gout (9, 14).

Neutrophils undergoing NETosis in lesional skin of SchS patients and their absence in CSU patients may explain the clinical observation of more solid and stable wheals with longer duration in autoinflammatory patients compared to urticarial lesions in CSU patients (15). In contrast to SchS, lesional skin of CSU patients usually shows rather sparse lymphocytic infiltrates and fewer neutrophils (4). The spectrum of UV varies from only mild urticarial lesions to severe disease with systemic manifestations which could explain the heterogeneity of UV patients regarding the occurrence of NETs in lesional skin. Clinical phenotypes of neutrophilic dermatoses include pustular, urticarial, plaque-like, and ulcerous lesions. All of them are commonly associated with systemic diseases such as hematologic, autoimmune and autoinflammatory entities (5). The presence of NETs in SwS and PG suggests that NETosis contributes to the pathogenesis of other neutrophilic dermatoses as well. This is underscored by a very recent publication showing that enhanced NET formation and decreased NET degradation contribute to the inflammation in the hereditary autoinflammatory disease Pyogenic arthritis, pyoderma gangrenosum and acne (PAPA) syndrome (16). Although neutrophilic dermatoses are clinically heterogenous disorders linked to either autoimmune or autoinflammatory pathways, they share the activation of neutrophils that could be elicited via alterations in homeostasis or chemotaxis of neutrophils (17).

NETosis was previously associated with skin inflammation in psoriasis and SLE (7, 8). Psoriasis is characterized by epidermal hyperproliferation and neutrophil infiltrates invading the epidermis. As expected, NETosis was primarily observed in the epidermis next to keratinocytes (7), whereas in SchS epidermal involvement is missing, and neutrophil infiltrates undergoing NETosis are dermally located as can also been seen in SLE (8).

A dual role for NETs was implicated in the pathophysiology of inflammatory diseases. In prototype autoimmune disease SLE, NETs induce the expression of double stranded DNA (dsDNA) and LL-37, resulting in externalization of autoantigens and immunostimulatory proteins (8). These may contribute to an antigenic source for autoantibodies that promote the inflammation and damage of endothelial cells by synthesis of proinflammatory cytokines or type I interferons in SLE (8). On the other hand, NETs may limit the inflammation as suggested for autoinflammatory disorders gout and FMF (9, 14). Aggregated NETs in gout were shown to contribute to the resolution of inflammation by degrading cytokines and chemokines via serine proteases (14). In FMF, neutrophils were demonstrated to release IL-1ß through NETs, but they also downregulated further NETosis and thereby resolved FMF attacks via a negative feedback mechanism (9).

NETosis rates in psoriasis patients correlated well with clinical disease activity (7). Although this was not the case in our study, we observed a positive correlation between high NETosis rates and increased inflammatory marker CRP in SchS. We hypothesize that the systemic inflammation drives NET formation in SchS. These NETs may exert both pro- and anti-inflammatory functions. NETosis could stimulate aberrant NLRP3 inflammasome activation in SchS monocytes and macrophages via cathelicidins and thereby enhance the release of inflammatory cytokines followed by further NETosis as shown for SLE (18). Also, NETs may support the resolution of inflammation by degrading cytokines locally in SchS (**Figure 6**). As in gout inflammation, high amounts of aggregated neutrophils were found in lesional tissue of SchS patients. The inflammation-limiting ability of NETosis via cytokine degradation could explain the observation that SchS patients with low NETosis rates suffer from persistent chronic joint and bone inflammation as degradation of cytokines may not be sufficient in these patients.

In lesional skin of patients with prototype autoinflammatory urticarial syndrome CAPS, we observed only single neutrophils undergoing NET formation. This finding may indicate a pathophysiological link of NET formation and SchS-specific paraproteinemia. Nevertheless, we could not show a significant correlation between NETosis rates and immunoglobulin levels, and there is no evidence for a link between paraproteinemia and NET formation in other diseases associated with paraproteinemia. However, aberrant

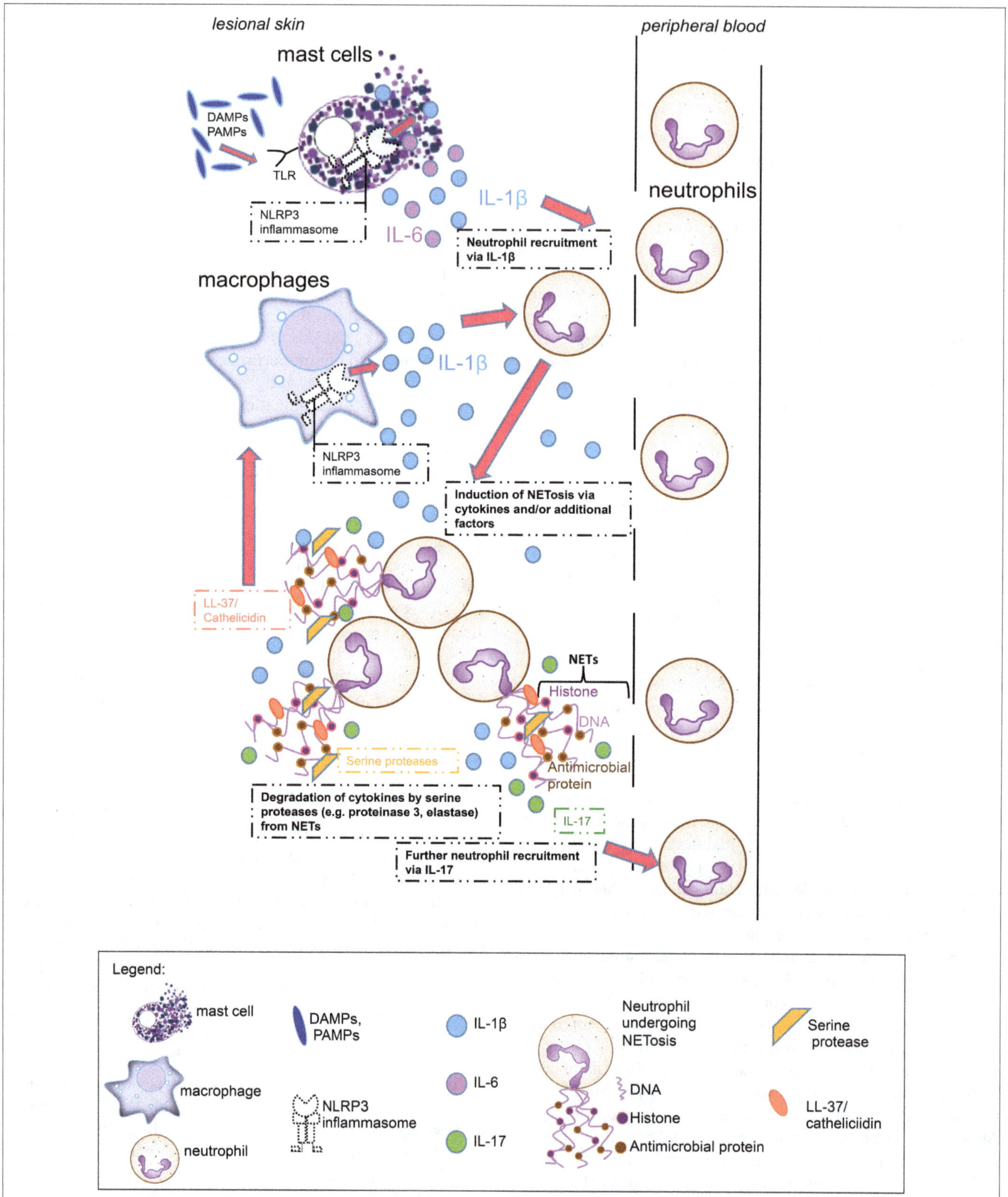

FIGURE 6 | Main hypothesis on the pathophysiological role of neutrophil extracellular traps (NETs) in Schnitzler's syndrome: Mast cells hypersensitive to damage-associated molecular patterns (DAMPs) or pathogen-associated molecular patterns (PAMPs), are activated via Toll-like receptors (TLRs) and

(Continued)

FIGURE 6 | produce Interleukin (IL)-1ß and IL-6. Cytokine production by mast cells is presumably mediated via the NLRP3 inflammasome. These proinflammatory cytokines lead to neutrophil recruitment from peripheral blood. Cytokines and other serum factors induce initial NET formation in the skin. During NETosis, IL-17 and LL-37 (cathelicidin) are secreted. IL-17 induces further neutrophil recruitment, while LL-37 activates the NLRP3 inflammasome in macrophages to produce further IL-1ß, which again recruits neutrophils. Additional NETting neutrophils aggregate and secrete serine proteases such as proteinase 3 and elastase which degrade cytokines (e.g., IL-1ß) and limit inflammation.

inflammasome component expression is described in both SchS and multiple myeloma (19, 20).

The pathophysiologic mechanisms of how neutrophils are activated to undergo NETosis locally in the lesional tissue as well as systemically in the peripheral blood of SchS patients, are unclear. Our results of higher NETosis of donor neutrophils induced by SchS serum compared to healthy serum are in line with the findings in psoriasis and support the existence of a potential serum factor inducing NETosis (7). Several proinflammatory cytokines, including IL-1ß, IL-6, and IL-17 were shown to be elevated in the serum of different inflammatory conditions such as sepsis, diabetes and rheumatoid arthritis and to induce enhanced NETosis of peripheral neutrophils in these disorders (12, 21, 22). These cytokines are known to be upregulated in SchS as well (3, 4). Interestingly, mast cells induce neutrophil recruitment and were shown to be a source of IL-1β and IL-6 in lesional skin of SchS patients (3, 4). Whether these proinflammatory cytokines e.g., produced by mast cells or even neutrophils themselves contribute to NET formation locally in lesional skin of SchS patients remains to be elucidated. However, none of these cytokines, whether alone or in combination, could induce NETosis of peripheral neutrophils in our study, and we are assuming that additional factors are needed to stimulate neutrophils to form NETs in SchS.

Limitations of our study comprise the relatively small patient number, which is explained by the rarity of SchS and the heterogeneity of individual experiments showing considerable variability.

In conclusion, our results suggest that skin and systemic inflammation in SchS are associated with neutrophils undergoing NETosis. These may exert pro-inflammatory or in the case of aggregated NETs anti-inflammatory properties. For the future, evaluation of drivers of NET formation in autoinflammatory diseases are essential in order to better understand disease mechanisms. Also, these studies may help to identify therapeutic targets that promote cytokine degradation and resolution of inflammation via enhancing aggregation of NETs.

AUTHOR CONTRIBUTIONS

HB designed and performed the experiments, analyzed the data, and prepared the manuscript. JS designed the experiments and provided intellectual assistance. JW performed the experiments. SH performed confocal microscopy. MM gave critical input to the manuscript. KK took care of the patients, designed the experiments and prepared, and revised the manuscript. All authors read, reviewed, and approved the final manuscript.

ACKNOWLEDGMENTS

We acknowledge support from the German Research Foundation (DFG) and the Open Access Publication Fund of Charité - Universitätsmedizin Berlin. The authors thank Dr. Volker Brinkmann for providing the subnucleosomal complex antibody and Evelin Hagen for excellent technical assistance.

SUPPLEMENTARY MATERIAL

Table S1 | Main clinical, biological, and therapeutic features of Schnitzler's syndrome patients included in this study. *Patients were untreated when NETosis rates were assessed. #NETosis rates were assessed in untreated and treated patients.

Figure S1 | Hematoxylin-Eosin staining of infiltrates in lesional skin of patients with Cryopyrin-associated periodic syndrome (CAPS), Schnitzler's syndrome (SchS), Sweet-Syndrome (SwS), Pyoderma gangrenosum (PG), chronic spontaneous urticaria (CSU), urticarial vasculitis (UV), and healthy controls (original magnification 50x, 200x). Images are published in part in Bonnekoh (13).

REFERENCES

1. Simon A, Asli B, Braun-Falco M, De Koning H, Fermand JP, Grattan C, et al. Schnitzler's syndrome: diagnosis, treatment, and follow-up. *Allergy.* (2013) 68:562–8. doi: 10.1111/all.12129
2. Krause K, Tsianakas A, Wagner N, Fischer J, Weller K, Metz M, et al. Efficacy and safety of canakinumab in schnitzler syndrome: a multicenter randomized placebo-controlled study. *J Allergy Clin Immunol.* (2017) 139:1311–20. doi: 10.1016/j.jaci.2016.07.041
3. de Koning HD, van Vlijmen-Willems IM, Rodijk-Olthuis D, van der Meer JW, Zeeuwen PL, Simon A, et al. Mast cell interleukin-1 beta, neutrophil interleukin-17 and epidermal antimicrobial proteins in the neutrophilic urticarial dermatosis in Schnitzler's syndrome. *Br J Dermatol.* (2015) 173:448–56. doi: 10.1111/bjd.13857
4. Bonnekoh H, Scheffel J, Maurer M, Krause K. Use of skin biomarker profiles to distinguish Schnitzler syndrome from chronic spontaneous urticaria: results of a pilot study. *Br J Dermatol.* (2018) 178:561–2. doi: 10.1111/bjd.15705
5. Alavi A, Sajic D, Cerci FB, Ghazarian D, Rosenbach M, Jorizzo J. Neutrophilic dermatoses: an update. *Am J Clin Dermatol.* (2014) 15:413–23. doi: 10.1007/s40257-014-0092-6
6. Brinkmann V, Reichard U, Goosmann C, Fauler B, Uhlemann Y, Weiss DS. Neutrophil extracellular traps kill bacteria. *Science.* (2004) 303:1532–5. doi: 10.1126/science.1092385

7. Hu SC, Yu HS, Yen FL, Lin CL, Chen GS, Lan CC. Neutrophil extracellular trap formation is increased in psoriasis and induces human β-defensin-2 production in epidermal keratinocytes. *Sci Rep.* (2016) 6:31119. doi: 10.1038/srep31119
8. Villanueva E, Yalavarthi S, Berthier CC, Hodgin JB, Khandpur R, Lin AM, et al. Netting neutrophils induce endothelial damage, infiltrate tissues, and expose immunostimulatory molecules in systemic lupus erythematosus. *J Immunol* (2011) 187:538–52. doi: 10.4049/jimmunol.1100450
9. Apostolidou E, Skendros P, Kambas K, Mitroulis I, Konstantinidis T, Chrysanthopoulou A, et al. Neutrophil extracellular traps regulate IL-1beta-mediated inflammation in familial Mediterranean fever. *Ann Rheum Dis* (2014) 5:269–77. doi: 10.1136/annrheumdis-2014-205958
10. Mitroulis I, Kambas K, Chrysanthopoulou A, Skendros P, Apostolidou E, Kourtzelis I, et al. Neutrophil extracellular trap formation is associated with IL-1β and autophagy-related signaling in gout. *PLoS ONE.* (2011) 6:e29318. doi: 10.1371/journal.pone.0029318
11. Brinkmann V, Laube B, Abu Abed U, Goosmann C, Zychlinsky A. Neutrophil extracellular traps: how to generate and visualize them. *J Vis Exp.* (2010) 1724. doi: 10.3791/1724
12. Brinkmann V, Goosmann C, Kühn LI, Zychlinsky A. Automatic quantification of *in vitro* NET formation. *Front Immunol.* (2012) 3:413. doi: 10.3389/fimmu.2012.00413
13. Bonnekoh H. *An Immunohistological charaCterization of Potential Diagnostic Biomarkers in Urticarial Vasculitis and Autoinflammatory Skin Diseases* (2016). Available online at: https://refubium.fu-berlin.de/handle/fub188/11977
14. Schauer C, Janko C, Munoz LE, Zhao Y, Kienhöfer D, Frey B, et al. Aggregated neutrophil extracellular traps limit inflammation by degrading cytokines and chemokines. *Nat Med.* (2014) 20:511–7. doi: 10.1038/nm.3547
15. Krause K, Grattan CE, Bindslev-Jensen C, Gattorno M, Kallinich T, de Koning HD, et al. How not to miss autoinflammatory diseases masquerading as urticaria. *Allergy.* (2012) 67:1465–74. doi: 10.1111/all.12030
16. Mistry P, Carmona-Rivera C, Ombrello AK, Hoffmann P, Seto NL, Jones A, et al. Dysregulated neutrophil responses and neutrophil extracellular trap formation and degradation in PAPA syndrome. *Ann Rheum Dis.* (2018) 77:1825–33. doi: 10.1136/annrheumdis-2018-213746
17. Maalouf D, Battistella M, Bouaziz JD. Neutrophilic dermatosis: disease mechanism and treatment. *Curr Opin Hematol.* (2015) 22:23–9. doi: 10.1097/MOH.0000000000000100
18. Kahlenberg JM, Carmona-Rivera C, Smith CK, Kaplan MJ. Neutrophil extracellular trap-associated protein activation of the NLRP3 inflammasome is enhanced in lupus macrophages. *J Immunol.* (2013) 190:1217–26. doi: 10.4049/jimmunol.1202388
19. Li Y, Li N, Yan Z, Li H, Chen L, Zhang Z, et al. Dysregulation of the NLRP3 inflammasome complex and related cytokines in patients with multiple myeloma. *Hematology.* (2016) 21:144–51. doi: 10.1179/1607845415Y.0000000029
20. Pizzirani C, Falzoni S, Govoni M, La Corte R, Donadei S, Di Virgilio F, et al. Dysfunctional inflammasome in Schnitzler's syndrome. *Rheumatology.* (2009) 48:1304–8. doi: 10.1093/rheumatology/kep222
21. Joshi MB, Lad A, Bharath Prasad AS, Balakrishnan A, Ramachandra L, Satyamoorthy K. High glucose modulates IL-6 mediated immune homeostasis through impeding neutrophil extracellular trap formation. *FEBS Lett.* (2013)587:2241–6. doi: 10.1016/j.febslet.2013.05.053
22. Khandpur R, Carmona-Rivera C, Vivekanandan-Giri A, Gizinski A, Yalavarthi S, Knight JS, et al. NETs are a source of citrullinated autoantigens and stimulate inflammatory responses in rheumatoid arthritis. *Sci Transl Med.* (2013) 5:178ra40. doi: 10.1126/scitranslmed.3005580

12

Systemic Lupus Erythematosus and DNA Degradation and Elimination Defects

*Borros Arneth**

Institute of Laboratory Medicine and Pathobiochemistry, Molecular Diagnostics, University Hospital of Giessen and Marburg, Justus Liebig University Giessen, Giessen, Germany

Correspondence:
Borros Arneth
borros.arneth@klinchemie.med.uni-giessen.de

Introduction: Systemic lupus erythematosus (SLE) is a chronic autoimmune disease that is characterized by the production of autoantibodies specific for components of the cell nucleus and that causes damage to body tissues and organs. The pathogenesis of SLE remains unclear, with numerous studies pointing to a combination of genetic and environmental factors. A critical stage in SLE development is cell necrosis, in which undegraded chromatin and nucleoproteins are released into the blood, resulting in circulating cell-free DNA and serum nucleoproteins that trigger anti-dsDNA autoantibody production. This systematic literature review aimed to examine whether SLE stems from a DNA degradation and elimination defect.

Materials and Methods: An advanced literature search was conducted in PubMed using the following keywords: [("SLE" OR "Systemic Lupus Erythematosus" OR "Lupus")] AND [("DNA" OR "DNA Degradation")] AND [("Defect Elimination")]. More articles were obtained from the references of the identified articles and basic Google searches. Twenty-five peer-reviewed articles published within the past 10 years (2007–2018) were included for review.

Results: The findings of each study are summarized in **Tables 1**, **2**.

Discussion and Conclusion: The etiopathogenesis of SLE remains controversial, which limits therapeutic inventions for this disease. However, SLE is a DNA degradation and elimination disorder caused by uncleared histones and nuclear material that leak into the extracellular space and form cell-free DNA, triggering an immune response that destroys tissues and organs. Under normal conditions, apoptosis allows DNA and other nuclear material to be efficiently cleared through degradation and additional complex mechanisms such that this material does not trigger the immune system to produce nuclear autoantibodies.

Keywords: SLE, DNA-degradation, DNA-elimination, SLE-Systemic Lupus Nephritis, DNA-anti DNA

INTRODUCTION

Systemic lupus erythematosus (SLE) is an autoimmune disorder characterized by the production of antinuclear antibodies (ANAs) specific for nuclear antigens originating from uncleared apoptotic cells. The disease affects several organs of the body. Globally, ~5 million people suffer from SLE, which has no cure to date (1). Evidence from previous studies shows that environmentally induced defects and genetic abnormalities in immune cells, mutations in regulatory components involved in cellular apoptosis and defects in mechanisms of cellular debris clearance are key contributors to SLE pathogenesis (2). More precise evidence from genome-wide studies shows that SLE patients have mutations in the three prime repair exonuclease 1 (TREX1), autophagy-related 5 (ATG5), RAD518, and deoxyribonuclease I (DNASE1) genes, which are involved in the degradation of DNA, cell apoptosis and the elimination of cellular debris (3).

Abnormalities in cell death processes have been implicated in the production of nuclear autoantigens, which result in a systemic autoimmune response if imperfectly cleared. This effect has been observed in SLE and many other chronic inflammatory diseases (4). These cell death processes include apoptosis, necrosis (primary and secondary), NETosis (a neutrophil-specific type of cell death), autophagy, necroptosis, and pyroptosis (5). Through a complex series of events, the production of autoantigens stimulates the immune system to produce autoantibodies that combine with uncleared cellular debris in the blood or tissues, leading to the formation of immune complexes (ICs). When dendritic cells, macrophages, and phagocytes clear ICs from the blood, proinflammatory cytokines are secreted, which subsequently leads to inflammation (4). The continued production of antibodies due to uncleared tissue debris in the blood and tissues results in perpetual inflammation and tissue damage, a characteristic of SLE (4).

Mitochondria hyperpolarization, ROS production, lysosomal membrane disintegration, organelle and cellular swelling, and plasma membrane rupture characterize necrotic cell death, which is often regarded as inflammatory since the loss of plasma membrane integrity stimulates the release of autoantigens and damage-associated molecular patterns (DAMPs), which act as chemoattractants for inflammatory cells (5).

Conversely, deoxyribonucleic acid (DNA) is an essential molecule for life; it carries hereditary information and is necessary for all organisms (6). Various events can trigger the degradation of DNA into nucleotides by DNase. Apoptosis is a classic example of such an event. This process has been well-known for years, but recent developments show that improper DNA degradation can result in various diseases, such as autoinflammation, cancer, and cataracts (7). SLE is characterized by the production of ANAs, which are autoantibodies specific for a variety of nuclear autoantigens. Anti-dsDNA autoantibodies are among the ANAs used to diagnose SLE (8). Normally, dsDNA is present in the nucleus and mitochondria, where it is shielded from recognition by the immune system. DNase I destroys DNA in the extracellular space, whereas DNAse II and III degrade endosomal and cytoplasmic DNA. Defective cell apoptosis, NETosis, and elimination processes result in elevated levels of cell-free dsDNA (cfDNA) in SLE patients (8). Therefore, understanding the complex pathways and processes involved in the formation of autoantigens and autoantibodies can help in the diagnosis and treatment of various diseases, such as cancer and SLE. Furthermore, these defects can be prevented effectively if proper DNA degradation is facilitated through extrinsic factors, such as drugs. In this paper, we review the connection between SLE and defective DNA degradation.

MATERIALS AND METHODS

An advanced literature search was conducted to retrieve the most relevant articles from the evidence base. Additional methods of identifying relevant literature were also employed, including looking up sources in the reference lists of other research reports, manual searching of relevant journals, and searching by author.

The advanced search was done using PubMed only because PubMed features top resources in chemicals and bioassays, DNA and RNA, and genes and expression, among other topics. Boolean connectors ("AND" and "OR") were used to connect keywords in the search boxes of PubMed. The following search terms were used: [("SLE" OR "Systemic Lupus Erythematosus" OR "Lupus")] AND [("DNA" OR "DNA Degradation")] AND [("Defect Elimination")]. When the search terms were applied, 2,728 results were retrieved, including 1,047 articles published within the last 10 years. Only articles with free full texts were selected (490 articles). After screening the relevance of these articles using the titles, 42 articles were selected. The selected articles were then emailed to the researcher directly from PubMed, and their abstracts were further screened for relevance; 23 articles were retrieved and included in this review.

However, before implementing the advanced search strategy, a basic Google search was conducted as a prescreen search, which yielded 144,000 results when the following keywords were used: "Systemic Lupus Erythematosus," "SLE," "DNA degradation," and "Defect elimination." Four articles were retrieved, of which two were excluded; one of the excluded articles discussed how circulating free DNA may signal SLE severity and be used to monitor therapy (9), and the other article was excluded because it was outdated despite being relevant (10). Regarding the articles that were retrieved and included, one was about the relationship between the presence of SLE and the failure of DNA degradation (11), whereas the other was about the important role of neutrophil extracellular traps (NETs) in SLE (12). Therefore, 25 articles were included in this review.

Abbreviations: ANAs, Antinuclear antibodies; ATG5, Autophagy related 5; BAF, Barrier-to-autointegration factor; CD3Z, Cluster of differentiation 3Z; CD40, Cluster of differentiation 40; CD40L, Cluster of differentiation 40 ligand (CD40L); cfDNA, Circulating free DNA; DAMPs, Damage associated molecular patterns; DNA, Deoxyribonucleic acid; DNASE II, Deoxyribonuclease II; DNASE III, Deoxyribonuclease III; DNASE I, Deoxyribonuclease I; DNMT1, DNA methyltransferase 1; DNMT3B, DNA methyltransferase 3 beta; DUSP23, Dual-specificity protein phosphatase 23; Gfi1, Growth factor independence 1; ICF, Immunodeficiency-centromeric instability-facial anomalies; ICs, Immune complexes; IFN-γ, Interferon gamma; IRF5, Interferon regulatory factor 5; MHC, Major histocompatibility complex; MMF, Mycophenolate mofetil; mtDNA, Mitochondrial DNA; NETs, Neutrophil extracellular traps; NIC, NF-κB-inducing kinase; NK, Natural killer; PDCs, Plasmacytoid dendritic cells; RNA, Ribonucleic acid; RVCL, Retinal vasculopathy with cerebral leukodystrophy; SLE, Systemic lupus erythematosus; SNP, Single-nucleotide polymorphism; STAT, Signal transducer and activator of transcription; STING, Stimulator of interferon genes; TLR, Toll-like receptor; TNFRSF, Tumor necrosis factor receptor superfamily; TNF-α, Tumor necrosis factor alpha; TREX1, Three prime repair exonuclease 1.

TABLE 1 | Retrieved articles selected for review.

References	Year of publication
Hendy et al. (9)	2016
Leffler (11)	2015
Wang et al. (12)	2015
Zhang et al. (13)	2014
Garcia-Romo et al. (14)	2011
Brightbill et al. (15)	2017
Niu et al. (16)	2017
Balada et al. (17)	2017
Nawrocki et al. (18)	2017
Yang et al. (19)	2015
Huang et al. (20)	2016
Gupta et al. (21)	2016
Hong et al. (22)	2017
Shu et al. (23)	2017
Zhu et al. (24)	2016
Sisirak et al. (25)	2016
Panza et al. (26)	2016
Yeung et al. (27)	2017
Steri et al. (28)	2017
Reddy et al. (29)	2017
Virdis et al. (30)	2015
Ikeda et al. (31)	2017
Li et al. (32)	2017
Sakai et al. (33)	2017
Stearns et al. (34)	2016

RESULTS

Twenty-five articles were retrieved for review by using the above search strategy (see **Table 1**). **Figure 1** shows a PRISMA diagram of the search strategy described above.

Findings

This subsection will summarize the findings of each study; the findings will then be coded and categorized in the Discussion section. **Tables 1, 2** summarize the retrieved studies considered in the discussion.

Several studies have been conducted in this field, with the most recent study reporting that NF-κB-inducing kinase (NIK) inhibition can improve outcomes in patients with SLE (35). Much remains unknown about SLE, and more studies are needed to explore more accurate and reliable ways of diagnosing and treating SLE. The following section of this paper will discuss these findings in the context of whether SLE is a DNA degradation defect.

DISCUSSION

Defective Cell Death and cfDNA

Programmed cell death, termed apoptosis, is essential for homeostasis during both development and aging. Under normal conditions, apoptotic cells are engulfed into lysosomes within phagocytes and destroyed; this process occurs without inflammation (36). Many studies have maintained that SLE originates from the defective clearance of apoptotic remnants and NETs from the circulation and tissues (37–41). Thus, there is a consensus that SLE begins to develop when the clearance of dying cells is impaired. The clearance of cellular debris involves many ligands and receptors, and there must be sufficient bridging molecules between phagocytes and dying cells (42). This process is closely controlled and very intricate, but some studies have elucidated the details (43–45). Understanding this complex process has therapeutic potential, mainly in the timely prevention of SLE (45). Dying cells that are not quickly and efficiently removed go through secondary necrosis and subsequently burst, releasing nuclear material upon loss of an intact cell membrane (44).

The impaired clearance of apoptotic cells in SLE is due to their failed recognition by phagocytes because (a) the phagocytes are smaller (4), (b) the phagocytes have diminished and delayed phagocytic activity (46), (c) the phagocytes have reduced adherence (47), or (d) the differentiation of phagocytes from CD34-positive hematopoietic stem cells is reduced (48–50). Therefore, professional and non-professional phagocytes in patients with SLE have reduced phagocytic activity and are thus unable to clear NETs, and apoptosis remains incomplete (51).

During NETosis, NETs are generated by neutrophils upon pathogen stimulation to kill invading pathogens (40, 44). Cellular and nuclear components, including dsDNA, histones, neutrophil elastase, and myeloperoxidase, are released during NETosis. Proinflammatory components, including tumor necrosis factor (TNF)-α, interleukin (IL)-17, IL-8, and interferon (IFN)-γ, also trigger the production of NETs (13). Additionally, low-density granulocytes among peripheral blood mononuclear cells in SLE patients have been shown to form NETs (13). The formed NETs are normally degraded by DNase I, which hydrolyzes dsDNA through its endonuclease activity, thus breaking down chromatin during apoptosis (13).

Incomplete degradation of NETs by DNase I results in the accumulation of the remaining NETs, which react with other proteins to form complexes that are involved in autoimmune SLE (9, 12–14, 35). Elevated levels of undegraded residual NETs are the major source of serum dsDNA, also called circulating cfDNA, in SLE patients (51). The clearance of NETs entirely depends on an efficient and active DNase I enzyme. Defective DNase I leads to undegraded chromatin, which is positively related to SLE disease activity (9, 12, 51). The presence of mitochondrial DNA (mtDNA) in NETs and its positive correlation with plasmacytoid dendritic cells (PDCs) and type 1 IFN-α imply that SLE is a disorder of defective DNA clearance. Studies have shown that NETs in SLE patients activate PDCs and the IFN pathway, triggering the production of autoantigens (14). Therefore, defective DNA degradation leads to defective chromatin breakdown and is thus etiopathogenically involved in SLE development.

NIK usually engages non-canonical NF-κB to signal downstream of several TNF family members, including TWEAK, BAF, OX40, and CD40, which are involved in SLE pathogenesis (15). In addition to type I IFN and Toll-like receptor (TLR), numerous members of the TNF receptor superfamily (TNFRSF) are involved in SLE pathophysiology. CD40 and B cell-activating

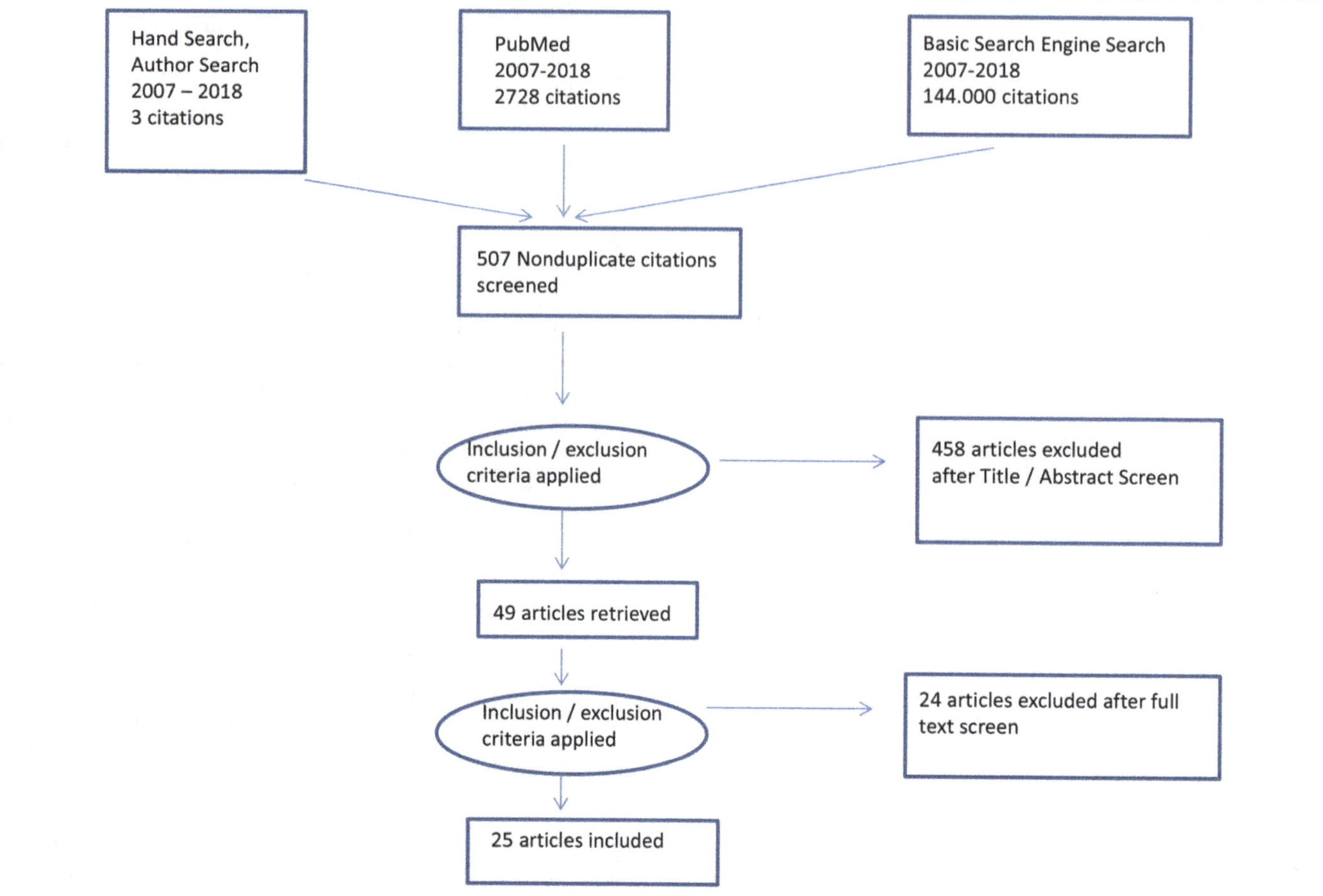

FIGURE 1 | PRISMA diagram of the search strategy.

factor (BAFF) are essential for B cell survival and differentiation into autoantibody-generating plasma cells. CD40 ligand (CD40L) blockade showed promise in initial clinical trials of lupus, although therapeutic development was halted because of thrombotic side effects. In contrast, blockade of BAFF via belimumab is moderately effective and is currently the only new approved treatment for lupus (15).

T Cell Activation and Defective DNA Degradation

Autoantigens that trigger the production of autoantibodies in SLE originate from cell death by apoptosis and NETosis. Dying cells usually undergo morphological changes, such as DNA fragmentation, shrinking, and blebbing of the plasma membrane; the nuclear autoantigens that are targeted in SLE are usually stored in these plasma membrane blebs (52). On the other hand, NETosis results in rupture of the plasma membrane, releasing the nuclear autoantigens that are targeted in SLE (53). These autoantigens resulting from apoptosis and NETosis trigger the production of antibodies that bind uncleared apoptotic material to form ICs. The mechanism through which these autoantibodies are produced is well-documented; T cells trigger B cells to differentiate, proliferate, and finally mature. Then, the T cells stimulate class switching of B cells to produce different classes of autoantibodies (16, 54). Due to alterations in T cells that modulate the production of autoantibodies specific for lupus autoantigens by B cells, lupus T cells have been categorized as abnormal (54).

Lupus has also been shown to be associated with reduced expression of DNA cytosine-5-methyltransferases, which have hypomethylation activity that might be responsible for the production of autoreactive antibodies. **Figure 2** gives an overview about the most important key-elements in the pathophysiology involved in systemic lupus erythematosus.

DNA methylation is essential for marking chromatin accessibility and regulating gene expression (55). DNA methylation involves the addition of a methyl group at the 5th carbon of cytosine residues in CG dinucleotides, and this process is usually involved in cell differentiation, X-chromosome inactivation, imprinting, and the suppression of transcriptional noise and parasitic DNA. Abnormalities in DNA methylation pathways have pathological consequences. For example, *de novo* mutation of the DNA methyltransferase DNMT3B leads to immunodeficiency-centromeric instability-facial anomalies syndrome (ICF syndrome). Complete DNMT1 deficiency is incompatible with life. Moreover, acquired defects in DNA

TABLE 2 | Findings from each study.

References	Findings
Hendy et al. (9)	SLE patients have elevated levels of serum circulating cfDNA compared to healthy individuals. The elevated levels of serum dsDNA in SLE patients correlate with disease activity (9).
Leffler et al. (11)	Serum from SLE patients exhibits a very limited ability to degrade DNA from NETs and primary and secondary necrotic cells (11).
Wang H et al. (12)	mtDNA was detected in NETs, and elevated levels of anti-mtDNA antibodies were detected in serum from SLE patients. High levels of mtDNA in NETs and serum anti-mtDNA antibodies correlate with PDCs and type 1 IFN-α (12).
Zhang et al. (13)	SLE patients have very high serum levels of circulating cfDNA, which positively correlate with lupus nephritis (LN) activity. Further analysis showed that SLE patients with high levels of low-density granulocytes in peripheral blood mononuclear cells have high serum cfDNA levels and severe disease. This finding was attributed to lower DNase 1 activity in SLE patients than in healthy individuals (13).
Garcia-Romo et al. (14)	IFN-α stimulates neutrophils in SLE patients to form NETs in the presence of anti-ribonucleoprotein (RNP) antibodies. The formed NETs contain non-engulfed chromatin that facilitates DNA uptake by PDCs. NETs are the source of the elevated cfDNA levels in SLE patients (14).
Brightbill et al. (15)	Selective inhibition of NF-κB-inducing kinase (NIK) leads to improved survival of SLE mice *in vivo*. NIK mediates the activation of TNF proteins that have been implicated in SLE pathogenesis (15).
Niu et al. (16)	PBX1 has a direct regulatory effect on genes associated with T cell activation, and the PBX1-d isoform is associated with lupus. PBX1–d lacks a DNA-binding domain, and its expression in SLE patients leads to the production of autoreactive CD4+ T cells (16).
Balada et al. (17)	DUSP23 is overexpressed in SLE, which is linked to the expression of DNA methyltransferases (DNMTs) in CD4+ T cells (17).
Nawrocki et al. (18)	SLE is associated with decreased DNA methyltransferase mRNA expression levels (18).
Yang et al. (19)	Severe nephropathy in SLE can be indicated by IgG and concurrent reactivity to anti-dsDNA, anti-nucleosome, and anti-histone antibodies (19).
Huang et al. (20)	T cell vaccination helps improve and regulate the manifestations of SLE (20).
Gupta et al. (21)	Anti-IFN-γ autoantibodies are linked to aggressive SLE (21).
Hong et al. (22)	The hypermethylation of CD3Z is linked to severe clinical manifestations of SLE. CD3Z and VHL hypermethylation is associated with SLE. CD3Z hypermethylation is potentially an environmentally induced epigenetic modification (22).
Shu et al. (23)	Histone deacetylase inhibitors (HDACi), such as trichostatin (TSA), repress IRF5 and hence have therapeutic potential in patients with SLE. TSA-mediated inhibition of IRF5 binding to RNA polymerase II, HDAC3, DNA Sp1, and p300 in children with SLE suggests that SLE is associated with DNA degradation abnormalities and elimination defects (23).
Zhu et al. (24)	Several differentially expressed genes in SLE are involved in the IFN and TLR signaling pathways. The presence of hypomethylated upregulated genes and hypermethylated downregulated genes in SLE patients indicates that DNA methylation plays a role in SLE development (24).
Sisirak et al. (25)	The tolerance mechanism for SLE is marked by the digestion of chromatin in microparticles from dying cells. Mice and patients without the DNASE1L3 enzyme produce anti-dsDNA antibodies specific for serum dsDNA; hence, defective DNA degradation is associated with SLE (25).
Panza et al. (26)	PK201/CAT plasmid (PK) DNA and histone 4 (H4) assays are reliable for the differential diagnosis of SLE. Anti-PK/H4 antigens correlate with the level of SLE disease activity, suggesting a DNA damage defect in this disease (26).
Yeung et al. (27)	Unfractionated white blood cells can be used to indicate abnormal DNA methylation in SLE (27).
Steri et al. (28)	A variant of TNFSF13B is associated with SLE. Serum TNFSF13B correlates with serum dsDNA autoantigens in patients with SLE (28).
Reddy et al. (29)	Lower baseline serum IgM levels and sequential therapy with mycophenolate mofetil can predict IgM hypogammaglobulinemia after rituximab treatment in patients with SLE. No significant change in anti-dsDNA antibodies was observed in patients with initially higher levels, even after treatment. This finding suggests that high SLE disease activity is associated with dsDNA autoantigens in serum (29).
Virdis et al. (30)	Early treatment with hydroxychloroquine can curb the development of endothelial dysfunction in SLE patients (30).
Ikeda et al. (31)	The increase in anti-dsDNA antibodies in mice with higher SLE disease activity suggests that abnormal DNA degradation occurs in SLE (31).
Li et al. (32)	Aconitine can inhibit disease evolution and improve pathologic lesions in SLE. Elevated levels of dsDNA, ANAs, and proliferating cell nuclear antigen in mice with SLE before therapy show that SLE is characterized by defective DNA degradation and abnormal elimination of cellular debris. Aconitine therapy significantly reduced dsDNA autoantigens in serum and improved quality of life, indicating that defective DNA degradation is associated with SLE (32).
Sakai et al. (33)	OST inhibition can suppress autoantibody production in mice with SLE. Mutations in TREX1, such as D272fs, result in an inactive DNase in mice with SLE (33).
Stearns et al. (34)	The use of poly-L-lysine as a capture agent enhances the detection of SLE autoantibodies by ELISA. The detection of dsDNA, histones, RNP, SSA, and SSB antigens in serum from SLE patients using this assay showed that SLE is associated with abnormal DNA damage and elimination (34).

methylation are related to diseases, including autoimmunity and cancer (55).

DNA methylation is principally a transcriptionally repressive epigenetic mark that renders chromatin inaccessible and promotes gene silencing through transcriptional repression; these events occur through different mechanisms, including the recruitment of methylcytosine binding domain-containing proteins that successively recruit histone deacetylases, which promote chromatin condensation (55).

Pbx1 is a member of the TALE family of homeodomain-containing transcription factors that regulates the DNA binding of Hox proteins. Pbx1 plays an essential role during organogenesis and development by integrating several signals via interactions with various partners, including Prep1 TALE

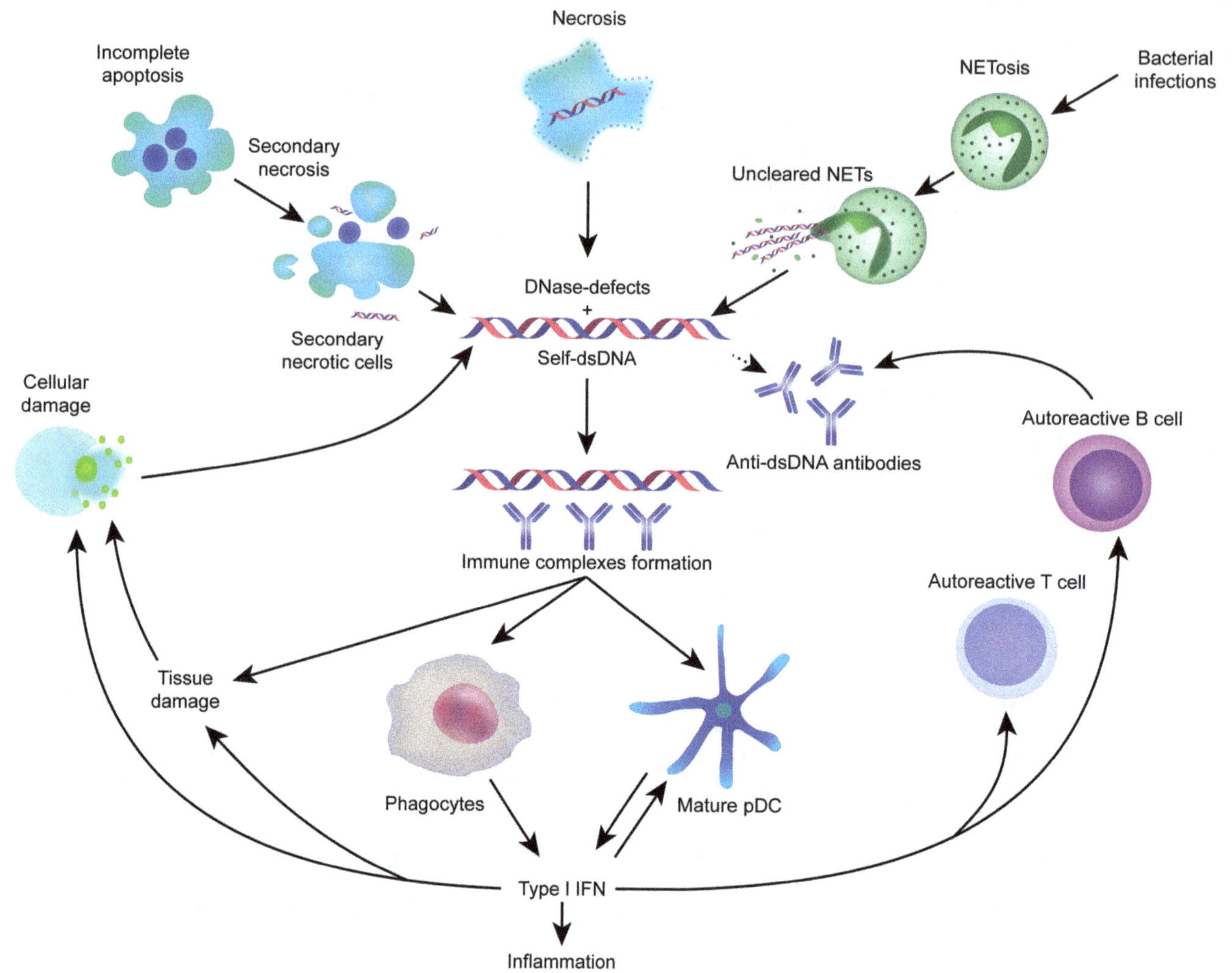

FIGURE 2 | Self-dsDNA released during cell death plays an important role in the pathogenesis of SLE.

proteins and Meis, that control chromatin remodeling and co-activator access. During immune system development, Pbx1 is vital for maintaining hematopoietic stem cell self-renewal and limiting myeloid maturation to preserve the differentiation ability of lymphoid progenitors. The absence of Pbx1 in embryonic stem cells leads to the failure to produce common lymphoid progenitors, the absence of NK and B cells, and the development of impaired T cells (16). In addition, Pbx1 regulates chromatin accessibility to various genes and is conserved between humans and mice. The Pbx1-d dominant-negative isoform is more commonly expressed in CD4$^+$ T cells from lupus patients than in those from healthy controls. Pbx1-d is related to autoreactive T cell production in mice with the Sle1a1 lupus vulnerability locus (56).

Dual-specificity protein phosphatase 23 (DUSP23) activates the IFN and IL pathways via dephosphorylation (17), and these pathways are responsible for the formation of NETs, which are sources of cfDNA (17, 18, 57). DUSP3, DUSP22, and VH1 participate in both the IL and IFN signaling pathways mainly by dephosphorylating signal transducer and activator of transcription (STAT) proteins (37, 38). High IFN-α activity is frequently detected in sera from SLE patients (39). Moreover, patients with SLE exhibit a particular mRNA expression profile of IFN-dependent genes in leucocytes known as the IFN signature (17, 40, 41).

The presence of hypomethylated DNA in SLE patients implies that the DNA will not be degraded; hence, SLE is a defective DNA degradation disorder. Additionally, simultaneously high levels of anti-dsDNA, anti-nucleosome, and anti-histone antibodies in serum suggest that defective DNA degradation marks the genesis of SLE (19) and can indicate severe nephropathy in SLE. In summary, these findings improve our understanding of the role of T cells in SLE (20). During SLE pathogenesis, autoreactive T cells trigger the differentiation, proliferation, and maturation of B cells, thus supporting the formation of autoantibodies. Moreover, attenuating T cells normally alleviates the manifestations of autoimmune diseases, such as clearing pathogenic autoreactive T cells in SLE.

Interferons and Defective DNA Degradation

The presence of pathogens, including lupus autoantigens, stimulates host cells to make and release a group of signaling proteins (cytokines) called IFNs through complex processes. There are three types of IFNs, namely, alpha, beta, and gamma IFNs. Gamma IFNs are known for the expansion of macrophages and inducing the class II major histocompatibility complex (MHC). Anti-IFN-γ autoantibodies are associated with amplified disease activity in patients with SLE (21). IFN-γ is commonly referred to as a type II IFN, whereas IFN-α and IFN-β are referred to as type I IFNs, a subtype of cytokines that help regulate the immune system.

Type I IFNs generated during a viral infection trigger the production of MCP-1, which is responsible for inducing the migration of inflammatory monocytes to the inflammation site. After recruitment, inflammatory monocytes are triggered by type I IFNs to generate IL-18, which then signals via IL-18R expressed by NK cells to induce the production of IFN-γ.

Abundant autoantibody production and IC formation cause tissue damage; hence, SLE is regarded as a B cell disorder. Conversely, the significance of helper T cells in inducing B cell immunity was identified based on defective CD3ζ function or expression. Reduced CD3ζ-chain expression has been identified in cancer patients and those with autoimmune illnesses. In contrast, decreased CD3ζ-chain levels are maintained during the course of SLE in most patients (22).

Moreover, IFN regulatory factor 5 (IRF5) plays a crucial role in the stimulation of type I IFNs, TNF-α, and the proinflammatory cytokines IL-6 and IL-12. It is also involved in adaptive and innate immunity. The first identified single-nucleotide polymorphism (SNP) in IRF5, Rs2004640, is closely related to the high expression of several IRF5 isoforms and is a valuable genetic risk factor for SLE (23).

Gene expression studies have identified hypomethylated upregulated genes and hypermethylated downregulated genes in SLE patients, indicating that DNA methylation plays a role in SLE development (24). Differentially expressed genes (differential gene co-expression) in SLE are involved in the IFN and TLR signaling pathways (24). The transcriptional repressor growth factor independence 1 (Gfi1) plays a critical role in myeloid cell regulation, as well as in the prevention of unprompted lupus autoimmunity, mainly by negatively regulating TLR7 signaling (58).

Before therapy with Gfi1, SLE mice showed high levels of serum autoantibodies specific for DNA and RNA, which are indicative of defective nucleic acid degradation in SLE. Hence, IFNs are involved in the etiopathogenesis of SLE by stimulating the formation of NETs, the main sources of cfDNA, and exploring their mechanisms of involvement has therapeutic potential (58).

The Role of DNA Degradation in SLE

Suurmond et al. (59) maintained that studying genetic risk alleles can improve our understanding of failed tolerance mechanisms for DNA-reactive B cells and B cell alterations in SLE. Understanding the complexity of interactions between immune disturbance in SLE and epigenetic mechanisms is a potential way to explore new therapeutic targets (60). In particular, the digestion of chromatin in apoptotic cell microparticles (25) marks a tolerance mechanism for SLE. The absence of DNASE1L3, a DNA degrading enzyme, results in the production of anti-dsDNA antibodies specific for serum dsDNA; hence, defective DNA degradation is associated with SLE (25). When this process reaches a point at which autoantibodies are produced because of defective clearance of NETs and apoptotic remnants, the person is said to have global loss of self-tolerance (25). This is the point at which impaired DNA degradation plays a role in the etiopathogenesis of SLE.

Nuclear autoantigens (e.g., antigens specific for DNA and histones) (61) and proteins from the cytoplasm of neutrophils (62) play a role in the etiopathogenesis of SLE when cellular material containing these components leaks to the extracellular space through apoptosis or NETosis, hence exposing these factors to the immune system. Histones, which are a group of chromatin proteins that are abundant in NETs and apoptotic blebs, are modified through various processes, such as methylation (63), acetylation (64), ubiquitination (65), and poly-ADP ribosylation (66), during apoptosis, and NETosis. When modified histones are exposed to the immune system in the extracellular space, they are recognized as foreign and dangerous by receptors of the innate immune system, such as TLRs. Therefore, the H4/PK assay is usually a reliable and simple test that is valuable for the differential diagnosis and evaluation of symptomatic activity in SLE patients (26).

On the other hand, DNA methylation, an epigenetic mechanism for controlling gene expression (67), plays a significant role in the etiopathogenesis of SLE. Abnormal DNA methylation in immune-related cells is associated with SLE and can be detected in unfractionated white blood cells, which has diagnostic implications (27). This abnormal DNA methylation in immune-related cells involves altered DNA methylation of cytokine genes, which makes the chromatin inaccessible for destruction (60).

Moreover, SLE is associated with decreased DNA methyltransferase mRNA expression levels (18), which is the exact mechanism through which abnormal DNA methylation occurs in immune-related cells. Therefore, DNA hypomethylation of immune-related cells plays a key role in the etiopathogenesis of SLE; however, little is known about hypermethylation in SLE.

Only one study examined the role of CD3Z (a T cell surface glycoprotein and component of the T cell antigen receptor) hypermethylation in SLE, and it was determined that this modification is a potential risk factor associated with severe SLE manifestations (28).

Hypermethylation of CD3Z could be an environmentally induced epigenetic modification (22). In particular, CD3Z hypermethylation could provide an important mechanism for CD3ζ-chain downregulation in SLE T cells. Furthermore, CD3Z DNA hypermethylation was connected to more severe clinical signs in persons with SLE; thus, CD3Z hypermethylation is a marker of disease severity (22).

Other Factors Related to Defective DNA Degradation

Many other factors have recently been associated with the etiopathogenesis, diagnosis, and treatment of SLE. There is extensive evidence for the association of IFNs and ILs with SLE; however, little is known about the role of TNFs (additional cytokines) in the etiopathogenesis of SLE. Variants of TNF ligand superfamily member 13B (TNFSF13B) are associated with defective DNA degradation in SLE disease development. Elevated serum levels of TNFSF13B correlate with serum dsDNA antigen levels, suggesting that TNF is associated with abnormal DNA degradation in SLE patients (28).

Moreover, recent studies have shown that some types of drugs can treat or contribute to the etiopathogenesis of SLE. Rituximab, which has proved efficacious in the treatment of diffuse alveolar hemorrhage in SLE, can cause IgM hypogammaglobulinemia, which can be predicted by lower baseline serum IgM levels and sequential therapy with mycophenolate mofetil (MMF) (29). This finding shows that high SLE disease activity is associated with dsDNA antigens in serum, suggesting defective DNA degradation. Early treatment with hydroxychloroquine can curb the development of endothelial dysfunction in SLE patients (30). Bortezomib, an anticancer drug, increases proinflammatory cytokine levels in mice, hence worsening SLE (31). Aconitine, a C19 norditerpenoid alkaloid, can inhibit disease progression and ameliorate pathologic lesions of SLE (32). This alkaloid, which is the key active component of *Aconitum*, has immunomodulatory properties and may be valuable for treating autoimmune diseases such as SLE (32).

TREX1 frame-shift mutations, such as V235fs and D272fs, trigger autoantibodies chiefly against non-nuclear antigens. Thus, patients who have such mutations are possibly ANA negative. High serum ANA levels are very rare among patients who have retinal vasculopathy with cerebral leukodystrophy (RVCL). Thus, diseases associated with such mutations may be under- or misdiagnosed. The oligosaccharyltransferase (OST) inhibitor aclacinomycin effectively suppressed the production of autoantibodies, confirming the possible therapeutic value of such medicines for treating phenotypes associated with the V235fs mutation. Moreover, the D272fs and V235fs mutations usually affect the DNase-independent roles of TREX1 and trigger serologic autoimmunity, which likely contributes to the development of autoimmune disease (33, 34).

In addition, IFN-α expression is positively related to IRF5 expression. Childhood-onset SLE normally follows a more aggressive course, with higher mortality and morbidity and a greater occurrence of serological and immunological abnormalities, than does adult-onset SLE, perhaps implicating dissimilar mechanisms in both clusters. Nonetheless, IRF5 plays an important role in childhood-onset SLE pathogenesis. Sp1 can increase IRF5 promoter activity and mRNA expression. Sp1 expression is increased in childhood-onset SLE and is positively related to IRF5 levels; thus, high Sp1 expression might contribute to high IRF5 levels, and the subsequent high IFN-α levels are a fundamental feature of SLE pathology (68).

DNase Defects Have Been Correlated to Lupus Erythematosus

DNase I, an endonuclease, is usually secreted to cleave extracellular DNA to tetranucleotides with 3′ hydroxyl DNA ends and 5′ monophosphate (68). Moreover, during apoptosis, DNase I is the specific endonuclease that facilitates chromatin breakdown. Together with the plasminogen system, DNase I enables prompt and efficient chromatin breakdown through the instantaneous degradation of DNA and DNA-binding proteins (68).

DNase I mutations have been associated with a familiar form of SLE (69).

DNase II is vital for self-dsDNA clearance in lysosomes to circumvent an immune response. Moreover, DNase II knockout is usually embryonically lethal in mice due to uncontrolled inflammation, whereas cGAS deletion in DNase II-deficient mice salvages this lethal phenotype. DNASEII defects are associated with autoinflammtion, but however have so far not been linked to the classical lupus phenotype.

TREX1, also known as **DNase III**, is a DNA exonuclease that engages in cytoplasmic dsDNA and ssDNA clearance. Loss-of-function mutations of TREX1 result in the accumulation of self-DNA and autoimmune diseases, such as SLE. **Mutations in DNase III/TREX1** have also been associated with a familiar form of lupus erythematosus (70–72).

TREX1-deficient mice display markedly reduced survival due to unprompted inflammatory myocarditis, increased circulatory failure and cardiomyopathy Trex1 prevents the cell-intrinsic initiation of autoimmunity in the mice model of TREX1-deficient mice (73–76).

Depletion of **STING**, IRF3, cGAS, or IFN-I receptor in TREX1-deficient mice protects against autoimmune disorders and death, indicating that cGAS–STING–IRF3 axis-regulated IFN-I production is responsible for autoimmune disorder development in TREX1-deficient mice. Nevertheless, in STING-deficient lupus mice, serum cytokine levels, autoantibody production, and lymphoid hypertrophy increase significantly in comparison to STING-adequate littermates.

Mutations leading to STING activation cause autoinflammation and can lead to an inflammatory vascular and pulmonary syndrome (77) and has also been linked to a familiar form of lupus erythematosus (78, 79).

But on the other hand STING deficiency can also lead to autoimmunity mediated by enhanced TLR activation in lupus prone mice (80). In this case STING potently suppresses inflammation in a model of SLE. This controversial behavior points out the complexity of regulation and is important to be considered for the development of targeted therapies directed against STING.

ANAs are considered the serological characteristic of SLE. These antibodies often bind various nuclear antigens, including DNA, histones, non-histone proteins and protein complexes with RNA and DNA. Due to the frequent manifestation of ANA abnormalities in SLE, ANA analysis is a vital element of clinical assessments and determinations of suitability for clinical tests or the use of particular therapies (34).

DNase I, an endonuclease, is usually secreted to cleave extracellular DNA to tetranucleotides with 3′ hydroxyl DNA ends and 5′ monophosphate (68). Moreover, during apoptosis, DNase I is the specific endonuclease that facilitates chromatin breakdown. Together with the plasminogen system, DNase I enables prompt and efficient chromatin breakdown by the instantaneous degradation of DNA and DNA-binding proteins (68).

Self-dsDNA is involved in SLE pathogenesis; these molecules are normally cleared in apoptosis, necrosis and NETs, but these processes are defective in SLE patients, thereby triggering the production of autoantibodies through unknown mechanisms. In addition, anti-dsDNA antibodies are formed by autoreactive B cells and autoreactive T cells. dsDNA ICs and autoantibodies stimulate robust IFN-I production via several intercellular DNA sensors, primarily in PDCs and phagocytes (81).

CONCLUSION

The etiopathogenesis of SLE is still controversial, and there are limited therapeutic inventions for this disease. However, this paper has demonstrated that SLE is a DNA degradation disorder. In normal apoptosis, DNA and other nucleic materials are efficiently cleared through degradation and other complex mechanisms, blocking the formation of nuclear autoantigens. Autoantibodies produced against cfDNA are responsible for tissue and organ damage in SLE patients.

AUTHOR CONTRIBUTIONS

The author confirms being the sole contributor of this work and has approved it for publication.

REFERENCES

1. Meas R, Burak M, Sweasy J. DNA repair and systemic lupus erythematosus. *DNA Repair.* (2017) 56:174–82. doi: 10.1016/j.dnarep.2017.06.020
2. Wu H, Fu S, Zhao M, Lu L, Lu Q. Dysregulation of cell death and its epigenetic mechanisms in systemic lupus erythematosus. *Molecules.* (2017) 2:30. doi: 10.3390/molecules22010030
3. Teruel M, Alarcón-Riquelme M. The genetic basis of lupus erythematosus: what are the risk factors and what we have learned. *J Autoimmun.* (2016) 74:161–75. doi: 10.1016/j.jaut.2016.08.001
4. Mahajan A, Herrmann M, Muñoz L. Clearance deficiency and cell death pathways: a model for the pathogenesis of SLE. *Front Immunol.* (2016) 7:35. doi: 10.3389/fimmu.2016.00035
5. Mistry P, Kaplan M. Cell death in the pathogenesis of systemic lupus erythematosus and lupus nephritis. *Clin Immunol.* (2016) 185:59–73. doi: 10.1016/j.clim.2016.08.010
6. Kawane K, Motani K, Nagata S. DNA degradation and its defects. *Cold Spring HarborPerspect Biol.* (2014) 6:a016394. doi: 10.1101/cshperspect.a016394
7. Jackson S, Bartek J. The DNA-damage response in human biology and disease. *Nature.* (2009) 461:1071–8. doi: 10.1038/nature08467
8. Rekvig OP. Anti-dsDNA antibodies as a classification criterion and a diagnostic markers for systemic lupus erythematosus: critical remarks. *Clin Exp Immunol.* (2015) 179:5–10. doi: 10.1111/cei.12296
9. Hendy O, Motalib T, El Shafie M, Khalaf F, Kotb S, Khalil A, et al. Circulating cell free DNA as a predictor of systemic lupus erythematosus severity and monitoring of therapy. *Egypt J Med Hum Genet.* (2016) 17:79–85. doi: 10.1016/j.ejmhg.2015.07.001
10. Lunec J, Herbert K, Blount S, Griffiths H, Emery P. 8-hydroxydeoxyguanosine: a marker of oxidative DNA damage in systemic lupus erythematosus. *FEBS Lett.* (1994) 348:131–8. doi: 10.1016/0014-5793(94)00583-4
11. Leffler J, Ciacma K, Gullstrand B, Bengtsson A, Martin M, Blom A. A subset of patients with systemic lupus erythematosus fails to degrade DNA from multiple clinically relevant sources. *Arthr Res Ther.* (2015) 17:1–10. doi: 10.1186/s13075-015-0726-y
12. Wang H, Li T, Chen S, Gu Y, Ye S. Neutrophil extracellular trap mitochondrial DNA and its autoantibody in systemic lupus erythematosus and a proof-of-concept trial of metformin. *Arthr Rheumatol.* (2015) 67:3190–200. doi: 10.1002/art.39296
13. Zhang S, Lu X, Shu X, Tian X, Yang H, Yang W, et al. Elevated plasma cfDNA may be associated with active lupus nephritis and partially attributed to abnormal regulation of neutrophil extracellular traps (NETs) in patients with systemic lupus erythematosus. *Inter Med.* (2014) 53:2763–71. doi: 10.2169/internalmedicine.53.2570
14. Garcia-Romo GS, Caielli S, Vega B, Connolly J, Allantaz F, Xu Z, et al. Netting neutrophils are major inducers of type I IFN production in pediatric systemic lupus erythematosus. *Sci Transl Med.* (2011) 3:73ra20. doi: 10.1126/scitranslmed.3001201
15. Brightbill H, Suto E, Blaquiere N, Ramamoorthi N, Sujatha-Bhaskar S, Gogol E, et al. NF-κB inducing kinase is a therapeutic target for systemic lupus erythematosus. *Nat Commun.* (2018) 9:179. doi: 10.1038/s41467-017-02672-0
16. Niu Y, Sengupta M, Titov A, Choi S, Morel L. The PBX1 lupus susceptibility gene regulates CD44 expression. *Mol Immunol.* (2017) 85:148–54. doi: 10.1016/j.molimm.2017.02.016
17. Balada E, Felip L, Ordi-Ros J, Vilardell-Tarrés M. DUSP23is over-expressed and linked to the expression ofDNMTsin CD4+T cells from systemic lupus erythematosus patients. *Clin Exp Immunol.* (2016) 187:242–50. doi: 10.1111/cei.12883
18. Nawrocki M, Majewski D, Puszczewicz M, Jagodzinski P. Decreased mRNA expression levels of DNA methyltransferases type 1 and 3A in systemic lupus erythematosus. *Rheumatol Int.* (2017) 37:775–83. doi: 10.1007/s00296-017-3711-8
19. Yang J, Xu Z, Sui M, Han J, Sun L, Jia X, et al. Co-positivity for Anti-dsDNA, -nucleosome and -histone antibodies in lupus nephritis is indicative of high serum levels and severe nephropathy. *PLoS ONE.* (2015) 10:e0140441. doi: 10.1371/journal.pone.0140441
20. Huang L, Yang Y, Kuang Y, Wei D, Li W, Yin Q, et al. The impact of T cell vaccination in alleviating and regulating systemic lupus erythematosus manifestation. *J Immunol Res.* (2016) 2016:1–9. doi: 10.1155/2016/5183686
21. Gupta S, Tatouli I, Rosen L, Hasni S, Alevizos I, Manna Z, et al. Distinct functions of autoantibodies against interferon in systemic lupus erythematosus: a comprehensive analysis of anticytokine autoantibodies in common rheumatic diseases. *Arthr Rheumatol.* (2016) 68:1677–87. doi: 10.1002/art.39607
22. Hong K, Kim H, Park S, Poojan S, Kim M, Sung J, et al. CD3Zhypermethylation is associated with severe clinical manifestations in systemic lupus erythematosus and reduces CD3ζ-chain expression in T cells. *Rheumatology.* (2016) 56:kew405. doi: 10.1093/rheumatology/kew405
23. Shu J, Li L, Zhou L, Qian J, Fan Z, Zhuang L, et al. IRF5 is elevated in childhood-onset SLE and regulated by histone acetyltransferase

and histone deacetylase inhibitors. *Oncotarget.* (2017) 8:47184–94. doi: 10.18632/oncotarget.17586

24. Zhu H, Mi W, Luo H, Chen T, Liu S, Raman I, et al. Whole-genome transcription and DNA methylation analysis of peripheral blood mononuclear cells identified aberrant gene regulation pathways in systemic lupus erythematosus. *Arthr Res Ther.* (2016) 18:162. doi: 10.1186/s13075-016-1050-x
25. Sisirak V, Sally B, D'Agati V, Martinez-Ortiz W, Özçakar Z, David J, et al. Digestion of chromatin in apoptotic cell microparticles prevents autoimmunity. *Cell.* (2016) 166:88–101. doi: 10.1016/j.cell.2016.05.034
26. Panza F, Alcaro M, Petrelli F, Angelotti F, Pratesi F, Rovero P, et al. A novel DNA/histone H4 peptide complex detects autoantibodies in systemic lupus erythematosus sera. *Arthr Res Ther.* (2016) 18:220. doi: 10.1186/s13075-016-1117-8
27. Yeung K, Chung B, Choufani S, Mok M, Wong W, Mak C, et al. Genome-wide DNA methylation analysis of chinese patients with systemic lupus erythematosus identified hypomethylation in genes related to the type I interferon pathway. *PLoS ONE.* (2017) 12:e0169553. doi: 10.1371/journal.pone.0169553
28. Steri M, Orrù V, Idda M, Pitzalis M, Pala M, Zara I, et al. Overexpression of the cytokine BAFF and autoimmunity risk. *N Engl J Med.* (2017) 376:1615–26. doi: 10.1056/NEJMoa1610528
29. Reddy V, Martinez L, Isenberg D, Leandro M, Cambridge G. Pragmatic treatment of patients with systemic lupus erythematosus with rituximab: long-term effects on serum immunoglobulins. *Arthr Care Res.* (2017) 69:857–66. doi: 10.1002/acr.22993
30. Virdis A, Tani C, Duranti E, Vagnani S, Carli L, Kühl A, et al. Early treatment with hydroxychloroquine prevents the development of endothelial dysfunction in a murine model of systemic lupus erythematosus. *Arthr Res Ther.* (2015) 17:277. doi: 10.1186/s13075-015-0790-3
31. Ikeda T, Fujii H, Nose M, Kamogawa Y, Shirai T, Shirota Y, et al. Bortezomib treatment induces a higher mortality rate in lupus model mice with a higher disease activity. *Arthr Res Ther.* (2017) 19:187. doi: 10.1186/s13075-017-1397-7
32. Li X, Gu L, Yang L, Zhang D, Shen J. Aconitine: a potential novel treatment for systemic lupus erythematosus. *J Pharmacol Sci.* (2017) 133:115–21. doi: 10.1016/j.jphs.2017.01.007
33. Sakai T, Miyazaki T, Shin D, Kim Y, Qi C, Fariss R, et al. DNase-active TREX1 frame- shift mutants induce serologic autoimmunity in mice. *J Autoimmun.* (2017) 81:13–23. doi: 10.1016/j.jaut.2017.03.001
34. Stearns N, Zhou S, Petri M, Binder S, Pisetsky D. The use of poly-L-lysine as a capture agent to enhance the detection of antinuclear antibodies by ELISA. *PLoS ONE.* (2016) 11:e0161818. doi: 10.1371/journal.pone.0161818
35. Elliott M, Ravichandran K. Clearance of apoptotic cells: implications in health and disease. *J Cell Biol.* (2010) 189:1059–70. doi: 10.1083/jcb.2010 04096
36. Biermann M, Maueroder C, Brauner JM, Chaurio R, Janko C, Herrmann M, et al. Surface code –biophysical signals for apoptotic cell clearance. *Phys Biol.* (2013) 10:065007. doi: 10.1088/1478-3975/10/6/065007
37. Shao W, Cohen P. Disturbances of apoptotic cell clearance in systemic lupus erythematosus. *Arthr Res Ther.* (2010) 13:202. doi: 10.1186/ar3206
38. Muñoz L, Lauber K, Schiller M, Manfredi A, Herrmann M. The role of defective clearance of apoptotic cells in systemic autoimmunity. *Nat Rev Rheumatol.* (2010) 6:280–9. doi: 10.1038/nrrheum.2010.46
39. Fadeel B, Xue D, Kagan V. Programmed cell clearance: molecular regulation of the elimination of apoptotic cell corpses and its role in the resolution of inflammation. *Biochem Biophy Res Commun.* (2010) 396:7–10. doi: 10.1016/j.bbrc.2010.02.106
40. Elliott M, Chekeni F, Trampont P, Lazarowski E, Kadl A, Walk S, et al. Nucleotides released by apoptotic cells act as a find-me signal to promote phagocytic clearance. *Nature.* (2009) 461:282–6. doi: 10.1038/nature08296
41. Muñoz L, Peter C, Herrmann M, Wesselborg S, Lauber K. Scent of dying cells: the role of attraction signals in the clearance of apoptotic cells and its immunological consequences. *Autoimmun Rev.* (2010) 9:425–30. doi: 10.1016/j.autrev.2009.11.016
42. Rahman Z, Shao W, Khan T, Zhen Y, Cohen P. Impaired apoptotic cell clearance in the germinal center by mer-deficient tingible body macrophages leads to enhanced antibody-forming cell and germinal center responses. *J Immunol.* (2010) 185:5859–68. doi: 10.4049/jimmunol.1001187
43. Ravichandran K. Find-me and eat-me signals in apoptotic cell clearance: progress and conundrums. *J Exp Med.* (2010) 207:1807–17. doi: 10.1084/jem.20101157
44. Röszer T. Transcriptional control of apoptotic cell clearance by macrophage nuclear receptors. *Apoptosis.* (2016) 22:284–94. doi: 10.1007/s10495-016-1310-x
45. Poon I, Lucas C, Rossi A, Ravichandran K. Apoptotic cell clearance: basic biology and therapeutic potential. *Nat Rev Immunol.* (2014) 14:166–80. doi: 10.1038/nri3607
46. Gaipl US, Munoz LE, Grossmayer G, Lauber K, Franz S, Sarter K, et al. Clearance deficiency and systemic lupus erythematosus (SLE). *J Autoimmun.* (2007) 28:114–21. doi: 10.1016/j.jaut.2007.02.005
47. Munoz LE, Chaurio RA, Gaipl US, Schett G, Kern P. MoMa from patients with systemic lupus erythematosus show altered adhesive activity. *Autoimmunity.* (2009) 42:269–71. doi: 10.1080/08916930902827983
48. Bradley S, Suarez-Fueyo A, Moss D, Kyttaris V, Tsokos G. T cell transcriptomes describe patient subtypes in systemic lupus erythematosus. *PLoS ONE.* (2015) 10:e0141171. doi: 10.1371/journal.pone.0141171
49. Munoz LE, Frey B, Appelt U, Janko C, Sarter K, Voll R, et al. Peripheral blood stem cells of patients with systemic lupus erythematosus show altered differentiation into macrophages. *Open Autoimmun J.* (2010) 2:11–6. doi: 10.2174/1876894601002010011
50. Szondy Z, Garabuczi Ã, JoÃs G, Tsay G, Sarang Z. Impaired clearance of apoptotic cells in chronic inflammatory diseases: therapeutic implications. *Front Immunol.* (2014) 5:1–8. doi: 10.3389/fimmu.2014.00354
51. Fernado MV, Eva B, Joseph O, MIquel V. DNase 1 and systemic lupus erythematosus. *Sci Direct.* (2008) 7:359–63. doi: 10.1016/j.autrev.2008.02.002
52. Pieterse E, van der Vlag J. Breaking immunological tolerance in systemic lupus erythematosus. *Front Immunol.* (2014) 5:1–8. doi: 10.3389/fimmu.2014.00164
53. Goldmann O, Medina E. The expanding world of extracellular traps: not only neutrophils but much more. *Front Immunol.* (2012) 3:420. doi: 10.3389/fimmu.2012.00420
54. Mak A, Kow NY. The pathology of T cells in systemic lupus erythematosus. *J Immunol Res.* (2014) 2014:419029. doi: 10.1155/2014/419029
55. Hughes T, Webb R, Fei Y, Wren JD, Sawalha AH. DNA methylome in human CD4+ T cells identifies transcriptionally repressive and non-repressive methylation peaks. *Genes Immun.* (2010) 11:554–60. doi: 10.1038/gene.2010.24
56. Choi SC, Hutchinson TE, Titov AA, Seay HR, Li S, Brusko TM, et al. The lupus susceptibility gene Pbx1 regulates the balance between follicular helper T cell and regulatory T cell differentiation. *J Immunol.* (2016) 197:458–69. doi: 10.4049/jimmunol.1502283
57. Hooks JJ, Moutsopoulos HM, Geis SA, Stahl NI, Decker JL, Notkins AL. Immune interferon in the circulation of patients with autoimmune disease. *N Engl J Med.* (1979) 301:5–8 doi: 10.1056/NEJM1979070530 10102
58. Desnues B, Macedo A, Ordoñez-Rueda D, Roussel-Queval A, Malissen B, Bruhns P, et al. The transcriptional repressor Gfi1 prevents lupus autoimmunity by restraining TLR7 signaling. *Eur J Immunol.* (2016) 46:2801–11. doi: 10.1002/eji.201646573
59. Suurmond J, Calise J, Malkiel S, Diamond B. DNA-reactive B cells in lupus. *Curr Opin Immunol.* (2016) 43:1–7. doi: 10.1016/j.coi.2016.07.002
60. Wang Z, Chang C, Peng M, Lu Q. Translating epigenetics into clinic: focus on lupus. *Clin Epigen.* (2017) 9:78. doi: 10.1186/s13148-01 7-0378-7
61. Herrmann M, Podolska M, Biermann M, Maueröder C, Hahn J. Inflammatory etiopathogenesis of systemic lupus erythematosus: an update. *J Inflamm Res.* (2015) 8:161–71. doi: 10.2147/JIR.S70325
62. Bouts Y, Wolthuis D, Dirkx M, Pieterse E, Simons E, Van Boekel A, et al. Apoptosis and NET formation in the pathogenesis of SLE. *Autoimmunity.* (2012) 45:597–601. doi: 10.3109/08916934.2012.719953
63. Liu C, Tangsombatvisit S, Rosenberg J, Mandelbaum G, Gillespie E, Gozani O, et al. Correction: specific post-translational histone modifications of neutrophil extracellular traps as immunogens and potential targets of lupus autoantibodies. *Arthr Res Ther.* (2012) 14:403. doi: 10.1186/ar3933

64. Long H, Huang W, Yin H, Zhao S, Zhao M, Lu Q. Abnormal expression pattern of histone demethylases in CD4 + T cells of MRL/lpr lupus-like mice. *Lupus.* (2009) 18:1327–8. doi: 10.1177/0961203309104869
65. Kawasaki A, Ito I, Ito S, Hayashi T, Goto D, Matsumoto I, et al. Association of TNFAIP3 polymorphism with susceptibility to systemic lupus erythematosus in a Japanese population. *J Biomed Biotechnol.* (2010) 2010:1–5. doi: 10.1155/2010/207578
66. Krukenberg K, Kim S, Tan E, Maliga Z, Mitchison T. Extracellular poly(ADP-Ribose) is a pro-inflammatory signal for macrophages. *Chem Biol.* (2015) 22:446–52. doi: 10.1016/j.chembiol.2015.03.007
67. Matzke M, Mosher R. RNA-directed DNA methylation: an epigenetic pathway of increasing complexity. *Nat Rev Genet.* (2014) 15:394–408. doi: 10.1038/nrg3683
68. Baranovskii AG, Buneva VN, Nevinsky GA. Human deoxyribonucleases. *Biochemistry.* (2004) 9:587–601. doi: 10.1023/B:BIRY.0000033731.50496.01
69. Al-Mayouf SM, Sunker A, Abdwani R, Abrawi SA, Almurshedi F, Alhashmi N, et al. Loss-of-function variant in DNASE1L3 causes a familial form of systemic lupus erythematosus. *Nat Genet.* (2011) 43:1186–8. doi: 10.1038/ng.975
70. Lee-Kirsch MA, Chowdhury D, Harvey S, Gong M, Senenko L, Engel K, et al. A mutation in TREX1 that impairs susceptibility to granzyme A-mediated cell death underlies familial chilblain lupus. *J Mol Med.* (2007) 85:531–7. doi: 10.1007/s00109-007-0199-9
71. Günther C, Berndt N, Wolf C, Lee-Kirsch MA. Familial chilblain lupus due to a novel mutation in the exonuclease III domain of 3' repair exonuclease 1 (TREX1). *JAMA Dermatol.* (2015) 151:426–31. doi: 10.1001/jamadermatol.2014.3438
72. Wolf C, Rapp A, Berndt N, Staroske W, Schuster M, Dobrick-Mattheuer M, et al. RPA and Rad51 constitute a cell intrinsic mechanism to protect the cytosol from self DNA. *Nat Commun.* (2016) 7:11752. doi: 10.1038/ncomms11752
73. Yang YG, Lindahl T, Barnes DE. Trex1 exonuclease degrades ssDNA to prevent chronic checkpoint activation and autoimmune disease. *Cell.* (2007) 131:873–86. doi: 10.1016/j.cell.2007.10.017
74. Lee-Kirsch MA, Gong M, Chowdhury D, Senenko L, Engel K, Lee YA. Mutations in the gene encoding the 3′-5′ DNA exonuclease TREX1 are associated with systemic lupus erythematosus. *Nat Genet.* (2007) 39:1065–7. doi: 10.1038/ng2091
75. Stetson DB, Ko JS, Heidmann T, Medzhitov R. Trex1 prevents cell-intrinsic initiation of autoimmunity. *Cell.* (2008)22:587–98. doi: 10.1016/j.cell.2008.06.032
76. Gall A, Treuting P, Elkon KB, Loo YM, Gale M Jr, Barber GN, et al. Autoimmunity initiates in nonhematopoietic cells and progresses via lymphocytes in an interferon-dependent autoimmune disease. *Immunity.* (2012) 36:120–31. doi: 10.1016/j.immuni.2011.11.018
77. Liu Y, Jesus AA, Marrero B, Yang D, Ramsey SE, Sanchez GA, et al. Activated STING in a vascular and pulmonary syndrome. *N Engl J Med.* (2014)371:507–18. doi: 10.1056/NEJMoa1312625
78. König N, Fiehn C, Wolf C, Schuster M, Cura Costa E, Tüngler V, et al. Familial chilblain lupus due to a gain-of-function mutation in STING. *Ann Rheum Dis.* (2017)76:468–72. doi: 10.1136/annrheumdis-2016-209841
79. Jeremiah N, Neven B, Gentili M, Callebaut I, Maschalidi S, Stolzenberg MC, et al. Inherited STING-activating mutation underlies a familial inflammatory syndrome with lupus-like manifestations. *J Clin Invest.* (2014)124:5516–20. doi: 10.1172/JCI79100
80. Sharma S, Campbell AM, Chan J, Schattgen SA, Orlowski GM, Nayar R, et al. Suppression of systemic autoimmunity by the innate immune adaptor STING. *Proc Natl Acad Sci USA.* (2015)112:E710–7. doi: 10.1073/pnas.14202 17112
81. Bai Y, Tong Y, Liu Y, Hu H. Self-dsDNA in the pathogenesis of systemic lupus erythematosus. *Clin Exp Immunol.* (2018) 191:1–0. doi: 10.1111/cei.13041

13

Assessing the Correlation Between Disease Severity Indices and Quality of Life Measurement Tools in Pemphigus

Rebecca L. Krain[1,2†], *Carolyn J. Kushner*[1,2†], *Meera Tarazi*[1,2], *Rebecca G. Gaffney*[1,2], *Andrea C. Yeguez*[1,2], *Danielle E. Zamalin*[1,2], *David R. Pearson*[1,2,3], *Rui Feng*[4], *Aimee S. Payne*[2] and *Victoria P. Werth*[1,2*†]

[1] Corporal Michael J. Crescenz VA Medical Center, Philadelphia, PA, United States, [2] Department of Dermatology, University of Pennsylvania, Philadelphia, PA, United States, [3] Department of Dermatology, University of Minnesota, Minneapolis, MN, United States, [4] Department of Biostatistics and Epidemiology, University of Pennsylvania, Philadelphia, PA, United States

***Correspondence:**
Victoria P. Werth
werth@pennmedicine.upenn.edu

† These authors have contributed equally to this work

Pemphigus, an autoimmune blistering disease that affects the skin and mucous membranes, adversely impacts patients' quality of life (QOL). While there are various QOL measurement tools that can be used in this disease, few studies have assessed how a patient's change in disease severity can affect their QOL. This study aims to identify which disease severity index correlates best with the change in QOL. Fifty pemphigus patients completed QOL surveys with disease severity scored over two visits. QOL was assessed with the Autoimmune Bullous Disease Quality of Life (ABQOL), Dermatology Life Quality Index (DLQI), Skindex-29, and Short Form Survey 36 (SF-36). Disease severity was scored with the Pemphigus Disease Area Index (PDAI) and Autoimmune Bullous Skin Disorder Intensity Score (ABSIS). Correlations between the change in QOL scores and change in disease severity were analyzed using Spearman's coefficient (r). The change in PDAI showed a strong correlation ($r = 0.60$–0.79) with changes in the ABQOL, Skindex-29 symptoms (Skindex-S), and Skindex-29 functioning (Skindex-F) subscales for all patients ($n = 50$). For patients with mucosal disease ($n = 24$), the change in PDAI showed a strong correlation with changes in the ABQOL and Skindex-S subscale. For patients without mucosal disease, the change in PDAI showed a strong correlation with the Skindex-S. The change in ABSIS showed a strong correlation with Skindex-S for all patients and patients with no mucosal involvement, but showed no strong correlations for patients with mucosal involvement. The changes in PDAI always had a stronger correlation than the changes in ABSIS scores to changes in the ABQOL, DLQI, and Skindex-29 subscales, except where the PDAI and ABSIS scores were about the same for the Skindex-S subscale in patients with no mucosal involvement ($r = 0.76$ and $r = 0.77$, respectively). PDAI is superior to ABSIS in its correlation with validated QOL tools. The QOL tools that appear to be of most use in clinical trials and patient management are the Skindex-S and ABQOL.

Keywords: pemphigus, disease severity, autoimmunity, dermatology, skin, outcome measures, autoimmune bullous disease

INTRODUCTION

Pemphigus is a rare but serious autoimmune blistering disease caused by autoantibodies against desmosomes (1, 2). Although a previously deadly diagnosis because of skin barrier breakdown leading to infection, the advent of steroids and steroid-sparing agents have allowed pemphigus to be considered a less-fatal, chronic disease (3). Therefore, assessing a pemphigus patient's quality of life (QOL) has become an important part of monitoring the disease (3). Despite the limited literature on QOL in pemphigus (3–12), it is clear that this disease greatly affects patients' emotions, physical health, and social functioning (12, 13). The number of clinical trials in pemphigus have increased immensely over the past decade (14), creating a growing need for objective measurements in both QOL and disease severity to monitor improvement.

Health related QOL outcomes are becoming important measurements when conducting clinical trials and assessing new pharmaceutical treatments (15). Therefore, multiple QOL measurement tools across all fields, including dermatology, have been created. QOL outcome measurements can also be useful for physicians, patients, and health insurers when deciding on therapeutic options and allowing for shared-decision making (15). In regard to QOL in pemphigus, dermatologists have used general health QOL measurement tools including the Short Form Survey 36 (SF-36), as well as dermatology specific tools such as the Dermatology Life Quality Index (DLQI) and the Skindex-29 (12, 16). An autoimmune blistering disease-specific QOL measurement tool has also been created, the Autoimmune Bullous Disease Quality of Life (ABQOL) (3, 6).

In addition to the various QOL assessment tools, there are also two commonly used validated objective disease severity indices: the Pemphigus Disease Area Index (PDAI) and the Autoimmune Bullous Skin Disorder Intensity Score (ABSIS) (17–19). Just as it is important to have a validated QOL measurement tool for clinical trials, there is a similar need for understanding the properties of QOL measures in blistering diseases and to have an established disease severity index to compare and assess results across the field.

The purpose of this study is to evaluate which disease severity score correlates best with the change in QOL scores. This may help in clinical trial design when choosing a measurement tool that captures both disease severity and QOL.

PATIENTS AND METHODS

Patients with the appropriate clinical presentation, histological findings on biopsy, and at least one positive immunochemical test consistent with pemphigus (direct or indirect immunofluorescence, and/or ELISA), provided written consent to study participation in a prospective autoimmune blistering disease database at the Hospital of the University of Pennsylvania (HUP) between April of 2016 and February of 2019. The study protocol was approved by the institutional review board. Of the 107 patients in our database who were diagnosed with pemphigus vulgaris (PV) or pemphigus foliaceus (PF), 50 patients completed both an enrollment and a follow-up visit. Patients with no disease activity at both enrollment and follow-up visits were not included in the study. Subcategorization was performed for patients with mucosal disease and patients without mucosal disease. Patients with mucosal disease had documented mucosal findings at enrollment and/or follow-up visits. Patients without mucosal disease did not have mucosal findings at both enrollment and follow-up visits, regardless of a prior history of mucosal involvement. At each visit, patients completed four QOL forms: the ABQOL, DLQI, Skindex-29, and SF-36. Patients' skin was examined and assessed during the visits using the PDAI and the ABSIS scoring systems. Patient demographics, including age, sex, and disease type, were recorded.

Pemphigus Disease Area Index (PDAI)

The PDAI scores disease activity based on anatomical location and the size of lesions. A maximum of 120 points are available to score skin activity excluding the scalp, 10 for scalp activity, and 120 points for mucosal activity, with a maximum score of 250 points (20–22). Damage or post-inflammatory hyperpigmentation is scored separately from the activity score, with a maximum of 13 points available (20–22). The PDAI has been validated and shown to have an intra-rater intra-class correlation coefficient (ICC) of 0.98 and an inter-rater ICC of 0.86 for skin activity (23–25).

Autoimmune Bullous Skin Disorder Intensity Score (ABSIS)

The ABSIS ranges from 0 (no activity or damage) to 206, with 150 points for skin activity or damage, 11 for mucosal involvement, and 45 for oral pain or bleeding (a subjective/patient reported measurement). The ABSIS score combines disease activity and damage together, by scoring the quality of the skin lesion (26). The ABSIS applies the "rule of nines," which measures amount of disease by body surface area (BSA), where the palm of the patient's hand is one BSA (26). The percent BSA is multiplied by whether the lesion is re-epithelialized (0.5), dry and erosive (1.0), or exudative and erosive (1.5) (21, 22, 26). The lowest BSA score that can be assigned is a 1, even if a patient only has one small lesion with a BSA of 0.1%. Therefore, using this example, if this patient had an exudative lesion with a BSA of 0.1%, then the score would be 1.5 (1% BSA × 1.5), rather than 0.15 (0.1% BSA × 1.5) (23).

Quality of Life Measurement Tools

Many QOL measurement tools have been developed to assess various diseases. The SF-36 is a form used for all disease entities, not limited to dermatology. It looks at eight different QOL categories: physical functioning, role limitations due to physical health, role limitations due to emotional problems, energy/fatigue, emotional well-being, social functioning, pain, and general health. Higher SF-36 scores indicate a more favorable QOL (27).

The DLQI and the Skindex-29 are both QOL measurement tools developed specifically for dermatologic diseases. The DLQI is a 10-question survey: scores range from 0 to 30, with a higher score indicating worse QOL. Questions concern topics such as patients' symptoms and feelings, daily activities, leisure, personal relationships, work and school, as well as treatment (12, 28). The Skindex-29 has 29 questions split into three subscales: Skindex-29 symptoms (Skindex-S), emotions (Skindex-E), and functioning (Skindex-F) (29, 30).

The ABQOL is a 17 question QOL measurement tool specific for autoimmune blistering diseases that was developed to capture issues related to the disease that may not be reflected in skin-specific instruments (31). The ABQOL has shown reliable internal constancy and test-retest reliability, with an intra-class correlation coefficient of 0.93 (95% confidence interval, 0.88–0.94) (3).

Statistical Analysis

The difference, or change, in score for each QOL measurement tool, as well as the difference in disease severity index scores, were calculated from enrollment to follow-up visits. The correlation between change in QOL scores and change in disease severity scores were analyzed using Spearman's correlation coefficient (r) for all combinations of the QOL measurement tools and the disease severity indices (PDAI and ABSIS). Spearman correlation coefficient cutoffs for very weak, weak, moderate, strong, and very strong were the absolute value of 0.0–0.19, 0.20–0.39, 0.40–0.59, 0.60–0.79, and 0.80–1.0 respectively, which has been classified by the *British Medical Journal* guidelines (32). This analysis was completed for all patients, as well as for the subcategorization of patients who had mucosal involvement at some point during their two visits and patients who did not have mucosal involvement during their visits. GraphPad Prism was used to conduct the analyses.

TABLE 1 | Patient characteristics.

	All (n = 50)
Age	
<45	8 (16%)
45-64.9	22 (44%)
≥65	20 (40%)
Sex	
Male	24 (48%)
Female	26 (52%)
Diagnosis	
Pemphigus Foliaceus	7 (14%)
Pemphigus Vulgaris	43 (86%)
Mucosal Involvement	
Yes	24 (48%)
No	26 (52%)
Race	
White	37 (74%)
African American or Black	3 (6%)
Asian	8 (16%)
Other	2 (4%)

RESULTS

A total of 50 patients, 43 (86%) with PV and 7 (14%) with PF completed both an enrollment and follow-up visit. Twenty-four (48%) patients had mucosal involvement at some point during their two visits, and 26 (52%) did not have mucosal involvement. Further patient characteristics are summarized in **Table 1**. Median time from disease onset to enrollment visit was 2.8 years (IQR = 0.8–5.4) for all patients, 1.9 years for patients with mucosal involvement, and 4.5 years for patients with no mucosal involvement. Median time from enrollment to follow-up visit was 0.45 years. Median PDAI scores at enrollment for all patients, patients with mucosal disease, and those without mucosal disease were 5.00, 5.30, and 3.50 respectively, while median PDAI scores during follow-up were 3.00 for all patients and patients with mucosal disease, and 4.30 for patients without mucosal disease. Median ABSIS scores at enrollment for all patients, patients with mucosal disease, and those without mucosal disease were 4.00, 6.28, and 1.50, while median ABSIS scores during follow-up were 2.00, 2.50, and 2.00, respectively (**Figure 1** and **Table 2**).

For all patients ($n = 50$), the change in PDAI showed a strong correlation ($r = 0.60–0.79$) with changes in the ABQOL ($r = 0.60$), Skindex-S ($r = 0.75$), and Skindex-F ($r = 0.61$) subscales. For patients with mucosal disease ($n = 24$), the change in PDAI showed a strong correlation with changes in the ABQOL ($r = 0.67$) and Skindex-S subscale ($r = 0.62$). For patients without mucosal disease during the two visits, the change in PDAI showed a strong correlation with the Skindex-S subscale ($r = 0.76$). The change in ABSIS displayed a strong correlation with Skindex-S for all patients ($r = 0.73$) and patients with no mucosal involvement ($r = 0.77$), but showed no strong correlations for patients with mucosal involvement (**Table 3**).

The eight different SF-36 subscales as well as the DLQI primarily displayed weak to moderate correlations to both the PDAI and ABSIS. For all patients ($n = 50$), the change in the SF-36 role limitations due to physical heath, energy/fatigue, and pain subscales showed weak to moderate correlations with the change in PDAI ($r = -0.38$, -0.41, and -0.33, respectively) and ABSIS ($r = -0.37$, -0.40, and -0.45, respectively). A weak correlation was also found with the change in the SF-36 emotional well-being subscale to the change in PDAI ($r = -0.33$). For patients with mucosal disease ($n = 24$), the change in the SF-36 energy/fatigue subscale showed moderate correlations with the change in PDAI ($r = -0.59$) and ABSIS ($r = -0.44$). For patients with no mucosal disease ($n = 26$), the change in SF-36 pain subscale showed a moderate correlation with the change in PDAI ($r = -0.58$), and a strong correlation with the change in ABSIS ($r = -0.63$) (**Table 3**). In regard to the change in PDAI, the DLQI showed moderate correlations to all patients, patients with mucosal involvement, and no mucosal involvement ($r = 0.58$, 0.50, and 0.58, respectively). Similarly, in regard to the ABSIS, all patients and patients with no mucosal involvement remained in the moderate range when correlating to the DLQI, however, patients with mucosal involvement had a weak correlation of the ABSIS to the DLQI ($r = 0.29$).

The Skindex-29, specifically the Skindex-S, and ABQOL displayed generally stronger correlations than the other

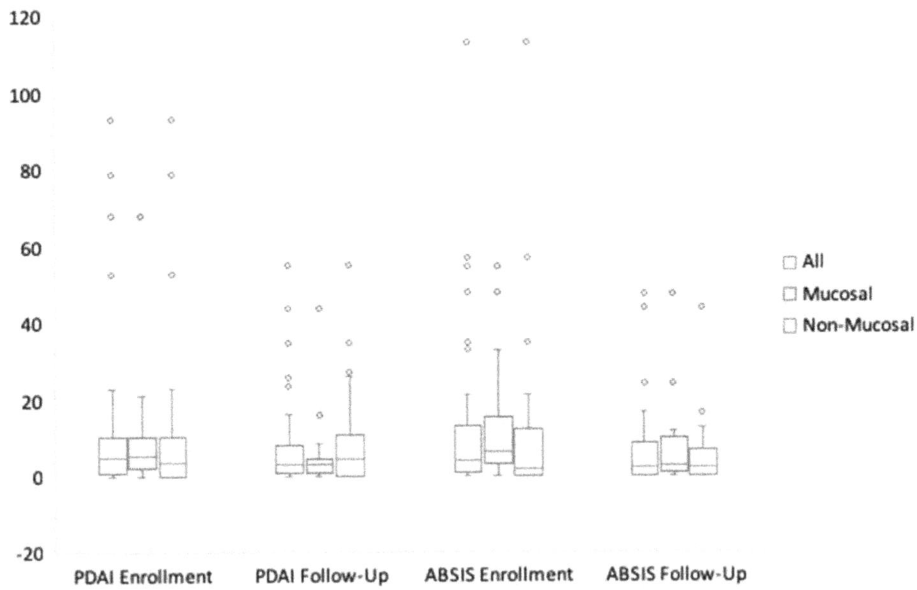

FIGURE 1 | Median PDAI and ABSIS with IQR from enrollment to follow-up visit.

TABLE 2 | Median PDAI score and IQR.

	All		Mucosal		Non-mucosal	
	Median score	IQR	Median score	IQR	Median score	IQR
PDAI Enrollment	5.00	1.25–10	5.30	2.98–10.15	3.50	0.00–9.33
PDAI Follow-up	3.00	1.00–8.00	3.00	1.00–4.08	4.30	0.50–9.58
ABSIS Enrollment	4.00	1.00–12.38	6.28	3.00–14.00	1.50	0.00–12.00
ABSIS Follow-up	2.00	0.10–7.50	2.50	1.00–9.56	2.00	0.00–5.75

PDAI, Pemphigus Disease Area Index; ABSIS, Autoimmune Bullous Skin Disorder Intensity Score; IQR, interquartile range.

measurement tools. Strong correlations were found with the change in Skindex-S to both the PDAI and ABSIS for all patients ($r = 0.75$ and $r = 0.73$, respectively), patients with no mucosal involvement ($r = 0.76$ and 0.77, respectively), and patients with mucosal involvement for PDAI only ($r = 0.62$) (**Table 3**). A moderate correlation was noted for the Skindex-S and ABSIS for patients with mucosal involvement ($r = 0.52$). The Skindex-E and Skindex-F showed weak and moderate correlations to the PDAI and ABSIS, except for a strong correlation with the change in Skindex-F and change in PDAI for all patients ($r = 0.61$) (**Table 3**). For the ABQOL, strong correlations were found with the change in PDAI for all patients ($r = 0.60$) and patients with mucosal involvement ($r = 0.67$). The change in ABQOL also showed moderate correlations with the change in ABSIS for all patients ($r = 0.51$) and patients with no mucosal involvement ($r = 0.49$), and with the change in PDAI in patients with no mucosal involvement ($r = 0.56$). A weak correlation was noted for patients with mucosal involvement in regard to the ABSIS ($r = 0.38$). There were no strong correlations found with the DLQI; however, moderate correlations were noted for each category, except for a weak correlation with the ABSIS for patients with mucosal involvement ($r = 0.29$) (**Table 3**).

DISCUSSION

Treatment options for pemphigus have greatly improved over the past two decades (13). Nonetheless, there is a high unmet need for FDA-approved therapies, and many agents have entered, or are entering, clinical trials for pemphigus. To optimize these trials, standard measurement tools should be used to assess skin disease severity as well as QOL. Assuming QOL decreases with skin severity, we conducted this study to identify which disease severity index correlates best with QOL.

Our data revealed that the SF-36 did not correlate strongly with the PDAI or ABSIS for the majority of analyses (**Table 3**). Most SF-36 and DLQI correlations were weak or moderate, except for the SF-36 pain subscale. We hypothesize that the SF-36 showed generally weak correlations because it addresses overall health rather than specific dermatologic symptoms. This relates to our patient population, where 40% are over the age of 65 and likely suffering from other health conditions or limitations of

TABLE 3 | Correlation using Spearman's correlation coefficient (*r*) of the change in quality of life score with the change in disease severity from enrollment to follow-up visit.

	PDAI			ABSIS		
	All (*n* = 50)	Mucosal Involvement (*n* = 24)	No Mucosal Involvement (*n* = 26)	All (*n* = 50)	Mucosal Involvement (*n* = 24)	No Mucosal Involvement (*n* = 26)
ABQOL	0.60	0.67	0.56	0.51	0.38	0.49
DLQI	0.58	0.50	0.58	0.46	0.29	0.51
Skindex-29						
Symptoms	0.75	0.62	0.76	0.73	0.52	0.77
Emotions	0.45	0.29	0.59	0.37	0.17	0.51
Functioning	0.61	0.40	0.56	0.49	0.28	0.44
SF-36						
General health	−0.14	−0.11	−0.19	−0.11	−0.0053	−0.25
Physical functioning	−0.23	−0.17	−0.25	−0.16	−0.0043	−0.33
Role limitations (physical health)	−0.38	−0.29	−0.37	−0.37	−0.15	−0.37
Role limitations (emotional problems)	−0.19	0.0093	−0.29	−0.27	−0.056	−0.38
Energy/fatigue	−0.41	−0.59	−0.24	−0.40	−0.44	−0.27
Emotional well-being	−0.33	−0.31	−0.23	−0.21	0.039	−0.24
Social functioning	−0.27	−0.10	−0.22	−0.28	−0.19	−0.17
Pain	−0.33	0.079	−0.58	−0.45	−0.16	−0.63

PDAI, Pemphigus Disease Area Index; ABSIS, Autoimmune Bullous Skin Disorder Intensity Score; ABQOL, Autoimmune Bullous Disease Quality of Life; DLQI, Dermatology Life Quality Index; SF-36, Short Form Survey 36.

older age (33, 34). The age group of our cohort (median age = 60) is consistent with the general pemphigus population, who tend to present in their fifth to sixth decade of life (35).

Assessment of the QOL measurement tools showed largely strong correlations with the Skindex-S subscale to both the PDAI and ABSIS for all patients as well as patients with and without mucosal disease, demonstrating its use, and potential preference, in patient management and clinical trials (**Table 3**). On the contrary, the Skindex-S unexpectedly showed only a moderate, rather than strong, correlation to the ABSIS for patients with mucosal disease (r = 0.52). This finding was surprising, as the ABSIS contains QOL questions regarding mucosal involvement (pain and bleeding). It was therefore believed that a score that addressed oral symptoms would show a strong correlation with the Skindex-S subscale score for patients with mucosal disease. However, of the 206 possible points in the ABSIS, only 56 of those points directly address mucosal involvement (11 points) as well as subjective oral pain and bleeding (45 points). In contrast, the PDAI allocates more points toward mucosal involvement (120 out of 250 total points). Therefore, although the ABSIS may include QOL questions, this aspect is only a minor part of the disease severity index.

The ABQOL was also found to show strong correlations with the PDAI in regard to all patients (r = 0.60) and patients with mucosal involvement (r = 0.67), and was the strongest correlation found in patients with mucosal disease. It is likely that the ABQOL correlated best with the PDAI for patients with mucosal disease because this disease-specific QOL measurement tool directly addresses painful erosions in the mouth. For instance, 3 of the 17 questions in the ABQOL assess for mucosal involvement, compared to the other QOL measurement tools, like the DLQI, that only emphasize skin disease, which patients often interpret as not including the mucosa. The ABQOL assessment may therefore be a useful tool in clinical trials for pemphigus patients with mucosal involvement, such as PV specific trials.

Correlations of the change in PDAI were superior to those of the ABSIS in regard to the change in the majority of QOL tools. Looking at all patients, those with mucosal involvement, and those without, there were a total of 13 analyses conducted for the ABQOL, DLQI, the three subscales of the Skindex-29, and the eight subscales of the SF-36 in correlation with the PDAI and ABSIS. Ten of the 13 (76.9%) analyses showed a stronger correlation with the PDAI over the ABSIS. The analysis that showed a stronger correlation with the ABSIS was the Skindex-S for patients without mucosal involvement, although the ABSIS and PDAI values were about the same (r = 0.77 and r = 0.76, respectively). While some correlations did not vary greatly between the two severity tools, the fact that the PDAI had largely stronger correlations suggests that the PDAI may be better at capturing disease activity that correlates with QOL. This finding is consistent with a prior study that showed ABSIS data to be skewed to the left (lower scores) as compared to the PDAI (23). The lower scores seen in the ABSIS support its limitation in its ability to evaluate changes in skin disease severity in patients with mild disease and, given the generally mild disease in our cohort, may be why this index did not correlate well with the changes in QOL measurement tools.

This study had several strengths as well as limitations. The strengths included data collection in a prospective manner and a relatively large pemphigus database, although the cohort size was small for the statistical analyses. Additionally, this study included a patient population similar to those who may be eligible to enter future pemphigus clinical trials. The limitations included a retrospective analysis, a cohort from a single institution that is a tertiary center, and the absence of data on comorbid conditions when assessing the QOL tools.

Our cohort had relatively mild disease, with low PDAI and ABSIS scores, which may have prevented our results from being fully applicable to patients with moderate to severe disease. Patients typically present with highly active disease for a short period of time because steroids are fast-acting and effective, lowering disease activity by their first follow-up visit. However, our first study visit was not always with new patients, and many may have been well-controlled by the time they were enrolled in our database. At initial visit for our database, 14 patients displayed a PDAI of ≥9 and 7 patients had a PDAI of ≥15, which are considered two different "moderate" disease cutoff points (17, 36). Only 4 patients displayed both a PDAI of ≥25 and ≥45, two different "severe" disease cutoff points (17, 36). Our results may therefore have been different if we gathered data at the peak of their disease. Often, however, patients who are enrolled in clinical trials have been initially controlled on steroids or other first-line treatments prior to receiving further therapy or interventions.

Our study identified disease severity index and QOL measurement tools that should be used in clinical trials and patient management. The PDAI and the Skindex-S subscale of the Skindex-29 showed excellent promise for use in such settings, in a patient population that is representative of those seen during routine practice at a tertiary referral medical center. Future studies of the ABQOL in patients with mucosal involvement and in those with higher disease activity scores may further elucidate the utility of the various QOL measurement tools in relation to disease activity.

AUTHOR CONTRIBUTIONS

RK, CK, and VW contributed to the conception and design of the study and wrote the manuscript. RK, CK, AY, and DZ organized the database. RK, CK, RG, MT, RF, DP, AP, and VW analyzed and interpreted the dataset. All authors contributed to manuscript revision, read, and approved the submitted version.

ACKNOWLEDGMENTS

This material was supported by the Veterans Health Administration, Office of Research and Development, Biomedical Laboratory Research and Development.

REFERENCES

1. Hammers CM, Stanley JR. Mechanisms of disease: pemphigus and bullous pemphigoid. *Annu Rev Pathol.* (2016) 11:175–97. doi: 10.1146/annurev-pathol-012615-044313
2. Kasperkiewicz M, Ellebrecht CT, Takahashi H, Yamagami J, Zillikens D, Payne AS, et al. Pemphigus. *Nat Rev Dis Prim.* (2017) 3:17026. doi: 10.1038/nrdp.2017.26
3. Sebaratnam DF, Okawa J, Payne A, Murrell DF, Werth VP. Reliability of the autoimmune bullous disease quality of life (ABQOL) questionnaire in the USA. *Qual Life Res.* (2015) 24:2257–60. doi: 10.1007/s11136-015-0965-z
4. Paradisi A, Sampogna F, Di Pietro C, Cianchini G, Didona B, Ferri R. et al. Quality-of-life assessment in patients with pemphigus using a minimum set of evaluation tools. *J Am Acad Dermatol.* (2009) 60:261–9. doi: 10.1016/j.jaad.2008.09.014
5. Paradisi A, Cianchini G, Lupi F, Di Pietro C, Sampogna F, Didona B. et al. Quality of life in patients with pemphigus receiving adjuvant therapy. *Clin Exp Dermatol.* (2012) 37:626–30. doi: 10.1111/j.1365-2230.2011.04282.x
6. Yang B, Chen G, Yang Q, Yan X, Zhang Z, Murrell DF. et al. Reliability and validity of the Chinese version of the autoimmune bullous disease quality of life (ABQOL) questionnaire. *Health Qual Life Outcomes.* (2017) 15:31. doi: 10.1186/s12955-017-0594-z
7. Mayrshofer F, Hertl M, Sinkgraven R, Sticherling M, Pfeiffer C, Zillikens D, et al. Significant decrease in quality of life in patients with pemphigus vulgaris. Results from the German Bullous Skin Disease (BSD) Study Group. *J Dtsch Dermatol Ges.* (2005) 3:431–5. doi: 10.1111/j.1610-0387.2005.05722.x
8. Terrab Z, Benchikhi H, Maaroufi A, Hassoune S, Amine M, Lakhdar H. Quality of life and pemphigus. *Ann Dermatol Venereol.* (2005) 132:321–8. doi: 10.1016/S0151-9638(05)79276-0
9. Sung JY, Roh MR, Kim SC. Quality of life assessment in korean patients with Pemphigus. *Ann Dermatol.* (2015) 27:492–8. doi: 10.5021/ad.2015.27.5.492
10. Chee SN, Murrell DF. Pemphigus and quality of life. *Dermatol Clin.* (2011) 29:521–5. doi: 10.1016/j.det.2011.03.009
11. Pena S, Payne A, Stanley J, Werth V. Quality of life in autoimmune blistering diseases (AIBD). *J Invest Dermatol.* (2017) 137:S67. doi: 10.1016/j.jid.2017.02.406
12. Ghodsi SZ, Chams-Davatchi C, Daneshpazhooh M, Valikhani M, Esmaili N. Quality of life and psychological status of patients with pemphigus vulgaris using dermatology life quality index and general health questionnaires. *J Dermatol.* (2012) 39:141–4. doi: 10.1111/j.1346-8138.2011.01382.x
13. Sebaratnam DF, McMillan JR, Werth VP, Murrell DF. Quality of life in patients with bullous dermatoses. *Clin Dermatol.* (2012) 30:103–7. doi: 10.1016/j.clindermatol.2011.03.016
14. Payne AS. Quantifying disease extent in pemphigus. *Br J Dermatol.* (2016) 175:18–9. doi: 10.1111/bjd.14562
15. Revicki DA, Osoba D, Fairclough D, Barofsky I, Berzon R, Leidy NK, et al. Recommendations on health-related quality of life research to support labeling and promotional claims in the United States. *Qual Life Res.* (2000) 9:887–900. doi: 10.1023/A:1008996223999
16. Rencz F, Gulácsi L, Tamási B, Kárpáti S, Péntek M, Baji P, et al. Health-related quality of life and its determinants in pemphigus: a systematic review and meta-analysis. *Br J Dermatol.* (2015) 173:1076–80. doi: 10.1111/bjd.13848
17. Boulard C, Duvert Lehembre S, Picard-Dahan C, Kern JS, Zambruno G, Feliciani C, et al. Calculation of cut-off values based on the autoimmune bullous skin disorder intensity score (ABSIS) and Pemphigus Disease Area Index (PDAI) pemphigus scoring systems for defining moderate, significant and extensive types of pemphigus. *Br J Dermatol.* (2016) 175:142–9. doi: 10.1111/bjd.14405
18. Hanna S, Kim M, Murrell DF. Validation studies of outcome measures in pemphigus. *Int J Womens Dermatol.* (2016) 2:128–39. doi: 10.1016/j.ijwd.2016.10.003
19. Pfütze M, Niedermeier A, Hertl M, Eming R. Introducing a novel Autoimmune Bullous Skin Disorder Intensity Score (ABSIS) in pemphigus. *Eur J Dermatol.* (2007) 17:4–11. doi: 10.1684/ejd.2007.0090

20. Murrell DF, Dick S, Ahmed AR, Amagai M, Barnadas MA, Borradori L, et al. Consensus statement on definitions of disease, end points, and therapeutic response for pemphigus. *J Am Acad Dermatol.* (2008) 58:1043–6. doi: 10.1016/j.jaad.2008.01.012
21. Rahbar Z, Daneshpazhooh M, Mirshams-Shahshahani M, Esmaili N, Heidari K, Aghazadeh N, et al. Pemphigus disease activity measurements: pemphigus disease area index, autoimmune bullous skin disorder intensity score, and pemphigus vulgaris activity score. *JAMA Dermatol.* (2014) 150:266–72. doi: 10.1001/jamadermatol.2013.8175
22. Hébert V, Boulard C, Houivet E, Duvert Lehembre S, Borradori L, Della Torre R, et al. Large international validation of ABSIS and PDAI pemphigus severity scores. *J Invest Dermatol.* (2019) 139:31–7. doi: 10.1016/j.jid.2018.04.042
23. Rosenbach M, Murrell DF, Bystryn JC, Dulay S, Dick S, Fakharzadeh S, et al. Reliability and convergent validity of two outcome instruments for pemphigus. *J Invest Dermatol.* (2009) 129:2404–10. doi: 10.1038/jid.2009.72
24. Hundley JL, Carroll CL, Lang W, Snively B, Yosipovitch G, Feldman SR, et al. Cutaneous symptoms of dermatomyositis significantly impact patients' quality of life. *J Am Acad Dermatol.* (2006) 54:217–20. doi: 10.1016/j.jaad.2004.12.015
25. Heald P, Mehlmauer M, Martin AG, Crowley CA, Yocum RC, Reich SD, et al. Topical bexarotene therapy for patients with refractory or persistent early-stage cutaneous T-cell lymphoma: results of the phase III clinical trial. *J Am Acad Dermatol.* (2003) 49:801–15. doi: 10.1016/S0190-9622(03)01475-0
26. Daniel BS, Hertl M, Werth VP, Eming R, Murrell DF. Severity score indexes for blistering diseases. *Clin Dermatol.* (2012) 30:108–13. doi: 10.1016/j.clindermatol.2011.03.017
27. Ware JE Jr, Sherbourne CD. The MOS 36-item short-form health survey (SF-36). I. Conceptual framework and item selection. *Med Care.* (1992) 30:473–83. doi: 10.1097/00005650-199206000-00002
28. Lewis VAY. Finlay, 10 years experience of the dermatology life quality index (DLQI). *J Investig Dermatol Symp Proc.* (2004) 9:169–80. doi: 10.1111/j.1087-0024.2004.09113.x
29. Gill TM, Feinstein AR. A critical appraisal of the quality of quality-of-life measurements. *JAMA.* (1994) 272:619–26. doi: 10.1001/jama.272.8.619
30. Abeni D, Picardi A, Pasquini P, Melchi CF, Chren MM. Further evidence of the validity and reliability of the Skindex-29: an Italian study on 2,242 dermatological outpatients. *Dermatology.* (2002) 204:43–9. doi: 10.1159/000051809
31. Chen SC. Dermatology quality of life instruments: sorting out the quagmire. *J Invest Dermatol.* (2007) 127:2695–6. doi: 10.1038/sj.jid.5701176
32. Punekar YS, Riley JH, Lloyd E, Driessen M, Singh SJ. Systematic review of the association between exercise tests and patient-reported outcomes in patients with chronic obstructive pulmonary disease. *Int J Chron Obstruct Pulmon Dis.* (2017) 12:2487–506. doi: 10.2147/COPD.S100204
33. Lee PG, Cigolle C, Blaum C. The co-occurrence of chronic diseases and geriatric syndromes: the health and retirement study. *J Am Geriatr Soc.* (2009) 57:511–6. doi: 10.1111/j.1532-5415.2008.02150.x
34. Chren MM, Lasek RJ, Quinn LM, Covinsky KE. Convergent and discriminant validity of a generic and a disease-specific instrument to measure quality of life in patients with skin disease. *J Invest Dermatol.* (1997) 108:103–7. doi: 10.1111/1523-1747.ep12285650
35. Cotell S, Robinson ND, Chan LS. Autoimmune blistering skin diseases. *Am J Emerg Med.* (2000) 18:288–99. doi: 10.1016/S0735-6757(00)90124-4
36. Shimizu T, Takebayashi T, Sato Y, Niizeki H, Aoyama Y, Kitajima Y, et al. Grading criteria for disease severity by pemphigus disease area index. *J Dermatol.* (2014) 41:969–73. doi: 10.1111/1346-8138.12649

14

Role of Regulatory Immune Cells and Molecules in Autoimmune Bullous Dermatoses

Tianyu Cao [1†], *Shuai Shao* [2†], *Hui Fang* [2†], *Bing Li* [2] *and Gang Wang* [2*]

[1] *Department of Dermatology, Tangdu Hospital, Fourth Military Medical University, Xi'an, China,* [2] *Department of Dermatology, Xijing Hospital, Fourth Military Medical University, Xi'an, China*

***Correspondence:**
Gang Wang
xjwgang@fmmu.edu.cn

† These authors have contributed equally to this work

Autoimmune bullous dermatoses (AIBD) include a series of typical organ-specific autoimmune diseases characterized by extensive mucocutaneous blisters. It is generally accepted to be caused by pathological autoantibodies that directly target specific adhesion components of the skin or the adjacent mucous membranes. Both innate and adaptive immune systems are critically involved in the misguided immune response against self-antigens. Recent studies have indicated that the dysfunction of regulatory T cells, regulatory B cells, and complement regulatory proteins that play essential roles in maintaining a healthy immune environment is also closely related to immune disorders in AIBD. It is important to summarize these studies, elucidate the changes in these regulatory immune cells and molecules for the pathogenesis of AIBD, and reveal the mechanisms by which they lose their ability to regulate immune disorders. In this review, we highlight the role of regulatory immune cells and molecules in the pathogenesis of pemphigus vulgaris and bullous pemphigoid, the two most representative forms of AIBD, and indicate issues that should be addressed in future investigations.

Keywords: regulatory T cells, regulatory B cells, complement regulating proteins, pemphigus vulgaris, bullous pemphigoid

INTRODUCTION

The immune system is guided by a series of regulatory mechanisms, the main components of which are a large number of immunoreactive and suppressor cells, that modulate the host response (1). Various immune cells and molecules that have been found to possess a regulatory capacity include regulatory T (Treg) cells, regulatory B (Breg) cells, macrophages, myeloid-derived suppressor cells (MDSCs), dendritic cells (DCs), mesenchymal stromal cells (MSCs), and complement regulatory proteins (CRPs) (2). Alteration or disruption of these immune regulatory mechanisms may lead to the survival and activation of autoreactive lymphocytes upon encountering appropriate self-antigens, which may cause corresponding tissue and organ damage (2). For instance, regulatory immune mechanisms have been implicated in the development of many autoimmune disorders, such as systemic lupus erythematosus (SLE), rheumatoid arthritis, and multiple sclerosis (3–5).

Autoimmune bullous dermatoses (AIBD) include a series of diseases that cause blistering of the skin and mucous membranes through autoantibody attacks on keratinocyte junction structures or on components of the dermal-epidermal junction (6). Based on the location of its formation, AIBD can be divided into two subgroups: pemphigus and pemphigoid diseases (7). Pemphigus diseases are characterized by the production of IgG autoantibodies against keratinocyte adhesion molecules, resulting in intraepidermal blistering, flaccid vesicles, and erosions of the skin and/or mucous membranes. Diseases in this group include pemphigus vulgaris (PV), pemphigus foliaceus, paraneoplastic pemphigus, and IgA pemphigus (6). In contrast, pemphigoid diseases are characterized by autoantibodies that directly attack structural proteins within the dermal-epidermal junction, leading to urticarial lesions, and tense blisters on the skin (8). This group includes bullous pemphigoid (BP), linear IgA bullous dermatosis, dermatitis herpetiformis, mucous membrane pemphigoids, herpes gestationis, and epidermolysis bullosa acquisita (7).

Recent studies have shown several regulatory immune cells and molecules to be involved in the progression of AIBD. In this review, we aim to elucidate the different mechanisms and roles of regulatory immune cells and molecules in AIBD by summarizing and discussing the findings of various clinical and experimental studies, and outline some of the challenges that lie ahead.

CLINICAL PRESENTATION AND PATHOPHYSIOLOGY OF AIBD

Clinical and Immunohistological Features

The pemphigus group of AIBD contains several rare organ specific autoimmune diseases that affect the skin and mucous membranes (9). PV, as the most common representative disease of the pemphigus group (10), is characterized by extremely painful erosions of the mucous membranes, and flaccid blisters localized mainly in the flexural areas, face, scalp, and extremities (**Figures 1A,B**). Typical lesional biopsy specimens of PV show acantholysis, which can progress to the formation of non-inflammatory intraepithelial blisters; however, a few eosinophils or neutrophils can be occasionally seen in the upper dermis and epidermis as well (**Figure 1C**). Meanwhile, direct immunofluorescence (DIF) of perilesional biopsy specimens from patients with PV shows IgG antibodies, and infrequently complement C3 protein, deposits on the surface of keratinocytes (**Figure 1D**). Whereas, DIF of normal skin shows no specific fluorescence (**Supplementary Figure 1**). Indirect immunofluorescence (IIF) using monkey or human normal skin as substrates enables a semiquantitative detection of circulating autoantibodies in serum. And IIF typically shows serum IgG autoantibodies from patients with PV bound to the surface of epithelium (**Figure 1E**).

BP is the most frequently occurring representative of the pemphigoid group, and is clinically characterized by tense, serous, or hemorrhagic bullae on erythematous or apparently normal skin (**Figures 1F,G**). The lesional biopsy specimens of BP typically reveal sub-epidermal blister formation with eosinophil and/or neutrophil-rich inflammatory infiltration in the superficial dermis (**Figure 1H**). In addition, DIF of BP lesions shows the deposits of IgG and/or C3 along the basement membrane zone (BMZ) (**Figure 1I**), and IgA and IgE were occasionally seen in a similar pattern (11). IIF also shows circulating IgG antibodies form patients with BP bound to the dermoepidermal junction (**Figure 1J**).

Genetic Factors

Although the genetic background of AIBD has not been precisely determined, a genetic predisposition in the etiology is evident. The human HLA class I and II molecules play a critical role in the recognition of antigenic peptides by T cells. Several HLA alleles, including HLA-DRB1*0402 (in Jewish people) and HLA-DQB1*0503 (in non-Jewish populations), have been found to be strongly associated with PV (12). Meanwhile, in BP, HLA-DQB1*03:01 is considered the most common HLA class II allele, associated with patients in multiple populations (13–15). Other HLA alleles, such as HLADRB1*04, DRB1*1101, and DQB1*0302, were more frequent in Japanese patients with BP (16), suggesting different HLA class II haplotypes to genetically influence susceptibility to BP across different populations.

Autoantibody Mediated Blister Formation

The binding of autoantibodies to antigens is universally known as the main cause of blister formation in AIBD. The autoantibodies in PV are against the members of cadherin family, desmoglein (Dsg) 1, and Dsg3, which maintain intercellular adhesion in stratified squamous epithelia (17, 18). The main mechanism of blister formation in PV is steric hindrance, since atomic force microscopy experiments had shown that PV IgG can directly inhibit Dsg3-mediated transinteraction (19). Besides this, several cell signaling pathways and factors are also involved in the blister formation in PV, including p38 mitogen-activated protein kinase (MAPK) (20), c-Myc (21), epidermal growth factor receptor (22), caspases (23), and mitochondria (24).

The autoantibodies in BP target two components of the hemidesmosome adhesion complex, BP180 (collagen XVII) and BP230 (dystonin-e), and the non-collagenous 16A (NC16A) domain of BP180 contains the major epitopes recognized by autoreactive T and B cells (25). In contrast to that in PV, the formation of sub-epidermal blisters in BP depends mainly on the autoantibody-induced inflammation, including activation of complement, degranulation of mast cells (MCs), and activation of neutrophils, since the knockdown of C4 (component of classical complement activation pathway), C5aR (expression on MCs), MC protease-4 (homolog of the human MC chymase), and FcγRIII (the main receptor on neutrophils) were, respectively, resistant to anti-BP180 antibody induced blistering in mice (26–30). Besides, neutrophil elastase, matrix metalloproteinase-9, and other proteolytic enzymes released by neutrophils could directly split the epidermis from the dermis (31).

Abbreviations: AIBD, autoimmune bullous dermatoses; ARG1, arginase-1; BP, bullous pemphigoid; Breg cells, regulatory B cells; B10eff cells, functional IL-10-secreting effector B cells; B10pro cells, IL-10-secreting progenitor B cells; CRPs, complement regulatory proteins; CTLA-4, cytotoxic T-lymphocyte associated protein 4; DCs, dendritic cells; DIF, direct immunofluorescence; Dsg, desmoglein; EAE, experimental autoimmune encephalomyelitis; H&E, haematoxylin and eosin; IDO, indoleamine 2,3-dioxygenase; IIF, indirect immunofluorescence; IL, interleukin; IVIG, intravenous immunoglobulin; mAb, monoclonal antibody; BMZ, basement membrane zone; MCs, mast cells; MDSCs, myeloid-derived suppressor cells; MSCs, mesenchymal stromal cells; NC16A, non-collagenous 16A; NK cells, natural killer cells; nTreg cells, natural Treg cells; PV, pemphigus vulgaris; SLE, systemic lupus erythematosus; TGF-β, transforming growth factor-β; TNF-α, tumor necrosis factor-α; Treg cells, regulatory T cells; Tr1 cells, regulatory type 1 cells.

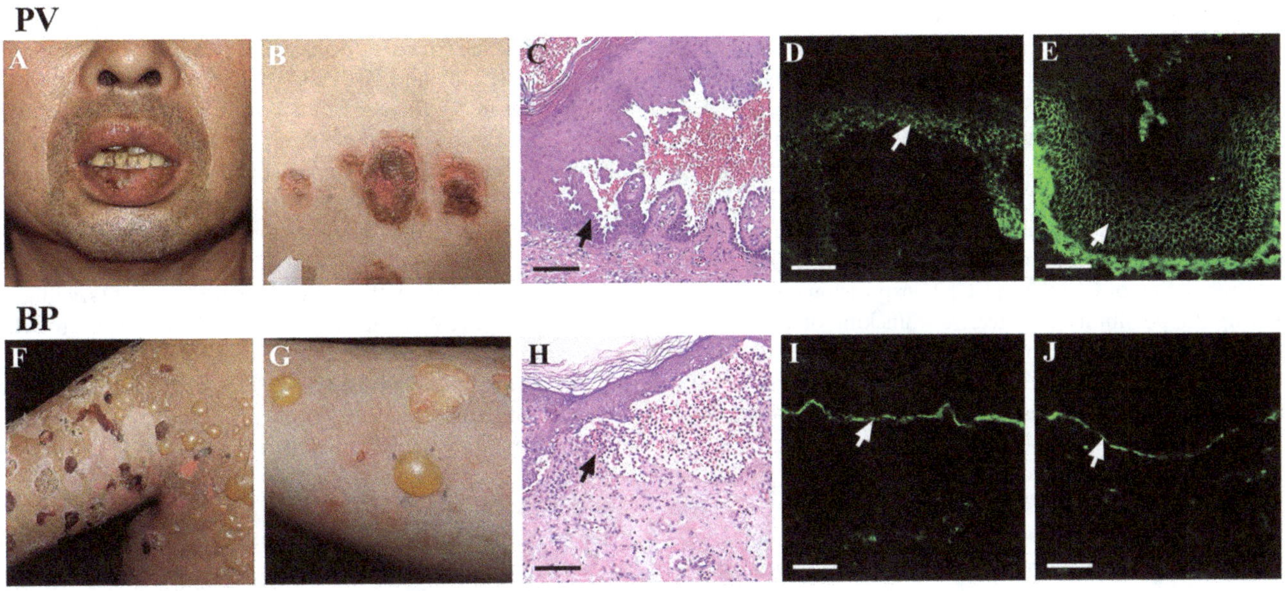

FIGURE 1 | Clinical and immunohistological features of AIBD. AIBD contains two groups: pemphigus group and pemphigoid group. The representative members of these two groups are PV and BP. PV can present with erosions on the mucous membranes **(A)**, and flaccid vesicles or erosion on the skin **(B)**. Haematoxylin and eosin (HandE) staining of PV lesions demonstrates an intraepithelial blister with acantholysis **(C)**. DIF of PV lesions shows IgG antibodies deposit on the surface of keratinocytes **(D)**. IIF using monkey esophagus shows serum IgG autoantibodies from patients with PV bind to the surface of epitheliums **(E)**. Whereas, BP presents with large, tense bullae, and erythematous patches on the skin **(F,G)**. H & E staining of BP lesions reveals an subepidermal blister with eosinophil-rich inflammatory infiltration in the superficial dermis **(H)**. DIF of BP lesions shows IgG antibodies deposit along the dermoepidermal junction **(I)**. IIF using normal skin shows the presence of serum IgG antibodies form BP patients bound to the dermoepidermal junction **(J)**. Bar = 100 μm.

Animal Models

Although no single animal model could completely simulate the entire process of PV and BP, several models have been developed for different areas of research. For PV, passive transfer with circulating IgG antibodies, from patients with PV, could induce a PV-like phenotype in neonatal mice (32), which can be used to study the function of autoantibodies. In addition, adoptive transfer of peripheral lymphocytes from Dsg3$^{-/-}$ mice to Rag-2$^{-/-}$ immunodeficient mice could also develop a PV-like phenotype (33). This model may be used to isolate anti-Dsg3 monoclonal antibodies, investigate the roles of T and B lymphocytes in perpetuating autoantibody production for autoimmune response, and evaluate immunosuppressive therapeutic strategies (34, 35).

On the other hand, passive transfer with IgG autoantibodies from patients with BP could not induce a BP-like disease in animals, since BP autoantibodies reacting with NC16A domain failed to cross-react with mouse BP180. In 1993, Liu et al. had reported an experimental BP model by transferring rabbit anti-mouse BP180 NC14A into neonatal mice, which developed the same clinical, histological, and immunopathological features of BP (36). This model has been widely used to investigate the roles of autoantibodies, complement, MCs, neutrophils, and FcγRs in BP (28, 30, 37). Additionally, in humanized mouse whose murine BP180NC14A is replaced with the homologous human BP180NC16A epitope cluster region, injection of anti-BP180NC16A autoantibodies result in the development of BP-like subepidermal blisters (25).

TREG CELLS IN AIBD

CD4$^+$ CD25^{Bright} FoxP3$^+$ Natural Treg (nTreg) Cells

The pathogenetic progress of AIBD includes a series of immune events, including activation of autoreactive T cells, T–B cell interaction, autoantibody production, and blister formation (38). Recent studies have indicated the involvement of regulatory immune cells and molecules as well in AIBD. Although a wealth of regulatory immune cells have been identified, CD4$^+$ CD25^{bright} FoxP3$^+$ natural Treg (nTreg) cells remain the most extensively studied cell-type (39). In 1995, Sakaguchi et al. firstly reported and defined a subset of CD4$^+$ cells showing stable expression of the lineage-specific transcription factor FoxP3 and high concentrations of the interleukin 2 (IL2) receptor α-chain (CD25) (40). CD4$^+$ CD25^{bright} FoxP3$^+$ Treg cells account for 10% of peripheral CD4$^+$ T cells and demonstrate the suppressing function, both in cell contact-dependent and -independent manner (41). CD4$^+$ CD25^{bright} FoxP3$^+$ Treg cells expressed cytotoxic T-lymphocyte associated protein 4 (CTLA-4), CD25, CD39, and CD73 ectoenzymes, which directly suppressed the production of CD8$^+$ T cells, DCs, myeloid cells, and possibly natural killer (NK) cells (42–44). Moreover, CD4$^+$ CD25^{bright} FoxP3$^+$ Treg cells can also produce a variety of immunomodulatory cytokines, such as IL-10, granzymes, and transforming growth factor-β (TGF-β), which suppress the proinflammatory responses of effector T cells, NK cells, B cells, DCs, and macrophages (45).

nTreg Cells in Pemphigus Vulgaris

The concentration and function of $CD4^+$ $CD25^{bright}$ $FoxP3^+$ Treg cells in patients with PV are abnormal. Sugiyama et al. (46) found that $CD4^+$ Treg cells were remarkably reduced in the blood of patients with PV (46). In addition, $CD4^+$ $CD25^{bright}$ Treg cells in such patients showed significantly higher CD45RO and lower CD45RA expression levels than in normal controls. Moreover, the expression of FoxP3 and CTLA-4 in $CD4^+$ $CD25^{bright}$ Treg cells was significantly down-regulated in patients with PV compared to that in healthy people, along with dysregulation of CCR4 and CCL22 expression (46, 47), thus suggesting the possibility of defective trafficking of Treg cells in skin lesions of patients with PV. Furthermore, the number of $CD4^+$ Treg cells was negatively correlated with that of Th17 cells, which is significantly increased in patients with PV (48). This imbalance might be an important factor in the progression of PV. Importantly, recent studies have indicated that increasing the number of $CD4^+$ $CD25^{bright}$ $FoxP3^+$ Treg cells, by adoptive transfer or use of the super-agonistic anti-CD28 antibody D665, could suppress antibody production in mouse models of PV, whereas depleting them enhanced the autoantibody production in the same model (49, 50). These results suggested that $CD4^+$ $CD25^{bright}$ $FoxP3^+$ Treg cell dysfunction promotes the progression of PV.

However, there have been several studies that showed inconsistent results for the change of nTreg cells after treatment. Bhattacharjee et al. found no obvious changes in $CD4^+$ $CD25^+$ $FoxP3^+$ T cell counts in patients with PV after monotherapy with rituximab, an anti-CD20 monoclonal antibody that could induce B cell depletion and is commonly used in autoimmune diseases (51, 52). El-Zawahry et al. however showed that the circulating $CD4^+$ $CD25^+$ T cells in patients with PV were reduced after treatment with rituximab (53). In several other autoimmune diseases, such as lupus nephritis, idiopathic thrombocytopenic purpura, myasthenia gravis, and rheumatoid arthritis, treatment with rituximab significantly increased the growth of $CD4^+$ $CD25^{bright}$ $FoxP3^+$ Treg cells (54–57). These discrepancies in the results may be due to the limited number of samples, or differences in the pathogenesis of each disease. Therefore, whether nTreg cells function as a therapy against PV is still debatable.

In brief, defects in the growth and function of nTreg cells, not only reduce the excessive response limit of Th cells, but also promote the production of autoantibodies, thus contributing to the development of PV (**Figure 2**). However, the molecular mechanism controlling the suppression of nTreg cells, as well as their therapeutic potential, warrants further investigations.

nTreg Cells in Bullous Pemphigoid

In patients with BP, the number of $CD4^+$ $CD25^{bright}$ $FoxP3^+$ Treg cells was found to be significantly reduced, both in the blood and skin (58, 59). In addition, the function of $CD4^+$ $CD25^{bright}$ $FoxP3^+$ Treg cells in BP has also been found to be abnormal. For instance, a study had shown that scurfy mice, which carry *FoxP3* gene mutations, lacked functional Treg cells, displayed severe erosive skin lesions similar to that in BP, and produced autoantibodies targeting murine BP230 and BP180. Moreover, the transfer of CD4+ T cells from scurfy mice to immunodeficient mice induced the expression of autoantibodies targeting BP230 and BP180, and this phenomenon was ameliorated in *STAT6* gene knockout mice (60). An additional study had discovered that the formation of sub-epidermal blisters in scurfy mice is caused by the monoclonal antibody (mAb) 20B12, which could cross-react with human BP230 (61). These studies together suggest that the absence of $FoxP3^+$ Treg cells leads to the BP phenotype in mice by inducing the expression of pathogenic autoantibodies targeting BP antigens (**Figure 2**). Further research is required to clarify the immunological mechanisms controlling the inhibition of autoantibody production by $CD4^+$ Treg cells and to understand why this function is lost in BP.

Another study had shown that $CD25^{high}$ Treg cells were in similar proportions to that of $CD4^+$ T cells in BP and healthy blood, and that the ability of $CD4^+$ $CD25^{high}$ Treg cells to suppress T cell proliferation and interferon-γ (IFN-γ) secretion in patients with BP was similar to that in normal individuals (62). Although the results seemed to be contradictory, CD4 and CD25, by themselves, are not sufficient to identify Treg cells. $CD4^+$ $CD25^{bright}$ cells may represent not only Treg cells, but also $FoxP3^-$activated T cells. The inconsistent results may have been caused by the different phenotypes of Treg cells.

Induced Treg (iTreg) Cells

Besides thymus-derived $FoxP3^+$ nTreg cells, there are several other types of Treg cells that can be induced from peripheral naive T lymphocytes in the periphery, including $FoxP3^+$ iTreg cells (63), IL-10-producing T regulatory type 1 (Tr1) cells (64), TGF-β-secreting Th3 cells (65), and B-cell-induced $Foxp3^-$ regulatory T cells (Treg-of-B cells) (66). Among them, Tr1 cells are the most extensively studied type. Tr1 cells were first reported in 1997 and could produce high levels of IL-10 and TGF-β, which played a key role in suppressing antigen-specific T cell responses (67).

Veldman et al. had shown that Dsg3-responsive Tr1 cells, isolated from healthy carriers of two PV-associated HLA class II alleles (DRB1*0402 and DQB1*0503), were present in significantly higher proportions than in patients with PV. This population of cells secreted IL-10, TGF-β, and IL-5 in response to Dsg-3, and inhibited the proliferation of Dsg3-reactive Th cells (68). The Dsg3-responsive Tr1 cells could be divided into two subpopulations based on their cell size and granularity. The smaller subset expressed FoxP3 and secreted IL-10 and TGF-β in response to Dsg3 stimulation. The larger subset, on the other hand, did not express FoxP3, exhibited a Th cell-like phenotype, and secreted IL-2 (69) (**Figure 2**). Inhibition of *FoxP3* mRNA in Tr1, using antisense oligonucleotides resulted in the cells showing features similar to those of Th2 cells, such as the secretion of IL-2 and loss of anergy in response to Dsg3 antigen stimulation (70). After treatment with rituximab, the mean count of Tr1 cells increased in 2 weeks, and gradually declined over the remaining period (51). In summary, alterations in the growth and function of Dsg3- responsive Tr1 cells in

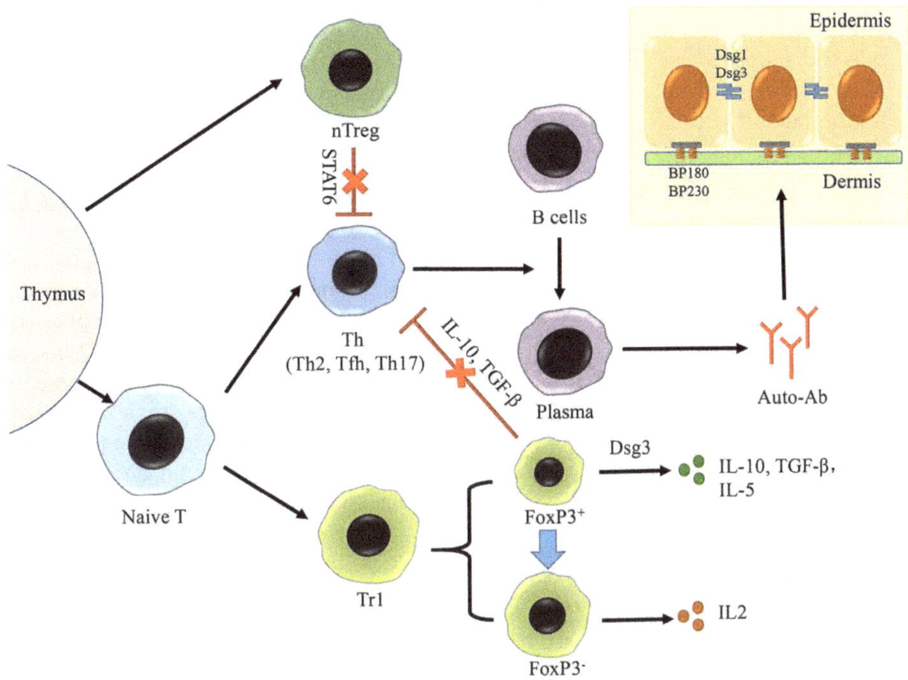

FIGURE 2 | Role of treg cells in AIBD. The production of autoantibodies by plasma cells is the crucial process in the pathogenesis of both PV and BP, in which Th–B cell interaction plays an important role. Treg cells can be divided into two groups: nTreg cells and iTreg cells. nTreg cells number is decreased in PV, which have a negative correlation with Th17 cells. nTreg cells could suppress the functions of Th2 and Tfh cells on activing B cells in an STAT6-dependent manner, but they lost this function in BP. Additionally, Tr1 cells, the most intensively studied cell type of iTreg cells, could be divided into two subpopulations based on the cell size and granularity in PV. The smaller subset achieves the suppressing function by secreting IL-10, TGF-β in response to Dsg3. The larger subset loses the ability in response to Dsg3, exhibits a Th cell-like phenotype, and secretes IL-2.

PV, as well as their inhibitory effect on Th cells, indicate their relevance in PV pathogenesis. Future studies should focus on the underlying mechanisms controlling phenotypic changes in Tr1 cells during PV pathogenesis, and the development of related PV treatment strategies.

Not enough evidence in AIBD accounts for the changes in other iTreg cell subsets. One study had shown that the proportion of TGF-β-secreting Th3 cells did not change in PV cases compared to that in normal individuals, although there was an increase in the mean value at 14 weeks after treatment with rituximab (51). Since the phenotypic identification on Treg cells has long been inconsistent, reliability of some studies of Treg cells remains debatable. Future studies should be based on the improved classification and identification of Treg cell subsets to further determine the changes in number and function of these cell subsets in AIBD.

CD8^{+} Treg Cells

While CD4^{+} Treg cells have attracted much attention for their important role in the regulation of immune homeostasis, recent findings have also identified a subset of CD8^{+} T cells with immunoregulatory functions, known as CD8^{+} Treg cells (71–73). Till date, three subsets of CD8^{+} Treg cells have been identified: CD8^{+} CD25^{+} T cells, CD8^{+} CD122^{+} T cells, and CD8^{+} CXCR3^{+} T cells. CD8^{+} CD25^{+} Treg cells express surface CTLA-4 and GITR, as well as intracellular FoxP3, similar to that observed in CD4^{+} Treg cells (74). Meanwhile, CD8^{+}CD25^{+} Treg cells could directly contact CD4^{+} CD25^{-} T cells and down-regulate the expression of IL-2Rα, thus suppressing the growth of target cells (74, 75). In addition, human CD8^{+} CXCR3^{+} T cells were found to suppress the expression of IFN-γ in immune cells by secreting IL-10, similar to the observed mechanism in murine CD8^{+} CD122^{+} Treg cells (76–78). CD8^{+} FoxP3^{+} Treg cells were also found to play an important role in the up-regulation of FoxP3 and proliferation of CD4^{+} CD25^{+} Treg cells (79). Although an association between CD8^{+} Treg cells and several autoimmune diseases, such as SLE and experimental autoimmune encephalomyelitis (EAE) has been identified (80, 81), evidence linking CD8^{+} Treg cells to AIBD is still lacking.

BREG CELLS IN AIBD

Breg cells were first identified as a subset of IL-10-producing B cells, and were first described by Mizoguchi and Bhan (82). The exact surface markers present in human Breg cells remain unclear. Different B cell subsets in circulation have suppressive regulatory functions that are dependent on IL-10, namely CD19^{+} CD24^{high} CD38^{high} Breg cells, CD19^{+} CD24^{high} CD27^{+} Breg cells, and CD25^{high} CD27^{high} CD86^{high} CD1^{high} Breg cells (83–85). Recently, other Breg subsets, known as TGF-β- expressing

Breg cells, have also been identified (86). In autoimmune diseases, such as SLE, multiple sclerosis, lupus nephritis, and type 1 diabetes mellitus, Breg cells are found to be dysfunctional in terms of immune suppression, leading to the breakdown of self-tolerance (87–92). In addition, adoptive transfer of Breg cells ameliorated inflammatory symptoms in animal models of many autoimmune diseases, including SLE, type I diabetes, and contact hypersensitivity (93–96).

Breg Cells in Pemphigus Vulgaris

Activated B cells are generally considered to be pathogenic regulators in patients with PV via the secretion of autoantibodies targeting Dsg3 (97). However, little attention has been paid to the function of Breg cells in the pathogenesis of PV. Several studies have shown that the frequency of $CD19^{+}$ $CD24^{high}$ $CD38^{high}$ Breg cells is significantly increased in the blood of patients with PV compared to that in healthy individuals, both in the active group and in remittent group (98, 99). Breg cells from patients with PV displayed impaired IL-10 expression, even when they were activated over a longer period of time, compared to the healthy Breg cells (98). Therefore, the Breg cells in PV did not directly regulate the humoral response, and rather lost their ability to down-regulate the production of IFN-γ in $CD4^{+}$ T cells (**Figure 3**). In addition, after being treated with rituximab or intravenous immunoglobulin (IVIG), patients with PV, showing complete remission, had a significantly higher proportion of IL-10-secreting Breg cells and increased levels of IL-10 compared to those who showed no response and incomplete remission (100, 101). Maturation of IL-10-secreting progenitor B ($B10_{pro}$) cells into functional IL-10-secreting effector B ($B10_{eff}$) cells has been confirmed to require IL-21- and CD40-dependent cognate interactions with T cells (102) (**Figure 3**). Whether patient-derived B10 cells in PV display a defective interaction with T cells, or fail to respond to IL-21 cytokines warrants further investigation.

Breg Cells in Bullous Pemphigoid

In 2007, Kabuto et al. had found no significant difference in the frequencies of $CD19^{+}$ $CD24^{high}$ $CD38^{high}$ B cells between patients with BP and healthy controls (99). However, in our recent research, we found the frequency of circulating $CD19^{+}$ $CD24^{high}$ $CD27^{+}$ Breg cells and IL-$10^{+}CD19^{+}$ Breg cells to be increased in patients with BP. In addition, these patient-derived Breg cells displayed impaired function regarding suppression of $CD4^{+}$ T cell activation and autoantibody production, despite secreting high levels of tumor necrosis factor-α (TNF-α) and IFN-γ (**Figure 3**). Moreover, the TNF inhibitor etanercept could inhibit autoantibody production *in vitro* (103). According to our results, Breg cells in patients with BP displayed increased production of inflammatory cytokines (mainly TNF-α). Although there is an apparent inconsistency between the pro-inflammatory phenotype and weaker immunosuppressive function of Breg cells in patients with BP, recent studies have proposed immunosuppression not be controlled by a devoted Breg cell lineage with a specific phenotype; rather, it is rather the result of a dynamic balance between multiple B cell subsets and other cells within the immune system (104). Therefore, functional flexibility of the Breg subset may be responsible for the difference in phenotypic vs. functional observations. Further analysis of the Breg phenotype will improve our understanding of its role in BP, and animal models should also be used to study the function of Breg cells in AIBD.

OTHER REGULATORY CELLS

In addition to the cells described above, there are several other cells that have been reported to possess immunomodulatory functions, including DCs, macrophages, MDSCs, and MSCs. Function of DCs is related to their maturation state: immature DCs promote tolerogenic response by expressing anti-inflammatory molecules, such as IL-10 and TGF-β, whereas mature DCs promote immunogenic responses (105, 106). In addition, macrophages can be divided into three populations: classically activated macrophages, wound-healing macrophages, and regulatory macrophages (107). Regulatory macrophages produce high levels of IL-10 and low levels of IL-12, thereby dampening the immune response and limiting inflammation (108, 109). Moreover, MDSCs could also produce a large array of anti-inflammatory molecules, including arginase-1 (ARG1), TGF-β, IL-10, and indoleamine 2,3-dioxygenase (IDO), and have the ability of suppressing T cell response and promoting the functions of Treg cells (110–112). Furthermore, MSCs have been proven to have immunoregulatory effect on innate (NK cells) and adaptive immune system (DCs, B cells, and T cells) by cellular contact and/or secretion of regulatory molecules, such as TGF-β1, HGF, IDO, Prostaglandin E2, and IL-10 (113–116). MSCs also possess the ability to promote the function of Treg cells, including $CD4^{+}$ $CD25^{bright}$ $FoxP3^{+}$ Treg cells and Tr1 cells (117).

Taken together, besides the Treg and Breg cells, many other kinds of cells also have regulatory functions on immune system, and are related to the pathology and/or treatment of autoimmune diseases. However, little is known about the role of these cells in AIBD. One case report had shown CTLA4-overexpressing adipose tissue-derived MSCs transplantation could improve the clinical symptoms of a dog with pemphigus foliaceus (118), suggesting the therapeutic potential of these regulatory cells in AIBD. Further studies are recommended to investigate the roles of these regulatory cells in AIBD, as well as for its treatment.

COMPLEMENT REGULATORY PROTEINS IN AIBD

CRPs refer to an important class of regulatory proteins in the complement system that controls enzymatic cascades, assembly of the membrane attack complex, and homeostasis of the complement system (119, 120); they include CD55 (decay accelerating factor), CD59 (membrane inhibitor of reactive lysis; MIRL), CD35 (type 1 complement receptor; CR1), and CD46 (membrane cofactor protein; MCP). Since the over-activation of the complement system could injure the host, effectors of complement activation need to be tightly

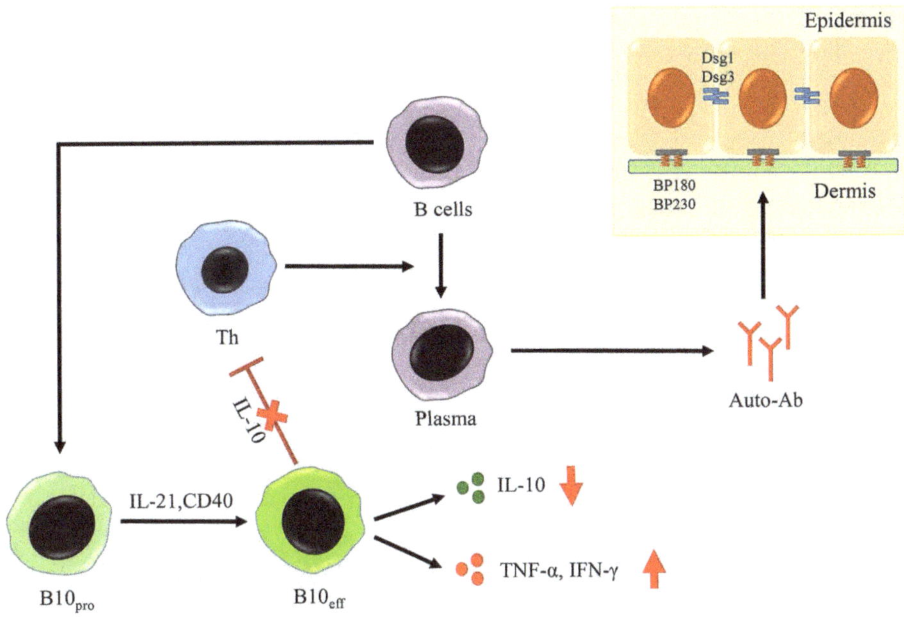

FIGURE 3 | Role of Breg cells in AIBD. The maturation of $B10_{pro}$ cells into $B10_{eff}$ cells requires IL-21- and CD40-dependent cognate interactions with T cells. In PV, $B10_{eff}$ cells is impaired in the functions of secreting IL-10 and down-regulating the production of IFN-γ in $CD4^+$ T cells. Moreover, Breg cells from BP patients acquire the function of producing TNF-α and IFN-γ, two important inflammatory cytokines in the pathogenesis of BP.

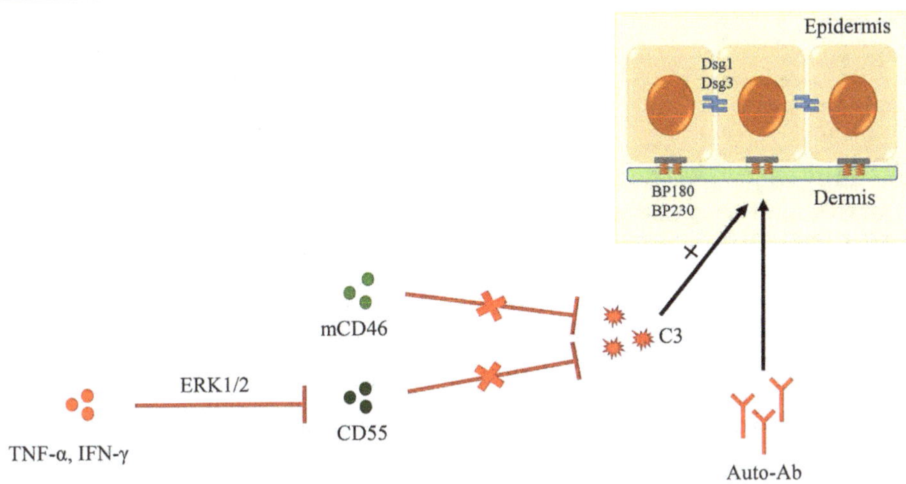

FIGURE 4 | Role of CRPs in AIBD. Complement activation is one of the pivotal steps in BP development. mCD46 and CD55, two important CRPs, could inhibit autoantibody-mediated complement activation. Additionally, CD55 is down-regulated by TNF-α and IFN-γ though ERK1/2 signaling pathway in BP lesions.

regulated by complement regulatory proteins to maintain the balance between efficient destruction of harmful factors and unwanted over-activation of host tissue (121). Dysregulation of these proteins is related to many autoimmune diseases, including SLE, autoimmune hemocytopenias, and rheumatoid arthritis (122–126).

Although DIF studies of patients with PV often show C3 deposits at the keratinocyte surface, blister formation in PV has been proven to be independent of complement (127). Complement activation via the classical pathway is one of the pivotal steps in BP development (27). However, little is known about the role and mechanism of CRPs in BP. In our latest study, we examined the role of CD46 and CD55 in the pathogenesis of BP; results showed that sCD46 was up-regulated in both serum and blister fluid of the patients, and that its expression was positively correlated with the levels of anti-BP180 antibody and C3a. Importantly, the levels of mCD46 and CD55 were decreased in skin lesions of patients with BP. While the depletion of CD46 or CD55 enhanced C3 deposition and autoantibody-mediated complement activation, exogenous CD46 or CD55 significantly inhibited this phenomenon (128, 129) (**Figure 4**). These data suggested CD46 and CD55 to be key inhibitors of complement activation and that their down-regulation is involved in the pathogenesis of BP.

CONCLUSION

According to the previous results and our recent investigations, it is clear that the components of immunoregulatory system, including Treg cells, Breg cells, and CRPs, are important for the development of autoimmune disorders in AIBD. Recently, pharmacological approaches targeting Treg cells to restore their impaired function have been considered viable therapeutic methods for some autoimmune diseases (130–133), clarifying the importance of immunoregulatory system in the pathogenesis of these diseases, and showing the latent capacity of regulatory immune cells and molecules in these diseases. However, present studies have relied on the identification of changes in cell counts and functions, without exploring its role in disease development and treatment of AIBD in depth. Since the animal models of AIBD have been well-developed, more studies based on animal models would be required to expound the role and possible therapeutic applications of these cells and molecules in AIBD. Studies exploiting their suppressive characteristics should also be carefully designed to obtain maximum clinical benefits.

ETHICS STATEMENT

All the patients gave written informed consent for the publication of the pictures.

AUTHOR CONTRIBUTIONS

TC and GW conceived the idea. TC, SS, HF, and BL contributed to the writing of the manuscript. TC contributed to figure preparation for the manuscript.

ACKNOWLEDGMENTS

We would like to thank Yu Ye, Juan Guo, Meihong Yu, and Wenjing Li for their help with histological analysis.

REFERENCES

1. Zhang Q, Vignali DA. Co-stimulatory and co-inhibitory pathways in autoimmunity. *Immunity.* (2016) 44:1034–51. doi: 10.1016/j.immuni.2016.04.017
2. Papp G, Boros P, Nakken B, Szodoray P, Zeher M. Regulatory immune cells and functions in autoimmunity and transplantation immunology. *Autoimmun Rev.* (2017) 16:435–44. doi: 10.1016/j.autrev.2017.03.011
3. Kleinewietfeld M, Hafler DA. Regulatory T cells in autoimmune neuroinflammation. *Immunol Rev.* (2014) 259:231–44. doi: 10.1111/imr.12169
4. Komatsu N, Takayanagi H. Regulatory T cells in Arthritis. *Prog Mol Biol Transl Sci.* (2015) 136:207–15. doi: 10.1016/bs.pmbts.2015.07.021
5. Tao JH, Cheng M, Tang JP, Liu Q, Pan F, Li XP. Foxp3, regulatory T cell, and autoimmune diseases. *Inflammation.* (2017) 40:328–39. doi: 10.1007/s10753-016-0470-8
6. Schmidt E, Zillikens D. Modern diagnosis of autoimmune blistering skin diseases. *Autoimmun Rev.* (2010) 10:84–9. doi: 10.1016/j.autrev.2010.08.007
7. Baum S, Sakka N, Artsi O, Trau H, Barzilai A. Diagnosis and classification of autoimmune blistering diseases. *Autoimmun Rev.* (2014) 13:482–9. doi: 10.1016/j.autrev.2014.01.047
8. Schmidt E, Zillikens D. Pemphigoid diseases. *Lancet.* (2013) 381:320–32. doi: 10.1016/S0140-6736(12)61140-4
9. Kridin K. Pemphigus group: overview, epidemiology, mortality, and comorbidities. *Immunol Res.* (2018) 66:255–70. doi: 10.1007/s12026-018-8986-7
10. Kasperkiewicz M, Ellebrecht CT, Takahashi H, Yamagami J, Zillikens D, Payne AS, et al. Pemphigus. *Nat Rev Dis Primers.* (2017) 3:17026. doi: 10.1038/nrdp.2017.26
11. Bagci IS, Horvath ON, Ruzicka T, Sardy M. Bullous pemphigoid. *Autoimmun Rev.* (2017) 16:445–55. doi: 10.1016/j.autrev.2017.03.010
12. Yan L, Wang JM, Zeng K. Association between HLA-DRB1 polymorphisms and pemphigus vulgaris: a meta-analysis. *Br J Dermatol.* (2012) 167:768–77. doi: 10.1111/j.1365-2133.2012.11040.x
13. Banfield CC, Wojnarowska F, Allen J, George S, Venning VA, Welsh KI. The association of HLA-DQ7 with bullous pemphigoid is restricted to men. *Br J Dermatol.* (1998) 138:1085–90
14. Esmaili N, Mortazavi H, Chams-Davatchi C, Daneshpazhooh M, Damavandi MR, Aryanian Z, et al. Association between HLA-DQB1*03:01 and Bullous pemphigoid in Iranian patients. *Iran J Immunol.* (2013) 10:1–9.
15. Chagury AA, Sennes LU, Gil JM, Kalil J, Rodrigues H, Rosales CB, et al. HLA-C*17, DQB1*03:01, DQA1*01:03 and DQA1*05:05 alleles associated to bullous pemphigoid in brazilian population. *Ann Dermatol.* (2018) 30:8–12. doi: 10.5021/ad.2018.30.1.8
16. Okazaki A, Miyagawa S, Yamashina Y, Kitamura W, Shirai T. Polymorphisms of HLA-DR and -DQ genes in Japanese patients with bullous pemphigoid. *J Dermatol.* (2000) 27:149–56. doi: 10.1111/j.1346-8138.2000.tb02141.x
17. Bystryn JC, Rudolph JL. Pemphigus. *Lancet.* (2005) 366:61–73. doi: 10.1016/S0140-6736(05)66829-8
18. Spindler V, Waschke J. Pemphigus-a disease of desmosome dysfunction caused by multiple mechanisms. *Front Immunol.* (2018) 9:136. doi: 10.3389/fimmu.2018.00136
19. Heupel WM, Zillikens D, Drenckhahn D, Waschke J. Pemphigus vulgaris IgG directly inhibit desmoglein 3-mediated transinteraction. *J Immunol.* (2008) 181:1825–34. doi: 10.4049/jimmunol.181.3.1825
20. Mao X, Sano Y, Park JM, Payne AS. p38 MAPK activation is downstream of the loss of intercellular adhesion in pemphigus vulgaris. *J Biol Chem.* (2011) 286:1283–91. doi: 10.1074/jbc.M110.172874
21. Williamson L, Hunziker T, Suter MM, Muller EJ. Nuclear c-Myc: a molecular marker for early stage pemphigus vulgaris. *J Invest Dermatol.* (2007) 127:1549–55. doi: 10.1038/sj.jid.5700735
22. Bektas M, Jolly PS, Berkowitz P, Amagai M, Rubenstein DS. A pathophysiologic role for epidermal growth factor receptor in pemphigus acantholysis. *J Biol Chem.* (2013) 288:9447–56. doi: 10.1074/jbc.M112.438010
23. Li N, Zhao M, Wang J, Liu Z, Diaz LA. Involvement of the apoptotic mechanism in pemphigus foliaceus autoimmune injury of the skin. *J Immunol.* (2009) 182:711–7. doi: 10.4049/jimmunol.182.1.711

24. Chen Y, Chernyavsky A, Webber RJ, Grando SA, Wang PH. Critical role of the neonatal Fc receptor (FcRn) in the pathogenic action of antimitochondrial autoantibodies synergizing with anti-desmoglein autoantibodies in pemphigus vulgaris. *J Biol Chem.* (2015) 290:23826–37. doi: 10.1074/jbc.M115.668061
25. Liu Z, Sui W, Zhao M, Li Z, Li N, Thresher R, et al. Subepidermal blistering induced by human autoantibodies to BP180 requires innate immune players in a humanized bullous pemphigoid mouse model. *J Autoimmun.* (2008) 31:331–8. doi: 10.1016/j.jaut.2008.08.009
26. Chen R, Ning G, Zhao ML, Fleming MG, Diaz LA, Werb Z, et al. Mast cells play a key role in neutrophil recruitment in experimental bullous pemphigoid. *J Clin Invest.* (2001) 108:1151–8. doi: 10.1172/JCI11494
27. Nelson KC, Zhao M, Schroeder PR, Li N, Wetsel RA, Diaz LA, et al. Role of different pathways of the complement cascade in experimental bullous pemphigoid. *J Clin Invest.* (2006) 116:2892–900. doi: 10.1172/JCI17891
28. Zhao M, Trimbeger ME, Li N, Diaz LA, Shapiro SD, Liu Z. Role of FcRs in animal model of autoimmune bullous pemphigoid. *J Immunol.* (2006) 177:3398–405. doi: 10.4049/jimmunol.177.5.3398
29. Heimbach L, Li Z, Berkowitz P, Zhao M, Li N, Rubenstein DS, et al. The C5a receptor on mast cells is critical for the autoimmune skin-blistering disease bullous pemphigoid. *J Biol Chem.* (2011) 286:15003–9. doi: 10.1074/jbc.M111.221036
30. Lin L, Bankaitis E, Heimbach L, Li N, Abrink M, Pejler G, et al. Dual targets for mouse mast cell protease-4 in mediating tissue damage in experimental bullous pemphigoid. *J Biol Chem.* (2011) 286:37358–67. doi: 10.1074/jbc.M111.272401
31. Liu Z, Zhou X, Shapiro SD, Shipley JM, Twining SS, Diaz LA, et al. The serpin alpha1-proteinase inhibitor is a critical substrate for gelatinase B/MMP-9 *in vivo*. *Cell.* (2000) 102:647–55. doi: 10.1016/s0092-8674(00)00087-8
32. Anhalt GJ, Labib RS, Voorhees JJ, Beals TF, Diaz LA. Induction of pemphigus in neonatal mice by passive transfer of IgG from patients with the disease. *N Engl J Med.* (1982) 306:1189–96. doi: 10.1056/NEJM198205203062001
33. Amagai M, Tsunoda K, Suzuki H, Nishifuji K, Koyasu S, Nishikawa T. Use of autoantigen-knockout mice in developing an active autoimmune disease model for pemphigus. *J Clin Invest.* (2000) 105:625–31. doi: 10.1172/JCI8748
34. Takahashi H, Amagai M, Nishikawa T, Fujii Y, Kawakami Y, Kuwana M. Novel system evaluating in vivo pathogenicity of desmoglein 3-reactive T cell clones using murine pemphigus vulgaris. *J Immunol.* (2008) 181:1526–35. doi: 10.4049/jimmunol.181.2.1526
35. Takae Y, Nishikawa T, Amagai M. Pemphigus mouse model as a tool to evaluate various immunosuppressive therapies. *Exp Dermatol.* (2009) 18:252–60. doi: 10.1111/j.1600-0625.2008.00776.x
36. Liu Z, Diaz LA, Troy JL, Taylor AF, Emery DJ, Fairley JA, et al. A passive transfer model of the organ-specific autoimmune disease, bullous pemphigoid, using antibodies generated against the hemidesmosomal antigen, BP180. *J Clin Invest.* (1993) 92:2480–8. doi: 10.1172/JCI116856
37. Lessey E, Li N, Diaz L, Liu Z. Complement and cutaneous autoimmune blistering diseases. *Immunol Res.* (2008) 41:223–32. doi: 10.1007/s12026-008-8028-y
38. Hammers CM, Stanley JR. Mechanisms of disease: pemphigus and bullous pemphigoid. *Annu Rev Pathol.* (2016) 11:175–97. doi: 10.1146/annurev-pathol-012615-044313
39. Plitas G, Rudensky AY. Regulatory T cells: differentiation and function. *Cancer Immunol Res.* (2016) 4:721–5. doi: 10.1158/2326-6066.CIR-16-0193
40. Sakaguchi S, Sakaguchi N, Asano M, Itoh M, Toda M. Immunologic self-tolerance maintained by activated T cells expressing IL-2 receptor alpha-chains (CD25). Breakdown of a single mechanism of self-tolerance causes various autoimmune diseases. *J Immunol.* (1995) 155:1151–64.
41. Sakaguchi S. Naturally arising Foxp3-expressing $CD25^+CD4^+$ regulatory T cells in immunological tolerance to self and non-self. *Nat Immunol.* (2005) 6:345–52. doi: 10.1038/ni1178
42. Wing K, Onishi Y, Prieto-Martin P, Yamaguchi T, Miyara M, Fehervari Z, et al. CTLA-4 control over $Foxp3^+$ regulatory T cell function. *Science.* (2008) 322:271–5. doi: 10.1126/science.1160062
43. Levine AG, Arvey A, Jin W, Rudensky AY. Continuous requirement for the TCR in regulatory T cell function. *Nat Immunol.* (2014) 15:1070–8. doi: 10.1038/ni.3004
44. Chinen T, Kannan AK, Levine AG, Fan X, Klein U, Zheng Y, et al. An essential role for the IL-2 receptor in Treg cell function. *Nat Immunol.* (2016) 17:1322–33. doi: 10.1038/ni.3540
45. Galgani M, De Rosa V, La Cava A, Matarese G. Role of Metabolism in the Immunobiology of Regulatory T Cells. *J Immunol.* (2016) 197:2567–75. doi: 10.4049/jimmunol.1600242
46. Sugiyama H, Matsue H, Nagasaka A, Nakamura Y, Tsukamoto K, Shibagaki N, et al. $CD4^+CD25^{high}$ regulatory T cells are markedly decreased in blood of patients with pemphigus vulgaris. *Dermatology.* (2007) 214:210–20. doi: 10.1159/000099585
47. Asothai R, Anand V, Das D, Antil PS, Khandpur S, Sharma VK, et al. Distinctive Treg associated CCR4-CCL22 expression profile with altered frequency of Th17/Treg cell in the immunopathogenesis of Pemphigus Vulgaris. *Immunobiology.* (2015) 220:1129–35. doi: 10.1016/j.imbio.2015.06.008
48. Xu RC, Zhu HQ, Li WP, Zhao XQ, Yuan HJ, Zheng J, et al. The imbalance of Th17 and regulatory T cells in pemphigus patients. *Eur J Dermatol.* (2013) 23:795–802. doi: 10.1684/ejd.2013.2177
49. Yokoyama T, Matsuda S, Takae Y, Wada N, Nishikawa T, Amagai M, et al. Antigen-independent development of $Foxp3^+$ regulatory T cells suppressing autoantibody production in experimental pemphigus vulgaris. *Int Immunol.* (2011) 23:365–73. doi: 10.1093/intimm/dxr020
50. Schmidt T, Willenborg S, Hunig T, Deeg CA, Sonderstrup G, Hertl M, et al. Induction of T regulatory cells by the superagonistic anti-CD28 antibody D665 leads to decreased pathogenic IgG autoantibodies against desmoglein 3 in a HLA-transgenic mouse model of pemphigus vulgaris. *Exp Dermatol.* (2016) 25:293–8. doi: 10.1111/exd.12919
51. Bhattacharjee R, De D, Handa S, Minz RW, Saikia B, Joshi N. Assessment of the effects of rituximab monotherapy on different subsets of circulating T-regulatory cells and clinical disease severity in severe pemphigus vulgaris. *Dermatology.* (2016) 232:572–7. doi: 10.1159/000448031
52. Franks SE, Getahun A, Hogarth PM, Cambier JC. Targeting B cells in treatment of autoimmunity. *Curr Opin Immunol.* (2016) 43:39–45. doi: 10.1016/j.coi.2016.09.003
53. El-Zawahry B, Bassiouny D, Hegazy R, Gawdat H, Shalaby S, Khorshied M, et al. Rituximab treatment in pemphigus vulgaris: effect on circulating Tregs. *Arch Dermatol Res.* (2017) 309:551–6. doi: 10.1007/s00403-017-1754-z
54. Cao D, Malmstrom V, Baecher-Allan C, Hafler D, Klareskog L, Trollmo C. Isolation and functional characterization of regulatory $CD25^{bright}CD4^+$ T cells from the target organ of patients with rheumatoid arthritis. *Eur J Immunol.* (2003) 33:215–23. doi: 10.1002/immu.200390024
55. Vigna-Perez M, Hernandez-Castro B, Paredes-Saharopulos O, Portales-Perez D, Baranda L, Abud-Mendoza C, et al. Clinical and immunological effects of Rituximab in patients with lupus nephritis refractory to conventional therapy: a pilot study. *Arthritis Res Ther.* (2006) 8:R83. doi: 10.1186/ar1954
56. Stasi R, Cooper N, Del Poeta G, Stipa E, Laura Evangelista M, Abruzzese E, et al. Analysis of regulatory T-cell changes in patients with idiopathic thrombocytopenic purpura receiving B cell-depleting therapy with rituximab. *Blood.* (2008) 112:1147–50. doi: 10.1182/blood-2007-12-1 29262
57. Catzola V, Battaglia A, Buzzonetti A, Fossati M, Scuderi F, Fattorossi A, et al. Changes in regulatory T cells after rituximab in two patients with refractory myasthenia gravis. *J Neurol.* (2013) 260:2163–5. doi: 10.1007/s00415-013-6987-y
58. Quaglino P, Antiga E, Comessatti A, Caproni M, Nardo T, Ponti R, et al. Circulating $CD4^+$ $CD25brightFOXP3^+$ regulatory T-cells are significantly reduced in bullous pemphigoid patients. *Arch Dermatol Res.* (2012) 304:639–45. doi: 10.1007/s00403-012-1213-9
59. Antiga E, Quaglino P, Volpi W, Pierini I, Del Bianco E, Bianchi B, et al. Regulatory T cells in skin lesions and blood of patients with bullous pemphigoid. *J Eur Acad Dermatol Venereol.* (2014) 28:222–30. doi: 10.1111/jdv.12091
60. Muramatsu K, Ujiie H, Kobayashi I, Nishie W, Izumi K, Ito T, et al. Regulatory T-cell dysfunction induces autoantibodies to bullous pemphigoid antigens in mice and human subjects. *J Allergy Clin Immunol.* (2018) 142:1818–1830.e6. doi: 10.1016/j.jaci.2018.03.014

61. Haeberle S, Wei X, Bieber K, Goletz S, Ludwig RJ, Schmidt E, et al. Regulatory T-cell deficiency leads to pathogenic bullous pemphigoid antigen 230 autoantibody and autoimmune bullous disease. *J Allergy Clin Immunol.* (2018) 142:1831–1842.e7. doi: 10.1016/j.jaci.2018.04.006
62. Rensing-Ehl A, Gaus B, Bruckner-Tuderman L, Martin SF. Frequency, function and CLA expression of $CD4^+CD25^+FOXP3^+$ regulatory T cells in bullous pemphigoid. *Exp Dermatol.* (2007) 16:13–21. doi: 10.1111/j.1600-0625.2006.00522.x
63. Curotto de Lafaille MA, Lafaille JJ. Natural and adaptive $foxp3^+$ regulatory T cells: more of the same or a division of labor? *Immunity.* (2009) 30:626–35. doi: 10.1016/j.immuni.2009.05.002
64. Roncarolo MG, Gregori S, Battaglia M, Bacchetta R, Fleischhauer K, Levings MK. Interleukin-10-secreting type 1 regulatory T cells in rodents and humans. *Immunol Rev.* (2006) 212:28–50. doi: 10.1111/j.0105-2896.2006.00420.x
65. Weiner HL. Induction and mechanism of action of transforming growth factor-beta-secreting Th3 regulatory cells. *Immunol Rev.* (2001) 182:207–14. doi: 10.1034/j.1600-065X.2001.1820117.x
66. Chien CH, Chiang BL. Regulatory T cells induced by B cells: a novel subpopulation of regulatory T cells. *J Biomed Sci.* (2017) 24:86. doi: 10.1186/s12929-017-0391-3
67. Groux H, O'Garra A, Bigler M, Rouleau M, Antonenko S, de Vries JE, et al. A $CD4^+$ T-cell subset inhibits antigen-specific T-cell responses and prevents colitis. *Nature.* (1997) 389:737–42. doi: 10.1038/39614
68. Veldman C, Hohne A, Dieckmann D, Schuler G, Hertl M. Type I regulatory T cells specific for desmoglein 3 are more frequently detected in healthy individuals than in patients with pemphigus vulgaris. *J Immunol.* (2004) 172:6468–75. doi: 10.4049/jimmunol.172.10.6468
69. Veldman C, Pahl A, Hertl M. Desmoglein 3-specific T regulatory 1 cells consist of two subpopulations with differential expression of the transcription factor Foxp3. *Immunology.* (2009) 127:40–9. doi: 10.1111/j.1365-2567.2008.02932.x
70. Veldman C, Pahl A, Beissert S, Hansen W, Buer J, Dieckmann D, et al. Inhibition of the transcription factor Foxp3 converts desmoglein 3-specific type 1 regulatory T cells into Th2-like cells. *J Immunol.* (2006) 176:3215–22. doi: 10.4049/jimmunol.176.5.3215
71. Billerbeck E, Thimme R. $CD8^+$ regulatory T cells in persistent human viral infections. *Hum Immunol.* (2008) 69:771–5. doi: 10.1016/j.humimm.2008.07.016
72. Sakaguchi S, Yamaguchi T, Nomura T, Ono M. Regulatory T cells and immune tolerance. *Cell.* (2008) 133:775–87. doi: 10.1016/j.cell.2008.05.009
73. Suzuki M, Konya C, Goronzy JJ, Weyand CM. Inhibitory $CD8^+$ T cells in autoimmune disease. *Hum Immunol.* (2008) 69:781–9. doi: 10.1016/j.humimm.2008.08.283
74. Cosmi L, Liotta F, Lazzeri E, Francalanci M, Angeli R, Mazzinghi B, et al. Human $CD8^+CD25^+$ thymocytes share phenotypic and functional features with $CD4^+CD25^+$ regulatory thymocytes. *Blood.* (2003) 102:4107–14. doi: 10.1182/blood-2003-04-1320
75. Jarvis LB, Matyszak MK, Duggleby RC, Goodall JC, Hall FC, Gaston JS. Autoreactive human peripheral blood $CD8^+$ T cells with a regulatory phenotype and function. *Eur J Immunol.* (2005) 35:2896–908. doi: 10.1002/eji.200526162
76. Rifa'I M, Kawamoto Y, Nakashima I, Suzuki H. Essential roles of $CD8^+CD122^+$ regulatory T cells in the maintenance of T cell homeostasis. *J Exp Med.* (2004) 200:1123–34. doi: 10.1084/jem.20040395
77. Endharti AT, Rifa IM, Shi Z, Fukuoka Y, Nakahara Y, Kawamoto Y, et al. Cutting edge: $CD8^+CD122^+$ regulatory T cells produce IL-10 to suppress IFN-gamma production and proliferation of $CD8^+$ T cells. *J Immunol.* (2005) 175:7093–7. doi: 10.4049/jimmunol.175.11.7093
78. Shi Z, Okuno Y, Rifa'I M, Endharti AT, Akane K, Isobe K, et al. Human $CD8^+CXCR3^+$ T cells have the same function as murine $CD8^+CD122^+$ Treg. *Eur J Immunol.* (2009) 39:2106–19. doi: 10.1002/eji.200939314
79. Lerret NM, Houlihan JL, Kheradmand T, Pothoven KL, Zhang ZJ, Luo X. Donor-specific $CD8^+$ $Foxp3^+$ T cells protect skin allografts and facilitate induction of conventional $CD4^+$ $Foxp3^+$ regulatory T cells. *Am J Transplant.* (2012) 12:2335–47. doi: 10.1111/j.1600-6143.2012.04120.x
80. Filaci G, Bacilieri S, Fravega M, Monetti M, Contini P, Ghio M, et al. Impairment of $CD8^+$ T suppressor cell function in patients with active systemic lupus erythematosus. *J Immunol.* (2001) 166:6452–7. doi: 10.4049/jimmunol.166.10.6452
81. Lee YH, Ishida Y, Rifa'I M, Shi Z, Isobe K, Suzuki H. Essential role of $CD8^+CD122^+$ regulatory T cells in the recovery from experimental autoimmune encephalomyelitis. *J Immunol.* (2008) 180:825–832. doi: 10.4049/jimmunol.180.2.825
82. Mizoguchi A, Bhan AK. A case for regulatory B cells. *J Immunol.* (2006) 176:705–10. doi: 10.4049/jimmunol.176.2.705
83. Blair PA, Norena LY, Flores-Borja F, Rawlings DJ, Isenberg DA, Ehrenstein MR, et al. $CD19(^+)$CD24(hi)CD38(hi) B cells exhibit regulatory capacity in healthy individuals but are functionally impaired in systemic Lupus Erythematosus patients. *Immunity.* (2010) 32:129–40. doi: 10.1016/j.immuni.2009.11.009
84. Kessel A, Haj T, Peri R, Snir A, Melamed D, Sabo E, et al. Human $CD19(^+)$CD25(high) B regulatory cells suppress proliferation of $CD4(^+)$ T cells and enhance Foxp3 and CTLA-4 expression in T-regulatory cells. *Autoimmun Rev.* (2012) 11:670–7. doi: 10.1016/j.autrev.2011.11.018
85. Zha B, Wang L, Liu X, Liu J, Chen Z, Xu J, et al. Decrease in proportion of $CD19^+$ CD24(hi) $CD27^+$ B cells and impairment of their suppressive function in Graves' disease. *PLoS ONE.* (2012) 7:e49835. doi: 10.1371/journal.pone.0049835
86. Lee JH, Noh J, Noh G, Choi WS, Cho S, Lee SS. Allergen-specific transforming growth factor-beta-producing $CD19^+CD5^+$ regulatory B-cell (Br3) responses in human late eczematous allergic reactions to cow's milk. *J Interferon Cytokine Res.* (2011) 31:441–9. doi: 10.1089/jir.2010.0020
87. Giannoukakis N, Trucco M. A role for tolerogenic dendritic cell-induced B-regulatory cells in type 1 diabetes mellitus. *Curr Opin Endocrinol Diabetes Obes.* (2012) 19:279–87. doi: 10.1097/MED.0b013e328355461b
88. Michel L, Chesneau M, Manceau P, Genty A, Garcia A, Salou M, et al. Unaltered regulatory B-cell frequency and function in patients with multiple sclerosis. *Clin Immunol.* (2014) 155:198–208. doi: 10.1016/j.clim.2014.09.011
89. Vadasz Z, Peri R, Eiza N, Slobodin G, Balbir-Gurman A, Toubi E. The Expansion of CD25 high IL-10 high FoxP3 high B regulatory cells is in association with SLE disease activity. *J Immunol Res.* (2015) 2015:254245. doi: 10.1155/2015/254245
90. Han J, Sun L, Fan X, Wang Z, Cheng Y, Zhu J, et al. Role of regulatory b cells in neuroimmunologic disorders. *J Neurosci Res.* (2016) 94:693–701. doi: 10.1002/jnr.23749
91. Heinemann K, Wilde B, Hoerning A, Tebbe B, Kribben A, Witzke O, et al. Decreased $IL\text{-}10(^+)$ regulatory B cells (Bregs) in lupus nephritis patients. *Scand J Rheumatol.* (2016) 45:312–6. doi: 10.3109/03009742.2015.1126346
92. Menon M, Blair PA, Isenberg DA, Mauri C. A regulatory feedback between plasmacytoid dendritic cells and regulatory B cells is aberrant in systemic lupus erythematosus. *Immunity.* (2016) 44:683–97. doi: 10.1016/j.immuni.2016.02.012
93. Matsushita T, Yanaba K, Bouaziz JD, Fujimoto M, Tedder TF. Regulatory B cells inhibit EAE initiation in mice while other B cells promote disease progression. *J Clin Invest.* (2008) 118:3420–30. doi: 10.1172/JCI36030
94. Matsushita T. Regulatory B cells in mouse models of systemic lupus erythematosus (SLE). *Methods Mol Biol.* (2014) 1190:195–205. doi: 10.1007/978-1-4939-1161-5_14
95. Ray A, Basu S. Regulatory B cells in experimental autoimmune encephalomyelitis (EAE). *Methods Mol Biol.* (2014) 1190:243–55. doi: 10.1007/978-1-4939-1161-5_17
96. Rosser EC, Mauri C. Regulatory B cells in experimental mouse models of arthritis. *Methods Mol Biol.* (2014) 1190:183–94. doi: 10.1007/978-1-4939-1161-5_13
97. DiMarco C. Pemphigus: pathogenesis to treatment. *R I Med J.* (2016) 99:28–31.
98. Zhu HQ, Xu RC, Chen YY, Yuan HJ, Cao H, Zhao XQ, et al. Impaired function of $CD19(^+)$ CD24(hi) CD38(hi) regulatory B cells in patients with pemphigus. *Br J Dermatol.* (2015) 172:101–10. doi: 10.1111/bjd.13192
99. Kabuto M, Fujimoto N, Takahashi T, Tanaka T. Decreased level of interleukin-10-producing B cells in patients with pemphigus but not

in patients with pemphigoid. *Br J Dermatol.* (2017) 176:1204–12. doi: 10.1111/bjd.15113
100. Colliou N, Picard D, Caillot F, Calbo S, Le Corre S, Lim A, et al. Long-term remissions of severe pemphigus after rituximab therapy are associated with prolonged failure of desmoglein B cell response. *Sci Transl Med.* (2013) 5:175ra130. doi: 10.1126/scitranslmed.3005166
101. Kabuto M, Fujimoto N, Tanaka T. Increase of interleukin-10-producing B cells associated with long-term remission after i.v. immunoglobulin treatment for pemphigus. *J Dermatol.* (2016) 43:815–8. doi: 10.1111/1346-8138.13295
102. Yoshizaki A, Miyagaki T, DiLillo DJ, Matsushita T, Horikawa M, Kountikov EI, et al. Regulatory B cells control T-cell autoimmunity through IL-21-dependent cognate interactions. *Nature.* (2012) 491:264–8. doi: 10.1038/nature11501
103. Liu Z, Dang E, Li B, Qiao H, Jin L, Zhang J, et al. Dysfunction of CD19(+)CD24(hi)CD27(+) B regulatory cells in patients with bullous pemphigoid. *Sci Rep.* (2018) 8:703. doi: 10.1038/s41598-018-19226-z
104. Rosser EC, Mauri C. Regulatory B cells: origin, phenotype, and function. *Immunity.* (2015) 42:607–12. doi: 10.1016/j.immuni.2015.04.005
105. Manicassamy S, Pulendran B. Dendritic cell control of tolerogenic responses. *Immunol Rev.* (2011) 241:206–27. doi: 10.1111/j.1600-065X.2011.01015.x
106. Liu J, Cao X. Regulatory dendritic cells in autoimmunity: a comprehensive review. *J Autoimmun.* (2015) 63:1–12. doi: 10.1016/j.jaut.2015.07.011
107. Mosser DM, Edwards JP. Exploring the full spectrum of macrophage activation. *Nat Rev Immunol.* (2008) 8:958–69. doi: 10.1038/nri2448
108. Gerber JS, Mosser DM. Reversing lipopolysaccharide toxicity by ligating the macrophage Fc gamma receptors. *J Immunol.* (2001) 166:6861–8. doi: 10.4049/jimmunol.166.11.6861
109. Fleming BD, Mosser DM. Regulatory macrophages: setting the threshold for therapy. *Eur J Immunol.* (2011) 41:2498–502. doi: 10.1002/eji.201141717
110. Gabrilovich DI, Ostrand-Rosenberg S, Bronte V. Coordinated regulation of myeloid cells by tumours. *Nat Rev Immunol.* (2012) 12:253–68. doi: 10.1038/nri3175
111. Luan Y, Mosheir E, Menon MC, Wilson D, Woytovich C, Ochando J, et al. Monocytic myeloid-derived suppressor cells accumulate in renal transplant patients and mediate CD4(+) Foxp3(+) Treg expansion. *Am J Transplant.* (2013) 13:3123–31. doi: 10.1111/ajt.12461
112. Gabrilovich DI. Myeloid-derived suppressor cells. *Cancer Immunol Res.* (2017) 5:3–8. doi: 10.1158/2326-6066.CIR-16-0297
113. Aggarwal S, Pittenger MF. Human mesenchymal stem cells modulate allogeneic immune cell responses. *Blood.* (2005) 105:1815–22. doi: 10.1182/blood-2004-04-1559
114. Jiang XX, Zhang Y, Liu B, Zhang SX, Wu Y, Yu XD, et al. Human mesenchymal stem cells inhibit differentiation and function of monocyte-derived dendritic cells. *Blood.* (2005) 105:4120–6. doi: 10.1182/blood-2004-02-0586
115. Castro-Manrreza ME, Montesinos JJ. Immunoregulation by mesenchymal stem cells: biological aspects and clinical applications. *J Immunol Res.* (2015) 2015:394917. doi: 10.1155/2015/394917
116. Najar M, Raicevic G, Fayyad-Kazan H, De Bruyn C, Bron D, Toungouz M, et al. Bone marrow mesenchymal stromal cells induce proliferative, cytokinic and molecular changes during the T cell response: the importance of the IL-10/CD210 Axis. *Stem Cell Rev.* (2015) 11:442–52. doi: 10.1007/s12015-014-9567-3
117. Yan Z, Zhuansun Y, Chen R, Li J, Ran P. Immunomodulation of mesenchymal stromal cells on regulatory T cells and its possible mechanism. *Exp Cell Res.* (2014) 324:65–74. doi: 10.1016/j.yexcr.2014.03.013
118. Han SM, Kim HT, Kim KW, Jeon KO, Seo KW, Choi EW, et al. CTLA4 overexpressing adipose tissue-derived mesenchymal stem cell therapy in a dog with steroid-refractory pemphigus foliaceus. *BMC Vet Res.* (2015) 11:49. doi: 10.1186/s12917-015-0371-3
119. Miwa T, Song WC. Membrane complement regulatory proteins: insight from animal studies and relevance to human diseases. *Int Immunopharmacol.* (2001) 1:445–59. doi: 10.1016/S1567-5769(00)00043-6
120. Noris M, Remuzzi G. Overview of complement activation and regulation. *Semin Nephrol.* (2013) 33:479–92. doi: 10.1016/j.semnephrol.2013.08.001
121. Merle NS, Church SE, Fremeaux-Bacchi V, Roumenina LT. Complement system part I - molecular mechanisms of activation and regulation. *Front Immunol.* (2015) 6:262. doi: 10.3389/fimmu.2015.00262
122. Garcia-Valladares I, Atisha-Fregoso Y, Richaud-Patin Y, Jakez-Ocampo J, Soto-Vega E, Elias-Lopez D, et al. Diminished expression of complement regulatory proteins (CD55 and CD59) in lymphocytes from systemic lupus erythematosus patients with lymphopenia. *Lupus.* (2006) 15:600–5. doi: 10.1177/0961203306071916
123. Ruiz-Arguelles A, Llorente L. The role of complement regulatory proteins (CD55 and CD59) in the pathogenesis of autoimmune hemocytopenias. *Autoimmun Rev.* (2007) 6:155–61. doi: 10.1016/j.autrev.2006.09.008
124. Alegretti AP, Mucenic T, Merzoni J, Faulhaber GA, Silla LM, Xavier RM. Expression of CD55 and CD59 on peripheral blood cells from systemic lupus erythematosus (SLE) patients. *Cell Immunol.* (2010) 265:127–32. doi: 10.1016/j.cellimm.2010.07.013
125. Piccoli AK, Alegretti AP, Schneider L, Lora PS, Xavier RM. Expression of complement regulatory proteins CD55, CD59, CD35, and CD46 in rheumatoid arthritis. *Rev Bras Reumatol.* (2011) 51:503–10. doi: 10.1590/S0482-50042011000500009
126. Das N. Complement and membrane-bound complement regulatory proteins as biomarkers and therapeutic targets for autoimmune inflammatory disorders, RA and SLE. *Indian J Exp Biol.* (2015) 53:701–13.
127. Dainichi T, Chow Z, Kabashima K. IgG4, complement, and the mechanisms of blister formation in pemphigus and bullous pemphigoid. *J Dermatol Sci.* (2017) 88:265–70. doi: 10.1016/j.jdermsci.2017.07.012
128. Qiao P, Dang E, Cao T, Fang H, Zhang J, Qiao H, et al. Dysregulation of mCD46 and sCD46 contribute to the pathogenesis of bullous pemphigoid. *Sci Rep.* (2017) 7:145. doi: 10.1038/s41598-017-00235-3
129. Qiao P, Dang EL, Fang H, Zhang JY, Li B, Shen SX, et al. Decreased expression levels of complement regulator CD55 contribute to the development of bullous pemphigoid. *Oncotarget.* (2018) 9:35517–27. doi: 10.18632/oncotarget.21216
130. Ochi H, Abraham M, Ishikawa H, Frenkel D, Yang K, Basso AS, et al. Oral CD3-specific antibody suppresses autoimmune encephalomyelitis by inducing $CD4^{+}$ CD25- LAP^{+} T cells. *Nat Med.* (2006) 12:627–35. doi: 10.1038/nm1408
131. Ishikawa H, Ochi H, Chen ML, Frenkel D, Maron R, Weiner HL. Inhibition of autoimmune diabetes by oral administration of anti-CD3 monoclonal antibody. *Diabetes.* (2007) 56:2103–9. doi: 10.2337/db06-1632
132. Yamashita T, Sasaki N, Kasahara K, Hirata K. Anti-inflammatory and immune-modulatory therapies for preventing atherosclerotic cardiovascular disease. *J Cardiol.* (2015) 66:1–8. doi: 10.1016/j.jjcc.2015.02.002
133. Fasching P, Stradner M, Graninger W, Dejaco C, Fessler J. Therapeutic potential of targeting the Th17/Treg axis in autoimmune disorders. *Molecules.* (2017) 22:134. doi: 10.3390/molecules22010134

15

Autoimmune Theories of Chronic Spontaneous Urticaria

*Sonali J. Bracken[1], Soman Abraham[2,3] and Amanda S. MacLeod[3,4]**

[1] Department of Internal Medicine, Duke University School of Medicine, Durham, NC, United States, [2] Department of Pathology, Duke University Medical Center, Durham, NC, United States, [3] Department of Immunology, Duke University Medical Center, Durham, NC, United States, [4] Department of Dermatology, Duke University Medical Center, Durham, NC, United States

***Correspondence:**
Amanda S. MacLeod (née Büchau)
amanda.macleod@duke.edu

Urticaria (hives) is a highly prevalent skin disorder that can occur with or without associated angioedema. Chronic spontaneous urticaria (CSU) is a condition which persists for more than 6 weeks in duration and occurs in the absence of an identifiable provoking factor. CSU results from pathogenic activation of mast cells and basophils, which gives rise to the release of proinflammatory mediators that support the generation of urticaria. Several theories have been put forth regarding the pathogenesis of CSU with much evidence pointing toward a potential autoimmune etiology in up to 50% of patients with this condition. In this review, we highlight the evidence surrounding the autoimmune pathogenesis of chronic urticaria including recent data which suggests that CSU may involve contributions from both immunoglobin G (IgG)-specific and immunoglobulin E (IgE)-specific autoantibodies against a vast array of antigens that can span beyond those found on the surface of mast cells and basophils.

Keywords: chronic spontaneous urticaria, chronic idiopathic urticaria, autoimmune urticaria, anti-IgE, anti-FcεR1, autoallergy, anti-TPO

INTRODUCTION

Urticaria, more commonly known as "hives", is a prevalent disorder that affects between 15 and 25% of the population at some point during their lifetimes (1). The condition tends to be more common in adults than in children and in woman than in men with peak occurrence in the third to fifth decades of life. This condition is marked by the onset of pruritic "wheals," which represent well-circumscribed areas of non-pitting edema with blanched centers and raised borders that involve only the superficial portions of the dermis and are seen in conjunction with surrounding erythema of the skin (2). Lesions can be as small as a few millimeters in diameter but can coalesce to form wheals as large as several centimeters wide. They often remit within 24 h since time of onset. Urticaria may be accompanied by the presence of angioedema, which is a similar process that occurs at submucosal surfaces of the upper respiratory and gastrointestinal tracts and deeper layers of the skin including subcutaneous tissue (3). Urticaria is classified as either acute or chronic depending on whether the onset of episodes lasts for less or >6 weeks in duration, respectively. In this review, we will focus specifically on the pathophysiology of chronic urticaria. Formerly referred to as chronic idiopathic urticaria, chronic spontaneous urticaria (CSU) refers to recurrent urticaria lasting more than 6 weeks that occur in the absence of an identifiable trigger. Urticaria that are incited by a well-defined eliciting factor (e.g., pressure, temperature, vibration) are referred to as inducible urticaria and will not be further discussed in this review. Prevalence of chronic urticaria is estimated to be anywhere from 0.5 to 5% in the general population but is not truly known, though incidence is thought to fall around 1.4% annually (4). Recent guidelines now include isolated idiopathic angioedema within the definition of CSU provided that other causes of angioedema, particularly those that are bradykinin mediated, have been excluded (5). Multiple studies have suggested that CSU may be an autoimmune condition in a substantial proportion of cases, but it is important to identify potential triggers of disease and exclude other differential conditions prior to making the diagnosis as outlined in **Figure 1**. In this article, we will discuss the pathophysiology of chronic urticaria and review the evidence surrounding its autoimmune etiology.

MAST CELLS AND BASOPHILS AS CENTRALIZED REGULATORS OF CHRONIC SPONTANEOUS URTICARIA

The pathophysiology of CSU is not well-understood, but it is clear that derangement of both mast cell and basophil activation and degranulation remains central to the process. Of these, mast cells are most widely accepted as the primary effectors of chronic urticaria. While other cell types including lymphocytes and polymononuclear cells (PMNs) have been observed within the inflammatory infiltrates of patients with CSU, it is well-established that histamine and other mast cell products are predominantly responsible for development of this condition [note that skin biopsies are seldom needed for the diagnosis but are occasionally useful to distinguish CSU from other inflammatory conditions such as urticarial vasculitis (5)]. The physical manifestation of urticaria can be attributed to the enhanced vascular permeability that results from the release of preformed mediators from mast cells (e.g., histamine, tryptase, leukotrienes) and their delayed generation of cytokines. Ongoing research continues to probe into the mechanisms by which mast cells are activated by blood-borne antigens, with recent data from murine *in vivo* studies suggesting that CD301b$^+$ dermal dendritic cells (DCs) are actually first to sample antigen and then relay it to nearby mast cells through secreted microvesicles (6). However, the vast majority of cases of chronic urticaria are not triggered by any identifiable substance and are in fact idiopathic. In these cases, anaphylaxis does not occur though angioedema may be present.

Two major mechanisms have been put forward with regards to the pathogenesis of chronic urticaria. The first is not autoimmune in nature, but involves dysregulation of intracellular signaling pathways within mast cells and basophils that lead to defects in trafficking or function of these cells. The second involves the development of autoantibodies to FcεRIα or IgE on both mast cells and basophils and will be discussed in more detail in the following sections (7). Both of these mechanisms will be further explored here and are outlined in **Figure 2**.

DYSREGULATION OF INTRACELLULAR SIGNALING PATHWAYS CAN PREDISPOSE TO PATHOLOGIC ACTIVATION OF MAST CELLS AND BASOPHILS

Activation of the high-affinity IgE receptor, FcεR1, is an important step in the development of allergic responses and in the development of urticaria. This receptor is composed of an α-, β-, and two γ subunits (8). Whereas the α-subunit binds to the Cε3 constant region of the IgE molecule, the β-, and γ- subunits contain cell immunoreceptor tyrosine-based activation motifs (ITAMs) which, when phosphorylated, promote activation of spleen tyrosine kinase (SYK) and downstream recruitment of a host of secondary molecules including those involved in the phosphoinositide-3 kinase (PI3K) pathway. This series of events is responsible for degranulation of mast cells and can predispose to pathologic mast cell activation when inappropriately upregulated. SYK is recruited to the FcεR1 upon antigen stimulation, and inhibition of this protein has been shown to inhibit mast cell degranulation and production of both lipid mediators and cytokine activity (9). When mast cells from CSU patients with active urticarial disease at the time of blood sample collection were compared to those from healthy human donors, they were unsurprisingly found to release significantly more histamine *in vitro* than their healthy counterparts (10). Yet when these CSU patients were further subdivided into responders vs. non-responders based on their ability to degranulate in response to anti-IgE (with responders showing >10% degranulation activity), SYK levels were shown to be higher in the responder group than in the non-responder group, suggesting that this protein is a major determinant of predilection toward spontaneous degranulation. SYK expression is highly variable among the general population and is thought to correlate with the degree of IgE-mediated degranulation. Intriguingly, the presence of autoantibodies to FcεRIα or IgE do not predispose to upregulation of basophil SYK expression (11).

Negative regulation of mast cell activation occurs through phosphoinositide lipid phosphatases which function as well-described negative regulators of hematopoietic cell activation and proliferation. Src homology 2 (SH2)-containing inositol phosphatases SHIP-1 and SHIP-2 associate with the FcεR1 β subunit and are activated upon stimulation with IgE or antigen (12). It is likely that dysregulation of these pathways that leads to an imbalance of positive signaling plays a pathogenic role in the development of CSU. One study demonstrated that when basophils from highly allergic IgE-positive donors (distinguished as having the ability to mount a response to human-recombinant histamine release factor, a complete stimulus for histamine release) were compared to those from healthy human donors, they contained lower levels of SHIP protein. As such, they demonstrated hyperresponsiveness (i.e., degranulation) in response to stimuli that did not appear to affect IgE-negative basophils (13). Similar results have been

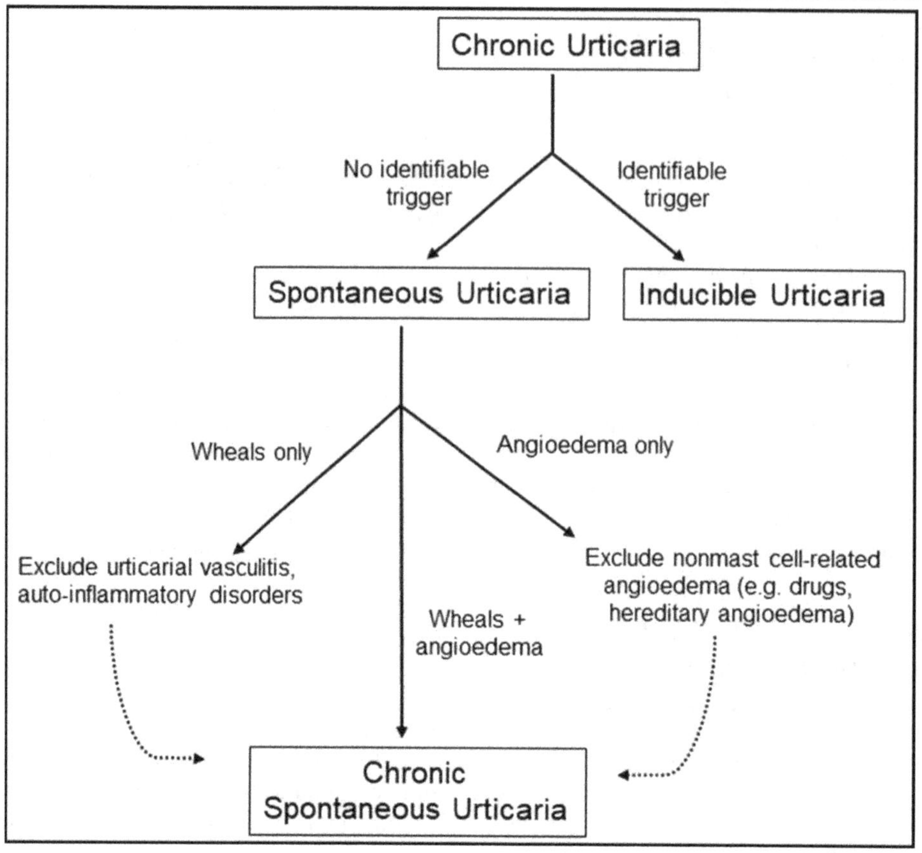

FIGURE 1 | Diagnostic workup of chronic urticaria.

shown in mast cells from CSU patients highly sensitive to degranulation, with responders showing significantly lower levels of SHIP protein than both non-responders and healthy human donors (10).

THE AUTOIMMUNE THEORY OF MAST CELL ACTIVATION IN CHRONIC SPONTANEOUS URTICARIA

While cellular signaling defects may account for some cases of CSU, the autoimmune theory is the more widely accepted hypothesis to explain the inappropriate activation of mast cells and basophils in patients with chronic spontaneous urticaria. Up to 45% of cases of CSU are thought to be autoimmune in etiology. In a sentinel study conducted by Grattan et al., 12 patients with chronic urticaria were subjected to intradermal autologous serum injection (14). Seven of the 12 subjects (of whom six were female) mounted a positive wheal-and-flare reaction to this test, and fewer of these patients described a history of disease exacerbation with application of pressure when compared to patients with a negative injection test. This suggested that these patients with a positive result were less likely to have an inducible urticarial syndrome. Additionally, only one patient described a personal history of atopy, suggesting an alternative etiology for urticaria in the majority of cases. When the same serum was re-injected into the same subjects 1 year later, most of the patients with an initial positive test demonstrated a second positive result, though the same was not necessarily true when fresh serum was injected. In the small number of serum-positive patients who did not mount a second reaction at 1 year, the authors noted that their urticaria had cleared. On the contrary, the two patients who continued to mount a reaction with both original and fresh serum at the 1 year interval were noted to have continued disease activity. Ultimately, the authors concluded that many patients with chronic urticaria contain a "circulating mediator" in their serum which is capable of inducing urticaria. Over the past 30 years, the search has been ongoing to identify the mysterious culprit; multiple theories have since been put forth. However, it was these initial findings that opened the floodgates to the autoimmune theory of chronic spontaneous urticaria.

Though theoretically performed by Grattan et al. (14), the autoimmune etiology of CSU was further supported by formal development of the autologous serum skin test (ASST), an *in vivo* assay of mast cell activation that is induced by intradermal injection of a patient's serum into self. It has now been accepted that nearly 50% of patients with CSU will have a positive test in response to factors present within their own serum within 30 min of injection. Additional groups have suggested that

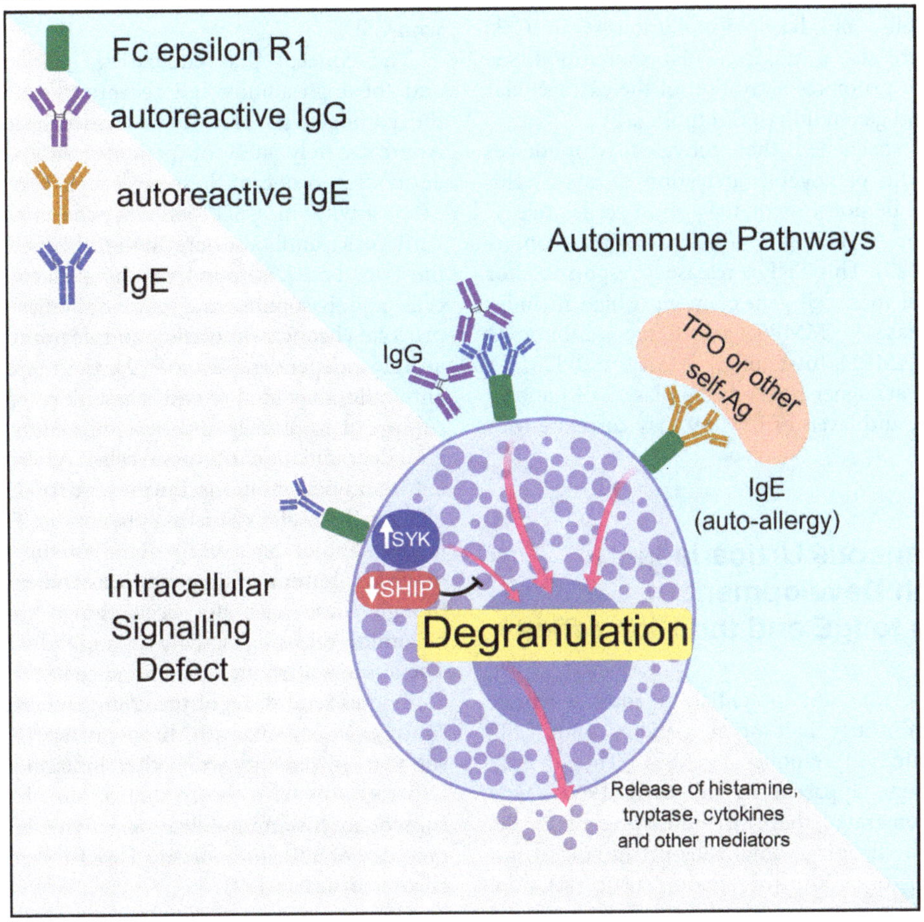

FIGURE 2 | Model of the mechanisms underlying chronic urticaria. Pathologic activation of mast cells and basophils in patients with chronic spontaneous urticaria is thought to occur via two major mechanisms: intracellular signaling defects and autoimmune mechanisms. In the former, inappropriate activation of molecules such a spleen tyrosine kinase (SYK) or inhibition of negative regulators including the Src homology 2 (SH2)-containing inositol phosphatases (SHIP) promotes spontaneous degranulation of mast cells/basophils with subsequent release of histamine and other protein and lipid mediators. The more commonly accepted theory of pathogenesis in CSU includes antibody-mediated mast cell and basophil activation, which can occur via IgG- or IgE- mediated pathways. In the former, IgG molecules directed against the Fc portion of IgE or the FcεR1 promote spontaneous cellular degranulation. In patients with autoallergy, crosslinking of Fc epsilon R1 (FcεR1) via autoreactive IgE molecules directed against self-antigens such as thyroid peroxidase (TPO) promote mast cell/basophil degranulation.

such "factors" are indeed autoantibodies or histamine-releasing factors that are capable of inducing mast cell degranulation. Unfortunately, these data have been somewhat difficult to interpret, as positive ASSTs are not unique to patients with CSU and have been noted in a substantial proportion of patients with allergic or non-allergic rhinitis, multiple drug allergy syndrome, and even in healthy control subjects (15). Furthermore, the positivity of the test has been shown to persist even when CSU patients are in clinical remission, particularly in subjects with autoimmune thyroiditis (16). Interestingly, it has been shown that levels of autoantibodies in CSU do not vary with disease activity which may, in part, explain this finding (17).

Some individuals have suggested that the autologous plasma skin test may be more sensitive than ASST for the diagnosis of CSU (18), though this result has not been reliably demonstrated (19). Since plasma and serum have similar levels of autoantibodies, additional mechanisms beyond autoantibody production have been put forth to explain the pathophysiology of the disease. One such theory states that factors that are uniquely present in plasma may be involved in the development of urticaria, and indeed it was shown that levels of the prothrombin fragment 1+2 (a marker of thrombin generation) were significantly higher in CSU patients than in control subjects (18). This suggests involvement of the clotting cascade in the development of the urticarial reaction. While the role of the coagulation cascade in the pathogenesis of urticaria is beyond the scope of this review, thrombin has been shown to directly increase mast cell degranulation, activate protease-activated receptors on mast cells, and enhance vascular permeability through actions on endothelial cells (20). It should also be noted that autoantibodies against the low affinity IgE receptor FcεRII (CD23) have been demonstrated in a large percentage of CSU patients (21). Anti-CD23 autoantibodies can activate eosinophils to release major basic protein, which in turn can trigger histamine release from mast cells, and basophils. Curiously, in CSU patients eosinophils are also a major cellular source of tissue factor, a protein which promotes activation of the extracellular coagulation cascade and generation of thrombin (22).

It has also been speculated that activated lymphocytes may play a role in the pathogenic activation of mast cells. Indeed it has been demonstrated that mast cells release inflammatory mediators including TNF-α upon direct contact with activated T cells (23). This TNF-α release is responsible for upregulation of several mast cell genes, among which includes matrix metalloproteinase 9 (MMP9) and tissue inhibitor of metalloproteinase 1 (TIMP1). Intriguingly, MMP9 and TIMP-1 have both been found at higher levels in the plasma of patients with chronic urticaria, and levels of MMP-9 may correlate with disease severity (24).

Chronic Spontaneous Urticaria Is Associated With Development of Autoantibodies to IgE and the High Affinity IgE Receptor

Circulating mediators with the potential to induce wheal-and-flare reactions in nearly half of all patients with CSU have been demonstrated in response to ASST. The identify of those factors became apparent in the early 1990s. One landmark study demonstrated that antibodies present in the serum of patients with chronic spontaneous urticaria (but not in patients with dermatographism or pressure urticaria) were able to elicit histamine release from healthy donor peripheral blood leukocytes with similar kinetics as anti-IgE antibodies (25). Intriguingly, the authors noted that preincubation of basophils with either anti-IgE or chronic urticarial serum abolished subsequent histamine release upon incubation with urticarial serum or anti-IgE, suggesting that both anti-IgE and chronic urticarial serum stimulate degranulation via a similar mechanism. Removing surface-bound IgE from leukocytes prior to incubation with urticarial serum or anti-IgE reduced histamine release. These important results suggested for the first time that histamine-releasing autoantibodies present in the serum of patients with chronic urticaria act by cross-linking cell surface IgE receptors.

In addition to the aforementioned findings, the authors astutely noted that histamine release could be elucidated when chronic urticarial serum was incubated with basophils from donors with very low serum IgE concentrations but not with anti-IgE (25). These data implied that non-IgE-dependent histamine releasing factors are present in the serum of patients with CSU. Shortly after the publication of this initial study, the same group determined the presence of IgG antibodies against the α subunit of the high-affinity FcεR1 in a group of patients with CSU (26). In this subset of patients, IgG anti-FcεR1α pathologically induced histamine release irrespective of the degree of IgE sensitization of the basophils. As proof of concept, histamine release was effectively neutralized in a concentration-dependent manner by preincubating donor basophils with soluble fragment of FcεR1α prior to the addition of purified IgG from sera of patients with CSU.

The concept that circulating IgG antibodies against IgE and the high-affinity IgE receptor FcεR1 likely contribute to the pathogenesis of CSU has since become widely accepted. Approximately 40% of patients with CSU have circulating antibodies to one of these targets (27) with a higher frequency of positivity in CSU patients who are ASST positive (28). Anti-FcεRI antibodies are thought to be the more common of the two. FcεRI is found on the surface of both dermal mast cells and basophils, and autoantibodies to this receptor can provoke chronic stimulation and degranulation of these cells in an IgE-independent fashion (2). On the contrary, IgG-anti IgE antibodies may bind to and crosslink receptor-bound IgE on the surface of mast cells and basophils, thus leading to activation and degranulation of these cells. As is the case with many autoimmune conditions, the presence of autoantibodies does not necessarily result in a disease phenotype. The presence of FcεR1α autoantibodies have been noted in the sera of patients with other autoimmune skin conditions and even in healthy subjects, though these have not been shown to display pronounced histamine-releasing activity in individuals without CSU (29). The authors attribute this difference to the fact that anti-FcεR1α antibodies tend to be of the complement-fixing IgG1 and IgG3 subtypes in patients with chronic urticaria but of IgG2 and IgG4 subtypes in patients with other inflammatory skin conditions. Other groups have shown that *in vitro* basophil activation and subsequent histamine-releasing activity fails to correlate with the presence of autoantibodies to FcεR1α even among patients with chronic urticarial (27).

The presence of autoantibodies to IgE and to FcεR1α infers the presence of antigen-specific lymphocytes in individuals with chronic urticarial disease. FcεR1α-specific T lymphocytes are detectable in a large percentage of patients with CSU and these cells more typically adopt a Th1 cytokine profile with the largest percentage being INF-γ secretors (30). Intriguingly, the relationship between INF-γ and autoantibody responses to FcεR1α has been found to be inversely related, similar to that which has been observed for T cell and autoantibody reactivity to glutamic acid decarboxylase antigen in individuals at risk for type 1 diabetes mellitus (31). It remains unclear how T cell reactivity vs. antibody reactivity to FcεR1α affects pathogenesis of CSU. However, it has been demonstrated that markers of T cell activation are directly proportional to markers of mast cell degranulation in chronic urticaria patients, particularly in patients known to have positive antibodies against FcεR1 (32). Further evidence for the involvement of T lymphocytes in the pathogenesis of CSU stems from observed variations in protein tyrosine phosphatase 22 (PTPN22) in patients with CSU (33). PTPN22 is a strong susceptibility gene for a variety of autoimmune disorders and encodes lymphoid specific tyrosine phosphatase (Lyp), which normally serves as an inhibitor of T cell activation.

An increased frequency of the HLA-DR4 allele has been found in patients with CSU (34). Intriguingly, the HLA-DR4 has been found at an increased frequency in a variety of other autoimmune disorders including rheumatoid arthritis, type 1 diabetes mellitus, and multiple sclerosis. Patients with autoimmunological subtypes of CSU have been noted to have a particularly high likelihood of carrying this HLA class II allele (35). However, these data have not been replicable across a wide spectrum of populations, with other studies noting increased frequencies of HLA-DR9 (30) and HLADR12 (30, 36) among patients with CSU. Heterogeneity in allelic association with this disease likely indicates that FcεR1α contains a number of different epitopes which act as targets of autoreactive T lymphocytes.

The Overlap Between Chronic Spontaneous Urticaria and Other Autoimmune Diseases

The concept of "overlapping autoimmune diseases" suggests that disorders which are autoimmune in nature occur at increased frequency in patients with known autoimmune disease. Numerous autoimmune conditions including systemic lupus erythematosus, polymyositis, dermatomyositis, and rheumatoid arthritis have been associated with chronic urticaria (2).

One large population study of over 12,000 subjects derived from a large health maintenance organization in Israel determined that female patients with CSU demonstrate a significantly higher incidence of rheumatoid arthritis, Sjögren syndrome, celiac disease, type I diabetes, and systemic lupus erythematosus than patients without CSU (37). While men also demonstrated higher odds of having these autoimmune conditions when compared with control subjects, these numbers did not reach statistical significance. When further investigation into serologic markers of autoimmune disease was performed, it was determined that patients with CSU as compared to control subjects had significantly higher levels of anti-thyroid peroxidase (anti-TPO) antibodies, antinuclear antibodies (ANA), antithyroglobulin (i.e., antimicrosomal) antibodies, rheumatoid factor, anti-transglutaminase IgA antibodies, and anti-parietal cell antibodies with anti-dsDNA, and anti-cardiolipin antibodies trending toward significance. Moreover, the mean platelet volume (MPV) was noted to be abnormally high in 29% of CSU patients and only in 1% of control subjects. Elevations in MPV occur when the body produces platelets at a more rapid rate and tend to correlate with levels of systemic inflammation.

As this study was the first of its kind to examine the relationship between CSU and other autoimmune diseases, it has shed some light on some intriguing commonalities between these two conditions. As is the case with most autoimmune conditions, CSU tends to affect women more commonly than it does men, and women with CSU tend to have much higher odds of developing other autoimmune conditions vs. men. This sex difference is also mirrored by the observation that both CSU and autoimmune diseases on the whole tend to occur more commonly in young adulthood as opposed to in older, post-menopausal adults. Additionally, the high prevalence of the aforementioned autoimmune conditions in CSU patients at much higher frequencies than occurs in the general population adds more strength to the theory that the underlying pathology of CSU is autoimmune in nature. When overlapping autoimmune conditions did occur, they were frequently diagnosed within the first 10 years after onset of CSU and quite commonly within the first 6 months. A recently conducted systematic review of autoimmune comorbidities in individuals with CSU also noted that organ-specific autoimmune disorders are more common than systemic autoimmune disorders in patients with urticaria, with endocrine, hematologic and skin disorders being among the most common (38). The reasons for this discrepancy remain largely unclear.

The common pathogenic mechanism between these conditions is the presence of autoantibodies on a background of chronic inflammation. However, autoimmune disorders are incredibly heterogenous in nature and thus it is difficult to extrapolate whether the link between chronic urticaria and the aforementioned conditions truly stems from a common pathologic tie or is merely reflective of detection bias. If a true connection does exist, one would imagine that CSU would be found at a higher frequency in patients with established autoimmune disease, but this link has been difficult to definitively make. For example, the prevalence of CSU in patients with SLE ranges from 0 to 22% depending on the individual study (39).

Autoallergy in Chronic Spontaneous Urticaria

With regards to the idea of overlapping autoimmune diseases, the well-established link between chronic urticaria and autoimmune thyroid disease deserves particular mention. Even among euthyroid subjects, many patients with CSU have detectable levels of antibodies against thyroglobulin or microsomal-derived antigen (40). Furthermore, an increased prevalence of clinical hypothyroidism (i.e., Hashimoto's thyroiditis) as well as hyperthyroidism has been found among patients with CSU, with one study estimating a 23 times and seven times greater odds for hypothyroidism in female and male patients with chronic urticaria compared to control subjects, respectively (37). In 80% of these cases, the diagnosis of thyroid disease was made within 10 years, of the diagnosis of urticaria. The occurrence of IgG anti-thyroid antibodies in patients with CSU documented in studies where more than 100 patients were enrolled was noted to be anywhere from 3.7 to 37.1% with two-thirds reporting increased anti-thyroid antibody levels in >10% of patients (41).

Patients with CSU also demonstrate higher levels of IgE anti-thyroid peroxidase (anti-TPO) antibodies relative to healthy controls, though this distribution was found to be bimodal with 39% of CSU patients exhibiting IgE anti-TPO levels similar to control subjects (IgE anti-TPO^{low}) (42). It is theorized that autoallergic mast cell activation may contribute to the pathophysiology in CSU patients with detectable levels of IgE anti-TPO. IgE has a well-established role in the defense against helminthic infections and in recognition of exogenous allergens, but it was not until very recently that its potential role in autoimmunity has emerged. The term "autoallergy" refers to a type I, IgE-mediated hypersensitivity reaction against self-antigens which can, in turn, promote degranulation of basophils and mast cells. It was first put forth by Rorsman et al. as an explanation for urticaria-induced basopenia (43). Rorsman theorized that unlike in physical causes of urticaria, antigen-antibody interactions in non-physical causes of urticaria are likely to occur in both the skin and within the circulation (44). Autoallergic mast cell activation has been shown to occur in a variety of skin disorders including atopic dermatitis (45, 46) and bullous pemphigoid (47). In such disorders, IgE directed against skin antigens may bind to these cognate antigens and activate mast cells residing within the skin. On the contrary, TPO can be released from the thyroid into circulation, where it is free to bind to the surface of FcεR1-expressing cells. This extracutaneous nature of TPO may be one reason why the manifestations of CSU are not simply limited to the skin as they are in many other autoimmune skin disorders. Indeed it has been shown that anti-IgE TPO antibodies have the ability to induce basophil degranulation *in vitro* in the presence of TPO antigen and likely play a role in the pathogenesis of CSU (48). Recent findings have demonstrated that IgE anti-TPO antibodies are present at higher frequency and amounts in patients with CSU and have greater potential to induce TPO-mediated skin reactions in these subjects vs. in healthy controls (49). These results were validated by increased upregulation of basophil activation markers in CSU subjects upon exposure to TPO and ability of anti-TPO IgE to induce positive skin reactions upon passive transfer of this antibody from a patient with CSU to the skin of a healthy subject. In addition to IgE anti-TPO antibodies, IgE anti-dsDNA antibodies have also been noted at higher frequency in patients with CSU (50). However, no significant difference in IgE anti-dsDNA levels were observed between ASST-positive vs. ASST-negative patients, which suggests that these antibodies may be correlated with but are not likely to be involved in the pathogenesis of CSU.

IgE-mediated autoimmunity is becoming increasingly recognized as a possible contributor to the pathogenesis of a variety of systemic conditions including systemic lupus erythematosus and rheumatoid arthritis (51). A multicenter study in patients with SLE showed over half of all subjects had detectable levels of IgE against at least one common nuclear autoantigen (dsDNA, SS-A, SS-B, Sm) (52). This frequency increased during active disease and was strongly associated with the presence of active nephritis. There is still much to learn about the fields of autoallergy and IgE-mediated autoimmunity, which currently remain in their infancy, but it is likely that this will reveal a host of novel, targetable autoantigens. Over 200 IgE autoantigens were recently demonstrated in CSU subjects that were not present in healthy controls, among which included IL-24, which were detected in all patients with CSU (53). Further *in vitro* analyses demonstrated that IL-24 contributes to histamine release from human mast cells sensitized with IgE from CSU but not control subjects and that IgE-anti-IL-24 levels have reasonable predictive value for disease activity. The questions of why and how IgE autoantibodies develop and to what degree they contribute to CSU pathogenesis when compared to IgG autoantibodies has yet to be determined and is likely to be the focus of many future studies in this field.

TREATMENT OF CHRONIC SPONTANEOUS URTICARIA

The primary treatment for chronic urticaria is to address the underlying pathology whenever possible and prevent mast cell activation. In any patient with chronic urticaria, elimination of potential triggers including drugs which can cause non-allergic hypersensitivity reactions (most commonly NSAIDs) should first be undertaken (5) Multiple guidelines have been put forth for management of CSU, though the EAACI/GA^{2}LEN/EDF/WAO remain the most popular among practicing clinicians (5). If cases where no triggers can be identified, antihistamines (particularly the modern 2nd-generation antihistamines) are recommended as the mainstay pharmacologic treatment modalities for this condition. In patients who are poorly responsive to antihistamine therapy, it is recommended that the dosage be increased up to four times the normal limit prior to initiating a new agent. In cases of severe urticaria not adequately controlled with antihistamines alone, the EAACI/GA^{2}LEN/EDF/WAO guidelines have recommended the addition of anti-IgE therapy, with cyclosporine being reserved for the most refractory cases of CSU. While short courses of prednisone do have a role in acute exacerbations of CSU, there is a strong recommendation against the use of long-term oral steroids given risk for adverse effects.

Evaluating the Use of Omalizumab for the Treatment of Chronic Spontaneous Urticaria

Omalizumab is an IgG monoclonal antibody against the Fc portion of the IgE antibody and prevents free IgE from binding to high-affinity FcεR1 receptors on mast cells and basophils. The first multicenter, placebo-controlled study evaluating omalizumab use in CSU examined efficacy of this therapy in subjects with IgE autoantibodies and found that 70% of omalizumab-treated patients who were otherwise refractory to standard antihistamine therapy were completely protected against wheal development (vs. 4.5% of placebo-treated subjects) (54). Another phase three study demonstrated that omalizumab given in three subcutaneous doses of either 150 or 300 mg over a 12 week period significantly reduced symptoms in antihistamine-refractory CSU patients without rebound of symptoms following discontinuation of the medication (55). Lack of relapse after discontinuation and very good safety profile have made omalizumab suitable for long-term therapy in patients with CSU, though cost still limits its use in many circumstances.

The mechanism by which omalizumab benefits patients with CSU has yet to be fully elucidated but the aforementioned results strongly argue for the contribution of IgE autoantibodies in the pathogenesis of CSU with rapid neutralization of these antibodies being an effective component of therapy. While the exact mechanisms by which omalizumab treatment benefits patients with CSU remain unclear, clearance of IgE autoantibodies is certainly likely to be of relevance. It has been well-established that omalizumab rapidly reduces levels of free IgE, which promotes downregulation of FcεR1 on basophils within the span of weeks and on mast cells within the span of months (56). The reason for this is because FcεR1 is effectively degraded when it is not stabilized by IgE binding (56, 57). Additionally, omalizumab has been shown to improve the genetic signature of lesional skin in patients with CSU to reflect non-lesional skin signatures by downregulating expression of genes involved in mast cell and leukocyte infiltration (FCER1G, C3AR1, CD93, S100A8), oxidative stress, vascularization (CYR61), and skin repair (KRT6A, KRT16) (56). Notably, non-responders to omalizumab do not demonstrate these genetic alterations. Basophils are also thought to be recruited to the urticarial lesions of patients with active CSU (58). *Post hoc* analysis of randomized clinical trial data have demonstrated that omalizumab increases peripheral blood basophil counts by likely reducing recruitment of these cells to the skin (59) and may also help to regulate defective basophil IgE receptor pathways (57). Clinical trials are currently underway to better characterize the effects of omalizumab on basophil responses.

Treatment with omalizumab has been shown to decrease levels of both FcεR1- and IgE- positive skin cells in skin of patients with CSU (60). In theory, omalizumab may reduce the autoimmune effects of self-antigen by mediating this decrease in pathogenic IgE levels and/or IgE receptors on the mast cell surface. Recently, a great deal of attention has been placed on the utility of IgE levels for predicting responses to omalizumab. Patients who have lower IgE levels prior to receiving omalizumab and lower IgE levels 4 weeks after undergoing treatment tend to respond less well to this therapy than those with higher baseline and post-treatment IgE levels (61), suggesting that these laboratory tests may help to guide management of CSU patients being considered for second- and third-line treatment options (61, 62). Interestingly, total IgE levels have been shown to positively correlate with basophil FcεR1 expression, the latter of which tends to be higher in those who respond quickly to omalizumab therapy (62). Despite our poor knowledge of the precise role of basophils in CSU pathophysiology, it is becoming clear that the time to effect for omalizumab in CSU appears to correlate with the expected time for reduction of FcεR1 on basophils (54) as opposed to on mast cells. Similar results were noted in prior studies examining use of omalizumab for cat allergy, which demonstrated that reduction of nasal symptoms correlated directly with a reduction in basophil responsiveness as opposed to mast cell responsiveness (63).

The question of how omalizumab benefits patients whose disease is mediated by a type I hypersensitivity reaction (autoallergy) vs. a type II hypersensitivity reaction (autoimmunity) is still largely unclear, however, it does appear that patients with autoallergy experience faster response times when treated with omalizumab. In one study, subjects refractory to standard antihistamine therapy with IgE anti-TPO antibodies were randomized to receive omalizumab in 2 or 4 week intervals for a span of 24 weeks. Patients with anti-IgE TPO antibodies experienced early responses to omalizumab, suggesting that rapid neutralization of IgE is the major mechanism by which omalizumab benefits this particular cohort (54). On the contrary, subjects who display a slow response to omalizumab are thought to have IgG antibodies against FcεRI since downregulation of this receptor occurs only after free IgE is first complexed by the drug (64). The authors validated this hypothesis by demonstrating a high correlation between length of time to the onset of omalizumab efficacy and positive basophil histamine release activity, with the latter predicting slower response times to treatment (64). Basophil activation, which is more specific for the detection of histamine-releasing autoantibodies in CSU patients than the ASST, may thus be a useful test in assessing patient responsiveness to omalizumab (64). As such, patients with refractory CSU may benefit from longer, more "personalized" courses of omalizumab (65). Further investigation on the mechanisms by which omalizumab benefits patients with CSU is certainly in need as are biomarkers to predict the efficacy of responsiveness and likelihood of relapse among patients with various subtypes of CSU.

CONCLUSION

Chronic spontaneous urticaria is a common and complex disorder that occurs in the absence of any identifiable provoking factor. While there are many aspects regarding CSU that have yet to be understood, it is becoming increasingly clear that both autoimmunity (IgG-mediated disease) and autoallergy (IgE-mediated disease) can contribute to the pathogenesis of this disorder and predispose subjects to the development of additional autoimmune diseases. Subjects with IgE autoantibody-mediated CSU appear to have a faster onset of improvement in response to omalizumab than those with IgG-mediated disease due to the unique mechanisms by which this drug sequentially affects IgE levels and FcεR1 status. Further investigation is required to determine how the presence of unique autoantibodies can predict the disease course and comorbidities associated with various subtypes of CSU as well as overall responsiveness to therapy.

AUTHOR CONTRIBUTIONS

SB and ASM conceptualized the topic of the review article and wrote the review. SA and ASM supervised the writing of this review.

REFERENCES

1. Poonawalla T, Kelly B. Urticaria : a review. *Am J Clin Dermatol.* (2009) 10:9–21. doi: 10.2165/0128071-200910010-00002
2. Kanani A, Betschel SD, Warrington R. Urticaria and angioedema. *Allergy Asthma Clin Immunol.* (2018) 14 (Suppl. 2):59. doi: 10.1186/s13223-018-0288-z
3. Haynes B, Soderberg KA, Fauci AS. *The Immune System in Health and Disease. Harrison's Principles of Internal Medicine.* Vol 2. 19 ed. McGraw Hill Education (2015).
4. Bernstein JA, Lang DM, Khan DA, Craig T, Dreyfus D, Hsieh F, et al. The diagnosis and management of acute and chronic urticaria: 2014 update. *J Allergy Clin Immunol.* (2014) 133:1270–7. doi: 10.1016/j.jaci.2014.02.036
5. Zuberbier T, Aberer W, Asero R, Abdul Latiff AH, Baker D, Ballmer-Weber B, et al. The EAACI/GA(2)LEN/EDF/WAO guideline for the

definition, classification, diagnosis and management of urticaria. *Allergy.* (2018) 73:1393–414. doi: 10.1111/all.13397

6. Choi HW, Suwanpradid J, Kim IH, Staats HF, Haniffa M, MacLeod AS, et al. Perivascular dendritic cells elicit anaphylaxis by relaying allergens to mast cells via microvesicles. *Science.* (2018) 362:eaao0666. doi: 10.1126/science.aao0666
7. Altman K, Chang C. Pathogenic intracellular and autoimmune mechanisms in urticaria and angioedema. *Clin Rev Allergy Immunol.* (2013) 45:47–62. doi: 10.1007/s12016-012-8326-y
8. Turner H, Kinet JP. Signalling through the high-affinity IgE receptor Fc epsilonRI. *Nature.* (1999) 402(6760 Suppl.):B24–30. doi: 10.1038/35037021
9. Rossi AB, Herlaar E, Braselmann S, Huynh S, Taylor V, Frances R, et al. Identification of the Syk kinase inhibitor R112 by a human mast cell screen. *J Allergy Clin Immunol.* (2006) 118:749–55. doi: 10.1016/j.jaci.2006.05.023
10. Saini SS, Paterniti M, Vasagar K, Gibbons SP, Sterba PM, Vonakis BM. Cultured peripheral blood mast cells from chronic idiopathic urticaria patients spontaneously degranulate upon IgE sensitization: relationship to expression of Syk and SHIP-2. *Clin Immunol.* (2009) 132:342–8. doi: 10.1016/j.clim.2009.05.003
11. MacGlashan D. Auto-antibodies to IgE and FceRI and the natural variability of SYK expression in basophils. *J Allergy Clin Immunol.* (2018) 143:1100–7.e11. doi: 10.1016/j.jaci.2018.05.019
12. Gimborn K, Lessmann E, Kuppig S, Krystal G, Huber M. SHIP down-regulates FcεR1-induced degranulation at supraoptimal IgE or antigen levels. *J Immunol.* (2005) 174:507–16. doi: 10.4049/jimmunol.174.1.507
13. Vonakis BM, Gibbons S, Sora R, Langdon JM, MacDonald SM. Src homology 2 domain-containing inositol 5' phosphatase is negatively associated with histamine release to human recombinant histamine-releasing factor in human basophils. *J Allergy Clin Immunol.* (2001) 108:822–31. doi: 10.1067/mai.2001.119159
14. Grattan CE, Wallington TB, Warin RP, Kennedy CT, Bradfield JW. A serological mediator in chronic idiopathic urticaria–a clinical, immunological and histological evaluation. *Br J Dermatol.* (1986) 114:583–590. doi: 10.1111/j.1365-2133.1986.tb04065.x
15. Taskapan O, Kutlu A, Karabudak O. Evaluation of autologous serum skin test results in patients with chronic idiopathic urticaria, allergic/non-allergic asthma or rhinitis and healthy people. *Clin Exp Dermatol.* (2008) 33:754–8. doi: 10.1111/j.1365-2230.2008.02819.x
16. Fusari A, Colangelo C, Bonifazi F, Antonicelli L. The autologous serum skin test in the follow-up of patients with chronic urticaria. *Allergy.* (2005) 60:256–8. doi: 10.1111/j.1398-9995.2005.00673.x
17. Eckman JA, Hamilton RG, Gober LM, Sterba PM, Saini SS. Basophil phenotypes in chronic idiopathic urticaria in relation to disease activity and autoantibodies. *J Invest Dermatol.* (2008) 128:1956–63. doi: 10.1038/jid.2008.55
18. Asero R, Tedeschi A, Riboldi P, Cugno M. Plasma of patients with chronic urticaria shows signs of thrombin generation, and its intradermal injection causes wheal-and-flare reactions much more frequently than autologous serum. *J Allergy Clin Immunol.* (2006) 117:1113–7. doi: 10.1016/j.jaci.2005.12.1343
19. Kocatürk E, Kavala M, Kural E, Sarigul S, Zindanci I. Autologous serum skin test vs. autologous plasma skin test in patients with chronic urticaria: evaluation of reproducibility, sensitivity and specificity and relationship with disease activity, quality of life and anti-thyroid antibodies. *Eur J Dermatol.* (2011) 21:339–43. doi: 10.1684/ejd.2011.1294
20. Cugno M, Tedeschi A, Asero R, Meroni PL, Marzano AV. Skin autoimmunity and blood coagulation. *Autoimmunity.* (2010) 43:189–94. doi: 10.3109/08916930903293086
21. Puccetti A, Bason C, Simeoni S, Millo E, Tinazzi E, Beri R, et al. In chronic idiopathic urticaria autoantibodies against Fc epsilonRII/CD23 induce histamine release via eosinophil activation. *Clin Exp Allergy.* (2005) 35:1599–607. doi: 10.1111/j.1365-2222.2005.02380.x
22. Cugno M, Marzano AV, Tedeschi A, Fanoni D, Venegoni L, Asero R. Expression of tissue factor by eosinophils in patients with chronic urticaria. *Int Arch Allergy Immunol.* (2009) 148:170–4. doi: 10.1159/000155748
23. Baram D, Vaday GG, Salamon P, Drucker I, Hershkoviz R, Mekori YA. Human mast cells release metalloproteinase-9 on contact with activated T cells: juxtacrine regulation by TNF-alpha. *J Immunol.* (2001) 167:4008–16. doi: 10.4049/jimmunol.167.7.4008
24. Tedeschi A, Asero R, Lorini M, Marzano AV, Cugno M. Plasma levels of matrix metalloproteinase-9 in chronic urticaria patients correlate with disease severity and C-reactive protein but not with circulating histamine-releasing factors. *Clin Exp Allergy.* (2010) 40:875–81. doi: 10.1111/j.1365-2222.2010.03473.x
25. Grattan CE, Francis DM, Hide M, Greaves MW. Detection of circulating histamine releasing autoantibodies with functional properties of anti-IgE in chronic urticaria. *Clin Exp Allergy.* (1991) 21:695–704.
26. Hide M, Francis DM, Grattan CE, Hakimi J, Kochan JP, Greaves MW. Autoantibodies against the high-affinity IgE receptor as a cause of histamine release in chronic urticaria. *N Engl J Med.* (1993) 328:1599–04. doi: 10.1056/NEJM199306033282204
27. Vasagar K, Vonakis BM, Gober LM, Viksman A, Gibbons SP, Saini SS. Evidence of *in vivo* basophil activation in chronic idiopathic urticaria. *Clin Exp Allergy.* (2006) 36:770–776. doi: 10.1111/j.1365-2222.2006.02494.x
28. Ulambayar B, Chen YH, Ban GY, Lee JH, Jung CG, Yang EM, et al. Detection of circulating IgG autoantibody to FcεRIα in sera from chronic spontaneous urticaria patients. *J Microbiol Immunol Infect.* (2017). doi: 10.1016/j.jmii.2017.10.003
29. Fiebiger E, Hammerschmid F, Stingl G, Maurer D. Anti-FcepsilonRIalpha autoantibodies in autoimmune-mediated disorders. Identification of a structure-function relationship. *J Clin Invest.* (1998) 101:243–51. doi: 10.1172/JCI511
30. Auyeung P, Mittag D, Hodgkin PD, Harrison LC. Autoreactive T cells in chronic spontaneous urticaria target the IgE Fc receptor Ialpha subunit. *J Allergy Clin Immunol.* (2016) 138:761–8.e764. doi: 10.1016/j.jaci.2016.04.036
31. Harrison LC, Honeyman MC, DeAizpurua HJ, Schmidli RS, Colman PG, Tait BD, et al. Inverse relation between humoral and cellular immunity to glutamic acid decarboxylase in subjects at risk of insulin-dependent diabetes. *Lancet.* (1993) 341:1365–9. doi: 10.1016/0140-6736(93)90940-I
32. Hidvégi B, Nagy E, Szabó T, Temesvári E, Marschalkó M, Kárpáti S, et al. Correlation between T-cell and mast cell activity in patients with chronic urticaria. *Int Arch Allergy Immunol.* (2003) 132:177–82. doi: 10.1159/000073719
33. Brzoza Z, Grzeszczak W, Rogala B, Trautsolt W, Moczulski D. PTPN22 polymorphism presumably plays a role in the genetic background of chronic spontaneous autoreactive urticaria. *Dermatology.* (2012) 224:340–5. doi: 10.1159/000339332
34. O'Donnell BF, O'Neill CM, Francis DM, Niimi N, Barr RM, Barlow RJ, et al. Human leucocyte antigen class II associations in chronic idiopathic urticaria. *Br J Dermatol.* (1999) 140:853–8. doi: 10.1046/j.1365-2133.1999.02815.x
35. Bozek A, Krajewska J, Filipowska B, Polanska J, Rachowska R, Grzanka A, et al. HLA status in patients with chronic spontaneous urticaria. *Int Arch Allergy Immunol.* (2010) 153:419–23. doi: 10.1159/000316354
36. Chen J, Tan Z, Li J, Xiong P. Association of HLA-DRB1, DQB1 alleles with chronic urticaria. *J Huazhong Univ Sci Technol Med Sci.* (2005) 25:354–6. doi: 10.1007/BF02828166
37. Confino-Cohen R, Chodick G, Shalev V, Leshno M, Kimhi O, Goldberg A. Chronic urticaria and autoimmunity: associations found in a large population study. *J Allergy Clin Immunol.* (2012) 129:1307–13. doi: 10.1016/j.jaci.2012.01.043
38. Kolkhir P, Borzova E, Grattan C, Asero R, Pogorelov D, Maurer M. Autoimmune comorbidity in chronic spontaneous urticaria: a systematic review. *Autoimmun Rev.* (2017) 16:1196–208. doi: 10.1016/j.autrev.2017.10.003
39. Kolkhir P, Pogorelov D, Olisova O, Maurer M. Comorbidity and pathogenic links of chronic spontaneous urticaria and systemic lupus erythematosus–a systematic review. *Clin Exp Allergy.* (2016) 46:275–87. doi: 10.1111/cea.12673
40. Rottem M. Chronic urticaria and autoimmune thyroid disease: is there a link? *Autoimmun Rev.* (2003) 2:69–72. doi: 10.1016/S1568-9972(02)00141-6
41. Kolkhir P, Metz M, Altrichter S, Maurer M. Comorbidity of chronic spontaneous urticaria and autoimmune thyroid diseases: a systematic review. *Allergy.* (2017) 72:1440–60. doi: 10.1111/all.13182

42. Altrichter S, Peter HJ, Pisarevskaja D, Metz M, Martus P, Maurer M. IgE mediated autoallergy against thyroid peroxidase–a novel pathomechanism of chronic spontaneous urticaria? *PLoS ONE.* (2011) 6:e14794. doi: 10.1371/journal.pone.0014794
43. Rorsman H. Basophilic leucopenia in different forms of urticaria. *Acta Allergol.* (1962) 17:168–84. doi: 10.1111/j.1398-9995.1962.tb02937.x
44. Rorsman H, Slatkin MW, Harber LC, Baer RL. The basophile leukocyte in urtincarial hypersensitivity to physical agents. *J Invest Dermatol.* (1962) 39:493–9. doi: 10.1038/jid.1962.148
45. Appenzeller U, Meyer C, Menz G, Blaser K, Crameri R. IgE-mediated reactions to autoantigens in allergic diseases. *Int Arch Allergy Immunol.* (1999) 118:193–6. doi: 10.1159/000024064
46. Valenta R, Duchêne M, Pettenburger K, Sillaber C, Valent P, Bettelheim P, et al. Identification of profilin as a novel pollen allergen; IgE autoreactivity in sensitized individuals. *Science.* (1991) 253:557–60. doi: 10.1126/science.1857985
47. Dimson OG, Giudice GJ, Fu CL, Van den Bergh F, Warren SJ, Janson MM, et al. Identification of a potential effector function for IgE autoantibodies in the organ-specific autoimmune disease bullous pemphigoid. *J Invest Dermatol.* (2003) 120:784–8. doi: 10.1046/j.1523-1747.2003.12146.x
48. Shin YS, Suh DH, Yang EM, Ye YM, Park HS. Serum specific IgE to thyroid peroxidase activates basophils in aspirin intolerant urticaria. *J Korean Med Sci.* (2015) 30:705–9. doi: 10.3346/jkms.2015.30.6.705
49. Sánchez J, Sánchez A, Cardona R. Causal relationship between anti-TPO IgE and chronic urticaria by *in vitro* and *in vivo* tests. *Allergy Asthma Immunol Res.* (2019) 11:29–42. doi: 10.4168/aair.2019.11.1.29
50. Hatada Y, Kashiwakura J, Hayama K, Fujisawa D, Sasaki-Sakamoto T, Terui T, et al. Significantly high levels of anti-dsDNA immunoglobulin E in sera and the ability of dsDNA to induce the degranulation of basophils from chronic urticaria patients. *Int Arch Allergy Immunol.* (2013) 161 (Suppl. 2):154–8. doi: 10.1159/000350388
51. Maurer M, Altrichter S, Schmetzer O, Scheffel J, Church MK, Metz M. Immunoglobulin E-mediated autoimmunity. *Front Immunol.* (2018) 9:689. doi: 10.3389/fimmu.2018.00689
52. Dema B, Pellefigues C, Hasni S, Gault N, Jiang C, Ricks TK, et al. Autoreactive IgE is prevalent in systemic lupus erythematosus and is associated with increased disease activity and nephritis. *PLoS ONE.* (2014) 9:e90424. doi: 10.1371/journal.pone.0090424
53. Schmetzer O, Lakin E, Topal FA, Preusse P, Freier D, Church MK, et al. IL-24 is a common and specific autoantigen of IgE in patients with chronic spontaneous urticaria. *J Allergy Clin Immunol.* (2018) 142:876–82. doi: 10.1016/j.jaci.2017.10.035
54. Maurer M, Altrichter S, Bieber T, Biedermann T, Bräutigam M, Seyfried S, et al. Efficacy and safety of omalizumab in patients with chronic urticaria who exhibit IgE against thyroperoxidase. *J Allergy Clin Immunol.* (2011) 128:202–9.e205. doi: 10.1016/j.jaci.2011.04.038
55. Maurer M, Rosen K, Hsieh HJ, Saini S, Grattan C, Gimenéz-Arnau A, et al. Omalizumab for the treatment of chronic idiopathic or spontaneous urticaria. *N Engl J Med.* (2013) 368:924–35. doi: 10.1056/NEJMoa1215372
56. Beck LA, Marcotte GV, MacGlashan D, Togias A, Saini S. Omalizumab-induced reductions in mast cell Fce psilon RI expression and function. *J Allergy Clin Immunol.* (2004) 114:527–30. doi: 10.1016/j.jaci.2004.06.032
57. Kaplan AP, Giménez-Arnau AM, Saini SS. Mechanisms of action that contribute to efficacy of omalizumab in chronic spontaneous urticaria. *Allergy.* (2017) 72:519–33. doi: 10.1111/all.13083
58. Grattan CE, Dawn G, Gibbs S, Francis DM. Blood basophil numbers in chronic ordinary urticaria and healthy controls: diurnal variation, influence of loratadine and prednisolone and relationship to disease activity. *Clin Exp Allergy.* (2003) 33:337–41.doi: 10.1046/j.1365-2222.2003.01589.x
59. Saini SS, Omachi TA, Trzaskoma B, Hulter HN, Rosén K, Sterba PM, et al. Effect of omalizumab on blood basophil counts in patients with chronic idiopathic/spontaneous urticaria. *J Invest Dermatol.* (2017) 137:958–61. doi: 10.1016/j.jid.2016.11.025
60. Metz M, Staubach P, Bauer A, Brehler R, Gericke J, Ashton-Chess J, et al. Omalizumab normalizes levels of high affinity immunoglobulin E receptor-positive skin cells in patients with chronic spontaneous urticaria: a randomized, double-blind, placebo-controlled study. In: *44th Annual Meeting of the European-Society-for-Dermatological-Research.* (2014). p. S30.
61. Ertas R, Ozyurt K, Atasoy M, Hawro T, Maurer M. The clinical response to omalizumab in chronic spontaneous urticaria patients is linked to and predicted by IgE levels and their change. *Allergy.* (2018) 73:705–12. doi: 10.1111/all.13345
62. Deza G, Bertolín-Colilla M, Sánchez S, Soto D, Pujol RM, Gimeno R, et al. Basophil FcvarepsilonRI expression is linked to time to omalizumab response in chronic spontaneous urticaria. *J Allergy Clin Immunol.* (2018) 141:2313-6.e2311. doi: 10.1016/j.jaci.2018.02.021
63. Eckman JA, Sterba PM, Kelly D, Alexander V, Liu MC, Bochner BS, et al. Effects of omalizumab on basophil and mast cell responses using an intranasal cat allergen challenge. *J Allergy Clin Immunol.* (2010) 125:889-895.e887. doi: 10.1016/j.jaci.2009.09.012
64. Gericke J, Metz M, Ohanyan T, Weller K, Altrichter S, Skov PS, et al. Serum autoreactivity predicts time to response to omalizumab therapy in chronic spontaneous urticaria. *J Allergy Clin Immunol.* (2017) 139:1059–61.e1051. doi: 10.1016/j.jaci.2016.07.047
65. Niemeyer-van der Kolk T, van Maaren MS, van Doorn MBA. Personalized omalizumab treatment improves clinical benefit in patients with chronic spontaneous urticaria. *J Allergy Clin Immunol.* (2018) 142:1992–4. doi: 10.1016/j.jaci.2018.07.032

16

IL-23/IL-17 Axis Activates IL-1β-Associated Inflammasome in Macrophages and Generates an Auto-Inflammatory Response in a Subgroup of Patients with Bullous Pemphigoid

Sébastien Le Jan[1*], *Céline Muller*[2], *Julie Plee*[2], *Anne Durlach*[3], *Philippe Bernard*[1] *and Frank Antonicelli*[1,4]

[1] *Laboratory of Dermatology, EA7509 IRMAIC, University of Reims-Champagne-Ardenne, Reims, France,* [2] *Department of Dermatology, University Hospital, University of Reims-Champagne-Ardenne, Reims, France,* [3] *Laboratory Pol Bouin, Hospital Maison Blanche, University Hospital, University of Reims-Champagne-Ardenne, Reims, France,* [4] *Department of Biological Sciences, Immunology, UFR Odontology, University of Reims-Champagne-Ardenne, Reims, France*

Correspondence:
Sébastien Le Jan
sebastien.le-jan@univ-reims.fr

Bullous Pemphigoid (BP) is a skin autoimmune blistering disease characterized by immune-mediated degradation of the dermo-epidermal junction and release of a large number of inflammatory cytokines. Interleukin-1β (IL-1β) is a pleiotropic pro-inflammatory cytokine associated with inflammasome activation and known to be pivotal in several auto-immune and auto-inflammatory diseases. We sought to clarify the presence of inflammasome-dependent IL-1β and to investigate its role in BP. Skin biopsy specimens (n = 13), serum (n = 60), blister fluid (n = 26), and primary inflammatory cells from patients with BP were used to investigate inflammasome activation and function. We here highlighted a differential occurrence of a functional *in situ* inflammasome in patients with BP, biologically distinguished by IL-1β and NLRP3 expression. Clinically, elevated IL-1β levels were associated with the presence of erythema and urticarial plaques reflecting the inflammatory phase preceding blister formation. We further identified IL-17 and IL-23 as important molecules favoring IL-1β expression in monocyte-derived macrophages from BP patients. Finally, we demonstrated the ability of IL-1β to stimulate the release of the matrix metalloproteinase-9 in those macrophages, reinforcing the role of IL-1β in the auto-amplification loop of the inflammatory response associated to BP. However, whether this inflammasome is an epiphenomenon associated with BP disease or constitutes an amplification inflammatory step in certain patients still need to be determined. In the context of a precision medicine approach, our findings allowed us to delineate a subgroup of patients with BP that showed similarities with auto-inflammatory diseases. Subsequently, this opens up alternative therapeutic strategies targeting IL-1β pathway in the aim to control the early, pre-blistering inflammatory phase. Ultimately, this could also help in reducing the detrimental effects associated with high doses of corticosteroids treatment.

Keywords: bullous pemphigoid, auto-inflammation, inflammasome, macrophages, IL-1β, IL-17

INTRODUCTION

Bullous pemphigoid (BP) is the most common auto-immune blistering skin disease, clinically characterized by urticarial erythema with tense blisters, and immunologically distinguished by the presence of autoantibodies directed against two structural proteins of the dermal-epidermal junction (DEJ), BP180, and BP230. Disease progression is related to a local autoantibody-induced inflammatory response that can be characteristically subdivided into an early non-bullous urticarial/erythematous phase and a later lesional phase with blisters and erosions (1). Although it has been shown that persistent elevated titer of anti-BP180 ELISA autoantibody was a good indicator of further relapse of BP (2), we also demonstrated that variation in the inflammatory response could affect both disease activity and relapse occurrence (3–6). We here further investigated whether self-directed inflammation driven *via* activation of innate immune pathways could be related to the auto-inflammation concept, and therefore to the expression of a functional *in situ* inflammasome in BP.

The "sterile" NLRP3 inflammasome has been increasingly involved in non-infectious inflammatory responses related to autoimmune diseases (7), leading to the production of bioactive IL-1β. Indeed, IL-1ß appears to be pivotal in connecting the innate immune response and the adaptive immune responses, particularly by driving lymphocyte polarization (8–11). "Sterile," i.e., non-infectious inflammation originates from endogenous factors including extracellular matrix (ECM) components released from tissue damage, which act as danger-associated molecular patterns (DAMPs) (12). In BP, we previously showed that elastase released in skin blisters induced BP180 fragmentation (13), and the presence of biological active peptide within the blister fluid (BF) (4). Those latter peptides were chemoattractant for neutrophils and favored the release of elastase, therefore creating an auto feedback loop (4). However, IL-1β reported concentrations in BF remain controversial (14–16) and could not be explained by IL-1β gene polymorphism in BP disease (17). Then, studies are still needed to define the molecular mechanisms leading to NLRP3 inflammasome activation and to the expression and activation of IL-1β, notably with respect to BP disease activity.

Activation of the NLRP3 inflammasome requires 2 signals: a priming signal that involves transcriptional upregulation of NLRP3 and of pro-inflammatory cytokines such as IL-1β; and an activating step that can be induced by various triggers leading to pro-caspase 1 expression and activation, and ultimately to IL-1β processing into its active form (18). Besides DAMPs, other inflammatory molecules classically associated with BP pathophysiological mechanisms, such as pro-inflammatory cytokines, complement, and reactive oxygen species (ROS) were shown to prime the NLRP3 inflammasome (19, 20). Notably, recent studies showed the implication of IL-17 in NLRP3 priming, IL-1ß release and activation through NF-kB and ROS pathways, respectively (21, 22). Besides, we previously demonstrated the presence of IL-17 in the serum of BP patients, but no direct correlation could be drawn with the extent of the disease (5). Additionally, BP autoantibodies could also participate to NLRP3 inflammasome activation, as demonstrated in monocyte/macrophages from SLE (23).

In this study we investigated in BP the concept of the inflammasome associated auto-inflammatory diseases being linked to the expression and activation of IL-1β. To that end, we measured the expression of several markers of inflammasome component, especially IL-1β and NLRP3, at the site of skin lesion and in biological fluids (serum and BFs) from patients with BP. We further assessed IL-1β clinical involvement by evaluating correlations between IL-1β levels and clinical activity of patients assessed by their BPDAI (bullous pemphigoid disease activity index). We then delineated the role of BF in regulating the auto-inflammatory response associated to BP through the involvement of several of its components including IL-17 and IL-23, as well as BP autoantibodies in NLRP3 inflammasome priming and activation. We finally evaluated the role of IL-1β in the amplification of the inflammatory response in BP.

MATERIALS AND METHODS

Study Design and Patients

This ancillary study is part of a main prospective, single-center study that was conducted in the Department of Dermatology at Reims University Hospital (French Referral Center for Autoimmune Bullous Diseases) between September 2013 and July 2017. Seventy-one consecutive patients with newly diagnosed BP were included in this ancillary study on the basis of clinical features typical of BP with the presence of at least 3 of 4 criteria by Vaillant et al. (24), subepidermal blistering on skin biopsy, and deposits of IgG, C3, or both in a linear pattern along the epidermal basement membrane zone by direct immunofluorescence (sex ratio F/H: 1,45; mean age, 81.7 years old; range, 55–98 years old). For the patients included, serum, BF and a skin biopsy specimen were collected at time of diagnosis, when possible. Clinical activity of the disease was evaluated for each patient using BPDAI score (25). The BPDAI measures separate scores for mucous membrane and skin activities, the latter evaluating separately both cutaneous urticarial/erythema (non-bullous phase) and cutaneous blisters/erosions (blistering phase). Serum samples used as controls were harvested from age- and sex-matched patients that were admitted to the Trauma Department of Reims University Hospital and that showed neither biological inflammatory syndrome (C-reactive protein levels lower than 10 mg/l) nor autoimmune diseases.

Ethics Statement

The investigation was conducted under the approval of the Ethic Committee of the University Hospital of Reims (CNIL authorization DR-2013-320), and all of the subjects gave their informed and written consent before participating in the study in accordance with the Helsinki Declaration.

Autoantibody and Cytokine Level Analysis

Anti-BP180 and anti-BP230 autoantibodies as well as IL-1β levels were measured in control and BP sera and in BF using specific commercially available enzyme-linked immunosorbent assays (ELISAs) according to the manufacturer's instructions (MBL,

Nagoya, Japan and Ebiosciences, Paris, France, respectively). IL-1β levels were also detected in supernatants issued from THP-1- and BP monocyte-derived macrophages. Finally, IL-17 and IL-23 levels were analyzed in BF using U-PLEX assay (MesoScale Diagnostics, Rockville, USA). U-PLEX technology allows multiplex cytokine measurement and is based on electro-chemiluminescence detection. Briefly biotinylated capture anti-IL17 and anti-IL-23 antibodies were coupled to U-PLEX Linkers. The U-PLEX Linkers then self-assembled onto unique spots on the U-PLEX plate. After binding to the capture antibodies, detection antibodies conjugated with electro-chemiluminescent labels (MSD GOLD SULFO-TAG) bound to the analytes to complete the sandwich immunoassay. The plate was then placed into an MSD instrument where the amounts of IL-17 and IL-23 present in BF were measured.

Cell Isolation and Cell Culture

The THP-1 (Tohoku Hospital Pediatrics-1) cell line, derived from the peripheral blood of a 1 year old human male with acute monocytic leukemia (26) and kindly provided by Dr S. Hart (University of Edinburgh, Scotland, UK), was cultured in RPMI 1640 medium (Life Technologies, NY, USA) supplemented with 10% FBS, 2 mmol/L glutamine, 25 U/mL penicillin, and 25 U/mL streptomycin at 37°C in a humidified 5% CO_2 incubator. For macrophage differentiation, THP-1 cells were incubated with phorbol myristate acetate (PMA) 50 nM for 68 h.

Peripheral Blood Mononuclear Cells (PBMCs) and polymorphonuclear (PMN) cells from control subjects and patients with BP were isolated using a density gradient technique from EDTA-treated whole blood (GranuloSep; Eurobio-Abcys, Courtaboeuf, France). Monocytes were then positively selected and purified from PBMCs by using CD14 immuno-magnetic beads according to the manufacturer's instructions (MACS; Miltenyi Biotec, Bergisch Gladbach, Germany). All leukocytes were cultured in RPMI 1640 medium (Life Technologies, NY, USA), 2 mmol/L glutamine, 25 U/mL penicillin, and 25 U/mL streptomycin at 378°C in a humidified 5% CO_2 incubator. Monocytes were differentiated into macrophages by culturing them for 7 days in the presence of autologous serum (10%).

In vitro Inflammasome Activation Assay

In order to analyze the priming of the NLRP3 inflammasome, THP-1- and BP monocyte-derived macrophages were stimulated with either lipopolysaccharide (LPS) (1 μg/ml) (Santa Cruz Biotechnology, Dallas, USA) or BF 25% for 3 h. Priming was also induced by recombinant IL-17 or recombinant IL-23 (Bio-Techne, Lille, France) in BP monocyte-derived macrophages. For IL-17 stimulation, a concentration of 1 ng/ml was chosen to be closer to the maximal BF concentration that was measured while staying in the range of the ED_{50} (3–15 ng/ml). While ED_{50} for recombinant human IL-23 was around 0.3 ng/ml, the concentration of IL-23 used for stimulation was also 1 ng/ml to remain in the same range of concentrations than the ones used for IL-17. Cells were then harvested for NLRP3 and IL-1β gene expression analysis. Activation of the inflammasome was induced by BF 25% for 30 min in either LPS-primed THP-1- and BP monocyte-derived macrophages or LPS-primed PMN cells. Supernatant were then collected for IL-1β concentration measurement. Nigericin 20 μM (Santa Cruz Biotechnology, Dallas, USA), by acting as a potassium ionophore, was used as a positive control of inflammasome activation. Added together with either Nigericin or BF to the cells, Glibenclamide 50 μM (Santa Cruz Biotechnology, Dallas, USA) was employed as an inhibitor of inflammasome activation.

Gene Expression Analysis

Total RNA from THP-1- and BP monocyte-derived macrophages was extracted with TRI Reagent (Euromedex, Souffelweyersheim, France). Reverse transcription was performed from 1 μg of total RNA by using the Maxima First Strand cDNA kit with dsDNAse (ThermoFisher Scientific, Waltham, USA), according to the manufacturer's instructions. *IL-1β* (Forward primer: 5′GGATATGGAGCAACAAGTGG 3′; Reverse primer: 5′ATG TACCAGTTGGGGAACTG 3′) and *NLRP3* (Forward primer: 5′CTTCTCTGATGAGGCCCAAG 3′; Reverse primer: 5′GCA GCAAACTGGAAAGGAAG 3') gene expression was analyzed by using real-time PCR with Power SYBR Green PCR Master mix (ThermoFisher Scientific, Waltham, USA) on the Stratagene Mx3005P system (Agilent Technologies, Santa Clara, USA). Relative quantification was performed with *GAPDH* as a reference gene.

Immunohistochemistry

Perilesional skin biopsy specimens from 13 patients with BP before the start of treatment were obtained. Tissues were fixed in paraformaldehyde, embedded in paraffin, and sectioned. Immunostaining with a mouse monoclonal anti-human NLRP3 antibody (clone Nalpy3-b, Enzo Life Sciences, Villeurbanne, France) or a mouse monoclonal anti-human CD163 antibody (Clone MRQ26, Roche Diagnostics, Meylan, France) was performed using routine methods with a biotinylated anti-mouse secondary antibody (BA-2000; Vector Laboratories, Burlingame, USA) and the ABC-peroxidase complex (Vector Laboratories, Burlingame, USA) with diaminobenzidine-H_2O_2 used as the chromogen for detection. In order to identify cells positive for both NLRP3 and CD163, immunohistochemistry for both markers was performed on 4 μm-thick serial BP skin section. Virtual slide images for NLRP3 and CD163 staining were taken using the VS120 Virtual Slide Microscope (Olympus France, Rungis, France). Virtual slide images corresponding to NLRP3 and CD163 staining were opened at the same time with OlyVIA software (Olympus France, Rungis, France) and synchronized for analysis.

Statistical Analysis

Descriptive statistics such as means and SEMs were conducted for all quantitative measures. The distribution of the variables was assessed using D'Agostino and Pearson omnibus normality test. As population could not be assumed to be normal and some of the groups examined were small, we used non-parametric testing to compare populations in this study. Comparisons between two groups were performed using the exact Wilcoxon signed-rank test for paired data and the Mann–Whitney test for unpaired data. Correlations were performed using non-parametric Spearman's correlation test. The results were considered significant if p-values were 0.05 or less.

RESULTS

Presence of IL-1β-Related Inflammasome in a Subgroup of Patients With Severe BP

We first looked for the presence of an *in situ* inflammasome in BP through the detection of NLRP3 by immunohistochemistry (IHC) on 13 BP skin biopsy specimens collected at baseline (**Figures 1A–H**). NLRP3 was highly expressed in 6/13 patients with BP (**Figure 1C**), slightly in 4/13 patients, and not detected in 3/13 patients (**Figure 1B**). When detected, NLRP3 was expressed by keratinocytes in the epidermis (**Figure 1D**). We further showed NLRP3 expression in the dermis and in the blister cavity, especially in skin resident cells (endothelial cells, fibroblasts; **Figure 1E**) and infiltrated inflammatory cells including PMN cells (**Figure 1F**) and macrophages (**Figure 1G**). Noteworthy, PMN cells also expressed NLRP3 in the lumen of the blood vessel at proximity of the lesion site (arrowhead in **Figure 1E**). Macrophages were further characterized by IHC performed on serial slides of BP skin biopsy specimen, which identified NLRP3-positive CD163$^+$ macrophage (**Figures 1G,H**) among the innate immune cell population observed at the vicinity of the blister.

Then, we determined the level of IL-1β in biological fluids of patients with BP and of control subjects. IL-1β was not detected or found at very low levels both in sera from patients with BP ($n = 60$; mean: 0.046 ± 0.024 pg/mL) and in sera from control subjects ($n = 28$; mean: 0.178 ± 0.107 pg/mL; **Figure 2A**). In contrast to BP sera, IL-1β levels were significantly enhanced in BF of patients with BP ($n = 26$; mean: 13.17 ± 4.553 pg/ml; $p < 0.001$; **Figure 2A**). However, IL-1β expression was heterogeneously distributed with 6 out of the 26 BF in which IL-1β was not detected, while IL-1β concentrations could raise up to 100 pg/ml in other BFs (**Figure 2A**). IL-1β concentration in the BF was correlated with the skin erythema/urticaria activity ($n = 25$; $r = 0.55$; $p = 0.0048$; **Figure 2D**), but neither with the total BPDAI score ($n = 25$; $r = 0.29$; $p = 0.15$; **Figure 2B**), nor with the skin BPDAI subscore associated with blisters and erosions ($n = 25$; $r = 0.11$; $p = 0.62$; **Figure 2C**). In order to further demonstrate the biological activity of IL-1β, we also measured the expression of its natural receptor antagonist IL-1ra, which works as a decoy receptor to limit IL-1β -associated inflammatory process. As IL-1β secretion was not correlated to IL-1ra production in BF of patients with BP (**Figure 2E**), we analyzed the ratio IL-1β vs. IL-1ra. The IL-1β/IL-1ra inflammatory ratio was associated with disease activity (**Figures 2F–H**). Indeed, the IL-1β /IL-1ra ratio was significantly correlated both with the total BPDAI score and with the erythema/urticaria BPDAI subscore (**Figures 2F–H**, $n = 20$; $r = 0.4545$, $p = 0.0441$ and $r = 0.5663$, $p = 0.0092$, respectively), but not with the blisters/erosions BPDAI subscore (**Figure 2G**, $n = 20$, $r = 0.06$, $p = 0.7977$).

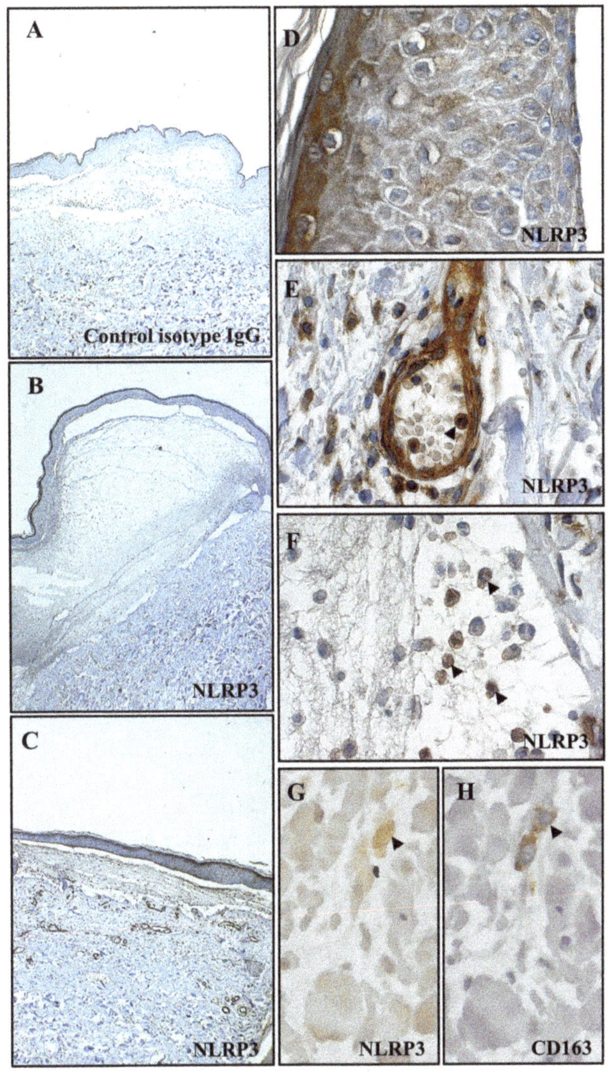

FIGURE 1 | NLRP3 was expressed at site of lesion in BP. Immunohistochemistry for NLRP3 was performed on skin biopsy specimen from 13 patients with BP. Representative pictures of technical negative control (with control isotype IgG), of BP skin negative for NLRP3 and of BP skin positive for NLRP3 were shown in **(A–C)** respectively (magnification x40). More precisely, immunohistochemistry for NLRP3 was analyzed in the epidermis **(D)**, in the dermis **(E)** and in the blister cavity **(F)** of BP skin. To note, arrowheads indicated polymorphonuclear cells in the lumen of a blood vessel in **(E)** and in the blister cavity in **(F)**. Serial staining for NLRP3 **(G)** and CD163 **(H)** was achieved in dermis and NLRP3-positive CD163$^+$ macrophage was indicated by an arrowhead (magnification x400).

BF Induced "Priming" and Activation of Inflammasome in Macrophages

To investigate whether enhanced IL-1β concentrations were related to the NLRP3 inflammasome activation, we then investigated whether the BF itself could favor the expression of IL-1β in macrophages. For this purpose, we first evaluated the effects of BF on the "priming" step of the inflammasome induction by measuring both NLRP3 and IL-1β mRNA expression in 2 different models of macrophages *in vitro*. In both THP-1- and serum-induced CD14$^+$ monocyte-derived macrophages stimulated with BF for 3 h, the increase of NLRP3 mRNA was associated with an increased expression of the IL-1β mRNA as demonstrated by a significant positive correlation between IL-1β and NLRP3 mRNA expressions under BF stimulation ($r = 0.94$, $p = 0.017$ and $r = 0.71$, $p = 0.05$, respectively; **Figures 3A,B**).

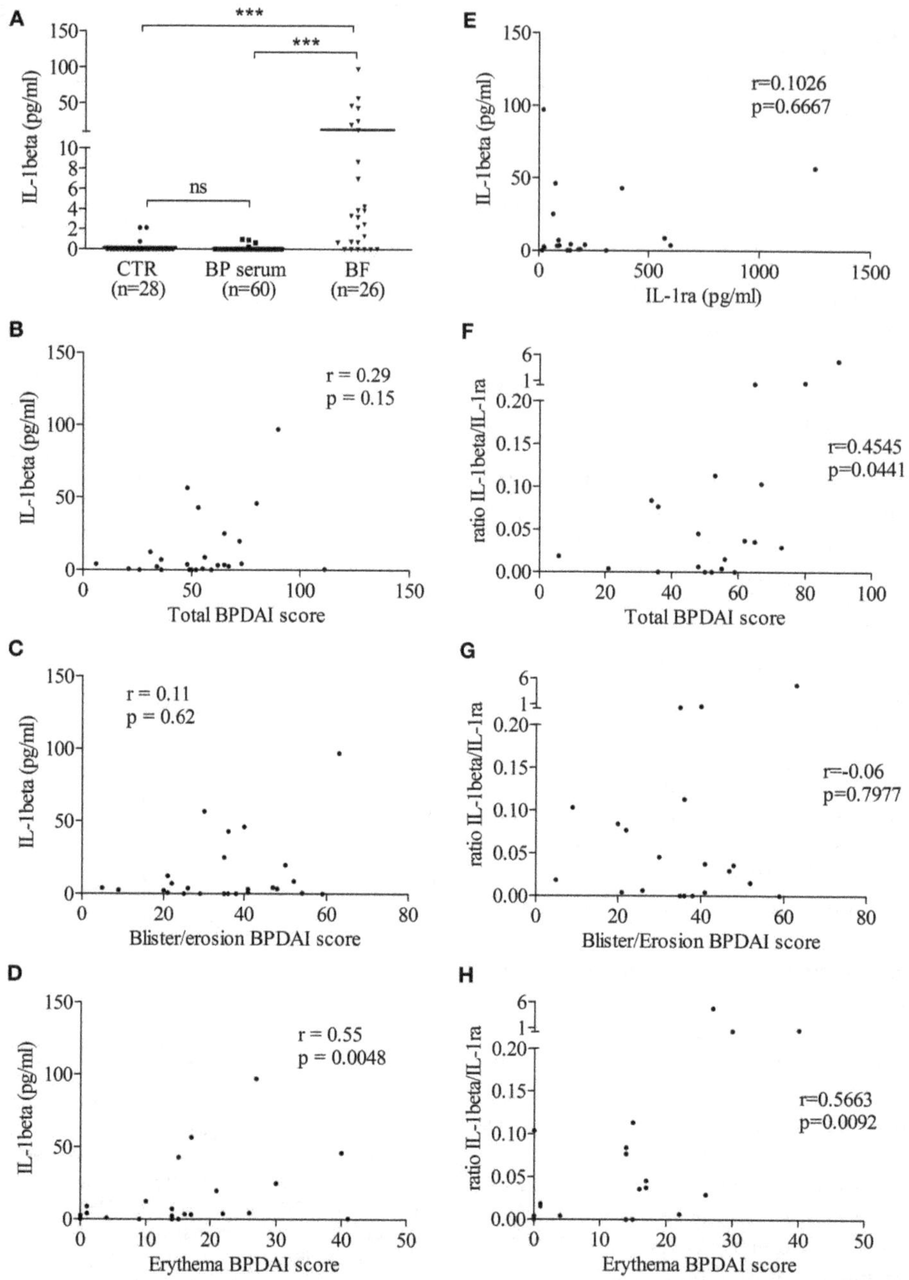

FIGURE 2 | *In situ* IL-1β levels were related to BP disease activity. **(A)** IL-1β levels were measured in biological fluids of control and BP patients using ELISA (Mann–Whitney test was used to compare populations; ns, not significant and ***$p < 0.001$). Correlations between total **(B,F)**, blister/erosion **(C,G)**, and erythema **(D,H)** BPDAI scores and both IL-1β **(B–D)** and the IL-1β/IL-1ra ratio, used as inflammatory marker **(F–H)**, were analyzed using the non-parametric Spearman's correlation test. **(E)** Levels of IL-1ra, the natural antagonist of IL-1β, were measured in BF of patients with BP and correlation between IL-1β and IL-1ra was analyzed using the non-parametric Spearman's correlation test.

Following the investigation of the "priming" step, we investigated whether factors within the BF could also participate to the "activation" step of the inflammasome characterized by the production of active IL-1β upon CASPASE-1 activation. In both THP-1- and monocyte-derived macrophages models, BF increased IL-1β secretion in LPS-primed macrophages (**Figures 3C,D**). Such activation was further confirmed by use of nigericin, a specific inducer of inflammasome activation, and glibenclamide a selective inhibitor of NLRP3 inflammasome activation, respectively. Indeed, both nigericin- and BF-induced IL-1β secretion was significantly inhibited by glibenclamide in THP-1-derived macrophages (**Figure 3E**). In contrast, BF did not increase IL-1β secretion in PMN cells originated from BP patients and primed with LPS for 3 h before BF stimulation (**Figure 3F**).

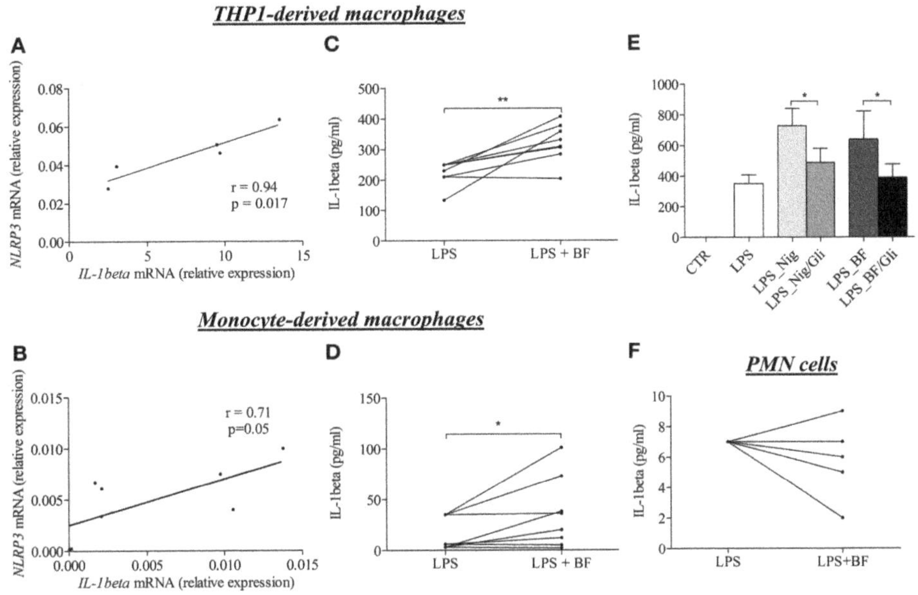

FIGURE 3 | BF of BP patients had the ability to induce "priming" and activation of NLRP3 inflammasome in macrophages. Using quantitative RT-PCR, NLRP3, and IL-1β mRNA relative expression were analyzed in both THP-derived macrophages **(A)** and in BP serum-induced CD14+ monocyte-derived macrophages **(B)** stimulated for 3 h with BF. Correlation between IL-1 and NLRP3 was then investigated using the non-parametric Spearman's correlation test. Activation of inflammasome was examined through IL-1β detection by ELISA in both THP-derived macrophages **(C)** and in serum-induced CD14+ monocyte-derived macrophages **(D)** primed with LPS for 3 h and stimulated with BF for 30 min ($n = 8$; Wilcoxon's test for paired data was applied for statistical analysis; *$p < 0.05$ and **$p < 0.01$). The effect of glibenclamide, a specific inhibitor of NLRP3 inflammasome, was studied on nigericin or BF-induced IL-1β secretion in LPS-primed THP-1-derived macrophages **(E)** ($n = 7$; Data are shown as the mean ± SEM; Wilcoxon's test for paired data was applied; *$p < 0.05$). Activation of inflammasome by BF was also examined in LPS-primed BP PMN cells through IL-1β detection by ELISA **(F)**.

IL-17 and IL-23 Had the Ability to Prime IL-1β-Related Inflammasome in BP Macrophages

Based on recent studies showing the ability of autoantibodies and cytokines such as IL-17 to induce "priming" and activation of the inflammasome, we sought correlation between immunological and biological data, such as the levels of anti-BP180 and anti-BP230 autoantibodies or pro-inflammatory cytokines IL-17 and IL-23, and levels of IL-1β in BF of patients with BP (**Figures 4A–D**). A positive and significant correlation was established between BF levels of IL-1β and the concentrations of both IL-17 and IL-23 in BF of patients with BP ($n = 22$; $r = 0.42$, $p = 0.05$ and $r = 0.43$, $p = 0.05$, respectively; **Figures 4C,D**).

To further clarify the contribution of the IL-17/IL-23 axis to the activation of inflammasome, we first looked for correlation between IL-1β expression and the concentration of IL-17 and IL-23 measured in BFs used to stimulate BP monocyte-derived macrophages in **Figure 3**. Our results showed a tendency for IL-1β expression to follow the BF concentration of IL-17 but not of IL-23 ($n = 6$; $r = 0.74$, $p = 0.09$ and $r = -0.30$, $p = 0.55$, respectively; **Figures 5A,B**). We further evaluated the direct capacity of IL-17 and IL-23 to induce the NLPR3-associated inflammasome in BP monocyte-derived macrophages. Priming of the NLRP3 inflammasome by IL-17 was demonstrated in macrophages by a significant increase of the expression of both IL-1β and NLRP3 mRNAs (**Figures 5C,D**). In contrast, IL-23 significantly induced IL-1β but not NLRP3 mRNA expression, although an increase of NLRP3 mRNA was observed in 5 cases out of 6 (**Figures 5E,F**). In contrast, inflammasome activation was affected by neither IL-17 nor IL-23, as these cytokines did not enhance IL-1β protein level from LPS primed monocyte-derived macrophages (data not shown).

IL-1β Induced MMP-9 Secretion in BP Monocyte-Derived Macrophages

Finally, to investigate the influence of NLRP3-associated IL-1β expression on disease activity of BP, we evaluated the potential role of IL-1β in matrix metalloproteinase-9 (MMP-9) release by macrophages and PMN cells. While PMN-released MMP-9 was not modified by IL-1β stimulation (**Figure 6A**), we showed a significant increase in MMP-9 secretion by IL-1β-stimulated monocyte-derived macrophages (**Figure 6B**).

DISCUSSION

In the context of a precision medicine approach, we defined in this study a subpopulation of patients with BP that displayed resemblances with auto-inflammatory diseases. Indeed, we provided evidence for a differential expression of a functional *in situ* "sterile" inflammasome in patients with BP, biologically characterized by the presence of NLRP3 and IL-1β. Clinically, IL-1β associated inflammasome was related to the presence of erythema and urticarial plaques, which are representative clinical signs of the early

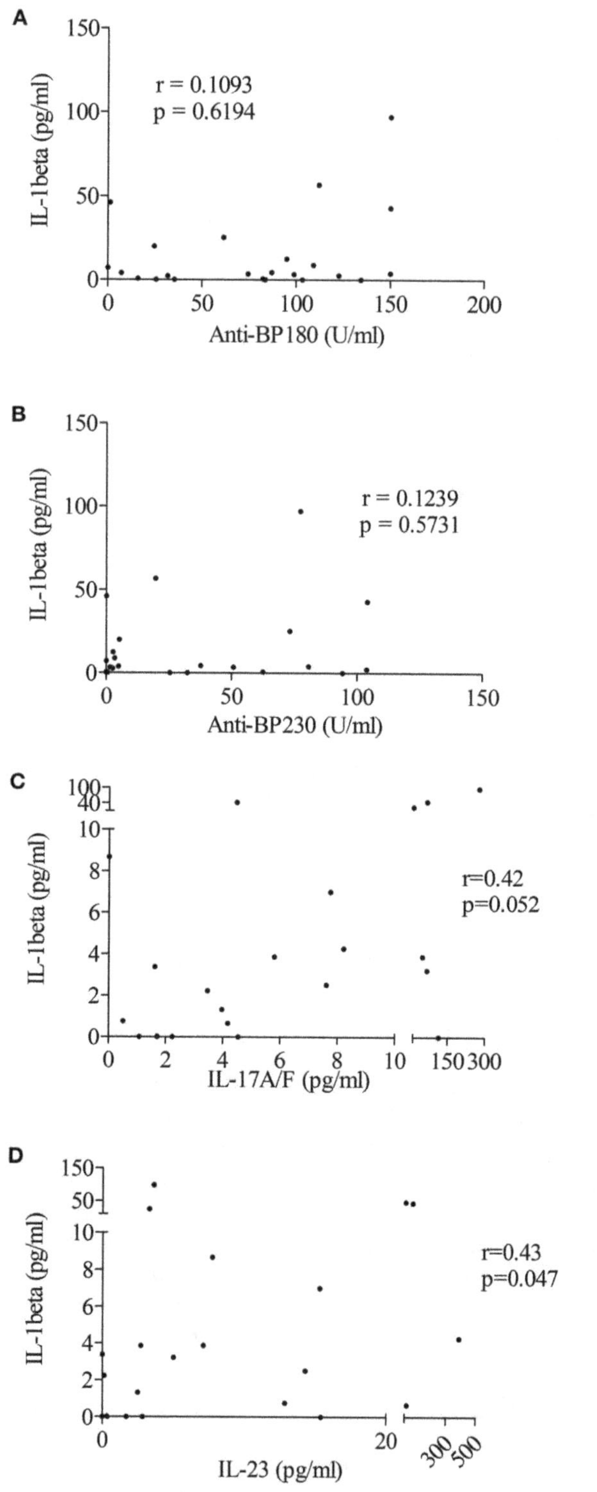

FIGURE 4 | IL-1β levels were associated with pro-inflammatory cytokines but not autoantibodies in BF of patients with BP. Levels of anti-BP180 **(A)** and anti-BP230 **(B)** autoantibodies but also of the pro-inflammatory cytokines IL-17 **(C)** and IL-23 **(D)** were measured in BF of BP patients using ELISA before testing any correlation with IL-1β levels (non-parametric Spearman's correlation test was used for statistical analysis with $n = 23$ for autoantibodies and $n = 22$ for cytokines).

inflammatory phase preceding blister formation. Biologically, we identified IL-17 and IL-23 as significant inflammatory mediators for inflammasome priming in BP monocyte-derived macrophages. Finally, the ability of IL-1β to induce macrophage-released MMP-9 supports its participation to the auto-amplification loop of the inflammatory response associated to BP (4).

At the active phase of the disease i.e., at time of diagnosis before treatment, IL-1β was detected at skin lesional site in BF of certain patients with BP but not in all of them, and not in the serum of BP patients. This observation is consistent with previous studies that showed the presence of IL-1β in a small series of BF but not in sera of BP patients (14, 16). Moreover, we also demonstrated a heterogeneous expression of NLRP3 in skin biopsy specimens originated from patients with BP. Corroborating IL-1β findings, some patients strongly expressed NLRP3 both in skin resident cells (keratinocytes, endothelial cells, fibroblasts) and in infiltrated innate immune cells including macrophages and PMN cells, while other showed very low or no expression of NLRP3. Notably, we observed NLRP3-positive PMN cells in the lumen of dermal blood vessels supporting the idea of an additional systemic inflammasome in BP patients that was recently demonstrated with the presence of IL-18 and NLRP3 in peripheral blood mononuclear cells (15). Altogether these results strongly suggest that NLRP3 inflammasome occurred only in certain BP patients, suggesting that either the inflammasome is an epiphenomenon involved in the amplification of the BP-related inflammatory response of the pathophysiological mechanism associated to BP, or that specific BP conditions are required. Accordingly, it was recently shown that expression of specific inflammasome gene module stratifies elderly individuals into two extreme clinical and immunological states (27): those without constitutive expression of IL-1β and the others with constitutive IL-1β that were more susceptible to age-related diseases. In addition, recent studies demonstrated the critical role of skin microbiota in the regulation of the inflammatory response in patients with atopic dermatitis or psoriasis (28). To know if such epiphenomena could have regulatory functions in the inflammasome-related BP pathophysiological mechanisms still needs further investigations and would be of great interest to better classify patients in a future precision medicine approach.

Although future investigations, notably with the use of a control group patients with autoimmune blistering disease sharing autoimmune/inflammation features such as dermatitis herpetiformis, could help to demonstrate whether inflammasome-related mechanisms are specific to BP disease or not, our results showed that such mechanisms are associated with BP activity. Indeed, IL-1β biological activity displayed a positive and significant correlation between the IL-1β levels in BF or the inflammatory ratio IL-1β/IL-1RA and the erythema/urticaria BPDAI subscore, suggesting its involvement in the early inflammatory phase. Notably, no correlation could be demonstrated either between IL-1β/IL-1ra ratio or IL-1β level and the blisters/erosions BPDAI subscore, reinforcing the significance of the "sterile" NLRP3 inflammasome in the early non-bullous urticaria/erythematous phase of the local

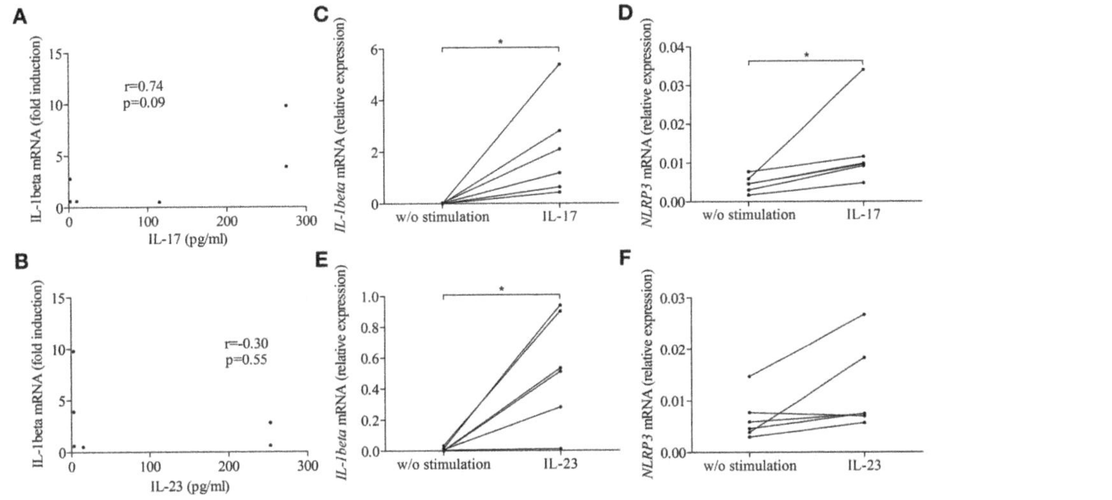

FIGURE 5 | IL-17 and IL-23 induced IL-1β expression in BP monocyte-derived macrophages. Correlations were tested between macrophage-expressed IL-1β and the concentrations of IL-17 **(A)** and IL-23 **(B)** measured in BFs used to prime BP monocyte-derived macrophages. IL-1β **(C,E)** and NLRP3 **(D,F)** mRNA expressions were investigated in CD14+ isolated monocytes originated from patients with BP, differentiated into macrophages in presence of BP serum for 7 days and stimulated for 3 h with IL-17 **(C,D)** and IL-23 **(E,F)** ($n = 6$, Wilcoxon's test for paired data was applied; $^*p \leq 0.05$).

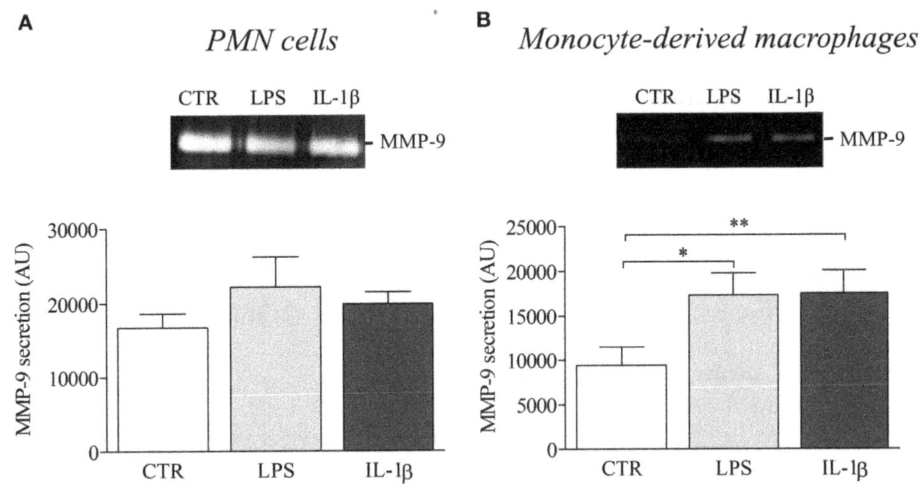

FIGURE 6 | IL-1β induced MMP-9 release in BP serum-differentiated macrophages. MMP-9 release was examined by gel zymography in PMN cells **(A)** and BP monocyte-derived macrophages **(B)** stimulated with LPS or IL-1β for 24 h ($n = 4$; Data are shown as the mean ± SEM; paired *T*-Test was applied for statistical analysis; $^*p \leq 0.05$; $^{**}p < 0.01$).

inflammatory response. Accordingly, no erythema was observed in 2 out 3 patients that did not show NLRP3 expression in skin biopsy specimen in contrast to all NLRP3-highly positive patients that exhibited numerous erythematous plaques (data not shown). Altogether these results highlighted the importance of considering these inflammasome-related mechanisms when initially treating patients with BP. In contrast, no significant relationship could be drawn between the presence of an NLRP3 inflammasome and IL-1β at skin lesional site and the specific auto-immune response defined by anti-BP180 and anti-BP230 serum autoantibodies, suggesting that the inflammasome in BP is rather associated with an auto-inflammatory than an auto-immune process. In our study, neither BF-related IL-1β nor NLRP3 could be identified as a predictive marker of relapse in patients with BP at diagnosis (data not shown).

BF of patients with BP contains all inflammatory molecules classically associated with the priming and the activation of the "sterile" NLRP3-related inflammasome, such as DAMPs (ECM components released from tissue damage), pro-inflammatory cytokines, complement and reactive oxygen species (ROS) (12, 19–22). Indeed, while IL-1β levels did not appeared to be correlated with the blisters/erosions BPDAI subscore, we showed here that BF has the ability to induce priming and activation of an NLRP3-dependent inflammasome in monocyte-derived macrophages through the concomitant regulation of IL-1β and NLRP3 mRNA expression and its increasing effects on IL-1β secretion in LPS-primed macrophage. This was further supported by the use of glibenclamide, a specific inhibitor of NLRP3 inflammasome activation. In line with the positive and significant correlations observed between the concentrations of the pro-inflammatory cytokines IL-17 or IL-23 and IL-1β in BF, we also demonstrated an increased expression of IL-1β mRNA expression in monocyte-derived macrophages primed with BF, especially with BF in which IL-17 concentrations were elevated, and in monocyte-derived macrophages primed with IL-17 or IL-23. These results suggest that IL-1β-dependent inflammation in BP could be at least partly linked to IL-17 and IL-23 but should not overshadow that other molecules contained in BF could also be involved either directly or indirectly in the activation of an inflammasome in BP. Meanwhile, NLRP3 mRNA expression was enhanced in response to IL-17 but not in response to IL-23 suggesting that IL-1β expression could also be regulated in an inflammasome-independent manner as recently highlighted in an experimental caspase-1/11-deficient mouse model of epidermolysis bullosa acquisita (29). We already highlighted discrepancies in the effects of IL-17 and IL-23 in a recent study showing that IL-23 was a more potent inductor of NETosis than IL-17 in BP (30). Release of immunomodulatory cytokines and chemokines during this process could play a role either in favoring the auto-immunity or the auto-inflammatory processes. Besides, although IL-17 induced NLRP3, neither IL-17 nor IL-23 induce the release of IL-1β by macrophage supporting the fact that these cytokines are not directly involved in the generation of the bioactive IL-1β. Thus, these results suggest that other molecules are required to IL-1β production, maybe through the cooperation between different immune cell types or inflammatory processes.

In BP, IL-1β production could involve MMP expression. Indeed MMPs, especially MMP-9, have the ability to cleave pro-IL-1β to generate biologically active IL-1β (31). Noteworthy, both IL-17 and IL-23 were shown to increase MMP-9 production in BP (4, 5). Besides cytokines and MMPs, DAMPs and ROS have also been largely involved in NLRP3 inflammasome activation by notably favoring the NLRP3/ASC complex assembly (20). Investigation of the redox status of BF from patients with BP showed a disturbance of the redox balance toward hyperoxidative status of all BF tested (data not shown), suggesting a potential role of ROS in the activation of the inflammasome in BP. However, ROS being present in all BF do not appear as the limiting factor in the generation of bioactive IL-1β in contrast to the pro-inflammatory cytokine IL-17 that is expressed only in a subpopulation of patients with BP as previously demonstrated (5).

In the present study, IL-1β had the ability to induce MMP-9 secretion in monocyte-derived macrophages but not in PMN cells. *In situ* MMP-9 release could degrade matrix molecules into peptides that could feed back the inflammatory and immune responses (12). Though, together with the pro-inflammatory cytokines IL-17, IL-23 and CXCL10 that we previously demonstrated to induce MMP-9 release in several types of cells (4–6), macrophage-released IL-1β could participate to the auto-amplification loop during the auto-inflammatory response associated with BP. Since IL-1ß plays a pivotal role in the pathogenesis of auto-inflammatory diseases, targeted therapies blocking IL-1 activity by different mechanisms were shown to result in a rapid and sustained reduction of disease severity, including anakinra (IL-1 receptor antagonist), canakinumab (neutralizing monoclonal anti-IL-1β antibody) or rilonacept (soluble decoy receptor) (32). Systemic or superpotent topical corticosteroids are the main effective first-line therapies in BP, but with low selectiveness. They are essentially symptomatic and associated with numerous adverse events. In the context of the precision medicine approach, our results open up new possibilities for therapeutic strategies potentially involving the combination of lower doses of corticosteroids and biotherapies targeting IL-1β pathway or maybe even better targeting pro-inflammatory cytokines such as IL-17 and IL-23 acting upstream of IL-1β to control the auto-inflammatory like process occurring in the early phase of the blister formation in BP.

AUTHOR CONTRIBUTIONS

SL, PB, and FA designed the study and wrote the manuscript. SL and CM performed experiments. CM, JP, and AD collected clinical data and biological material. SL, CM, JP, PB, and FA analyzed clinical and biological data. All authors critically evaluated the data and approved the final version for publication.

ACKNOWLEDGMENTS

We thank Christine Terryn and the Plateforme IBiSA Imagerie Cellulaire et Tissulaire for providing microscopy equipment.

REFERENCES

1. Bernard P, Antonicelli F. Bullous pemphigoid: a review of its diagnosis, associations and treatment. *Am J Clin Dermatol.* (2017) 18:513–28. doi: 10.1007/s40257-017-0264-2
2. Fichel F, Barbe C, Joly P, Bedane C, Vabres P, Truchetet F, et al. Clinical and immunologic factors associated with bullous pemphigoid relapse during the first year of treatment: a multicenter, prospective study. *JAMA Dermatol* (2014) 25–33. doi: 10.1001/jamadermatol.2013.5757
3. Giusti D, Gatouillat G, Le Jan S, Plée J, Bernard P, Antonicelli F, et al. Eosinophil Cationic Protein (ECP), a predictive marker of bullous pemphigoid severity and outcome. *Sci Rep.* (2017) 7:4833. doi: 10.1038/s41598-017-04687-5
4. Le Jan S, Plée J, Vallerand D, Dupont A, Delanez E, Durlach A, et al. Innate

immune cell-produced IL-17 sustains inflammation in bullous pemphigoid. *J Invest Dermatol.* (2014) 134:2908–17. doi: 10.1038/jid.2014.263

5. Plée J, Le Jan S, Giustiniani J, Barbe C, Joly P, Bedane C, et al. Integrating longitudinal serum IL-17 and IL-23 follow-up, along with autoantibodies variation, contributes to predict bullous pemphigoid outcome. *Sci Rep.* (2015) 5:18001. doi: 10.1038/srep18001
6. Riani M, Le Jan S, Plée J, Durlach A, Le Naour R, Haegeman G, et al. Bullous pemphigoid outcome is associated with CXCL10-induced matrix metalloproteinase 9 secretion from monocytes and neutrophils but not lymphocytes. *J Allergy Clin Immunol.* (2017) 139:863–72. doi: 10.1016/j.jaci.2016.08.012
7. Shen H-H, Yang Y-X, Meng X, Luo X-Y, Li X-M, Shuai Z-W, et al. NLRP3: a promising therapeutic target for autoimmune diseases. *Autoimmun Rev.* (2018) 17:694–702. doi: 10.1016/j.autrev.2018.01.020
8. Ben-Sasson SZ, Hogg A, Hu-Li J, Wingfield P, Chen X, Crank M, et al. IL-1 enhances expansion, effector function, tissue localization, and memory response of antigen-specific CD8 T cells. *J Exp Med.* (2013) 210:491–502. doi: 10.1084/jem.20122006
9. Chung Y, Chang SH, Martinez GJ, Yang XO, Nurieva R, Kang HS, et al. Critical regulation of early Th17 cell differentiation by interleukin-1 signaling. *Immunity.* (2009) 30:576–87. doi: 10.1016/j.immuni.2009.02.007
10. Ghiringhelli F, Apetoh L, Tesniere A, Aymeric L, Ma Y, Ortiz C, et al. Activation of the NLRP3 inflammasome in dendritic cells induces IL-1β - dependent adaptive immunity against tumors. *Nat Med.* (2009) 15:1170–8. doi: 10.1038/nm.2028
11. Koyama N, Harada N, Takahashi T, Mita S, Okamura H, Tominaga A, et al. Role of recombinant interleukin-1 compared to recombinant T-cell replacing factor/interleukin-5 in B-cell differentiation. *Immunology.* (1988) 63:277–83.
12. Frevert CW, Felgenhauer J, Wygrecka M, Nastase MV, Schaefer L. Danger-associated molecular patterns derived from the extracellular matrix provide temporal control of innate immunity. *J Histochem Cytochem.* (2018) 66:213–27. doi: 10.1369/0022155417740880
13. Verraes S, Hornebeck W, Polette M, Borradori L, Bernard P. Respective contribution of neutrophil elastase and matrix metalloproteinase 9 in the degradation of BP180 (Type XVII Collagen) in human bullous pemphigoid. *J Invest Dermatol.* (2001) 117:1091–6. doi: 10.1046/j.0022-202x.2001.01521.x
14. Ameglio F, D'Auria L, Bonifati C, Ferraro C, Mastroianni A, Giacalone B. Cytokine pattern in blister fluid and serum of patients with bullous pemphigoid: relationships with disease intensity. *Br J Dermatol.* (1998) 138:611–4. doi: 10.1046/j.1365-2133.1998.02169.x
15. Fang H, Shao S, Cao T, Lei J, Dang E, Zhang J, et al. Increased expression of NLRP3 inflammasome components and interleukin-18 in patients with bullous pemphigoid. *J Dermatol Sci.* (2016) 83:116–23. doi: 10.1016/j.jdermsci.2016.04.009
16. Schmidt E, Mittnacht A, Schömig H, Dummer R, Bröcker EB, Zillikens D. Detection of IL-1 alpha, IL-1 beta and IL-1 receptor antagonist in blister fluid of bullous pemphigoid. *J Dermatol Sci.* (1996) 11:142–7. doi: 10.1016/0923-1811(95)00435-1
17. Tabatabaei-Panah P-S, Moravvej H, Sadaf Z, Babaei H, Geranmayeh M, Hajmanouchehri S, et al. Proinflammatory Cytokine Gene Polymorphisms in Bullous Pemphigoid. *Front Immunol.* (2019) 10:636. doi: 10.3389/fimmu.2019.00636
18. Latz E, Xiao TS, Stutz A. Activation and regulation of the inflammasomes. *Nat Rev Immunol.* (2013) 13:397–411. doi: 10.1038/nri3452
19. Patel MN, Carroll RG, Galván-Peña S, Mills EL, Olden R, Triantafilou M, et al. Inflammasome priming in sterile inflammatory disease. *Trends Mol Med.* (2017) 23:165–80. doi: 10.1016/j.molmed.2016.12.007
20. Rubartelli A. Redox control of NLRP3 inflammasome activation in health and disease. *J Leukoc Biol.* (2012) 92:951–8. doi: 10.1189/jlb.0512265
21. Cho K-A, Suh JW, Lee KH, Kang JL, Woo S-Y. IL-17 and IL-22 enhance skin inflammation by stimulating the secretion of IL-1β by keratinocytes via the ROS-NLRP3-caspase-1 pathway. *Int Immunol.* (2012) 24:147–58. doi: 10.1093/intimm/dxr110
22. Zhang S, Yu N, Zhang R, Zhang S, Wu J. Interleukin-17A Induces IL-1β Secretion From RPE Cells Via the NLRP3 Inflammasome. *Invest Ophthalmol Vis Sci.* (2016) 57:312–9. doi: 10.1167/iovs.15-17578
23. Zhang H, Fu R, Guo C, Huang Y, Wang H, Wang S, et al. Anti-dsDNA antibodies bind to TLR4 and activate NLRP3 inflammasome in lupus monocytes/macrophages. *J Transl Med.* (2016) 14:156. doi: 10.1186/s12967-016-0911-z
24. Vaillant L, Bernard P, Joly P, Prost C, Labeille B, Bedane C, et al. Evaluation of clinical criteria for diagnosis of bullous pemphigoid. French Bullous Study Group. *Arch Dermatol.* (1998) 134:1075–80. doi: 10.1001/archderm.134.9.1075
25. Murrell DF, Daniel BS, Joly P, Borradori L, Amagai M, Hashimoto T, et al. Definitions and outcome measures for bullous pemphigoid: recommendations by an international panel of experts. *J Am Acad Dermatol.* (2012) 66:479–85. doi: 10.1016/j.jaad.2011.06.032
26. Tsuchiya S, Yamabe M, Yamaguchi Y, Kobayashi Y, Konno T, Tada K. Establishment and characterization of a human acute monocytic leukemia cell line (THP-1). *Int J Cancer.* (1980) 26:171–6. doi: 10.1002/ijc.2910260208
27. Furman D, Chang J, Lartigue L, Bolen CR, Haddad F, Gaudilliere B, et al. Expression of specific inflammasome gene modules stratifies older individuals into two extreme clinical and immunological states. *Nat Med.* (2017) 23:174–84 doi: 10.1038/nm.4267
28. Dainichi T, Kitoh A, Otsuka A, Nakajima S, Nomura T, Kaplan DH, et al. The epithelial immune microenvironment (EIME) in atopic dermatitis and psoriasis. *Nat Immunol.* (2018) 19:1286–98. doi: 10.1038/s41590-018-0256-2
29. Sadeghi H, Lockmann A, Hund A-C, Samavedam UKSRL, Pipi E, Vafia K, et al. Caspase-1-independent IL-1 release mediates blister formation in autoantibody-induced tissue injury through modulation of endothelial adhesion molecules. *J Immunol Baltim.* (2015) 194:3656–63. doi: 10.4049/jimmunol.1402688
30. Giusti D, Bini E, Terryn C, Didier K, Le Jan S, Gatouillat G, et al. NET formation in bullous pemphigoid patients with relapse is modulated by IL-17 and IL-23 interplay. *Front Immunol.* (2019) 10:701. doi: 10.3389/fimmu.2019.00701
31. Schönbeck U, Mach F, Libby P. Generation of biologically active IL-1 beta by matrix metalloproteinases: a novel caspase-1-independent pathway of IL-1 beta processing. *J Immunol Baltim.* (1998) 161:3340–6.
32. Dinarello CA, Simon A, van der Meer JWM. Treating inflammation by blocking interleukin-1 in a broad spectrum of diseases. *Nat Rev Drug Discov.* (2012) 11:633–52. doi: 10.1038/nrd3800

17

Complement Activation in Autoimmune Bullous Dermatoses: A Comprehensive Review

Gareth Edwards [1], Gilles F. H. Diercks [2], Marc A. J. Seelen [3], Barbara Horvath [1], Martijn B. A. van Doorn [4] and Jeffrey Damman [5]*

[1] Department of Dermatology, University Medical Center Groningen, Groningen, Netherlands, [2] Department of Pathology, University Medical Center Groningen, Groningen, Netherlands, [3] Department of Nephrology, University Medical Center Groningen, Groningen, Netherlands, [4] Department of Dermatology, Erasmus Medical Center Rotterdam, Rotterdam, Netherlands, [5] Department of Pathology, Erasmus Medical Center Rotterdam, Rotterdam, Netherlands

Correspondence:
Jeffrey Damman
j.damman@erasmusmc.nl

Autoimmune bullous dermatoses (AIBD) are characterized by circulating autoantibodies that are either directed against epidermal antigens or deposited as immune complexes in the basement membrane zone (BMZ). The complement system (CS) can be activated by autoantibodies, thereby triggering activation of specific complement pathways. Local complement activation induces a pathogenic inflammatory response that eventually results in the formation of a sub- or intraepidermal blister. Deposition of complement components is routinely used as a diagnostic marker for AIBD. Knowledge from different animal models mimicking AIBD and deposition of complement components in human skin biopsies provides more insight into the role of complement in the pathogenesis of the different AIBD. This review outlines the role of the CS in several AIBD including bullous pemphigoid, epidermolysis bullosa acquisita, mucous membrane pemphigoid (MMP), pemphigus, linear IgA-disease, and dermatitis herpetiformis. We also discuss potential therapeutic approaches targeting key complement components, pathways and pathogenic complement-mediated events.

Keywords: complement, auto-immune bullous dermatosis, bullous pemphigod, epidermolysis bullosa acquisita, mucus membrane pemphigoid, pemphigus, linear IgA bullous dermatoses, dermatitis herpetiformis

INTRODUCTION

The development of autoimmune bullous dermatoses (AIBD) is a complex interaction between multiple parts of the innate and adaptive immune system. Bullous pemphigoid (BP) is the most frequently encountered AIBD with an annual incidence estimated between 2.4 and 21.7 new cases per million population in different populations worldwide (1). In AIBD, autoantibodies are either directed against epidermal antigens or deposited as immune complexes in the basement membrane zone (BMZ). Besides deposition of immunoglobulins as part of the adaptive immune system, complement components can be found as part of the innate immune system. Secondary tissue injury and blistering can be initiated by complement-dependent and complement-independent mechanisms. Local complement activation triggers the release of cytokines and chemokines that results in the recruitment of inflammatory cells, including neutrophils and eosinophils. This pathogenic inflammatory response eventually results in the formation of sub- or intra-epidermal blisters that will reveal its unique clinical features of the specific disease.

The complement system (CS) is an important arm of the innate immune system. It functions as a defense system against pathogens and plays a major role in tissue homeostasis. The CS has three distinct activation routes: the classical pathway (CP), the alternative pathway (AP), and the lectin pathway (LP) (**Figure 1**). Activation and regulation of the complement system has been extensively outlined before by our group and therefore we refer to our previous publication by Giang et al. for a more detailed description (2).

BULLOUS PEMPHIGOID

Bullous pemphigoid (BP) is an AIBD characterized by autoantibodies against BP180 and/or BP230. Most antibodies in BP are directed against the NC16A domain of BP180, which is a major non-collagenous extracellular antigenic site. Clinically, patients present with tense pruritic dome-shaped, fluid-filled blisters measuring up to several centimeters in diameter. Histology reveals a subepidermal blister that is most often accompanied by an infiltrate of lymphocytes, eosinophils, neutrophils, mast cells, and monocytes/macrophages. Deposition of immunoglobulins and complement factor C3c are routinely used for diagnostic purposes (**Figure 2**). In addition, deposition of other complement factors of different complement pathways has been demonstrated by direct immunofluorescence (DIF) and immunoperoxidase staining on formalin-fixed paraffin-embedded tissue (3–10). Besides the diagnostic use of complement factors, mouse models have demonstrated an important role for complement in the pathogenesis of BP. In mice, Liu et al. passively transferred a rabbit-antibody against murine BP180NC14A, a homolog of human BP180NC16A. These mice developed a subepidermal blistering disease with a phenotype closely mimicking human BP. Using this model, serum complement depletion by cobra venom factor or C5-deficiency protected against the development of BP. Also, transfer of F(ab′)2-fragments derived from the anti-murine BP180 antibody failed to induce a BP phenotype (11). These findings indicate a crucial role for the IgG-Fc portion and likely the CP, since the FC tail bears the C1q binding region. In line with these findings, C4-KO mice as well as wildtype mice treated with anti-mC1q were resistant to develop BP. Besides a role for the CP, FB-deficient mice developed delayed and less intense blisters, indicating involvement of the AP. It is likely both the CP and AP act in concert when the amplification loop is activated upon CP activation (12, 13). So far, no role has been attributed to activation of the LP. It is questionable whether the previously cited findings can be translated into clinical practice, since BP180NC14a is poorly preserved in mice. For this reasons, humanized mice models were developed replacing mouse BP180NC14A by human BP180NC16A and introducing the human COL17 cDNA transgene into Col17-null mice (14). Importantly, Liu et al. also showed protection against BP in their humanized BP-model after complement depletion with cobra venom factor (15). Also, transfer of humanized IgG1 mutated at the C1q binding site has shown lower pathogenicity in COL17-humanized neonatal mice compared to unmutated humanized IgG1 (16). Although these experiments confirm the complement-dependent blister formation in BP, evidence emerges that also complement-independent mechanisms exist. Karsten et al. have recently demonstrated that the extent of skin lesions decreased with only 50% when C5-deficient mice were injected with anti-COL17 IgG in a humanized mouse model (17). This is in contrast with the previously cited findings in the non-humanized BP-model that showed full protection (11). The differences might be explained by the use of the humanized model by Karsten et al. or the existence of complement-independent mechanisms. Natsuga et al. have demonstrated that rabbit auto-antibodies specifically against the R7 domain within human NC16A induced subepidermal blister formation in COL17-humanized neonatal mice. It was found that the auto-antibody after immunoadsorption against R7, or decoying of R7 with BSA, significantly reduced skin fragility, despite ongoing complement activation. Moreover, F(ab′)2 fragments of anti-BP180 IgG antibodies from BP patients or rabbit IgG against humanized NC16A induced (in part) skin fragility in neonatal humanized mice (18). Lastly, Ujiie et al. found that passive transfer of human BP auto-antibodies induced blister formation in neonatal C3-deficient COL17 humanized mice (19). Altogether, these studies indicate that it is highly likely that also complement independent mechanisms play a role in the pathogenesis of BP. One hypothesis is the direct pathogenic effect of auto-antibodies against NC16A via macropinocytic internalization, ubiquitination and degradation of BP180 leading to impairment of hemidesmosome formation (19, 20). *In vitro* studies indeed demonstrated direct pathogenic effects of auto-antibodies and F(ab′)2 fragments leading to depletion of BP180 in cultured keratinocytes (18, 19, 21). Although complement-independent mechanisms are likely to exist, the contradictory results between different studies could also be explained by the differences in target epitopes on COL17 in the models used, antibody concentration, antibody affinity, or the clonality of antibodies in each experiment (19). Importantly, conflicting results are observed between the humanized and non-humanized models and could (in part) be explained by the lower murine complement fixating and activating capacities of the transferred human auto-antibodies compared to mouse and/or rabbit antibodies (22).

Liu et al. further characterized complement in BP and found that neutrophil depletion protected against the development of BP in wildtype mice, while injection of C5a or IL-8 in C5-KO mice regained susceptibility for BP (23). Moreover, absence of C5aR1-expression on mast cells demonstrated similar protection against BP development, despite complement activation and the presence of neutrophils. It was found that in the BP mouse model, extensive mast cell degranulation occurs that precedes the influx of neutrophil infiltration and subepidermal blister formation.

Abbreviations: AP, alternative pathway; AIBD, autoimmune bullous dermatoses; BMZ, basement membrane zone; BP, bullous pemphigoid; C5aR1, C5a receptor 1; C5aR2, C5a receptor 2; CP, classical pathway; CS, complement system; DH, dermatitis herpetiformis; DIF, direct immunofluorescence; KO, knock-out; LAD, Linear IgA disease; LP, lectin pathway; MAC, membrane attack complex; MBL, mannan binding lectin; MMP, mucous membrane pemphigoid.

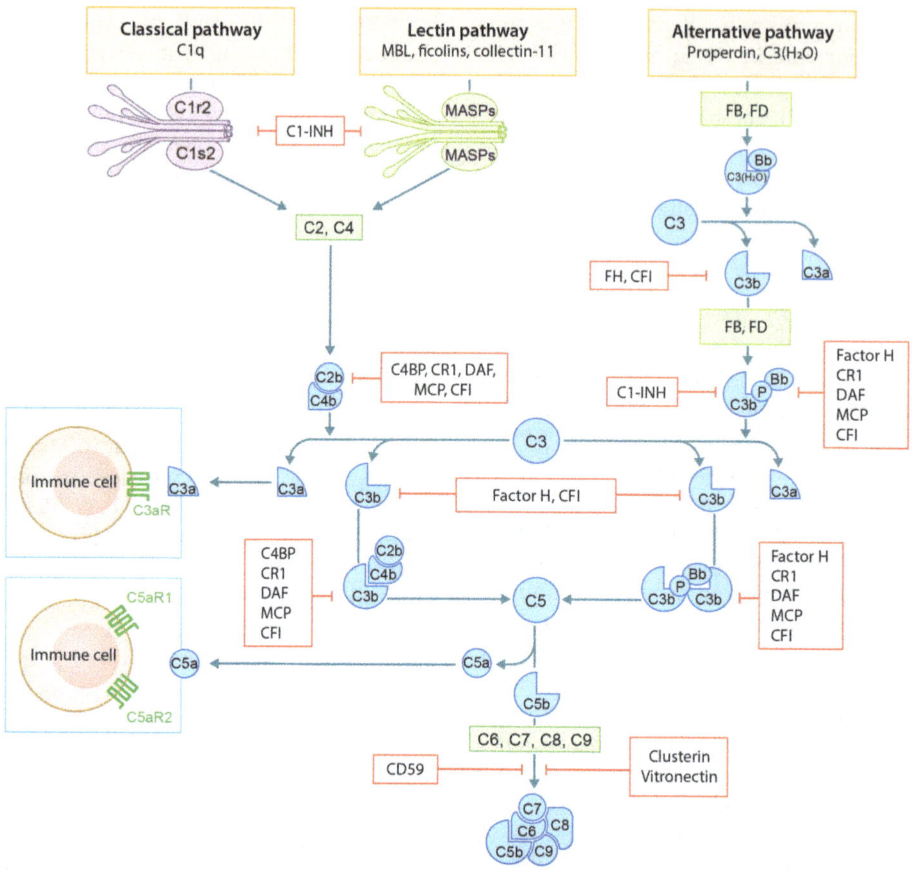

FIGURE 1 | Schematic overview of the complement system. Figure adapted from Giang et al. (2).

These findings reveal that complement-dependent neutrophil recruitment in BP acts, at least in part, via C5aR1-induced mast cell degranulation (12, 24). Recently, this hypothesis was further investigated by Karsten et al. who confirmed the protection of C5aR1-KO mice against BP, whereas C5aR2-KO animals were more susceptible for disease development. As a proof of principle, prophylactic treatment with a C5aR1-inhibitor PMX53 in mice also led to reduced disease activity (17). Altogether, these results indicate an important role for C5a-C5aR1-axis activation in the development of BP and could be an interesting target for intervention.

Although previous pre-clinical studies are encouraging, these experiments were all performed in mice which makes it difficult to translate these data to humans. However, Romeijn et al. showed in a large patient study comprising 300 patients with BP, that complement C3c was deposited in the majority of (peri)lesional skin biopsies. More interestingly, the extent of deposition was correlated with clinical and serological disease activity, strengthening the crucial role of complement in this disease (25). Besides the deposition of complement in the skin, Chiorean et al. recently found that functional complement-activation capacity of autoantibodies *ex-vivo* in BP also correlates with severity of skin disease and autoantibody titers (26).

MUCOUS MEMBRANE PEMPHIGOID

Mucous membrane pemphigoid (MMP) is an AIBD. The disease represents a spectrum, which affects both skin and mucosa, especially the oral and ocular mucous membranes. Cutaneous lesions manifest as tense blisters that, when ruptured, heal slowly and usually result in scarring. Histopathology reveals a subepidermal blister and a lymphocytic infiltrate in the upper dermis with eosinophils and sometimes neutrophils. DIF shows IgG- and C3c-deposition along the BMZ, but also IgA-, IgM-, and fibrin-deposition can be found (27, 28). Various autoantigens have been found in MMP including BP180 (BPAG2), BP230 (BPAG1), laminin 332, α6/β4 integrin, and laminin 6 (29). Early DIF studies have found deposition of C3, C1q, C4, FB, and properdin along the BMZ (28).

Experimental models that passively transferred rabbit anti-laminin 5 (laminin 332) produced subepidermal blisters with the same clinical, histologic, and immunopathologic features of MMP. However, blistering could not be prevented in C5-deficient mice, indicating that the terminal complement pathway is not involved in blister formation in this experimental model of MMP (30). Also, mice injected with F(ab')2-fragments instead of intact IgG, developed subepidermal blistering and a clinical

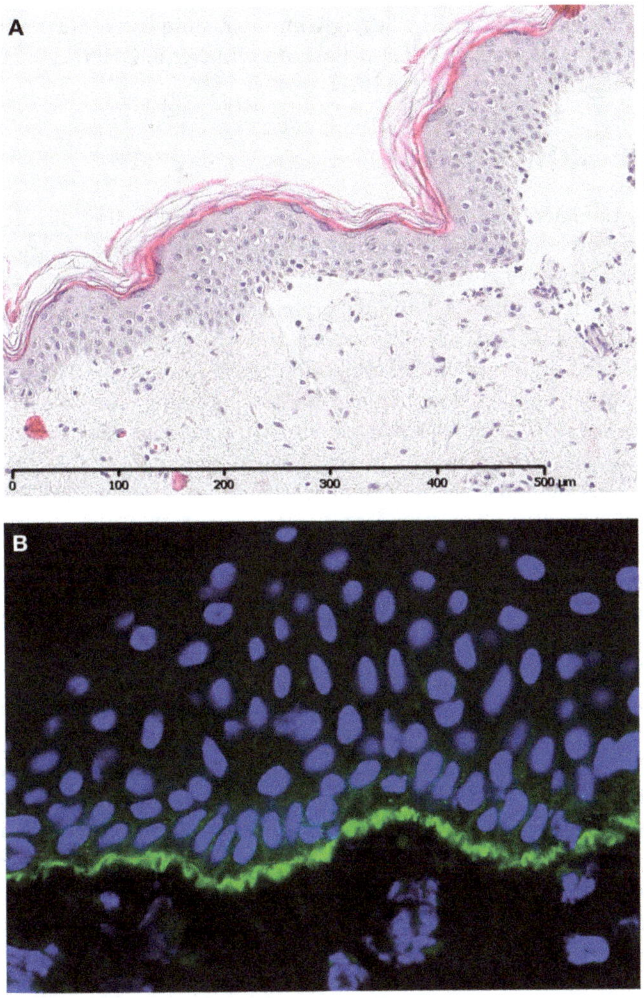

FIGURE 2 | A case of bullous pemphigoid. Histology shows a subepidermal blister **(A)** accompanied by specific linear C3c deposition along the BMZ visualized by direct immunofluorescence **(B)**. Figure (in part) adapted from Giang et al. (2).

MMP phenotype comparable to wildtype mice. These results strongly argue against a complement-dependent mechanism of blister formation in MMP (31). In a recent study by Heppe et al. a mouse MMP model was developed by passive transfer of rabbit anti-laminin 332 specifically against 2 immunodominant regions of LAMα3 in adult mice. The model reflects major clinical and immunopathological characteristics of the human disease. In contrast to the previously described model by Lazarova et al. mice in this model also developed conjunctival lesions and therefore might reflect the clinical situation more accurately. Importantly, clear differences were observed between the two models concerning complement activation. In contrast to Lazarova et al. development of MMP in the model of Heppe et al. was complement-dependent. Mice deficient in C5aR1 or FCqR showed reduced or no signs of MMP. Differences could be explained by the use of IgG against LAMa3 and the use of adult mice by Heppe et al. compared to the use of IgG against all subunits of human laminin 332 and neonatal mice by Lazarova et al. (29, 31).

EPIDERMOLYSIS BULLOSA ACQUISITA

Epidermolysis bullosa acquisita is a rare chronic subepidermal AIBD affecting skin and/or mucous membranes. It usually manifests in adults with lesions resembling dystrophic epidermolysis bullosa and is diagnosed after exclusion of all other acquired bullous dermatoses. The disease is characterized by tissue-bound and circulating IgG-autoantibodies against type VII collagen as well as linear u-serrated deposition of complement components along the BMZ (32, 33). In the mechanobullous variant, light microscopy reveals a subepidermal blister, a cell-free subepidermal vesicle, and usually no dermal inflammation. The inflammatory variant frequently resembles histological features of BP.

Experimental mouse models have demonstrated a subepidermal blistering phenotype upon passive administration of rabbit-anti-mouse collagen VII. Moreover, passive transfer of human epidermolysis bullosa acquisita-autoantibodies caused subepidermal blistering and induction of epidermolysis bullosa acquisita skin lesions in mice, proving the pathogenicity of these autoantibodies (34). Similar results were found in an *active* model of epidermolysis bullosa acquisita in which mice developed subepidermal blisters after immunization with collagen VII (35). These mice showed deposition of IgG as well as complement C3 along the BMZ. Comparable to BP, the findings in experimental epidermolysis bullosa acquisita models were also C5 and rabbit IgG-Fc portion dependent and suggests a role for the CP via C1q-FC-receptor binding (34, 36, 37). However, C1q-KO and MBL-KO mice were still susceptible for epidermolysis bullosa acquisita development, comparable to wildtype mice. To further unravel the complement pathways involved, Mihai et al. demonstrated that FB-deficient or wildtype-mice treated with anti-FB developed a delayed and less severe blistering disease compared to wildtype-mice (37, 38). These results attribute an important role to AP activation in the pathogenesis of epidermolysis bullosa acquisita (38). It was hypothesized that the AP serves as an amplification loop upon CP or LP activation, which are likely to compensate for each other. Notably, a role for ficolins in complement activation and amplification loop initiation cannot be fully excluded. Alternatively, AP might be activated upon binding of autoantibodies against complement regulator proteins.

More downstream, epidermolysis bullosa acquisita is likely to be C5aR1-dependent, since C5aR1-deficient animals were protected against development of epidermolysis bullosa acquisita (37, 39). Moreover, animals pretreated with anti-C5aR1 antibody developed a less severe blistering phenotype compared to controls. No protection was found in C6-deficient animals, excluding a major role for MAC formation in epidermolysis bullosa acquisita. In summary, these experimental models demonstrate involvement of CP- and AP-activation and C5a-C5aR1-axis activation in the development of epidermolysis bullosa acquisita.

LINEAR IGA DISEASE

Linear IgA disease (LAD) is defined as a rare group of subepidermal bullous diseases where IgA-autoantibodies target the epidermal BMZ. Patients present with pruritic blisters consisting of grouped vesicles on erythematous bases. The most common antigen targets are LAD-1 and LABD97, which are cleavage products of the extracellular domain of BP180. Histologically, a subepidermal blister is seen with neutrophils aligned along the dermal-epidermal junction or filling up the dermal papillae. DIF shows linear deposition of IgA along the BMZ.

The pathogenesis of LAD can be complement-dependent and -independent. Recent studies have shown that crosslinking of FcαRI on neutrophils by IgA-immune-complexes can directly initiate immune responses and activation and migration of neutrophils in LAD, independent of complement (40, 41). Although IgA is a weak activator of complement in comparison to IgM and IgG, in practice, deposition of C3 can be found in LAD up to 30% (42, 43). Since IgA does not have a C1q-binding site, it cannot activate the CP, but it can activate both the AP and LP (44, 45). It is known from patients with IgA-vasculitis and IgA-nephropathy that particularly the LP can be activated upon binding of MBL and ficolins to IgA deposits in vessel walls or glomeruli (45–47) Whether AP and LP are also involved in the pathogenesis of LAD remains to be investigated. Although complement is deposited in LAD, further research is needed to determine the contribution of complement to the pathogenesis of LAD.

DERMATITIS HERPETIFORMIS

Dermatitis herpetiformis (DH) is a rare cutaneous manifestation of celiac disease that mostly manifests in adults. Patients with DH present with highly pruritic papulovesicular eruptions on various extensor surfaces. Celiac disease is characterized by IgA-autoantibodies against tissue transglutaminase while DH also shows antibodies against epidermal transglutaminase. The tissue transglutaminase modifies a fraction of gluten, gliadin, to an antigen which binds to an HLA-DQ2 or HLA-DQ8 molecule, provoking an autoimmune reaction. The IgA autoantibodies against epidermal transglutaminase are deposited as granular immune-complexes in the dermis. Histology shows characteristic micro-abscesses and granular IgA-deposits in papillary dermis while C3-deposition can be found in up to 89% (48). Seah et al. suggested that complement is activated via the AP since no deposits of C1q were found in DH biopsies (48). Although IgA does not activate the CP of complement, the mere absence of C1q does not exclude CP activation since C1q has a relatively low half-life in tissue. For definitive proof of AP activation, Provost et al. demonstrated specific deposition of FB and properdin as markers of AP activation in DH (49). Also, the role of the LP cannot be ruled out and remains to be investigated. In addition to granular C3-deposition in DH, Preisz and colleagues also found vascular immune precipitates and C3-deposition in DH that strongly co-localized with epidermal transglutaminase (50). As previously discussed in the segment about LAD, the immune reaction in DH can also be complement-independent due to crosslinking of FcαRI with IgA-immune-complexes. However, since the percentage of C3-deposition is higher in DH, this likely to occur less often than in LAD.

PEMPHIGUS

Pemphigus includes a group of rare chronic blistering diseases characterized by IgG-autoantibodies directed against a variety of desmosomal transmembrane glycoproteins. Patients with pemphigus vulgaris typically present with lesions of the oral mucosa followed by skin-involvement and autoantibodies are directed against epithelial adhesion protein desmoglein 3 and/or desmoglein 1. In pemphigus foliaceus the lesions are localized on the skin, without involvement of the mucous membranes, and autoantibodies are directed against desmoglein 1. DIF studies demonstrate intercellular deposition of IgG and C3c, which suggests involvement of complement activation in the pathogenesis of pemphigus. Furthermore, components of all complement activation pathways can be found in the intercellular substance (ICS) including C1q, properdin, C3, C5, MBL, ficolins, and the MAC (51–53). Nevertheless, animal models have shown that blister formation in pemphigus can be independent of complement activation. In an experimental passive IgG-transfer mouse model, pathogenic patient pemphigus vulgaris IgG and F(ab′)2 were equally pathogenic, while the latter failed to induce complement C3-deposition. In the same model using only pemphigus vulgaris IgG, C5-deficient, or cobra venom factor pretreated neonatal mice also developed pemphigus blisters (54). Although this data indicates a minor role for complement in pemphigus, the results should be interpreted with caution. In contrast to high-dose pemphigus vulgaris IgG, complement-depleted animals transferred with low-dose pemphigus vulgaris IgG showed more limited and delayed onset of disease. Thus, complement activation might not be essential, but potentiates the pathogenicity of autoantibodies in experimental pemphigus. Whether complement plays a role in the initiation and or propagation of pemphigus in humans remains to be investigated.

TARGETING THE COMPLEMENT SYSTEM IN AUTOIMMUNE BULLOUS DERMATOSES

The greatest challenge in targeting complement activation, is to find the optimal balance between sufficient blocking and preservation of complement activity. Complete blocking of complement activation is undesirable since this is highly associated with infections. At this moment, no complement targeting drugs have been approved for clinical use in AIBD.

Recently, Kasprick et al. found that treatment with a mouse monoclonal anti-C1s antibody (TNT003) significantly reduced C3c-deposition and production of C4a and C5a, as well as neutrophil chemoattraction in an *ex-vivo* human skin cryosection assay (55). These results show that early inhibition of the CP can prevent IgG-induced complement activation *in-vitro*. Although the *in vivo* effect on inflammation or blistering is unknown, this data provides rationale to test Sutimlimab, a humanized monoclonal of TNT003, which was shown to be safe and well-tolerated in humans (56, 57). Selective CP inhibition without interfering in AP and LP opens new and safe opportunities for interventions in BP, thereby leaving important arms of the CS intact.

Other possible ways to inhibit the CS includes the inhibition of the C5a-C5aR axis. The anti-C5 monoclonal antibody Eculizumab binds to C5, thereby preventing cleavage into its active components, but has been associated with a thousand-fold increased risk of meningococcal disease (58). Coversin (a recombinant small protein) is another anti-C5 drug that is currently in phase IIA of clinical trials in BP-patients. In addition of binding C5, it also inhibits leukotriene B4, another powerful inflammatory mediator (https://adisinsight.springer.com/trials/700284185). Although C5-blocking drugs are interesting, it will also interfere with C5a-C5aR2-axis activation, which has recently shown protective effects in BP (17). Therefore, inhibition of C5a-C5aR1 axis might be more interesting, leaving C5a-C5aR2 interaction intact. Avacopan is an oral small molecule C5aR1-inhibitor and has shown promising results in clinical trials by having a long half-life and showing limited side effects (59).

Further studies are needed to investigate the mechanisms of complement activation in humans which provides a basis for developing more specific therapeutic approaches targeting key complement component, pathways and pathogenic events.

CONCLUSION

It has been shown through various experimental and clinical studies that the CS plays a role in several AIBD. In animals models using complement-deficient mice, different complement pathways are involved in the pathogenesis of different AIBD. Although recent clinical studies in BP found association of complement with disease activity, it still remains to be investigated how important the CS is in the pathogenesis of other AIBD. In the last few years multiple drugs targeting specific parts of the CS are in clinical development and some of these have shown promising results in preclinical studies. Selective neutralization of pathway-specific or terminal cascade specific components is promising, since this leaves most other parts of the CS intact. As with all new drugs, the ratio of risk to benefit for the patient must be assessed in future clinical trials.

AUTHOR CONTRIBUTIONS

GE, GD, MvD, and JD: wrote the review. MS and BH: edited and approved the manuscript.

REFERENCES

1. Kridin K, Ludwig RJ. The growing incidence of bullous pemphigoid: overview and potential explanations. *Front Med.* (2018) 5:220. doi: 10.3389/fmed.2018.00220
2. Giang J, Seelen MAJ, van Doorn MBA, Rissmann R, Prens EP, Damman J. Complement activation in inflammatory skin diseases. *Front Immunol.* (2018) 9:639. doi: 10.3389/fimmu.2018.00639
3. Dahl MV, Falk RJ, Carpenter R, Michael AF. Deposition of the membrane attack complex of complement in bullous pemphigoid. *J Investig Dermatol* (1984) 82:132–5. doi: 10.1111/1523-1747.ep12259679
4. Jordon RE, Day NK, Sams WM Jr, Good RA. The complement system in bullous pemphigoid. I. Complement and component levels in sera and blister fluids. *J Clin Investig.* (1973) 52:1207–14. doi: 10.1172/JCI107288
5. Jordon RE, Kawana S, Fritz KA. Immunopathologic mechanisms in pemphigus and bullous pemphigoid. *J Investig Dermatol.* (1985) 85(1 Suppl):72s–8s. doi: 10.1111/1523-1747.ep12275497
6. Chandler W, Zone J, Florell S. C4d immunohistochemical stain is a sensitive method to confirm immunoreactant deposition in formalin-fixed paraffin-embedded tissue in bullous pemphigoid. *J Cutan Pathol.* (2009) 36:655–9. doi: 10.1111/j.1600-0560.2008.01129.x
7. Kassaby SS, Hicks A, Leicht S, Youngberg GA. Bullous pemphigoid: use of C4d immunofluorescent staining in a case with repeated negative conventional direct immunofluorescence studies. *Am J Dermatopathol.* (2017) 39:932–4. doi: 10.1097/DAD.0000000000000943
8. Magro CM, Dyrsen ME. The use of C3d and C4d immunohistochemistry on formalin-fixed tissue as a diagnostic adjunct in the assessment of inflammatory skin disease. *J Am Acad Dermatol.* (2008) 59:822–33. doi: 10.1016/j.jaad.2008.06.022
9. Pfaltz K, Mertz K, Rose C, Scheidegger P, Pfaltz M, Kempf W. C3d immunohistochemistry on formalin-fixed tissue is a valuable tool in the diagnosis of bullous pemphigoid of the skin. *J Cutan Pathol.* (2010) 37:654–8. doi: 10.1111/j.1600-0560.2009.01450.x
10. Villani AP, Chouvet B, Kanitakis J. Application of C4d immunohistochemistry on routinely processed tissue sections for the diagnosis of autoimmune bullous dermatoses. *Am J Dermatopathol.* (2016) 38:186–8. doi: 10.1097/DAD.0000000000000333
11. Liu Z, Giudice GJ, Swartz SJ, Fairley JA, Till GO, Troy JL, et al. The role of complement in experimental bullous pemphigoid. *J Clin Investig.* (1995) 95:1539–44. doi: 10.1172/JCI117826
12. Heimbach L, Li Z, Berkowitz P, Zhao M, Li N, Rubenstein DS, et al. The C5a receptor on mast cells is critical for the autoimmune skin-blistering disease bullous pemphigoid. *J Biol Chem.* (2011) 286:15003–9. doi: 10.1074/jbc.M111.221036
13. Nelson KC, Zhao M, Schroeder PR, Li N, Wetsel RA, Diaz LA, et al. Role of different pathways of the complement cascade in experimental bullous pemphigoid. *J Clin Investig.* (2006) 116:2892–900. doi: 10.1172/JCI17891
14. Nishie W, Sawamura D, Goto M, Ito K, Shibaki A, McMillan JR, et al. Humanization of autoantigen. *Nat Med.* (2007) 13:378–83. doi: 10.1038/nm1496
15. Liu Z, Sui W, Zhao M, Li Z, Li N, Thresher R, et al. Subepidermal blistering induced by human autoantibodies to BP180 requires innate immune players in a humanized bullous pemphigoid mouse model. *J Autoimmun.* (2008) 31:331–8. doi: 10.1016/j.jaut.2008.08.009
16. Li Q, Ujiie H, Shibaki A, Wang G, Moriuchi R, Qiao HJ, et al. Human IgG1 monoclonal antibody against human collagen 17 noncollagenous 16A domain induces blisters via complement activation in experimental bullous pemphigoid model. *J Immunol.* (2010) 185:7746–55. doi: 10.4049/jimmunol.1000667
17. Karsten CM, Beckmann T, Holtsche MM, Tillmann J, Tofern S, Schulze FS, et al. Tissue destruction in bullous pemphigoid can be complement independent and may be mitigated by C5aR2. *Front Immunol.* (2018) 9:488. doi: 10.3389/fimmu.2018.00488
18. Natsuga K, Nishie W, Shinkuma S, Ujiie H, Nishimura M, Sawamura D, et al. Antibodies to pathogenic epitopes on type XVII collagen cause skin fragility in a complement-dependent and -independent manner. *J Immunol.* (2012) 188:5792–9. doi: 10.4049/jimmunol.1003402
19. Ujiie H, Sasaoka T, Izumi K, Nishie W, Shinkuma S, Natsuga K, et al. Bullous pemphigoid autoantibodies directly induce blister formation without complement activation. *J Immunol.* (2014) 193:4415–28. doi: 10.4049/jimmunol.1400095

20. Hiroyasu S, Ozawa T, Kobayashi H, Ishii M, Aoyama Y, Kitajima Y, et al. Bullous pemphigoid IgG induces BP180 internalization via a macropinocytic pathway. *Am J Pathol.* (2013) 182:828–40. doi: 10.1016/j.ajpath.2012.11.029
21. Iwata H, Kamio N, Aoyama Y, Yamamoto Y, Hirako Y, Owaribe K, et al. IgG from patients with bullous pemphigoid depletes cultured keratinocytes of the 180-kDa bullous pemphigoid antigen (type XVII collagen) and weakens cell attachment. *J Invest Dermatol.* (2009) 129:919–26. doi: 10.1038/jid.2008.305
22. Sesarman A, Oswald E, Chiriac MT, Csorba K, Vuta V, Feldrihan V, et al. Why human pemphigoid autoantibodies do not trigger disease by the passive transfer into mice? *Immunol Lett.* (2012) 143:92–100. doi: 10.1016/j.imlet.2012.01.006
23. Liu Z, Giudice GJ, Zhou X, Swartz SJ, Troy JL, Fairley JA, et al. A major role for neutrophils in experimental bullous pemphigoid. *J Clin Investig.* (1997) 100:1256–63. doi: 10.1172/JCI119639
24. Chen R, Ning G, Zhao M-L, Fleming MG, Diaz LA, Werb Z, et al. Mast cells play a key role in neutrophil recruitment in experimental bullous pemphigoid. *J Clin Investig.* (2001) 108:1151–8. doi: 10.1172/JCI11494
25. Romeijn TR, Jonkman MF, Knoppers C, Pas HH, Diercks GF. Complement in bullous pemphigoid: results from a large observational study. *Br J Dermatol.* (2017) 176:517–9. doi: 10.1111/bjd.14822
26. Chiorean RM, Baican A, Mustafa MB, Lischka A, Leucuta DC, Feldrihan V, et al. Complement-activating capacity of autoantibodies correlates with disease activity in bullous pemphigoid patients. *Front Immunol.* (2018) 9:2687. doi: 10.3389/fimmu.2018.02687
27. Griffith MR, Fukuyama K, Tuffanelli D, Silverman S Jr. Immunofluorescent studies in mucous membrane pemphigoid. *Arch Dermatol.* (1974) 109:195–9. doi: 10.1001/archderm.109.2.195
28. Rogers RS, Perry HO, Bean SF, Jordon RE. Immunopathology of cicatricial pemphigoid: studies of complement deposition. *J Investig Dermatol.* (1977) 68:39–43. doi: 10.1111/1523-1747.ep12485162
29. Heppe EN, Tofern S, Schulze FS, Ishiko A, Shimizu A, Sina C, et al. Experimental laminin 332 mucous membrane pemphigoid critically involves C5aR1 and reflects clinical and immunopathological characteristics of the human disease. *J Investig Dermatol.* (2017) 137:1709–18. doi: 10.1016/j.jid.2017.03.037
30. Lazarova Z, Yee C, Darling T, Briggaman RA, Yancey KB. Passive transfer of anti-laminin 5 antibodies induces subepidermal blisters in neonatal mice. *J Clin Investig.* (1996) 98:1509–18. doi: 10.1172/JCI118942
31. Lazarova Z, Hsu R, Briggaman RA, Yancey KB. Fab fragments directed against laminin 5 induce subepidermal blisters in neonatal mice. *Clin Immunol.* (2000) 95(1 Pt 1):26–32. doi: 10.1006/clim.2000.4845
32. Cho HJ, Lee IJ, Kim SC. Complement-fixing abilities and IgG subclasses of autoantibodies in epidermolysis bullosa acquisita. *Yonsei Med J.* (1998) 39:339–44. doi: 10.3349/ymj.1998.39.4.339
33. Mooney E, Falk RJ, Gammon WR. Studies on complement deposits in epidermolysis bullosa acquisita and bullous pemphigoid. *Arch Dermatol.* (1992) 128:58–60. doi: 10.1001/archderm.1992.01680110068008
34. Woodley DT, Ram R, Doostan A, Bandyopadhyay P, Huang Y, Remington J, et al. Induction of epidermolysis bullosa acquisita in mice by passive transfer of autoantibodies from patients. *J Invest Dermatol.* (2006) 126:1323–30. doi: 10.1038/sj.jid.5700254
35. Sitaru C, Chiriac MT, Mihai S, Buning J, Gebert A, Ishiko A, et al. Induction of complement-fixing autoantibodies against type VII collagen results in subepidermal blistering in mice. *J Immunol.* (2006) 177:3461–8. doi: 10.4049/jimmunol.177.5.3461
36. Sitaru C, Mihai S, Otto C, Chiriac MT, Hausser I, Dotterweich B, et al. Induction of dermal-epidermal separation in mice by passive transfer of antibodies specific to type VII collagen. *J Clin Investig.* (2005) 115:870–8. doi: 10.1172/JCI200521386
37. Mihai S, Hirose M, Wang Y, Thurman JM, Holers VM, Morgan BP, et al. Specific inhibition of complement activation significantly ameliorates autoimmune blistering disease in mice. *Front Immunol.* (2018) 9:535. doi: 10.3389/fimmu.2018.00535
38. Mihai S, Chiriac MT, Takahashi K, Thurman JM, Holers VM, Zillikens D, et al. The alternative pathway of complement activation is critical for blister induction in experimental epidermolysis bullosa acquisita. *J Immunol.* (2007) 178:6514–21. doi: 10.4049/jimmunol.178.10.6514
39. Karsten CM, Pandey MK, Figge J, Kilchenstein R, Taylor PR, Rosas M, et al. Anti-inflammatory activity of IgG1 mediated by Fc galactosylation and association of FcgammaRIIB and dectin-1. *Nat Med.* (2012) 18:1401–6. doi: 10.1038/nm.2862
40. Aleyd E, Heineke MH, van Egmond M. The era of the immunoglobulin A Fc receptor FcalphaRI; its function and potential as target in disease. *Immunol Rev.* (2015) 268:123–38. doi: 10.1111/imr.12337
41. van der Steen LP, Bakema JE, Sesarman A, Florea F, Tuk CW, Kirtschig G, et al. Blocking Fcalpha receptor I on granulocytes prevents tissue damage induced by IgA autoantibodies. *J Immunol.* (2012) 189:1594–601. doi: 10.4049/jimmunol.1101763
42. Wilson BD, Beutner EH, Kumar V, Chorzelski TP, Jablonska S. Linear IgA bullous dermatosis. An immunologically defined disease. *Int J Dermatol.* (1985) 24:569–74. doi: 10.1111/j.1365-4362.1985.tb05575.x
43. Monia K, Aida K, Amel K, Ines Z, Becima F, Ridha KM. Linear IgA bullous dermatosis in tunisian children: 31 cases. *Indian J Dermatol.* (2011) 56:153–9. doi: 10.4103/0019-5154.80406
44. Hiemstra PS, Gorter A, Stuurman ME, Van Es LA, Daha MR. Activation of the alternative pathway of complement by human serum IgA. *Eur J Immunol.* (1987) 17:321–6. doi: 10.1002/eji.1830170304
45. Roos A, Bouwman LH, van Gijlswijk-Janssen DJ, Faber-Krol MC, Stahl GL, Daha MR. Human IgA activates the complement system via the mannan-binding lectin pathway. *J Immunol.* (2001) 167:2861–8. doi: 10.4049/jimmunol.167.5.2861
46. Endo Y, Takahashi M, Fujita T. Lectin complement system and pattern recognition. *Immunobiology.* (2006) 211:283–93. doi: 10.1016/j.imbio.2006.01.003
47. Roos A, Rastaldi MP, Calvaresi N, Oortwijn BD, Schlagwein N, van Gijlswijk-Janssen DJ, et al. Glomerular activation of the lectin pathway of complement in IgA nephropathy is associated with more severe renal disease. *J Am Soc Nephrol.* (2006) 17:1724–34. doi: 10.1681/ASN.2005090923
48. Seah PP, Fry L, Mazaheri MR, Mowbray JF, Hoffbrand AV, Holborow EJ. Alternate-pathway complement fixation by IgA in the skin in dermatitis herpetiformis. *Lancet.* (1973) 2:175–7. doi: 10.1016/S0140-6736(73)93006-7
49. Provost TT, Tomasi TB Jr. Evidence for complement activation via the alternate pathway in skin diseases, I. Herpes gestationis, systemic lupus erythematosus, and bullous pemphigoid. *J Clin Invest.* (1973) 52:1779–87. doi: 10.1172/JCI107359
50. Preisz K, Sardy M, Horvath A, Karpati S. Immunoglobulin, complement and epidermal transglutaminase deposition in the cutaneous vessels in dermatitis herpetiformis. *J Eur Acad Dermatol Venereol.* (2005) 19:74–9. doi: 10.1111/j.1468-3083.2004.01132.x
51. de Messias-Reason IJ, Nisihara RM, Mocelin V. Mannan-binding lectin and ficolin deposition in skin lesions of pemphigus. *Arch Dermatol Res.* (2011) 303:521–5. doi: 10.1007/s00403-011-1132-1
52. Jordon RE, Schroeter AL, Rogers RS III, Perry HO. Classical and alternate pathway activation of complement in pemphigus vulgaris lesions. *J Investig Dermatol.* (1974) 63:256–9. doi: 10.1111/1523-1747.ep12680098
53. Kawana S, Geoghegan WD, Jordon RE, Nishiyanu S. Deposition of the membrane attack complex of complement in pemphigus vulgaris and pemphigus foliaceus skin. *J Investig Dermatol.* (1989) 92:588–92. doi: 10.1111/1523-1747.ep12709624
54. Anhalt GJ, Till GO, Diaz LA, Labib RS, Patel HP, Eaglstein NF. Defining the role of complement in experimental pemphigus vulgaris in mice. *J Immunol.* (1986) 137:2835–40.
55. Kasprick A, Holtsche MM, Rose EL, Hussain S, Schmidt E, Petersen F, et al. The anti-C1s antibody TNT003 prevents complement activation in the skin induced by bullous pemphigoid autoantibodies. *J Invest Dermatol.* (2018) 138:458–61. doi: 10.1016/j.jid.2017.08.030
56. Muhlbacher J, Jilma B, Wahrmann M, Bartko J, Eskandary F, Schorgenhofer C, et al. Blockade of HLA antibody-triggered classical complement activation in sera from subjects dosed with the anti-C1s monoclonal antibody TNT009-results from a randomized first-in-human phase 1 trial. *Transplantation.* (2017) 101:2410–8. doi: 10.1097/TP.0000000000001804
57. Bartko J, Schoergenhofer C, Schwameis M, Firbas C, Beliveau M, Chang C, et al. A randomized, first-in-human, healthy volunteer trial of

sutimlimab, a humanized antibody for the specific inhibition of the classical complement pathway. *Clin Pharmacol Ther.* (2018) 104:655–63. doi: 10.1002/cpt.1111

58. McNamara LA, Topaz N, Wang X, Hariri S, Fox L, MacNeil JR. High risk for invasive meningococcal disease among patients receiving eculizumab (Soliris) despite receipt of meningococcal vaccine. *Am J Transplant.* (2017) 17:2481–4. doi: 10.1111/ajt.14426
59. Jayne DRW, Bruchfeld AN, Harper L, Schaier M, Venning MC, Hamilton P, et al. Randomized trial of C5a receptor inhibitor avacopan in ANCA-associated vasculitis. *J Am Soc Nephrol.* (2017) 28:2756–67. doi: 10.1681/ASN.2016111179

18

Pemphigus Vulgaris: Short Time to Relapse in Patients Treated in a Danish Tertiary Referral Center

Aheen Faisal Mohamad[1], *Lars Iversen*[2] *and Rikke Bech*[2*]

[1] *Aalborg University Hospital, Aalborg, Denmark,* [2] *Department of Dermatology, Aarhus University Hospital, Aarhus, Denmark*

Correspondence:
Rikke Bech
rikkebecha@gmail.com

Pemphigus vulgaris is an autoimmune skin disorder with development of blisters in the skin and mucosa, and it can be a life-threatening disease if not treated. Corticosteroids have been a cornerstone for treating PV, but because of side effects the treatment is combined with other conventional immune modulating drugs and rituximab. The Danish treatment protocol for pemphigus vulgaris is similar to the other Scandinavian countries, and therefore this study is of importance for clinicians in the Scandinavian countries as well as other European countries. We retrospectively identified all patients with Pemphigus vulgaris in our tertiary center over a 7-year period in order to register patient characteristics, treatment, adverse events, comorbidities and the effect of prednisolone dose on remission. In this study 19 patients met the inclusion criteria and remission was seen after a mean of 19.9 weeks, and relapse was seen in 50% after the mean time of 15 weeks. Time to relapse in our study is relatively short compared to studies in which rituximab is used as a first-line drug in treating pemphigus vulgaris.

Keywords: prednisolone, mortality, comorbidity, treatment, pemphigus vulgaris

INTRODUCTION

Pemphigus vulgaris (PV) is an autoimmune skin disorder with development of blisters in the skin and in mucosa. PV is caused by autoantibodies attacking desmoglein 1 (Dsg1) and 3 (Dsg3), which are responsible for cell-cell adhesion. Binding of autoantigens to the intercellular connections leads to disruption of cell-cell adhesion, called acantholysis (1, 2).

Clinical features of PV consist of blisters in the oral cavity and cutaneous flaccid blisters that easily rupture, leaving the skin with painful erosions that easily become infected (3). Immunofluorescence is used to detect immunoglobulin (IgG) or C3 deposition on the basement membrane.

PV is a chronic disorder and can be fatal if not treated (3). Systemic treatment with high doses of corticosteroids is regularly given. Because of the severe side effects of corticosteroids, treatment is combined with other immune modulating drugs and/or rituximab to keep the steroid dose as low as possible (1, 4–6).

BACKGROUND

From former studies of bullous pemphigoid (7), we know that high dose prednisolone (>45 mg/day) treatment is associated to longer admission time. However, no association between high/low corticosteroid dose and remission rate, relapse rate and treatment length was found.

We considered whether corticosteroid treatment regimen was associated to remission, relapse and/or comorbidities in patients with pemphigus vulgaris? Therefore, the aim of the present study was to record total doses of prednisolone given to patients with PV either solely or in combination with other immunosuppressants. Additionally, comorbidities acquired before, during, or after diagnosis of PV were listed and a mortality rate was calculated (8–10).

METHODS

The medical records were retrieved for all patients admitted with a diagnosis of PV at the Department of Dermatology and Venereology at Aarhus University Hospital, Aarhus, Denmark, in the timespan 2011–2018. The project was approved by the Danish Data Protection Agency. Patients were included if they had had a biopsy that verified a diagnosis of PV according to the Danish pathology database, Patoweb. Patients younger than 18 years were excluded. A biopsy was considered diagnostic for PV if direct immunofluorescence showed deposits of IgG or C3 on the basement membrane.

Treatment was based on the department of dermatology's guidelines for patients with PV.

SPSS package software was used for statistical analysis. Graphpad Prism and Excel were used for figures. The descriptive analysis is made on the basis of continuous variables given as means with 95% confidence intervals (CI) and standard deviations (SDs) and categorical variables given in percentages. Treatment outcomes were categorical and compared using *p*-values computed from Fisher's exact test. *p*-values <0.05 were considered statistically significant.

RESULTS

In the period 2011–2018, 64 patients were identified, and 19 of these fulfilled the inclusion criteria. Ten patients were excluded because they appeared twice. A total of 15 patients did not fulfill the diagnostic criteria for PV and were all excluded. Due to limited access to patients' medical records before 2011, this research was limited to the time period 2011–2018. Nineteen patients were excluded because they were diagnosed with PV before 2011. Furthermore, one patient diagnosed with PV was below 18 years of age and was therefore excluded.

The age of PV onset ranged from 21 to 101 years, with a mean of 57.8, 95% CI (48.4–67.3), SD 21.06. Female: male ratio was 0.82. Five patients were of other ethnic origin than Danish, 14 patients were ethnically Danish. There was no significant difference in age at PV onset between male and female patients (56.3 ± 20.7 vs. 60.0 ± 22.8 years, respectively; $p = 0.7$).

A DXA (dual-energy X-ray absorptiometry) was performed in 9/19 patients. Four patients developed osteopenia and one patient was diagnosed with osteoporosis during the first 12-month period (**Figure 2**). Seven patients never had a DXA scan even though they met the national guideline criteria for being in a special risk category for developing osteoporosis. At the time of diagnosis of PV nine patients had no comorbidities but two of them developed osteopenia. Two patients did not receive any prednisolone and one patient died within 2 months of diagnosis (**Supplementary Figure 1**).

One patient became diabetic and had many prednisolone side effects, including moon face, buffalo hump, and myopathy. The same side effects appeared in another patient, presumably caused by very high doses of prednisolone.

Some of the patients had comorbidities before being diagnosed with PV, see **Table 1**. Three patients had hypertension, and two of these also had hypercholesterolemia. One patient had chronic heart failure, one had aorta insufficiency, one had migraine, and one patient had epilepsy. Two patients had previously been treated for cancer: one for breast cancer and the other for colorectal cancer. Two of the nineteen (2/19) PV patients were treated with ACE inhibitors (Enalapril) at PV diagnosis. ACE inhibitors are known to be able to elicit or maintain PV. However, one of the two patients discontinued Enalapril when PV had been diagnosed. Yet, the PV disease was unaffected by the discontinuation of ACE inhibitor in this patient.

Prednisolone was the most widely used treatment. Seventeen of the 19 patients received prednisolone. One patient refused to receive prednisolone because of obesity and was treated with cyclosporine, and the other patient was well treated on azathioprine and topical corticosteroids. The remaining 17 patients received prednisolone along with other adjuvants.

The primary treatment regimen was prednisolone and azathioprine, some were also given rituximab later in their course

TABLE 1 | Treatment specifications and comorbidities.

Treatment	Patients
Oral prednisolone	17
Oral prednisolone and rituximab	13
Oral prednisolone and azathioprine	7
Oral prednisolone and MTX	3
Oral prednisolone and dapsone	2
Oral prednisolone and plasmapheresis	2
Comorbidities	
Hypertension	3
Hypercholesterolemia	2
Chronic heart failure	1
Aorta insufficiency	1
Migraine	1
Epilepsy	1
Dermatitis herpitiformis	1
Celiac disease	1
Breast cancer	1
Colorectal cancer	1

Abbreviations: PV, Pemphigus vulgaris; IF, Direct immunofluorescence; Dsg1, Desmoglein 1; Dsg3, Desmoglein 3; PDAI, Pemphigus Disease Area Index; SD, Standard deviation; CI, Confidence interval; Pt, Patient; DXA, Dual-energy X-ray absorptiometry; SEM, Standard error of mean; mg/d, milligrams per day; ABSIS, Autoimmune Bullous Skin Disorder Intensity Score.

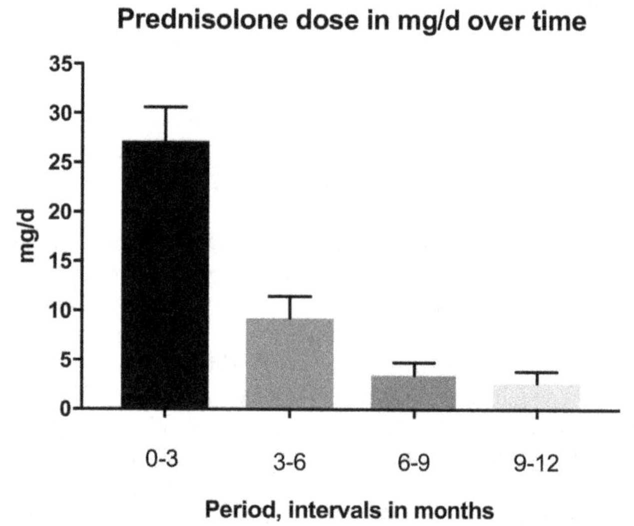

FIGURE 1 | Mean dose prednisolone per interval with the standard error of mean SEM.

of treatment. Rituximab was used only for recalcitrant patients, for patients with very severe PV disease and for patients with contraindications to other immunosuppresants, e.g., patients with a history of malignant disease. The mean prednisolone doses (mg/d) were at baseline 0–3 months 27.15 mg/d SD 14.9 (19 patients), 3–6 months 9.26 mg/d SD 9.3 (18 patients), 6–9 months 3.46 mg/d SD 5.4 (18 patients), and 9–12 months 2.71 mg/d SD 49 (18 patients). A comparison of baseline prednisolone doses to the other time periods revealed that the dose of prednisolone decreased significantly over time. The changes in prednisolone dose are shown in **Figure 1**.

In the 19 included PV patients, none were exclusively mucosal dominant. Four patients had cutaneous PV, and 14 patients had mucocutaneous PV. Most of the patients (10/19) with mucocutaneous PV had affection of skin and oral mucosa. Three patients with mucocutaneous PV had affection of skin, oral mucosa, and genital (vagina or penis, respectively) mucosa.

No patients had deposition of C3 only in DIF. Eight patients had IgG only in DIF, seven of these DIFs were done on a skin biopsy and two were done on a mucosal biopsy from gingiva and vagina, respectively. Five patients had C3 as well as IgG deposition in DIF on a skin biopsy, and one patient had C3 and IgG deposition in DIF on a mucosal biopsy from gingiva. In only one patient of the nineteen included patients DIF was done on both a skin and a mucosal biopsy. In this patient DIF showed IgG deposition on the skin biopsy but no specific reactions in DIF on mucosal (gingiva) biopsy. For additional information of DIF data, please see **Supplementary Table 1**.

Almost every patient started treatment with an adjuvant within the 1st week after onset of prednisolone treatment or 1 week later. Rituximab (1,000 mg) was given as an I:V: infusion two times at an interval of 2 weeks. This treatment was initiated after approximately 2 months of treatment with prednisolone and other adjuvants.

One patient had recalcitrant PV and was also treated with plasmapheresis once a month. Despite this, the patient never achieved remission.

By dividing patients into two groups, treatment outcomes could be compared. The groups were classified as receiving more than or <3,782 mg prednisone (mean total dose) during the first 12 months of treatment. Treatment outcome was measured as remission or no remission during the 12 months of follow-up time. Remission was defined as healing of blisters and no appearance of new blisters. The *p*-value was >0.05 and therefore prednisolone dose did not have any statistically significant effect on remission.

Remission was achieved in 16 patients at a mean of 19.9 weeks. Relapse was defined as appearance of new bullae. Remission followed by relapse was seen in nine patients (50%). We calculated mean time to relapse for the whole studied group (19 patients). The mean time from remission to the appearance of new bullae (relapse) was 15 weeks.

Minor adverse events like scalp infection, candida albicans in the oral cavity, diarrhea, urinary tract infection, and skin infection with *Staphylococci aureus* were seen in 9/19 (47%) patients during the first 12-month period.

Three patients (16%) had major adverse events. One patient had a single incidence of pneumonia. Another had pneumonia followed by septicemia, and a third patient had a reactivation of herpes zoster followed by pneumonia and septicemia and died. Thus, the mortality rate among our patients with PV was 5.3% (1/19) during the first 12 months of follow-up. The mortality rate was calculated to be 37 patients per 1,000 person years.

A PDAI score was found for 18 of the 19 patients. For one patient, it was not possible because of the poor quality of the description in the medical record. The majority of patients had a moderate PV according to PDAI score. Four patients had a significant PV, and only one had an extensive disease.

Results did not show a significant correlation between PDAI status and prednisolone dose.

DISCUSSION

We found no association between prednisolone dose (mean total dose more than or <3,782 mg) and time to remission. The patients in this study were down-regulated in prednisolone dose if they experienced clinical improvement. This makes remission and prednisolone dose dependent variables, and can explain why no association between the two variables was found. A prospective study in which patients are randomized to either low- or a high-dose prednisolone treatment could contribute with valuable information on prednisolone's role in inducing remission.

The mean time to relapse was relatively short in this study compared to other studies of patients with PV. This might be due to the fact that Prednisolone treatment was tapered too fast and before the patient achieved maximum effect of the Rituximab treatment. It is our clinical experience that most patients do not achieve maximum effect of the Rituximab infusion until 8–12 weeks after Rituximab infusion.

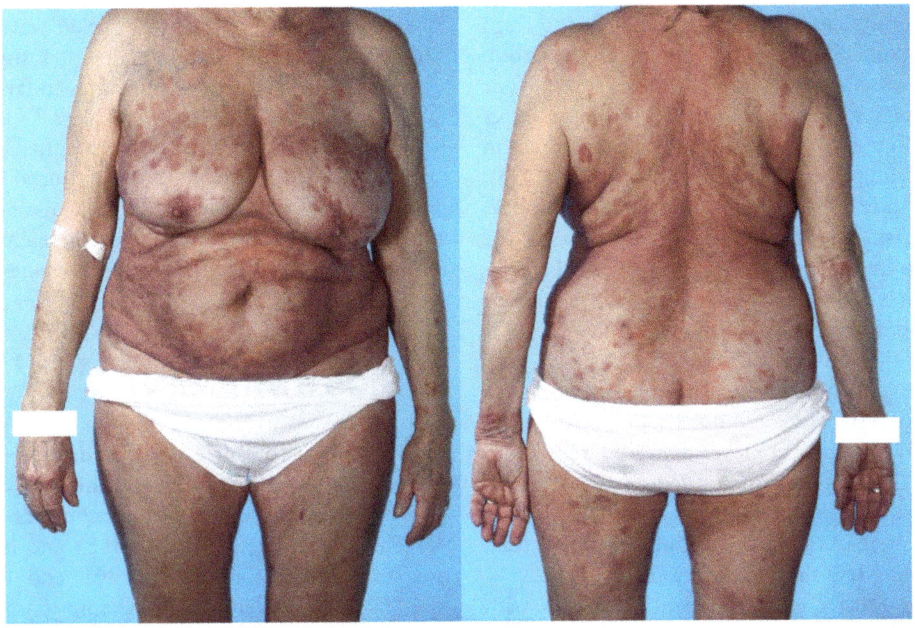

FIGURE 2 | Seventy six years old (at diagnosis of PV) ethnically danish woman with mucocutaneous PV, celiac disease, and former dermatitis herpetiformis as well as essential hypertension. The patient did not receive treatment with ACE inhibitor. Skin biopsy showed acantholysis. DIF on the skin biopsy showed intercellular deposition of IgG. The patient was treated with oral prednisolon, Methotrexate and two times Rituximab. Time to remission was 20.7 weeks which is close to mean time to remission (19.9 weeks) in the 19 included patients. The patient received a total dose of 2,495 mg prednisolone, which placed her in the "low dose prednisolone" group. This patient was later diagnosed with osteoporosis on DXA scan.

We attempted to determine the severity of PV disease by calculating PDAI based on information from the patient record (11). The ability to perform precise PDAI ranging was difficult. In a few cases, the clinician had thoroughly described size, number, and placement of the blisters. But in the vast majority, the information lacked precise details on location and total number of the blisters. In particular, blisters in the oral cavity were not described as located to a particular region of the oral cavity. This complicated the ranging of patients according to the PDAI and may possibly have underestimated the real PDAI score. In a prospective study, clinicians can be educated to register objective findings and comorbidities precisely so that the clinical data can be used in research.

The strengths of this study are the long study period and the validation of all PV diagnoses with direct immunofluorescence. The Danish civil registration number register in Denmark ensures that all procedures, administered medicine, and consultations are systematically documented. Furthermore, all patients' medical records were reviewed individually.

Selection bias may have had an influence on outcomes because the most severe cases in the region are referred to the Department of Dermatology and Venereology at Aarhus University Hospital. Also, the lack of patients with exclusive mucosal PV in this study group might reflect that these patients may primarily be referred to other departments in the hospital such as the oral surgeon unit.

The limitation of this study was the small sample size, hence the limited use of statistics. It should be taken into consideration that this is a retrospective study; the associations are therefore not conclusive.

Tavakolpour et al. report that relapse of disease is expected 6–10 months after infusion of rituximab (12). In this study, we found that 50% of the patients had a relapse after a mean of 15 weeks. This is a markedly shorter time period than expected. Relapse was assessed on clinical features alone and by different clinicians every time. In the future, it could be intriguing to also observe the serologic response in the same way as Horváth et al. did. In Horváth et al.'s study CD20+ B cells and specific antibodies against Dsg1 and Dsg3 were measured at the beginning of therapy and at every scheduled visit. Horváth et al. showed that a single course of two infusions of rituximab (500 mg each) at an interval of 2 weeks had a great effect on B-cell number and less on Dsg3 levels (13).

Knowledge of the serologic aspects of PV could clarify the disease process and elucidate how remission is accomplished and maintained.

In a multiprotocol for treatment of patients with pemphigus vulgaris or pemphigus foliaceus, Grando showed that repeated cycles with immunoglobulin (IVIg) infusion and Rituximab treatment combined with mitochondrion protecting drugs resulted in rapid disease control (0.2 months), short time to remission (1.7 months), and long time to relapse (mean time to relapse off drugs, 15.8 months). This seems to be a very efficient and safe treatment regimen for pemphigus vulgaris. However, the treatment is very expensive and hence will not be applicable to all patients or health care systems. In comparison the mean time to relapse in our study group was 15 weeks (14).

A study by Kanwar et al. investigated the clinical and serological difference between patients receiving two doses of

1,000 mg rituximab or 500 mg rituximab 14 days apart. Their results showed a statistically significant decline in Dsg1 and Dsg3 antibodies and a greater fall in clinical scoring in the group receiving 1,000 mg rituximab (15).

The above-mentioned studies enhance the serologic effect of rituximab on PV. Joly et al. showed a significant reduction in prednisolone dose in patients treated with rituximab (4). The patients in the study by Joly et al. had recalcitrant PV. Results showed that a single cycle of rituximab decreased the prednisolone dose required from 94 to 12 mg per day. Patients in this study were down-regulated in prednisolone dose to approximately 3.46 mg/d after only 6 months. This dose is considered a low dose with limited side effects.

In this study, one patient had recalcitrant PV and was treated with plasmapheresis once a month along with other adjuvants. Despite this, the patient never achieved remission. Kridin et al. states that immunoadsorption is superior to plasmapheresis. Plasmapheresis unselectively and inadvertently removes all plasma proteins in contrast to immunoadsorption, which removes circulating IgG autoantibodies (7).

In the study by Pfütze et al. patients treated with immunoadsorption had lower Dsg1 and Dsg3 antibody titres and a decrease in both skin and mucosal ABSIS (Autoimmune Bullous Skin Disorder Intensity Score). ABSIS and PDAI are the most often used scoring system to determine PV severity (11). In Pfütze's study, prednisolone was also reduced within 12 months (16). This points at immunoadsorption as a relevant treatment option for patients with recalcitrant PV. There are, however, some disadvantages associated with immunoadsorption because it is expensive and not generally available.

CONCLUSION

In conclusion, patients in this study showed clinical improvement and remission after a mean period of 19.9 weeks. Remission did not seem to correlate with prednisolone dose. The time to relapse (15 weeks) was relatively short in the studied PV group compared to other studies. This calls for a revision of our treatment guidelines in favor of more liberal use of Rituximab and IVIg treatment. The PV treatment in this study was primarily a combination of prednisolone and azathioprine or rituximab. Prednisolone was reduced considerably after 12 months, and consequently the risk of side effects was lowered over time. DXA scans must be used systematically in the clinical setting to reduce the risk of prednisolone-induced osteoporosis in patients with PV.

ETHICS STATEMENT

This study was conducted in accordance with the World Medical Association's Declaration of Helsinki. We consulted the national (Datatilsynet, Danmark) and local ethics committee (Styrelsen for Patientsikkerhed, Region Midt) and learned that the study was exempt from ethics approval and written consent from the included patients. This exemption from ethics approval was motivated by the fact that the study was retrospective, based on journal information and without identifiable-to-a-person data, and thus the study was considered a quality assurance study.

AUTHOR CONTRIBUTIONS

AM did the initial data collection, statistical analysis, and wrote the first manuscript draft. LI contributed to design of the study and all revisions of the manuscript. RB assisted AM in all phases of data collection, statistical analysis, the writing process, and revisions of the manuscript.

REFERENCES

1. Zhao CY, Murrell DF. Pemphigus vulgaris: an evidence-based treatment update. *Drugs.* (2015) 75:271–84. doi: 10.1007/s40265-015-0353-6
2. Pollmann R, Schmidt T, Eming R, Hertl M. Pemphigus: a comprehensive review on pathogenesis, clinical presentation and novel therapeutic approaches. *Clin Rev Allergy Immunol.* (2018) 54:1–25. doi: 10.1007/s12016-017-8662-z
3. Kridin K. Pemphigus group: overview, epidemiology, mortality, and comorbidities. *Immunol Res.* (2018) 66:255–70. doi: 10.1007/s12026-018-8986-7
4. Joly P, Mouquet H, Roujeau JC, D'Incan M, Gilbert D, Jacquot S, et al. A single cycle of rituximab for the treatment of severe pemphigus. *N Engl J Med.* (2007) 357:545–52. doi: 10.1056/NEJMoa067752
5. Kridin K. Emerging treatment options for the management of pemphigus vulgaris. *Ther Clin Risk Manage.* (2018) 14:757–78. doi: 10.2147/TCRM.S142471
6. Balighi K, Daneshpazhooh M, Khezri S, Mahdavi-nia M, Hajiseyed-javadi M, Chams-Davatchi C. Adjuvant rituximab in the treatment of pemphigus vulgaris: a phase II clinical trial. *Int J Dermatol.* (2013) 52:862–7. doi: 10.1111/j.1365-4632.2012.5847.x
7. Kibsgaard L, Bay B, Deleuran M, Vestergaard C. A retrospective consecutive case-series study on the effect of systemic treatment, length of admission time, and co-morbidities in 98 bullous pemphigoid patients admitted to a tertiary centre. *Acta Dermato Venereol.* (2015) 95:307–11. doi: 10.2340/00015555-1925
8. Hall RP III, Fairley J, Woodley D, Werth VP, Hannah D, Streilein RD, et al. A multicentre randomized trial of the treatment of patients with pemphigus vulgaris with infliximab and prednisone compared with prednisone alone. *Br J Dermatol.* (2015) 172:760–8. doi: 10.1111/bjd.13350
9. Balighi K, Daneshpazhooh M, Mahmoudi H, Badakhsh M, Teimourpour A, Ehsani AH, et al. Comparing early and late treatments with rituximab in pemphigus vulgaris: which one is better? *Arch Dermatol Res.* (2019) 311:63–9. doi: 10.1007/s00403-018-1881-1
10. Joly P, Maho-Vaillant M, Prost-Squarcioni C, Hebert V, Houivet E, Calbo S, et al. First-line rituximab combined with short-term prednisone versus prednisone alone for the treatment of pemphigus (Ritux 3): a prospective, multicentre, parallel-group, open-label randomised trial. *Lancet.* (2017) 389:2031–40. doi: 10.1016/S0140-6736(17)30070-3

11. Boulard C, Duvert Lehembre S, Picard-Dahan C, Kern JS, Zambruno G, Feliciani C, et al. Calculation of cut-off values based on the autoimmune bullous skin disorder intensity score (ABSIS) and pemphigus disease area index (PDAI) pemphigus scoring systems for defining moderate, significant and extensive types of pemphigus. *Br J Dermatol.* (2016) 175:142–9. doi: 10.1111/bjd.14405
12. Tavakolpour S, Mahmoudi H, Balighi K, Abedini R, Daneshpazhooh M. Sixteen-year history of rituximab therapy for 1085 pemphigus vulgaris patients: a systematic review. *Int Immunopharmacol.* (2018) 54:131–8. doi: 10.1016/j.intimp.2017.11.005
13. Horváth B, Huizinga J, Pas HH, Mulder AB, Jonkman MF. Low-dose rituximab is effective in pemphigus. *Br J Dermatol.* (2011) 166:405–12. doi: 10.1111/j.1365-2133.2011.10663.x
14. Grando SA. Retrospective analysis of a single-center clinical experience toward development of curative treatment of 123 pemphigus patients with a long-term follow-up: efficacy and safety of the multidrug protocol combining intravenous immunoglobulin with the cytotoxic immunosuppressorand mitochondrion-protecting drugs. *Int J Dermatol.* (2019) 58:114–25. doi: 10.1111/ijd.14143
15. Kanwar AJ, Vinay K, Sawatkar GU, Dogra S, Minz RW, Shear NH, et al. Clinical and immunological outcomes of high- and low-dose rituximab treatments in patients with pemphigus: a randomized, comparative, observer-blinded study. *Br J Dermatol.* (2014) 170:1341–9. doi: 10.1111/bjd.12972
16. Pfutze M, Eming R, Kneisel A, Kuhlmann U, Hoyer J, Hertl M. Clinical and immunological follow-up of pemphigus patients on adjuvant treatment with immunoadsorption or rituximab. *Dermatology.* (2009) 218:237–45. doi: 10.1159/000187431

19

Skin Barrier and Autoimmunity—Mechanisms and Novel Therapeutic Approaches for Autoimmune Blistering Diseases of the Skin

*Natalie E. Stevens, Allison J. Cowin and Zlatko Kopecki**

Regenerative Medicine Laboratory, Future Industries Institute, University of South Australia, Adelaide, SA, Australia

***Correspondence:**
Zlatko Kopecki
zlatko.kopecki@unisa.edu.au

One of the most important functions of the skin besides regulating internal body temperature includes formation of the barrier between the organism and the external environment, hence protecting against pathogen invasion, chemical and physical assaults and unregulated loss of water and solutes. Disruption of the protective barrier is observed clinically in blisters and erosions of the skin that form in autoimmune blistering diseases where the body produces autoantibodies against structural proteins of the epidermis or the epidermal-dermal junction. Although there is no cure for autoimmune skin blistering diseases, immune suppressive therapies currently available offer opportunities for disease management. In cases where no treatment is sought, these disorders can lead to life threatening complications and current research efforts have focused on developing therapies that target autoantibodies which contribute to disease symptoms. This review will outline the involvement of the skin barrier in main skin-specific autoimmune blistering diseases by describing the mechanisms underpinning skin autoimmunity and review current progress in development of novel therapeutic approaches targeting the underlying causes of autoimmune skin blistering diseases.

Keywords: skin barrier, autoimmunity, autoantibody, skin blistering diseases, therapy, pemphigus, pemphigoid, epidermolysis bullosa acquisita

INTRODUCTION

The stratified squamous epithelium of the human epidermis forms a continuous barrier against the external environment and impairments in epithelial adhesions lead to disorders characterized by significant morbidity and/or mortality (1). The hallmark feature of autoimmune blistering diseases (AIBDs) is the disruption of the intact skin barrier as a consequence of blistering and erosions caused by production of autoantibodies against structural proteins in the epidermis or at the epidermal-dermal junction. AIBDs generally occur in the elderly, and often have substantial clinical and immunopathological overlap and polymorphic clinical presentation which can make diagnosis challenging (2). Immunologically, these conditions are driven by humoral and cellular autoimmune responses directed against distinct target antigens and can be classed in three main groups including pemphigoid and pemphigus diseases as well as dermatitis herpetiformis (DH) (3).

Over the past four decades, our knowledge of the pathophysiology of AIBDs has been greatly advanced by demonstrating that passive transfer of antibodies against skin antigens can disrupt the skin barrier and induce blisters in experimental animals models with clinical, histologic, and immunopathogenic responses similar to those observed in human disease (1). Each AIBD is characterized by the presence of specific autoantibodies targeting distinct antigens in the epidermis or at the dermal-epidermal junction. Intraepidermal blistering found in pemphigus disorders are caused by autoantibodies targeting cadherin proteins in desmosomes; subtypes pemphigus vulgaris and pemphigus foliaceus are associated with antibodies against desmoglein (dsg)-3 and−1, respectively. In bullous pemphigoid (BP), autoantibodies target two hemidesmosome components BP180 and BP230; and in epidermolysis bullosa acquisita (EBA) patients have autoantibodies target type VII collagen anchoring fibrils. In DH patients, autoantibodies target tissue and epidermal transglutaminase (eTG) proteins (3) however recently a case was reported where autoimmune intraepidermal and subepidermal blistering disease coexisted with a patient who was reported to have autoantibodies to both desmoglein (Dsg) 1 and BP230 (4).

AIBDs typically present with generalized blister eruption associated with itch however atypical presentations are often encountered. For example, 20% of BP patients present with "non-bullous" presentations, while anti-p200 pemphigoid patients that normally present with tense blisters with erythematosus often show normal skin resembling BP. Additionally, epidermolysis bullosa acquisita, an autoimmune disease associated with autoantibodies against type VII collagen, has several phenotypes including a classical form that mimics dystrophic epidermolysis bullosa, an inflammatory form that mimics BP, or a form more similar to mucous membrane pemphigoid-like lesions (2).

Diagnosis of AIBDs relies on direct immunofluorescence microscopy studies and immunoserological assays (5, 6). Multiple mechanisms of skin barrier disruption and blister formation in AIBDs have been described: in pemphigus disorders steric hindrance (the direct inhibition of protein-protein binding by autoantibodies) and cell signaling events cause desmosomal instability, while complement and inflammatory cell activation mediated through Fc-signaling cause keratinocyte death and blister formation in pemphigoid and epidermolysis bullosa acquisita (7–9). Development of targeted therapies and management of affected patients is often challenging due to frequent relapses, lack of efficacy and number of adverse events (10, 11). Current standard treatment options rely on non-specific immunosuppression, highlighting the need for development of targeted therapeutic approaches (12, 13). In this review we will focus on skin barrier involvement in mechanisms underpinning autoimmunity and describe the latest approaches for development of targeted therapeutics for the treatment of AIBDs.

SKIN BARRIER AND MECHANISMS UNDERPINNING AUTOIMMUNE SKIN BLISTERING

More than 2.5% of the world's population is affected by autoantibody driven autoimmune disease, including AIBDs (7). The principles of autoantibody generation and detection in AIBDs have been reviewed extensively (7). Technological advancement in the last two decades have allowed us to identify the sequence of specific nanostructural and functional changes in the skin barrier following the binding of autoantibodies and define critical pathways and processes responsible for autoimmune pathology (14). The pathogenesis of AIBDs can be divided into three phases: (i) the *induction* phase (loss of self-tolerance or the initiation of autoimmunity to the target antigen), (ii) the *maintenance* phase (maintained production of autoantibodies) and (iii) the *effector* phase (autoantibody-mediated tissue damage). Specific mechanisms relating to these phases have been described for AIBDs, including pemphigus disorders, BP, EBA, and DH.

INDUCTION OF AUTOIMMUNITY AGAINST SKIN ANTIGENS

There are multiple theories that explain how the loss of tolerance to self-antigens initially occurs and it is understood that the majority of AIBDs are a product of several aberrant processes which disrupt skin barrier homeostasis. Genetic factors play an important role, as specific skin blistering diseases have varying prevalence in different populations and inherited human leukocyte antigen (HLA) types are associated with autoreactivity to specific autoantigens (15). Multiple HLA alleles have been identified which are associated with pemphigus vulgaris (15, 16), BP (17, 18), and EBA (19, 20). Genetic susceptibility is not limited to HLA types, as pemphigus vulgaris has been associated with mutations in *ST18* (a gene encoding a pro-apoptotic transcription factor) in certain populations (21) and experimental models of EBA have identified non-HLA murine gene loci that confer susceptibility to disease development (22), however further studies are required to extrapolate these findings to clinical populations.

Cell damage has been proposed as a common "triggering factor" which causes development of pathogenic adaptive autoimmune reactions—cell damage due to surgical trauma (23), UV radiation (24), neurological disorders and other pre-existing conditions (25–29), viral infection (30–33), and radiotherapy (34–36) have all been associated with disrupted skin barrier function and development of AIBDs (37). Cell damage via necrosis or necroptosis releases a complex intracellular milieu into the extracellular space which serves as a source of sensitizing autoantigens (38); additionally cell death results in the release of damage associated molecular patterns which stimulate localized inflammation and wound healing processes (39, 40). Normal healing responses following trauma aiming to re-establish the skin barrier cause infiltration of dendritic cells and other antigen presenting cells which may also participate in autoimmune sensitization (41, 42) of AIBDs.

Epitope spreading is an inbuilt mechanism of the adaptive immune system that aids in protecting against changing pathogens (43), however spreading from pathogenic to autologous epitopes and molecular mimicry of similar epitopes may also contribute to the formation of AIBDs (44). Fogo selvage, an endemic form of pemphigus foliaceus found in Brazilian populations, is associated with a history of sand fly bites and characterized by autoantibodies against Dsg1. These autoantibodies have shown cross reactivity to proteins present in sand fly saliva (45), which may represent epitope spreading from foreign proteins to similar autoantigens. Epitope spreading is also thought to be involved in paraneoplastic (PNP) pemphigus (46) where tumor-associated antigens may become targeted in an effort to destroy the tumor, however similar antigens may also be shared by keratinocytes (47). PNP pemphigus is most commonly associated with lymphatic malignancies, including non-Hodgkin's lymphoma and chronic lymphocytic leukemia. These malignancies are associated with the production and release of cytokines which can lead to over-stimulation of humoral immunity and autoimmune reactions, including disruption of skin barrier and development of AIBDs. Findings of autoimmune skin blistering in carcinoma patients has fuelled speculation that these diseases may be triggered by an anti-tumor immune response (48–50), however further studies are required to determine the relationship between these findings (51, 52). Coeliac-disease associated skin blistering, known as DH, is caused by antibodies against gluten-induced digestive enzyme tissue transglutaminase which undergo epitope spreading to cross-react with epidermal transglutaminase (eTG) leading to the disruption of the skin barrier and subsequent skin blistering (53, 54). Epitope spreading may also contribute to the diversity of and disease progression of AIBDs, as epitope spreading to related autoantigens has been associated with atypical or altered disease presentations (53, 55, 56).

AIBDs have been associated with the use of certain drugs which trigger pathogenesis through a variety of mechanisms. One of the most well-described etiologies is BP in diabetic patients taking dipeptidyl-peptidase 4 (DPP-4) inhibitors (57–59) which present with antibodies against the mid-portion of BP180. It has been suggested that DPP-4 inhibition reduces plasmin production and alters BP180 cleavage, resulting in altered antigenicity of BP180 (60) which is supported by the finding that symptoms generally subside after drug discontinuation. The use of immune checkpoint inhibitors for cancer therapy has been linked to secondary development of AIBD including mucous membrane pemphigoid and BP (61, 62), likely a consequence of nonspecific immune activation.

MAINTAINED AUTOANTIBODY PRODUCTION

Autoantibodies are often present in healthy individuals but are generally non-pathogenic IgM antibodies with low affinity present in low levels and do not alter skin barrier homeostasis. For autoantibodies to gain pathogenicity, class-switching to IgG or IgA subtypes, somatic mutation and increased production occur after exposure to self-antigen. Glycosylation and sialylation patterns on autoantibodies also contribute to pathogenicity and antibodies stimulated via T-cell interaction within germinal centers exhibit reduced sialyation patterns and are pro-inflammatory (63). In the context of AIBDs, the presence of self-antigen released by damaged keratinocytes may stimulate production of autoantibodies, which in turn bind to healthy tissue to stimulate skin barrier disruption and further tissue damage and promote more autoantibody generation in a self-perpetuating cycle. Continued production of pathogenic autoantibodies may be achieved by ongoing B cell activation and production of short-lived plasma cells (64, 65) or the production of long-lived plasma cells which are challenging to target (66–68). T-cell driven education within the germinal center appears to be a requirement for the development of long-lived plasma cells, which gives rise to both lasting immunity against pathogens and chronic autoimmunity. Murine models of EBA have also demonstrated the presence of plasma cells with "intermediate" lifespans which contribute to autoantibody persistence (69). Alterations in cellular immune networks also contribute to maintained autoantibody production and disease chronicity: Increased Th1 and Th17 cytokines and chemokines have been reported in patients with pemphigus disorders (70, 71), BP (72, 73), and DH (74) and changes in Treg populations are also associated with AIBDs (75, 76), with Tregs thought to be protective against pathogenic autoantibody production (77, 78). Higher frequencies of Th17 cells secreting IL-21 have been reported in pemphigus lesions which form a tertiary lymph node like structure within the skin and promote autoantibody production (79). Further investigation into cellular contributions to autoantibody production may reveal additional therapeutic targets which can be used to control AIBDs.

AUTOANTIBODY-INDUCED TISSUE DAMAGE

Autoimmune diseases of the skin are the result of pathological processes caused by autoantibodies against skin antigens. A number of common antigens targeted by disease-associated autoantibodies have been discovered, including antigens present on desmosomes, hemidesmosomes and proteins expressed by keratinocytes. Transfer of patient autoantibodies against Dsg 1 (80, 81) and Dsg 3 (82) and type VII collagen (83) is sufficient to cause skin barrier disruption and epidermal blistering in mice consistent with the associated clinical disease, thus autoantibodies are considered instrumental to pathogenesis in many AIBDs. **Figure 1** provides a diagram summary of blistering mechanisms and skin barrier disruption in prototypic AIBDs pemphigus disorders, BP, EBA, and DH. Inflammation triggered by autoantibody binding recruits and activates a number of myeloid and lymphoid cell subsets that participate in blister development and damage to the skin barrier, however these vary with specific disease and clinical context. Previous reviews have in details described the preclinical animal studies and some clinical evidence elucidating the contributions of eosinophils (84, 85), mast cells (86, 87), Th17 (70, 88), and Treg (89–91) cells to AIBD's, and these may represent novel therapeutic targets. Here we focus on contributions of autoantibodies to skin barrier disruption in different disease settings.

Unraveling the precise mechanisms of autoantibody-induced pathology has been the focus of much research in recent

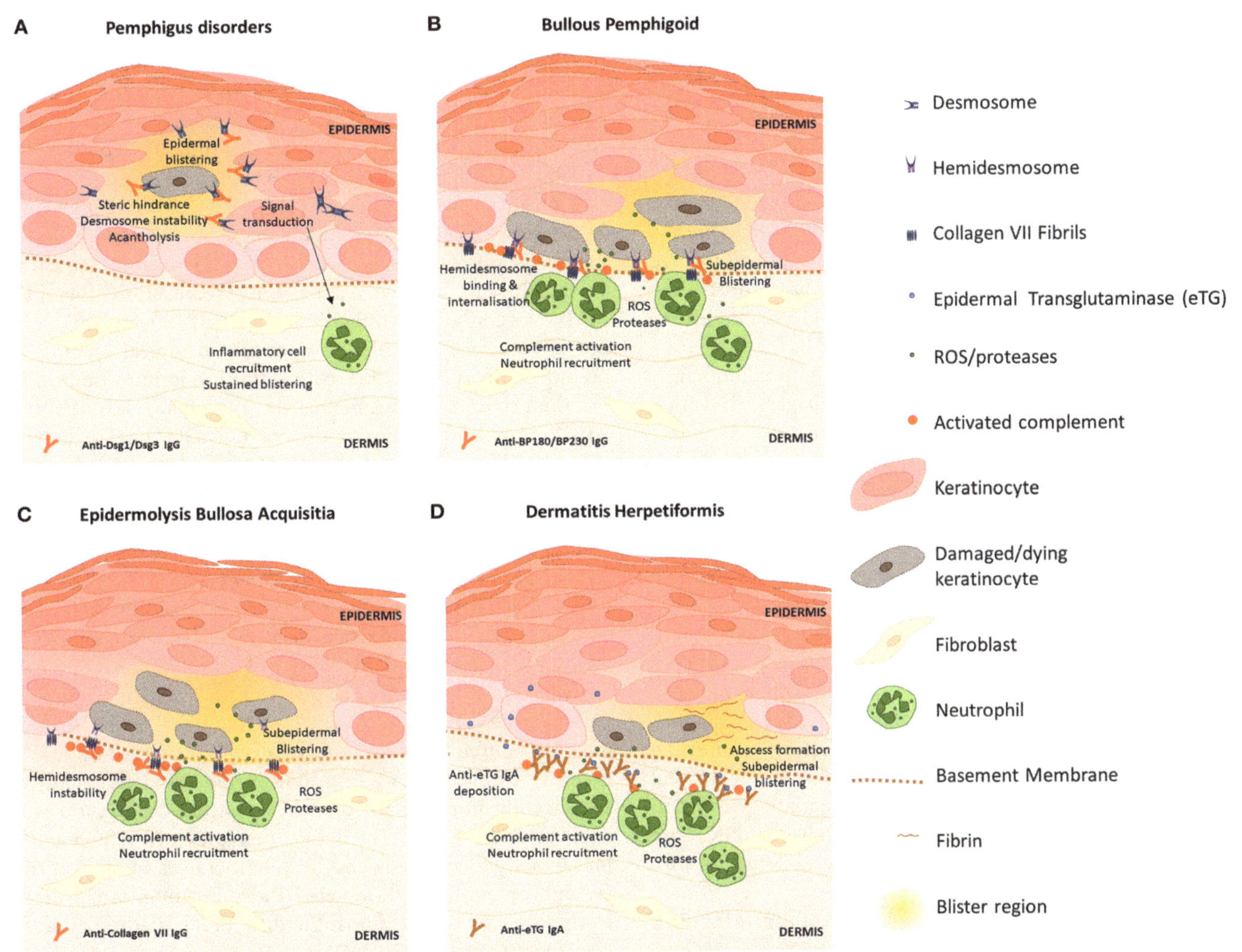

FIGURE 1 | Blistering mechanisms of prototypic autoimmune skin blistering disorders result in skin barrier disruption. **(A)** Pemphigus disorders are caused by autoantibodies against desmoglein (Dsg) proteins Dsg1 and Dsg3. Binding of anti-Dsg destabilizes desmosomes to cause acantholysis of keratinocytes within the epidermis and triggers keratinocyte signal transduction events which promote inflammation, skin barrier disruption and further skin blistering. **(B)** Blisters in bullous pemphigoid are caused by anti-BP180 antibodies which bind hemidesmosomes on basal keratinocytes and trigger complement activation and inflammatory responses including ROS and protease release by neutrophils which directly kill keratinocytes. Skin barrier disruption and skin blistering is caused by keratinocyte death and sustained localized inflammation. **(C)** Epidermolysis bullosa acquisita is caused by anti-Collagen VII antibodies which bind fibrils that anchor hemidesmosomes to the basement membrane. Deposition of IgG induces complement activation via the classical pathway and activation of neutrophils. Basal keratinocytes sustain damage via action of neutrophil-derived ROS and proteases resulting in splitting at the dermal-epidermal junction and skin barrier disruption. **(D)** Dermatitis hepetiformis (DH) is caused by cross-reactive antibodies that bind epidermal transglutaminase (eTG). eTG is produced by keratinocytes and accumulates in the papillary dermis where it forms immunogenic immune complexes with anti-eTG IgA that trigger complement activation. Fibrin deposition and influx of leukocytes (which damage keratinocytes via release of ROS and proteases) cause the formation of neutrophilic abscesses which develop into fluid-filled subepidermal blisters that disrupt the intact skin barrier.

years. Autoantibodies against Dsg proteins, as found in pemphigus diseases, were initially thought to interfere with Dsg-Dsg interactions in desmosomes by steric hindrance (92) however evidence for direct effects of Dsg-anti-Dsg binding on intracellular signaling events was later discovered, including the p38 mitogen-activated protein kinase pathway leading to acantholysis (93, 94). Anti-Dsg may also reduce the number of desmosomes by clustering Dsg on the cell surface and interfering with normal turnover of desmosomal proteins, thereby depleting desmosomes of Dsg (95) and promoting acantholysis. In more recent years, other autoantibody species (96–98) and non-Dsg interactions (99) have been identified as contributing to pemphigus pathology and have prompted the hypothesis that multiple pathways may act synergistically (100) to cause classical pemphigus disease pathology (101).

In BP, autoantibodies against BP180 and BP230 components of hemidesmosomes produce blistering at the dermal-epidermal junction. Activation of the complement cascade via classical and alternative pathways has been demonstrated to contribute to skin barrier disruption and BP pathology (102) and C3 deposition at the epidermal basement membrane is a common clinical finding (103). Complement activation induces inflammation and damages keratinocytes via cytotoxic action of neutrophils leading to skin blistering and barrier disruption (104). Though complement-independent mechanisms of BP pathology have been since described (105, 106) including direct activation of neutrophils via immune complex-FcγR binding, complement activation is still a prevalent target for novel BP therapeutics (103, 107). Autoreactive IgE and eosinophilia are common findings in BP patients and IgE immune complexes binding and activating eosinophils thereby contributing to blister formation has been shown in *in vitro* and *in vivo* studies (108), implicating eosinophils as potential therapeutic targets in BP.

Disease pathology in EBA is caused by predominantly IgG1 and IgG3 autoantibodies that bind Collagen VII within anchoring fibrils at the dermal-epidermal junction. As a rare disease, much of what is known about EBA pathogenesis has been elucidated with experimental models. Like BP, complement activation is considered key to EBA pathogenesis (109), however the alternative pathway appears to be the dominant pathway behind experimental EBA pathology (110). Activation of complement induces inflammation, leukocyte extraversion, complement activation and subsequent tissue damage and disruption of skin barrier via release of ROS and proteases from neutrophils and other myeloid cells. *Ex-vivo* studies of patient serum incubated with healthy skin and donor neutrophils exhibit loss of epidermal adherence, hence clearly indicating that antibodies mediate clinical EBA blistering via neutrophil activation (111). The role of T cells in EBA pathology is yet to be fully elucidated, however murine studies show that NKT and γδT cells likely amplify tissue damage in EBA via interaction with immune complexes and neutrophils (112).

DH is characterized by accumulation of ant-eTG IgA antibodies within the papillary dermis, however eTG is primarily expressed within superficial epidermal layers (113). It is hypothesized that eTG may be released into the blood, where interaction with IgA occurs in nearby dermal vessels; alternatively eTG may be deposited along the basement membrane as a result of trauma (54, 114), however further research is required to confirm these hypotheses. Following IgA deposition, papillary abscesses characterized by a neutrophilic infiltrate and fibrin accumulation form which develop into a split at the basement membrane and subepidermal blistering. Patients with DH show reduced levels of anti-inflammatory IL-10 and reduced Treg cell numbers in lesional skin compared to healthy skin (115) which indicates the role of Tregs in modulating local inflammatory responses in DH and represents an attractive therapeutic target.

TARGETED APPROACHES FOR TREATMENT OF AIBDS

The use of different *in-vitro* systems and experimental animal models in recent years has significantly improved our understanding of AIBDs ultimately leading to novel diagnostic tools and differentiated therapeutic approaches for these disorders (6, 7, 75, 89, 109, 116–123). These approaches can be broadly grouped into: traditional and topical therapies; rituximab and intravenous immunoglobulins and other treatments in pre-clinical and clinical trials. In this review, we will provide a broad summary of traditional treatments and novel emerging therapies which are also summarized in **Table 1**.

First line therapies for AIBDs generally include systemic oral or intravenous corticosteroids (0.5–2.0 mg/kg/day) such as prednisolone (12, 29). Topical high potency corticosteroids such as clobetasol propionate have also been demonstrated to be efficient alternatives to oral prednisolone therapy in BP by reducing autoantibodies against BP180 and BP230 (2). For more severe patients unresponsive to topical therapy, oral prednisolone is combined with adjuvant immunosuppressant (azathioprine, mycophenolate, or rituximab). Unlike other AIBDs, oral corticosteroids do not normally have a dramatic effect in EBA and to date there are no randomized controlled trials providing level 1 evidence for EBA treatment (4). Milder forms of EBA and DH may respond well to topical steroids including dapsone or sulfapyridine, while rituximab has been reported to be effective for severe patients (12, 61, 124, 140, 141). Combining conventional systemic corticosteroids with rituximab treatment has also showed beneficial clinical outcomes in mucous membrane pemphigoid diseases (142).

Second line therapies include corticosteroid-sparing agents azathioprine, mycophenolate mofetil, or rituximab, which may be combined with intravenous immunoglobulin (IVIG) therapy. Clinically, IVIG administration has been shown to significantly improve BP disease symptoms for several weeks after infusion (129). Third line therapies are dependent on individual patient needs and include therapies in clinical trials: cyclophosphamide, IgE-targeted therapies, immunoadsorption to remove pathogenic autoantibodies, IVIG, methotrexate, and plasma exchange.

Preclinical studies have identified potential emerging therapies which target immunological mechanisms in AIBDs, which aim to reduce damaging inflammatory processes. Direct targeting of antibody-producing B cells is efficacious, as anti-CD20 antibody (Rituximab) has been successfully used in the clinic for multiple AIBDs, however not all patients respond equally. Targeting other B cell markers including anti-CD19 and anti-CD22, or antigen-specific B cell receptors may improve targeting of long-lived plasma cells which produce pathogenic autoantibody in patients that are refractory to rituximab. Therapies targeting components of the complement cascade have exhibited success in preclinical and clinical trials, however concerns with side effects associated with existing complement targeting therapies may limit the clinical utility of these approaches (143, 144). Previous studies have highlighted the roles of cytokines in mediating AIBD tissue damage and have identified multiple therapeutic targets including TNFα (130, 145), IL-5 (84), IL-17A(117), and IL-1 blockade (146) and administration of anti-inflammatory IL-10 (147). Immunomodulatory anti-cytokine therapies are in various stages of development, with existing TNF-α inhibitors showing efficacy in treating AIBDs and antibodies against IL-5 and eotaxin-1 having entered clinical trials for BP treatment (148–150).

TABLE 1 | Current and emerging therapeutic approaches in autoimmune skin blistering diseases.

Approach	Therapeutic agents	Stage of development	Disease
Corticosteroids (oral or topical)	Prednisolone (12, 124, 125) Clobetasol propionate Dapsone, Sulfapyridine	First-line therapies	BP, PD, EBA, DH
Immuno-suppressant	Azathioprine (125) Mycophenolate mofetil Chlorambucil	Second-line therapies	BP, PD, EBA, DH
Antibody removal	Immunoadsorption Plasma exchange	Third-line therapies	BP, PD, EBA, DH
B-cell targeting	Anti-CD20 (Rituximab) (126)	Second-line therapy	BP, PD, EBA, DH
	Anti-CD19 (68)	Preclinical	PD
	Anti-CD22 (68)	Preclinical	PD
	Antigen-mediated targeting (127)	Preclinical	PD
	BCR signaling inhibition (128)	Phase III trials	PD
Immuno-modulatory	IVIG (129)	Second-line therapy	BP, PD, EBA
	Anti-TNFα (130)	Off-label use	BP, PD, MMP
	Anti-IL-17A (117)	Preclinical	BP
	Anti-IL-5 (131, 132)	Completed Phase II	BP
	Anti-Eotaxin-1 (133, 134)	Completed Phase II	BP
	HSP-90 inhibition (135, 136)	Preclinical	EBA
	SYK inhibition (137)	Preclinical	EBA
	Vitamin D (122, 138)	Preclinical	PD, EBA
Complement targeting	Anti-C1s (107)	Preclinical	BP
	Anti-C5 (103, 109)	Preclinical	EBA
	Anti-factor B (109)	Preclinical	EBA
	C5aR1 antagonist (109)	Preclinical	EBA
Wound healing therapies	Anti-Flii (139)	Preclinical	EBA

BCR, B-cell receptor; BP, Bullous pemphigoid; DH, dermatitis herpetiformis; EBA, epidermolysis bullosa acquisita; HSP, Heat-shock protein; IVIG, intravenous immunoglobulin; MMP, mucous membrane pemphigoid; PD, pemphigus disorders; SYK, spleen tyrosine kinase.

Like immunomodulatory therapies for other autoimmune diseases, these approaches are likely to be associated with known side effects of immunosuppression (151) thus further trials are needed to identify the safest and most efficacious dose regimens for specific diseases. Preclinical studies have identified cellular populations which may be exploited as therapeutic targets, such as Langerhans cells (152), dendritic cells (153), granulocytes (104, 111, 133, 154), and multiple T cell subsets including Th17 (117, 155), Treg (75), NKT (112), γδT (112), and CD8+ (156). Approaches to target specific immune cell functions are currently in preclinical development, including small molecule inhibition of spleen tyrosine kinase (137), an enzyme involves in proinflammatory Fc-receptor signal transduction in myeloid cells, and metabolites of Vitamin D which reduce myeloid cell activation and ROS production (122).

Understanding the mechanisms of autoantibody mediated tissue damage is critical in development of novel targeted therapies, however understanding the mechanisms behind resolution of blistering and inflammation in AIBDs can also offer insights into potential novel treatment modalities. Unresolved blistering can impact patient quality of life and increase risk of bleeding, infection and tumor development (157). Optimal healing is especially important for patients with extensive cutaneous blistering, or mucosal blistering which affects feeding, digestion and function of other organs (158, 159). Studies surrounding the role of Flightless protein (Flii) in skin blistering have revealed the first mechanism leading to the resolution of blistering and inflammation in antibody transfer induced EBA (8), and further research into similar pathways may reveal more potential therapeutic strategies where wound healing therapies may offer opportunities for decreasing the clinical symptoms associated with AIBDs.

In summary, there is a high unmet need for new targeted therapeutic approaches focussed on restoring the integrity of the skins' barrier 22and address both blistering mechanisms and clinical symptoms in systemic AIBDs. Innovative designs of randomized controlled trials using validated scales of assessment are needed to drive the development of novel therapeutic strategies for patients with AIBDs. Additionally, research efforts should focus on adapting immunomodulatory approaches that have been shown to be effective in other autoimmune diseases in order to target common pathogenic mechanisms and developing a better understanding of blister resolution and healing to improve patient symptoms.

CONCLUSION

As highlighted in this review, the contribution of the skin barrier to the mechanisms underpinning autoimmunity has greatly improve our understanding of AIBDs. Development of novel targeted therapeutics restoring skin barrier function and homeostasis will lead to improved treatment of patients with AIBDs.

CONTRIBUTION TO THE FIELD STATEMENT

Autoimmune skin blistering diseases are caused by pathogenic autoantibodies which trigger cellular, biochemical and immunological processes that disrupt the skin barrier and cause chronic blistering in patients. Understanding the mechanisms behind these processes has lead to the development of new targeted therapeutics which are in various stages of preclinical and clinical development. Current therapeutic approaches rely heavily on immunosuppressants and corticosteroids which are associated with adverse effects including risk of infection. Thus, new therapeutics are necessary to effectively control skin blistering and restore the skin barrier with fewer side effects. In this review, we highlight the different mechanisms behind autoimmune skin blistering disease development including initiation, maintenance and tissue damage. Additionally, we summarize current treatment and emerging therapeutics for autoimmune skin blistering diseases and highlight blistering mechanisms which may be exploited for development of novel targeted therapeutics.

AUTHOR CONTRIBUTIONS

All authors listed have made a substantial, direct and intellectual contribution to the work, and approved it for publication.

ACKNOWLEDGMENTS

AC is supported by NHMRC Senior Research Fellowship (GNT#1102617) and ZK is supported by a Future Industries Institute Foundation Fellowship.

REFERENCES

1. Yancey KB. The pathophysiology of autoimmune blistering diseases. *J Clin Invest.* (2005) 115:825–8. doi: 10.1172/JCI200524855
2. Amber KT, Murrell DF, Schmidt E, Joly P, Borradori L. Autoimmune subepidermal bullous diseases of the skin and mucosae: clinical features, diagnosis, and management. *Clin Rev Allergy Immunol.* (2018) 54:26–51. doi: 10.1007/s12016-017-8633-4
3. Vorobyev A, Ludwig RJ, Schmidt E. Clinical features and diagnosis of epidermolysis bullosa acquisita. *Expert Rev Clin Immunol.* (2017) 13:157–69. doi: 10.1080/1744666X.2016.1221343
4. Sugai T, Ujiie H, Nakamura H, Kikuchi K, Iwata H, Shimizu H. Case of autoimmune intraepidermal and subepidermal blistering disease in which autoantibodies to desmoglein 1 and BP230 coexist. *J Dermatol.* (2018). doi: 10.1111/1346-8138.14734. [Epub ahead of print].
5. Kopecki Z, Ludwig RJ, Cowin AJ. Cytoskeletal regulation of inflammation and its impact on skin blistering disease epidermolysis bullosa acquisita. *Int J Mol Sci.* (2016) 17:1116. doi: 10.3390/ijms17071116
6. Witte M, Zillikens D, Schmidt E. diagnosis of autoimmune blistering diseases. *Front Med (Lausanne).* (2018) 5:296. doi: 10.3389/fmed.2018.00296
7. Ludwig RJ, Vanhoorelbeke K, Leypoldt F, Kaya Z, Bieber K, McLachlan SM, et al. Mechanisms of autoantibody-induced pathology. *Front Immunol.* (2017) 8:603. doi: 10.3389/fimmu.2017.00603
8. Ludwig R. Immune mechanism-targeted treatment of experimental epidermolysis bullosa acquisita. *Expert Rev Clin Immunol.* (2015) 11:1365–78. doi: 10.1586/1744666X.2015.1085801
9. Kamaguchi M, Iwata H. The diagnosis and blistering mechanisms of mucous membrane pemphigoid. *Front Immunol.* (2019) 10:34. doi: 10.3389/fimmu.2019.00034
10. Murrell DF. Autoimmune diseases of the skin. *Immunol Allerg Clin North Am.* (2012) 32:xiii–iv. doi: 10.1016/j.iac.2012.04.015
11. Kasprick A, Bieber K, Ludwig RJ. Drug discovery for pemphigoid diseases. *Curr Protoc Pharmacol.* (2019) 84:e55. doi: 10.1002/cpph.55
12. Koga H, Prost-Squarcioni C, Iwata H, Jonkman MF, Ludwig RJ, Bieber K. Epidermolysis bullosa acquisita: the 2019 update. *Front Med (Lausanne).* (2018) 5:362. doi: 10.3389/fmed.2018.00362
13. Kasperkiewicz M, Schmidt E, Zillikens D. Current therapy of the pemphigus group. *Clin Dermatol.* (2012) 30:84–94. doi: 10.1016/j.clindermatol.2011.03.014
14. Seiffert-Sinha K, Yang R, Fung CK, Lai KW, Patterson KC, Payne AS, et al. Nanorobotic investigation identifies novel visual, structural and functional correlates of autoimmune pathology in a blistering skin disease model. *PLoS ONE.* (2014) 9:e106895. doi: 10.1371/journal.pone.0106895
15. Vodo D, Sarig O, Sprecher E. The genetics of pemphigus vulgaris. *Front Med (Lausanne).* (2018) 5:226. doi: 10.3389/fmed.2018.00226
16. Li S, Zhang Q, Wang P, Li J, Ni J, Wu J, et al. Association between HLA-DQB1 polymorphisms and pemphigus vulgaris: a meta-analysis. *Immunol Invest.* (2018) 47:101–12. doi: 10.1080/08820139.2017.1385622
17. Fang H, Shen S, Zheng X, Dang E, Zhang J, Shao S, et al. Association of HLA class I and class II alleles with bullous pemphigoid in Chinese Hans. *J Dermatol Sci.* (2018) 89:258–62. doi: 10.1016/j.jdermsci.2017.11.014
18. Ujiie H, Muramatsu K, Mushiroda T, Ozeki T, Miyoshi H, Iwata H, et al. HLA-DQB1*03:01 as a biomarker for genetic susceptibility to bullous pemphigoid induced by DPP-4 inhibitors. *J Invest Dermatol.* (2018) 138:1201–4. doi: 10.1016/j.jid.2017.11.023
19. Zumelzu C, Le Roux-Villet C, Loiseau P, Busson M, Heller M, Aucouturier F, et al. Black patients of African descent and HLA-DRB1*15:03 frequency overrepresented in epidermolysis bullosa acquisita. *J Invest Dermatol.* (2011) 131:2386–93. doi: 10.1038/jid.2011.231
20. Lee CW, Kim SC, Han H. Distribution of HLA class II alleles in Korean patients with epidermolysis bullosa acquisita. *Dermatology.* (1996) 193:328–9. doi: 10.1159/000246282
21. Vodo D, Sarig O, Geller S, Ben-Asher E, Olender T, Bochner R, et al. Identification of a functional risk variant for pemphigus vulgaris in the ST18 gene. *PLoS Genet.* (2016) 12:e1006008. doi: 10.1371/journal.pgen.1006008
22. Ludwig RJ, Muller S, Marques A, Recke A, Schmidt E, Zillikens D, et al. Identification of quantitative trait loci in experimental epidermolysis bullosa acquisita. *J Invest Dermatol.* (2012) 132:1409–15. doi: 10.1038/jid.2011.466
23. Sen BB, Ekiz O, Rifaioglu EN, Sen T, Atik E, Dogramaci AC. Localized bullous pemphigoid occurring on surgical scars. *Indian J Dermatol Venereol Leprol.* (2013) 79:554. doi: 10.4103/0378-6323.113111
24. Sanchez-Palacios C, Chan LS. Development of pemphigus herpetiformis in a patient with psoriasis receiving UV-light treatment. *J Cutan Pathol.* (2004) 31:346–9. doi: 10.1111/j.0303-6987.2004.0188.x
25. Khosravani S, Handjani F, Alimohammadi R, Saki N. Frequency of neurological disorders in bullous pemphigoid patients: a cross-sectional study. *Int Sch Res Notices.* (2017) 2017:6053267. doi: 10.1155/2017/6053267
26. Gambichler T, Segert H, Hoxtermann S, Schmitz L, Altmeyer P, Teegen B. Neurological disorders in patients with bullous pemphigoid: clinical and experimental investigations. *J Eur Acad Dermatol Venereol.* (2015) 29:1758–62. doi: 10.1111/jdv.12995

27. Bastuji-Garin S, Joly P, Lemordant P, Sparsa A, Bedane C, Delaporte E, et al. Risk factors for bullous pemphigoid in the elderly: a prospective case-control study. *J Invest Dermatol.* (2011) 131:637–43. doi: 10.1038/jid.2010.301
28. Varpuluoma O, Jokelainen J, Forsti AK, Timonen M, Huilaja L, Tasanen K. Dermatitis herpetiformis and celiac disease increase the risk of bullous pemphigoid. *J Invest Dermatol.* (2019) 139:600–4. doi: 10.1016/j.jid.2018.10.010
29. Bech R, Kibsgaard L, Vestergaard C. Comorbidities and treatment strategies in bullous pemphigoid: an appraisal of the existing litterature. *Front Med (Lausanne).* (2018) 5:238. doi: 10.3389/fmed.2018.00238
30. Baroero L, Coppo P, Bertolino L, Maccario S, Savino F. Three case reports of post immunization and post viral Bullous Pemphigoid: looking for the right trigger. *BMC Pediatr.* (2017) 17:60. doi: 10.1186/s12887-017-0813-0
31. Jang H, Jin YJ, Yoon CH, Kim CW, Kim L. Bullous pemphigoid associated with chronic hepatitis C virus infection in a hepatitis B virus endemic area: a case report. *Medicine (Baltimore).* (2018) 97:e0377. doi: 10.1097/MD.0000000000010377
32. Fernandes NC, Rampinelli H, Souza LM, Guimaraes M. Refractory pemphigus foliaceus associated with herpesvirus infection: case report. *Rev Inst Med Trop Sao Paulo.* (2017) 59:e41. doi: 10.1590/s1678-9946201759041
33. Gee SN, Velez NF, Sepehr A, Burgin S. Two distinct viral infections complicating pemphigus foliaceus. *Dermatol Online J.* (2012) 18:3.
34. Furukawa F, Ozaki M, Imamura S, Hirose S. Bullous pemphigoid associated with radiotherapy for esophageal carcinoma. *Dermatologica.* (1981) 162:451–4. doi: 10.1159/000250316
35. Melani L, Giomi B, Antiga E, Torchia D, Caproni M, Fabbri P. Radiation therapy as a trigger factor for initially localized bullous pemphigoid. *Breast J.* (2005) 11:485–6. doi: 10.1111/j.1075-122X.2005.00150.x
36. Nguyen T, Kwan JM, Ahmed AR. Relationship between radiation therapy and bullous pemphigoid. *Dermatology.* (2014) 229:88–96. doi: 10.1159/000362208
37. Fujinami RS, von Herrath MG, Christen U, Whitton JL. Molecular mimicry, bystander activation, or viral persistence: infections and autoimmune disease. *Clin Microbiol Rev.* (2006) 19:80–94. doi: 10.1128/CMR.19.1.80-94.2006
38. MacKay IR, Leskovsek NV, Rose NR. Cell damage and autoimmunity: a critical appraisal. *J Autoimmun.* (2008) 30:5–11. doi: 10.1016/j.jaut.2007.11.009
39. Land WG. The role of damage-associated molecular patterns in human diseases: part I - promoting inflammation and immunity. *Sultan Qaboos Univ Med J.* (2015) 15:e9–21.
40. Sachet M, Liang YY, Oehler R. The immune response to secondary necrotic cells. *Apoptosis.* (2017) 22:1189–204. doi: 10.1007/s10495-017-1413-z
41. Saadeh D, Kurban M, Abbas O. Update on the role of plasmacytoid dendritic cells in inflammatory/autoimmune skin diseases. *Exp Dermatol.* (2016) 25:415–21. doi: 10.1111/exd.12957
42. Ma L, Chan K, Trendell-Smith N, Lo C, To C, Huang F. Necrotic cells induce systemic autoimmune disease *in vivo* by activation of dendritic cells (DCs). *J Allergy Clin Immunol.* (2005) 115:891. doi: 10.1016/j.jaci.2005.01.047
43. Powell AM, Black MM. Epitope spreading: protection from pathogens, but propagation of autoimmunity? *Clin Exp Dermatol.* (2001) 26:427–33. doi: 10.1046/j.1365-2230.2001.00852.x
44. Aoki V, Millikan RC, Rivitti EA, Hans-Filho G, Eaton DP, Warren SJ, et al. Environmental risk factors in endemic pemphigus foliaceus (fogo selvagem). *J Investig Dermatol Symp Proc.* (2004) 9:34–40. doi: 10.1111/j.1087-0024.2004.00833.x
45. Qian Y, Jeong JS, Maldonado M, Valenzuela JG, Gomes R, Teixeira C, et al. Cutting Edge: Brazilian pemphigus foliaceus anti-desmoglein 1 autoantibodies cross-react with sand fly salivary LJM11 antigen. *J Immunol.* (2012) 189:1535–9. doi: 10.4049/jimmunol.1200842
46. Wieczorek M, Czernik A. Paraneoplastic pemphigus: a short review. *Clin Cosmet Investig Dermatol.* (2016) 9:291–5. doi: 10.2147/CCID.S100802
47. Chan LS. Epitope spreading in paraneoplastic pemphigus: autoimmune induction in antibody-mediated blistering skin diseases. *Arch Dermatol.* (2000) 136:663–4. doi: 10.1001/archderm.136.5.663
48. Fernandes J, Barad P, Shukla P. Association of bullous pemphigoid with malignancy: a myth or reality? *Indian J Dermatol.* (2014) 59:390–3. doi: 10.4103/0019-5154.135493
49. Das A, Das S, Das SK, Basuthakur S. A case of paraneoplastic bullous pemphigoid in association with squamous cell carcinoma of lung. *J Postgrad Med.* (2015) 61:197–9. doi: 10.4103/0022-3859.150906
50. Noguchi K, Kawamura H, Ishizu H, Okada K. Dramatic resolution of bullous pemphigoid after surgery for gastric cancer: a case report. *Int J Surg Case Rep.* (2014) 5:212–4. doi: 10.1016/j.ijscr.2014.02.008
51. Balestri R, Magnano M, La Placa M, Patrizi A, Angileri L, Tengattini V, et al. Malignancies in bullous pemphigoid: a controversial association. *J Dermatol.* (2016) 43:125–33. doi: 10.1111/1346-8138.13079
52. Cai SC, Allen JC, Lim YL, Tan SH, Tang MB. Association of bullous pemphigoid and malignant neoplasms. *JAMA Dermatol.* (2015) 151:665–7. doi: 10.1001/jamadermatol.2014.5263
53. Didona D, Di Zenzo G. Humoral epitope spreading in autoimmune bullous diseases. *Front Immunol.* (2018) 9:779. doi: 10.3389/fimmu.2018.00779
54. Clarindo MV, Possebon AT, Soligo EM, Uyeda H, Ruaro RT, Empinotti JC. Dermatitis herpetiformis: pathophysiology, clinical presentation, diagnosis and treatment. *An Bras Dermatol.* (2014) 89:865–75; quiz: 76–7. doi: 10.1590/abd1806-4841.20142966
55. Jonkman MF, Schuur J, Dijk F, Heeres K, de Jong MC, van der Meer JB, et al. Inflammatory variant of epidermolysis bullosa acquisita with IgG autoantibodies against type VII collagen and laminin alpha3. *Arch Dermatol.* (2000) 136:227–31. doi: 10.1001/archderm.136.2.227
56. Di Zenzo G, Thoma-Uszynski S, Calabresi V, Fontao L, Hofmann SC, Lacour JP, et al. Demonstration of epitope-spreading phenomena in bullous pemphigoid: results of a prospective multicenter study. *J Invest Dermatol.* (2011) 131:2271–80. doi: 10.1038/jid.2011.180
57. Kridin K, Bergman R. Association of bullous pemphigoid with dipeptidyl-peptidase 4 inhibitors in patients with diabetes: estimating the risk of the new agents and characterizing the patients. *JAMA Dermatol.* (2018) 154:1152–8. doi: 10.1001/jamadermatol.2018.2352
58. Kridin K, Ludwig RJ. The growing incidence of bullous pemphigoid: overview and potential explanations. *Front Med (Lausanne).* (2018) 5:220. doi: 10.3389/fmed.2018.00220
59. Mendonca FM, Martin-Gutierrez FJ, Rios-Martin JJ, Camacho-Martinez F. Three cases of bullous pemphigoid associated with dipeptidyl peptidase-4 inhibitors - one due to linagliptin. *Dermatology.* (2016) 232:249–53. doi: 10.1159/000443330
60. Izumi K, Nishie W, Mai Y, Wada M, Natsuga K, Ujiie H, et al. Autoantibody profile differentiates between inflammatory and noninflammatory bullous pemphigoid. *J Invest Dermatol.* (2016) 136:2201–10. doi: 10.1016/j.jid.2016.06.622
61. Sibaud V. Dermatologic reactions to immune checkpoint inhibitors : skin toxicities and immunotherapy. *Am J Clin Dermatol.* (2018) 19:345–61. doi: 10.1007/s40257-017-0336-3
62. Zumelzu C, Alexandre M, Le Roux C, Weber P, Guyot A, Levy A, et al. Mucous membrane pemphigoid, bullous pemphigoid, and anti-programmed death-1/ programmed death-ligand 1: a case report of an elderly woman with mucous membrane pemphigoid developing after pembrolizumab therapy for metastatic melanoma and review of the literature. *Front Med (Lausanne).* (2018) 5:268. doi: 10.3389/fmed.2018.00268
63. Hess C, Winkler A, Lorenz AK, Holecska V, Blanchard V, Eiglmeier S, et al. T cell-independent B cell activation induces immunosuppressive sialylated IgG antibodies. *J Clin Invest.* (2013) 123:3788–96. doi: 10.1172/JCI65938
64. Hoyer BF, Moser K, Hauser AE, Peddinghaus A, Voigt C, Eilat D, et al. Short-lived plasmablasts and long-lived plasma cells contribute to chronic humoral autoimmunity in NZB/W mice. *J Exp Med.* (2004) 199:1577–84. doi: 10.1084/jem.20040168
65. Colliou N, Picard D, Caillot F, Calbo S, Le Corre S, Lim A, et al. Long-term remissions of severe pemphigus after rituximab therapy are associated with prolonged failure of desmoglein B cell response. *Sci Transl Med.* (2013) 5:175ra30. doi: 10.1126/scitranslmed.3005166
66. Hiepe F, Dorner T, Hauser AE, Hoyer BF, Mei H, Radbruch A. Long-lived autoreactive plasma cells drive persistent autoimmune inflammation. *Nat Rev Rheumatol.* (2011) 7:170–8. doi: 10.1038/nrrheum.2011.1
67. Hiepe F, Radbruch A. Plasma cells as an innovative target in autoimmune disease with renal manifestations. *Nat Rev Nephrol.* (2016) 12:232–40. doi: 10.1038/nrneph.2016.20

68. Musette P, Bouaziz JD. B cell modulation strategies in autoimmune diseases: new concepts. *Front Immunol.* (2018) 9:622. doi: 10.3389/fimmu.2018.00622
69. Tiburzy B, Szyska M, Iwata H, Chrobok N, Kulkarni U, Hirose M, et al. Persistent autoantibody-production by intermediates between short-and long-lived plasma cells in inflamed lymph nodes of experimental epidermolysis bullosa acquisita. *PLoS ONE.* (2013) 8:e83631. doi: 10.1371/journal.pone.0083631
70. Timoteo RP, da Silva MV, Miguel CB, Silva DA, Catarino JD, Rodrigues Junior V, et al. Th1/Th17-related cytokines and chemokines and their implications in the pathogenesis of pemphigus vulgaris. *Mediators Inflamm.* (2017) 2017:7151285. doi: 10.1155/2017/7151285
71. Lee SH, Hong WJ, Kim SC. Analysis of serum cytokine profile in pemphigus. *Ann Dermatol.* (2017) 29:438–45. doi: 10.5021/ad.2017.29.4.438
72. Pickford WJ, Gudi V, Haggart AM, Lewis BJ, Herriot R, Barker RN, et al. T cell participation in autoreactivity to NC16a epitopes in bullous pemphigoid. *Clin Exp Immunol.* (2015) 180:189–200. doi: 10.1111/cei.12566
73. Gounni Abdelilah S, Wellemans V, Agouli M, Guenounou M, Hamid Q, Beck LA, et al. Increased expression of Th2-associated chemokines in bullous pemphigoid disease. Role of eosinophils in the production and release of these chemokines. *Clin Immunol.* (2006) 120:220–31. doi: 10.1016/j.clim.2006.03.014
74. Makino T, Yoshihisa Y, Mizawa M, Tsutsui K, Nishijima C, Inaoki M, et al. Increased serum levels of Th2-type cytokines and eotaxin in fibrillar-type dermatitis herpetiformis. *Acta Derm Venereol.* (2017) 97:642–3. doi: 10.2340/00015555-2604
75. Bieber K, Sun S, Witte M, Kasprick A, Beltsiou F, Behnen M, et al. Regulatory T cells suppress inflammation and blistering in pemphigoid diseases. *Front Immunol.* (2017) 8:1628. doi: 10.3389/fimmu.2017.01628
76. Sugiyama H, Matsue H, Nagasaka A, Nakamura Y, Tsukamoto K, Shibagaki N, et al. CD4+CD25high regulatory T cells are markedly decreased in blood of patients with pemphigus vulgaris. *Dermatology.* (2007) 214:210–20. doi: 10.1159/000099585
77. Veldman C, Hohne A, Dieckmann D, Schuler G, Hertl M. Type I regulatory T cells specific for desmoglein 3 are more frequently detected in healthy individuals than in patients with pemphigus vulgaris. *J Immunol.* (2004) 172:6468–75. doi: 10.4049/jimmunol.172.10.6468
78. Yokoyama T, Matsuda S, Takae Y, Wada N, Nishikawa T, Amagai M, et al. Antigen-independent development of Foxp3+ regulatory T cells suppressing autoantibody production in experimental pemphigus vulgaris. *Int Immunol.* (2011) 23:365–73. doi: 10.1093/intimm/dxr020
79. Yuan H, Zhou S, Liu Z, Cong W, Fei X, Zeng W, et al. Pivotal role of lesional and perilesional T/B lymphocytes in pemphigus pathogenesis. *J Invest Dermatol.* (2017) 137:2362–70. doi: 10.1016/j.jid.2017.05.032
80. Anhalt GJ, Labib RS, Voorhees JJ, Beals TF, Diaz LA. Induction of pemphigus in neonatal mice by passive transfer of IgG from patients with the disease. *N Engl J Med.* (1982) 306:1189–96. doi: 10.1056/NEJM198205203062001
81. Ding X, Diaz LA, Fairley JA, Giudice GJ, Liu Z. The anti-desmoglein 1 autoantibodies in pemphigus vulgaris sera are pathogenic. *J Invest Dermatol.* (1999) 112:739–43. doi: 10.1046/j.1523-1747.1999.00585.x
82. Amagai M, Nishikawa T, Nousari HC, Anhalt GJ, Hashimoto T. Antibodies against desmoglein 3 (pemphigus vulgaris antigen) are present in sera from patients with paraneoplastic pemphigus and cause acantholysis *in vivo* in neonatal mice. *J Clin Invest.* (1998) 102:775–82. doi: 10.1172/JCI3647
83. Woodley DT, Ram R, Doostan A, Bandyopadhyay P, Huang Y, Remington J, et al. Induction of epidermolysis bullosa acquisita in mice by passive transfer of autoantibodies from patients. *J Invest Dermatol.* (2006) 126:1323–30. doi: 10.1038/sj.jid.5700254
84. Amber KT, Valdebran M, Kridin K, Grando SA. The role of eosinophils in bullous pemphigoid: a developing model of eosinophil pathogenicity in mucocutaneous disease. *Front Med (Lausanne).* (2018) 5:201. doi: 10.3389/fmed.2018.00201
85. de Graauw E, Sitaru C, Horn M, Borradori L, Yousefi S, Simon HU, et al. Evidence for a role of eosinophils in blister formation in bullous pemphigoid. *Allergy.* (2017) 72:1105–13. doi: 10.1111/all.13131
86. Fang H, Zhang Y, Li N, Wang G, Liu Z. The autoimmune skin disease bullous pemphigoid: the role of mast cells in autoantibody-induced tissue injury. *Front Immunol.* (2018) 9:407. doi: 10.3389/fimmu.2018.00407
87. Yu X, Kasprick A, Hartmann K, Petersen F. The role of mast cells in autoimmune bullous dermatoses. *Front Immunol.* (2018) 9:386. doi: 10.3389/fimmu.2018.00386
88. Eyerich K, Dimartino V, Cavani A. IL-17 and IL-22 in immunity: driving protection and pathology. *Eur J Immunol.* (2017) 47:607–14. doi: 10.1002/eji.201646723
89. Haeberle S, Wei X, Bieber K, Goletz S, Ludwig RJ, Schmidt E, et al. Regulatory T-cell deficiency leads to pathogenic bullous pemphigoid antigen 230 autoantibody and autoimmune bullous disease. *J Allergy Clin Immunol.* (2018) 142:1831–42.e7. doi: 10.1016/j.jaci.2018.04.006
90. Hashimoto T, Takahashi H, Sakaguchi S. Regulatory T-cell deficiency and autoimmune skin disease: Beyond the scurfy mouse and immune dysregulation, polyendocrinopathy, enteropathy, X-linked syndrome. *J Allergy Clin Immunol.* (2018) 142:1754–6. doi: 10.1016/j.jaci.2018.08.028
91. Yang CH, Tian L, Ling GS, Trendell-Smith NJ, Ma L, Lo CK, et al. Immunological mechanisms and clinical implications of regulatory T cell deficiency in a systemic autoimmune disorder: roles of IL-2 versus IL-15. *Eur J Immunol.* (2008) 38:1664–76. doi: 10.1002/eji.200838190
92. Amagai M. Autoimmunity against desmosomal cadherins in pemphigus. *J Dermatol Sci.* (1999) 20:92–102. doi: 10.1016/S0923-1811(99)00016-X
93. Waschke J, Bruggeman P, Baumgartner W, Zillikens D, Drenckhahn D. Pemphigus foliaceus IgG causes dissociation of desmoglein 1-containing junctions without blocking desmoglein 1 transinteraction. *J Clin Invest.* (2005) 115:3157–65. doi: 10.1172/JCI23475
94. Berkowitz P, Chua M, Liu Z, Diaz LA, Rubenstein DS. Autoantibodies in the autoimmune disease pemphigus foliaceus induce blistering via p38 mitogen-activated protein kinase-dependent signaling in the skin. *Am J Pathol.* (2008) 173:1628–36. doi: 10.2353/ajpath.2008.080391
95. Aoyama Y, Kitajima Y. Pemphigus vulgaris-IgG causes a rapid depletion of desmoglein 3 (Dsg3) from the Triton X-100 soluble pools, leading to the formation of Dsg3-depleted desmosomes in a human squamous carcinoma cell line, DJM-1 cells. *J Invest Dermatol.* (1999) 112:67–71. doi: 10.1046/j.1523-1747.1999.00463.x
96. Chen Y, Chernyavsky A, Webber RJ, Grando SA, Wang PH. Critical role of the neonatal Fc receptor (FcRn) in the pathogenic action of antimitochondrial autoantibodies synergizing with anti-desmoglein autoantibodies in pemphigus vulgaris. *J Biol Chem.* (2015) 290:23826–37. doi: 10.1074/jbc.M115.668061
97. Saleh MA, Salem H, El Azizy H. Autoantibodies other than anti-desmogleins in pemphigus vulgaris patients. *Indian J Dermatol.* (2017) 62:47–51. doi: 10.4103/0019-5154.198032
98. Amber KT, Valdebran M, Grando SA. Non-desmoglein antibodies in patients with pemphigus vulgaris. *Front Immunol.* (2018) 9:1190. doi: 10.3389/fimmu.2018.01190
99. Nguyen VT, Ndoye A, Grando SA. Novel human alpha9 acetylcholine receptor regulating keratinocyte adhesion is targeted by Pemphigus vulgaris autoimmunity. *Am J Pathol.* (2000) 157:1377–91. doi: 10.1016/S0002-9440(10)64651-2
100. Grando SA. Pemphigus autoimmunity: hypotheses and realities. *Autoimmunity.* (2012) 45:7–35. doi: 10.3109/08916934.2011.606444
101. Sajda T, Sinha AA. Autoantibody signaling in pemphigus vulgaris: development of an integrated model. *Front Immunol.* (2018) 9:692. doi: 10.3389/fimmu.2018.00692
102. Chiorean RM, Baican A, Mustafa MB, Lischka A, Leucuta DC, Feldrihan V, et al. Complement-activating capacity of autoantibodies correlates with disease activity in bullous pemphigoid patients. *Front Immunol.* (2018) 9:2687. doi: 10.3389/fimmu.2018.02687
103. Kushner CJ, Payne AS. Increasing the complement of therapeutic options in bullous pemphigoid. *J Invest Dermatol.* (2018) 138:246–8. doi: 10.1016/j.jid.2017.09.026
104. Lin L, Hwang BJ, Culton DA, Li N, Burette S, Koller BH, et al. Eosinophils mediate tissue injury in the autoimmune skin disease bullous pemphigoid. *J Invest Dermatol.* (2018) 138:1032–43. doi: 10.1016/j.jid.2017.11.031
105. Ujiie H, Sasaoka T, Izumi K, Nishie W, Shinkuma S, Natsuga K, et al. Bullous pemphigoid autoantibodies directly induce blister formation without complement activation. *J Immunol.* (2014) 193:4415–28. doi: 10.4049/jimmunol.1400095

106. Iwata H, Kamio N, Aoyama Y, Yamamoto Y, Hirako Y, Owaribe K, et al. IgG from patients with bullous pemphigoid depletes cultured keratinocytes of the 180-kDa bullous pemphigoid antigen (type XVII collagen) and weakens cell attachment. *J Invest Dermatol.* (2009) 129:919–26. doi: 10.1038/jid.2008.305
107. Kasprick A, Holtsche MM, Rose EL, Hussain S, Schmidt E, Petersen F, et al. The anti-C1s antibody TNT003 prevents complement activation in the skin induced by bullous pemphigoid autoantibodies. *J Invest Dermatol.* (2018) 138:458–61. doi: 10.1016/j.jid.2017.08.030
108. Hammers CM, Stanley JR. Mechanisms of disease: pemphigus and bullous pemphigoid. *Annu Rev Pathol.* (2016) 11:175–97. doi: 10.1146/annurev-pathol-012615-044313
109. Mihai S, Hirose M, Wang Y, Thurman JM, Holers VM, Morgan BP, et al. Specific inhibition of complement activation significantly ameliorates autoimmune blistering disease in mice. *Front Immunol.* (2018) 9:535. doi: 10.3389/fimmu.2018.00535
110. Mihai S, Chiriac MT, Takahashi K, Thurman JM, Holers VM, Zillikens D, et al. The alternative pathway of complement activation is critical for blister induction in experimental epidermolysis bullosa acquisita. *J Immunol.* (2007) 178:6514–21. doi: 10.4049/jimmunol.178.10.6514
111. Sitaru C, Kromminga A, Hashimoto T, Brocker EB, Zillikens D. Autoantibodies to type VII collagen mediate Fcgamma-dependent neutrophil activation and induce dermal-epidermal separation in cryosections of human skin. *Am J Pathol.* (2002) 161:301–11. doi: 10.1016/S0002-9440(10)64182-X
112. Bieber K, Witte M, Sun S, Hundt JE, Kalies K, Drager S, et al. T cells mediate autoantibody-induced cutaneous inflammation and blistering in epidermolysis bullosa acquisita. *Sci Rep.* (2016) 6:38357. doi: 10.1038/srep38357
113. Valencia-Guerrero A, Dresser K, Cornejo K. The utility of tissue and epidermal transglutaminase immunohistochemistry in dermatitis herpetiformis. *Indian J Dermatopathol Diagn Dermatol.* (2018) 5:97–100. doi: 10.4103/ijdpdd.ijdpdd_22_18
114. Collin P, Salmi TT, Hervonen K, Kaukinen K, Reunala T. Dermatitis herpetiformis: a cutaneous manifestation of coeliac disease. *Ann Med.* (2017) 49:23–31. doi: 10.1080/07853890.2016.1222450
115. Antiga E, Quaglino P, Pierini I, Volpi W, Lami G, Bianchi B, et al. Regulatory T cells as well as IL-10 are reduced in the skin of patients with dermatitis herpetiformis. *J Dermatol Sci.* (2015) 77:54–62. doi: 10.1016/j.jdermsci.2014.11.003
116. Nigam R, Levitt J. Where does rituximab fit in the treatment of autoimmune mucocutaneous blistering skin disease? *J Drugs Dermatol.* (2012) 11:622–5.
117. Chakievska L, Holtsche MM, Kunstner A, Goletz S, Petersen BS, Thaci D, et al. IL-17A is functionally relevant and a potential therapeutic target in bullous pemphigoid. *J Autoimmun.* (2019) 96:104–12. doi: 10.1016/j.jaut.2018.09.003
118. Kasperkiewicz M, Sadik CD, Bieber K, Ibrahim SM, Manz RA, Schmidt E, et al. Epidermolysis bullosa acquisita: from pathophysiology to novel therapeutic options. *J Invest Dermatol.* (2016) 136:24–33. doi: 10.1038/JID.2015.356
119. Koga H, Kasprick A, Lopez R, Auli M, Pont M, Godessart N, et al. Therapeutic effect of a novel phosphatidylinositol-3-kinase delta inhibitor in experimental epidermolysis bullosa acquisita. *Front Immunol.* (2018) 9:1558. doi: 10.3389/fimmu.2018.01558
120. Lee J, Werth VP, Hall RP III, Eming R, Fairley JA, Fajgenbaum DC, et al. Perspective from the 5th international pemphigus and pemphigoid foundation scientific conference. *Front Med (Lausanne).* (2018) 5:306. doi: 10.3389/fmed.2018.00306
121. Ludwig RJ. Signalling and targeted therapy of inflammatory cells in epidermolysis bullosa acquisita. *Exp Dermatol.* (2017) 26:1179–86. doi: 10.1111/exd.13335
122. Tukaj S, Bieber K, Witte M, Ghorbanalipoor S, Schmidt E, Zillikens D, et al. Calcitriol treatment ameliorates inflammation and blistering in mouse models of epidermolysis bullosa acquisita. *J Invest Dermatol.* (2018) 138:301–9. doi: 10.1016/j.jid.2017.09.009
123. Witte M, Koga H, Hashimoto T, Ludwig RJ, Bieber K. Discovering potential drug-targets for personalized treatment of autoimmune disorders - what we learn from epidermolysis bullosa acquisita. *Expert Opin Ther Targets.* (2016) 20:985–98. doi: 10.1517/14728222.2016.1148686
124. Harman KE, Brown D, Exton LS, Groves RW, Hampton PJ, Mohd Mustapa MF, et al. British Association of Dermatologists' guidelines for the management of pemphigus vulgaris 2017. *Br J Dermatol.* (2017) 177:1170–201. doi: 10.1111/bjd.15930
125. Venning VA, Taghipour K, Mohd Mustapa MF, Highet AS, Kirtschig G. British Association of Dermatologists' guidelines for the management of bullous pemphigoid 2012. *Br J Dermatol.* (2012) 167:1200–14. doi: 10.1111/bjd.12072
126. Joly P, Maho-Vaillant M, Prost-Squarcioni C, Hebert V, Houivet E, Calbo S, et al. First-line rituximab combined with short-term prednisone versus prednisone alone for the treatment of pemphigus (Ritux 3): a prospective, multicentre, parallel-group, open-label randomised trial. *Lancet.* (2017) 389:2031–40. doi: 10.1016/S0140-6736(17)30070-3
127. Proby CM, Ota T, Suzuki H, Koyasu S, Gamou S, Shimizu N, et al. Development of chimeric molecules for recognition and targeting of antigen-specific B cells in pemphigus vulgaris. *Br J Dermatol.* (2000) 142:321–30. doi: 10.1046/j.1365-2133.2000.03328.x
128. Kridin K. Emerging treatment options for the management of pemphigus vulgaris. *Therap Clin Risk Manage.* (2018) 14:757–78. doi: 10.2147/TCRM.S142471
129. Amagai M, Ikeda S, Hashimoto T, Mizuashi M, Fujisawa A, Ihn H, et al. A randomized double-blind trial of intravenous immunoglobulin for bullous pemphigoid. *J Dermatol Sci.* (2017) 85:77–84. doi: 10.1016/j.jdermsci.2016.11.003
130. Hirose M, Kasprick A, Beltsiou F, Dieckhoff Schulze K, Schulze FS, Samavedam UK, et al. Reduced skin blistering in experimental epidermolysis bullosa acquisita after anti-TNF treatment. *Mol Med.* (2017) 22:918–26. doi: 10.2119/molmed.2015.00206
131. Diny NL, Rose NR, Cihakova D. Eosinophils in autoimmune diseases. *Front Immunol.* (2017) 8:484. doi: 10.3389/fimmu.2017.00484
132. Jaunzems AE, Woods AE, Staples A. Electron microscopy and morphometry enhances differentiation of epidermolysis bullosa subtypes. With normal values for 24 parameters in skin. *Arch Dermatol Res.* (1997) 289:631–9. doi: 10.1007/s004030050252
133. Gunther C, Wozel G, Meurer M, Pfeiffer C. Up-regulation of CCL11 and CCL26 is associated with activated eosinophils in bullous pemphigoid. *Clin Exp Immunol.* (2011) 166:145–53. doi: 10.1111/j.1365-2249.2011.04464.x
134. Koivukangas V, Oikarinen A. Suction blister model of wound healing. *Methods Mol Med.* (2003) 78:255–61. doi: 10.1385/1-59259-332-1:255
135. Tukaj S, Bieber K, Kleszczynski K, Witte M, Cames R, Kalies K, et al. Topically applied Hsp90 blocker 17AAG inhibits autoantibody-mediated blister-inducing cutaneous inflammation. *J Invest Dermatol.* (2017) 137:341–9. doi: 10.1016/j.jid.2016.08.032
136. Kasperkiewicz M, Muller R, Manz R, Magens M, Hammers CM, Somlai C, et al. Heat-shock protein 90 inhibition in autoimmunity to type VII collagen: evidence that nonmalignant plasma cells are not therapeutic targets. *Blood.* (2011) 117:6135–42. doi: 10.1182/blood-2010-10-314609
137. Samavedam UK, Mitschker N, Kasprick A, Bieber K, Schmidt E, Laskay T, et al. Whole-genome expression profiling in skin reveals SYK As a key regulator of inflammation in experimental epidermolysis bullosa acquisita. *Front Immunol.* (2018) 9:249. doi: 10.3389/fimmu.2018.00249
138. Costa Arantes DA, Guimarães JM, Batista AC. Therapeutic success of vitamin D replacement in oral pemphigus vulgaris: a case report. *Oral Surg Oral Med Oral Pathol Oral Radiol.* (2018) 126:e52. doi: 10.1016/j.oooo.2018.02.085
139. Kopecki Z, Ruzehaji N, Turner C, Iwata H, Ludwig RJ, Zillikens D, et al. Topically applied flightless i neutralizing antibodies improve healing of blistered skin in a murine model of epidermolysis bullosa acquisita. *J Invest Dermatol.* (2012) 133:1008–16. doi: 10.1038/jid.2012.457
140. Albers LN, Zone JJ, Stoff BK, Feldman RJ. Rituximab treatment for recalcitrant dermatitis herpetiformis. *JAMA Dermatol.* (2017) 153:315–8. doi: 10.1001/jamadermatol.2016.4676
141. Antiga E, Caproni M. The diagnosis and treatment of dermatitis herpetiformis. *Clin Cosmet Investig Dermatol.* (2015) 8:257–65. doi: 10.2147/CCID.S69127
142. Maley A, Warren M, Haberman I, Swerlick R, Kharod-Dholakia B, Feldman R. Rituximab combined with conventional therapy versus conventional

therapy alone for the treatment of mucous membrane pemphigoid (MMP). *J Am Acad Dermatol.* (2016) 74:835–40. doi: 10.1016/j.jaad.2016.01.020
143. Benamu E, Montoya JG. Infections associated with the use of eculizumab: recommendations for prevention and prophylaxis. *Curr Opin Infect Dis.* (2016) 29:319–29. doi: 10.1097/QCO.0000000000000279
144. Rathbone J, Kaltenthaler E, Richards A, Tappenden P, Bessey A, Cantrell A. A systematic review of eculizumab for atypical haemolytic uraemic syndrome (aHUS). *BMJ Open.* (2013) 3:e003573. doi: 10.1136/bmjopen-2013-003573
145. Berookhim B, Fischer HD, Weinberg JM. Treatment of recalcitrant pemphigus vulgaris with the tumor necrosis factor alpha antagonist etanercept. *Cutis.* (2004) 74:245-7.
146. Sadeghi H, Lockmann A, Hund AC, Samavedam UK, Pipi E, Vafia K, et al. Caspase-1-independent IL-1 release mediates blister formation in autoantibody-induced tissue injury through modulation of endothelial adhesion molecules. *J Immunol.* (2015) 194:3656–63. doi: 10.4049/jimmunol.1402688
147. Toto P, Feliciani C, Amerio P, Suzuki H, Wang B, Shivji GM, et al. Immune modulation in pemphigus vulgaris: role of CD28 and IL-10. *J Immunol.* (2000) 164:522–9. doi: 10.4049/jimmunol.164.1.522
148. Konig A, Bruckner-Tuderman L. Transforming growth factor-beta promotes deposition of collagen VII in a modified organotypic skin model. *Lab Invest.* (1994) 70:203–9.
149. Ryynanen J, Sollberg S, Olsen DR, Uitto J. Transforming growth factor-beta up-regulates type VII collagen gene expression in normal and transformed epidermal keratinocytes in culture. *Biochem Biophys Res Commun.* (1991) 180:673–80. doi: 10.1016/S0006-291X(05)81118-0
150. Sawamura D, McMillan JR, Akiyama M, Shimizu H. Epidermolysis bullosa: directions for future research and new challenges for treatment. *Arch Dermatol Res.* (2003) 295(Suppl. 1):S34–42. doi: 10.1007/s00403-002-0370-7
151. Rider P, Carmi Y, Cohen I. Biologics for targeting inflammatory cytokines, clinical uses, and limitations. *Int J Cell Biol.* (2016) 2016:9259646. doi: 10.1155/2016/9259646
152. Kitashima DY, Kobayashi T, Woodring T, Idouchi K, Doebel T, Voisin B, et al. Langerhans cells prevent autoimmunity via expansion of keratinocyte antigen-specific regulatory T cells. *EBioMedicine.* (2018) 27:293–303. doi: 10.1016/j.ebiom.2017.12.022
153. Iwata H, Bieber K, Tiburzy B, Chrobok N, Kalies K, Shimizu A, et al. B cells, dendritic cells, and macrophages are required to induce an autoreactive CD4 helper T cell response in experimental epidermolysis bullosa acquisita. *J Immunol.* (2013) 191:2978–88. doi: 10.4049/jimmunol.1300310
154. Samavedam UK, Iwata H, Muller S, Schulze FS, Recke A, Schmidt E, et al. GM-CSF modulates autoantibody production and skin blistering in experimental epidermolysis bullosa acquisita. *J Immunol.* (2014) 192:559–71. doi: 10.4049/jimmunol.1301556
155. Zebrowska A, Wozniacka A, Juczynska K, Ociepa K, Waszczykowska E, Szymczak I, et al. Correlation between IL36alpha and IL17 and Activity of the disease in selected autoimmune blistering diseases. *Mediators Inflamm.* (2017) 2017:8980534. doi: 10.1155/2017/8980534
156. Giurdanella F, Fania L, Gnarra M, Toto P, Di Rollo D, Sauder DN, et al. A possible role for CD8+ T lymphocytes in the cell-mediated pathogenesis of pemphigus vulgaris. *Mediators Inflamm.* (2013) 2013:764290. doi: 10.1155/2013/764290
157. Roujeau JC, Lok C, Bastuji-Garin S, Mhalla S, Enginger V, Bernard P. High risk of death in elderly patients with extensive bullous pemphigoid. *Arch Dermatol.* (1998) 134:465–9. doi: 10.1001/archderm.134.4.465
158. Zhao CY, Murrell DF. Autoimmune blistering diseases in females: a review. *Int J Womens Dermatol.* (2015) 1:4–12. doi: 10.1016/j.ijwd.2015.01.002
159. Saccucci M, Di Carlo G, Bossu M, Giovarruscio F, Salucci A, Polimeni A. Autoimmune diseases and their manifestations on oral cavity: diagnosis and clinical management. *J Immunol Res.* (2018) 2018:6061825. doi: 10.1155/2018/6061825

20

Targeting the Janus Kinase Family in Autoimmune Skin Diseases

Michael D. Howell†, Fiona I. Kuo† and Paul A. Smith†*

Incyte Corporation, Wilmington, DE, United States

***Correspondence:**
Paul A. Smith
psmith@incyte.com

†These authors have contributed equally to this work

Autoimmune skin diseases are characterized by significant local and systemic inflammation that is largely mediated by the Janus kinase (JAK)–signal transducer and activator of transcription (STAT) pathway. Advanced understanding of this pathway has led to the development of targeted inhibitors of Janus kinases (JAKinibs). As a class, JAK inhibitors effectively treat a multitude of hematologic and inflammatory diseases. Growing evidence suggests that JAK inhibitors are efficacious in atopic dermatitis, alopecia areata, psoriasis, and vitiligo. Additional evidence suggests that JAK inhibition might be broadly useful in dermatology, with early reports of efficacy in several other conditions. JAK inhibitors can be administered orally or used topically and represent a promising new class of medications. Here we review the evolving data on the role of the JAK-STAT pathway in inflammatory dermatoses and the potential therapeutic benefit of JAK-STAT antagonism.

Keywords: Janus kinase, cytokines, skin barrier, dermatology, autoimmunity

JAK-STAT SIGNALING PATHWAY

The mammalian Janus kinase (JAK) family contains three JAKs (JAK1–3) and tyrosine kinase 2 (TYK2), which selectively bind different receptor chains (1). Upon binding of ligand to its cognate cytokine receptor, associated JAKs become activated and undergo autophosphorylation and transphosphorylate the intracellular tail of their receptors. This creates docking sites for the SH2 domain of the cytoplasmic transcription factors termed signal transducers and activators of transcription (STATs). The human STAT family contains seven STATs: STAT1, STAT2, STAT3, STAT4, STAT5A, STAT5B, and STAT6. Following phosphorylation, STATs are translocated to the nucleus, dimerize, and bind to specific DNA sequences to regulate gene transcription (2). The JAK-STAT pathway is pivotal for the downstream signaling of inflammatory cytokines, including interleukins (ILs), interferons (IFNs), and multiple growth factors (3, 4). Overall, the selective use of JAKs by different receptors coupled to downstream STAT signal transduction results in an elegant mechanism to achieve exquisite *in vivo* specificity for more than 60 cytokines and growth factors (**Figure 1**).

Identification of selective pharmacologic JAK inhibitors (JAKinibs) has been an ongoing research and development goal. The first JAKinib to gain FDA approval in 2011 was ruxolitinib for intermediate or high-risk myelofibrosis, thereby showing that JAK inhibition was not only possible, but safe and effective for its intended uses. More recently, selective JAK inhibitors have been explored for specific inflammatory disease indications (**Table 1**).

THE JAK-STAT PATHWAY AND T HELPER SUBSETS

The differential fate of naive T cells into committed T helper (Th) subsets is orchestrated under the instruction of professional antigen-presenting cells within a JAK-STAT–dependent cytokine milieu (**Figure 2**). *In vivo* Th1 differentiation depends on JAK-mediated signaling through the IFNγ receptor (IFNGR), the IL-12 receptor (IL-12R), and downstream STAT1/4 phosphorylation culminating with T-bet gene transcription (5). Ultimately, IFNγ signaling initiates the Th1 differentiation program and IL-12 perpetuates it. In contrast, Th2 cells arise after occupancy of the IL-4Rα by its ligands IL-4 and IL-13, triggering JAK1/3 and subsequent activation of STAT6 (6), and leading to transcriptional regulation of the GATA3 target gene (5). More recently, the critical role of IL-17–producing Th cells (termed Th17 cells) in host defense against extracellular bacteria, maintenance of epithelium barrier integrity, and autoimmune pathogenesis has become increasingly clear. Within the immunologic microenvironment, IL-6 produced by activated dendritic cells (DCs) is a key factor in promoting Th17 differentiation via STAT3 and retinoic acid receptor–related orphan receptor γ (RORγt) induction (7) with IL-23 critical for memory Th17 *in vivo* function (3, 8).

ATOPIC DERMATITIS

Atopic dermatitis (AD) is a chronic, inflammatory skin disease that typically begins in early childhood and occurs more frequently in families with a history of other atopic diseases (bronchial asthma and/or allergic rhinoconjunctivitis). Overall, the prevalence of AD is up to 20% in children and 10% in adults, with rates varying geographically (9, 10). AD clinically manifests as recurrent eczematous lesions that negatively affect quality of life through sleep disturbances due to chronic itch (pruritus) (11, 12), increased likelihood of developing depression (13), and significant economic burden (14).

The cellular infiltrate of AD lesions mainly consist of $CD4^+$ T cells, which are considered key drivers of inflammation (15). Lesional skin is characterized by an overexpression of inflammatory Th2-cytokines (IL-4, IL-13, IL-31), and Th22-cytokines (IL-22) (16). Crucially, the cytokines IL-4, IL-13, IL-31, and IL-22 require JAK-STAT downstream signaling (3) for their biological function (**Figure 3**). Spontaneous and induced rodent dermatitis models have been extensively used to explore the effectiveness of small-molecule JAK inhibitors on reducing inflammation. Delgocitinib (pan-JAK) inhibited skin inflammation in hapten-induced chronic dermatitis in mice, as evidenced by reduced levels of inflammatory cytokines in the skin and IgE in serum (17). In addition, momelotinib (JAK1/JAK2) downregulated IL-4 expression, reduced the skin severity scores and reduced total serum IgE levels in the 2,4-dinitrochlorobenzene (DNCB)-induced AD mice (18). Similarly, tofacitinib (JAK1/3) and oclacitinib (JAK1) inhibited the production of proinflammatory Th2 cytokines, including IL-4, in the toluene-2,4-diisocyanate (TDI) dermatitis model (19). Moreover, tofacitinib demonstrated anti-inflammatory activity in the oxazolone-induced chronic allergic contact dermatitis model (20).

Interleukin-22 is elevated in AD lesions and is associated with epidermal thickening, skin barrier disruption, and increased expression of thymic stromal lymphopoietin (TSLP) and IL-33 cytokines (21). In addition, IL-22 potently induces the expression of gastrin-releasing peptide, a neuropeptide pruritogen, in dermal cells, dermal afferent fibers, and skin innervating ganglion neurons that positively correlate with the scratching behavior (22). The relevance of IL-22 in AD pathogenesis was emphasized by the observation of sustained clinical improvements in patients with moderate to severe AD receiving anti–IL-22 therapy (23). IL-22 binds its cognate receptor comprising a heterodimeric complex of IL-22RA1 and IL-10R2 subunits, leading to activation of JAK1 and TYK2 and phosphorylation of STAT3 (24).

Thymic stromal lymphopoietin and IL-31 cytokines also significantly contribute to triggering of inflammatory itch, under the control of IL-4, IL-13, and IL-33 (25). Crucially, pruritogenic cytokines IL-31 and TSLP use JAK1 and JAK2 downstream signaling (26, 27). Additionally, preclinical evidence has confirmed that pharmacologic inhibition of the JAK-STAT pathway is sufficient for the amelioration of pruritus-associated dermatitis. Examples include oclacitinib, which is licensed for pruritus associated with allergic dermatitis in dogs (28). Similarly, topical application of ruxolitinib (JAK1/JAK2) ameliorated TSLP-induced inflammation in mice (29). In the TDI-induced mouse model of dermatitis, oclacitinib and tofacitinib inhibited itch symptoms and significantly reduced IL-31, tumor necrosis factor–α (TNFα), and TSLP cytokine secretions (19). Moreover, TSLP can activate tissue resident dendritic cells that promote the transformation of Th-naïve lymphocytes to the Th2 phenotype thereby facilitating tissue inflammation (30). Finally, neuronal IL-4Rα acting via JAK1 signaling can also significantly contribute to chronic itch (31).

Skin barrier disruption and the resulting continuous exposure to allergens are presumed to be responsible for the development of atopic dermatitis (AD). JAK1-mediated Th2 cytokines IL-4 and IL-13 acting in a STAT-dependent manner (32) negatively affect skin barrier integrity by inhibiting the expression of filaggrin, loricrin, and involucrin, resulting in destabilization of tight junctions (33, 34). JAK inhibition restored filaggrin and loricrin expression following *in vitro* pretreatment with IL-4 /IL-13 cytokines of human keratinocyte. Moreover, mice harboring a point mutation leading to JAK1-specific hyperactivation develop spontaneous skin barrier disruption and a dermatitis phenotype

Abbreviations: AA, Alopecia areata; ACT, Nuclear factor NF-kappa-B activator 1; AD, Atopic dermatitis; BID, Twice daily; CD, Cluster of differentiation; CXCL, Chemokine (C-X-C motif) ligand; CXCR, Chemokine (C-X-C motif) receptor; DC, Dendritic cell; DNCB, 2,4-dinitrochlorobenzene; EASI, Eczema Area Severity Index; EPO, Erythropoietin; FDA, US Food and Drug Administration; FLG, Filaggrin; GATA-3, GATA transcription factor 3; GH, Growth hormone; GM-CSF, Granulocyte-macrophage colony-stimulating factor; IFN, Interferon; Ig, Immunoglobulin; IL, Interleukin; ILC2, Type 2 innate lymphoid cells; IGA, Investigator global assessment; INV, Involucrin; JAK, Janus kinase; JAKinibs, Janus kinase inhibitors; LOR, Loricrin; MHC, Major histocompatibility complex; NK, Natural killer cell; NKD2D, Natural Killer Group 2D; NKD2DL3, Natural Killer Group 2D ligand 3; PASI, Psoriasis Area and Severity Index; pDC, Plasmacytoid dendritic cell; PGA, Physician Global Assessment; QD, Once daily; OSM, Oncostatin M; OSMRβ, Oncostatin M receptor β; PI3K, Phosphoinositide 3-kinases; RAET1L, Retinoic acid early transcript 1L; RORγt, Retinoic acid receptor-related orphan receptor γ; SALT, Severity of Alopecia Tool; STAT, Signal transducer and activator of transcription; T-bet, T-box transcription factor TBX21; TGF, Transforming growth factor; Th, T helper; TNFα, Tumor necrosis factor alpha; TPO, Thrombopoietin; TSLP, Thymic stromal lymphopoietin; TYK2, Tyrosine kinase 2; VASI, Vitiligo Area Scoring Index.

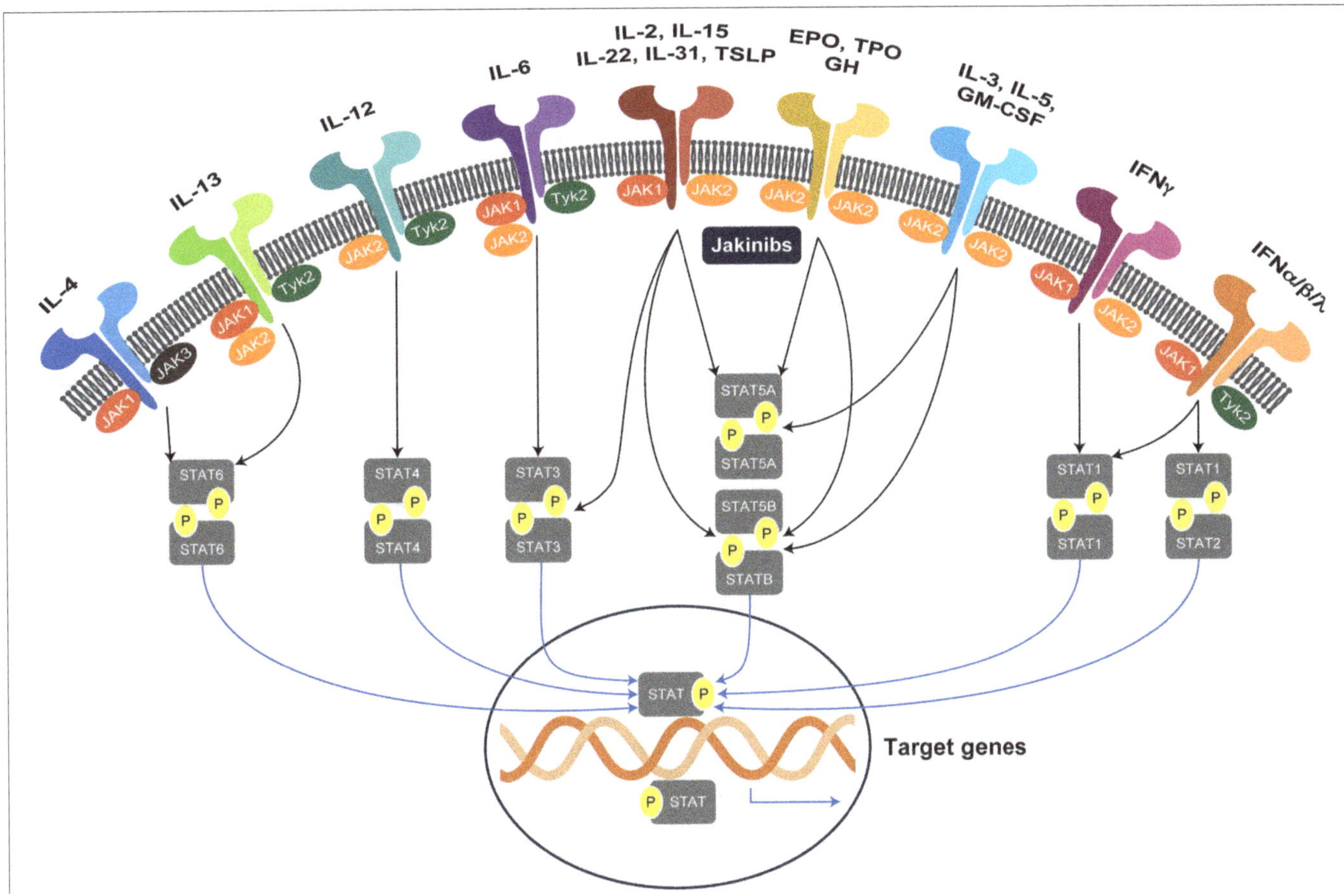

FIGURE 1 | JAK-STAT signaling pathways. Janus kinases (JAK1-3, TYK2) are activated by more than 60 extracellular stimuli and phosphorylate downstream STAT proteins, which translocate to the nucleus and activate target genes. EPO, erythropoietin; GH, growth hormone; GM-CSF, granulocyte-macrophage colony-stimulating factor; IFN, interferon; IL, interleukin; JAK, Janus kinases; JAKinibs, Janus kinase inhibitors; STAT, signal transducer and activator of transcription; TPO, thrombopoietin; TSLP, thymic stromal lymphopoietin; TYK2, tyrosine kinase.

(35). Topical application of delgocitinib ameliorated spontaneous AD-like skin inflammation and barrier disruption in an NC/Nga "dry skin" mouse model and restored filaggrin levels in an experimental human skin graft model leading to improved barrier function (36). Moreover, downstream signaling of IL-4 and IL-13 also suppresses the induction of innate immune response genes, such as β-defensins (33), thereby facilitating skin microbiome dysbiosis, including aberrant *Staphylococcus aureus* colonization (37).

The role and activation of Th1 and Th17 cell-mediated responses require further elucidation, but these pathways appear to be overexpressed in chronic disease stages, children, and people of Asian ethnicity (38, 39).

Targeting the JAK family of kinases in AD has proven, in recent years, to be therapeutically beneficial. Oral tofacitinib administration was evaluated in 6 patients with moderate to severe AD and showed a promising reduction in skin severity (40). The next generation of orally administered JAKinibs includes baricitinib (JAK1/2) along with two JAK1 selective molecules, upadacitinib (JAK1) and abrocitinib (JAK1). In clinical trials in moderate to severe AD patients, oral administration of these JAKinibs significantly reduced the eczema area severity index (EASI) scores by more than 50%. More specifically, in one clinical trial (ClinicalTrials.gov identifier, NCT02925117), oral administration of upadacitinib (JAK1) resulted in 90% improvement in the eczema area severity index (EASI) score for ~50% of enrolled participants after 16 weeks of treatment (41). Results from two baricitinib phase 3 studies showed that more patients achieved an investigator global assessment (IGA) 0/1 with barcitinib 4 mg once daily (QD) and 2 mg QD than with placebo (42). Significant improvements in EASI and patient-reported outcomes were observed as early as Week 1 (**Table 2**) (53). In a recent phase 1b study (NCT03139981), ASN002, a pan JAK inhibitor that also inhibits spleen tyrosine kinase (SYK), showed a 50% improvement in EASI in 100% of participants within 4 weeks (56).

Topical administration of tofacitinib to patients with mild to moderate AD in a clinical trial (NCT02001181) demonstrated significant improvement in EASI scores at Week 4 (43) and improvement in pruritus as early as Day 2. In a phase 2 study (NCT03011892) involving patients with mild to moderate AD receiving ruxolitinib cream, mean percentage change

TABLE 1 | Selectivity profiles of clinically active JAKinibs.

Inhibitor	JAK1	JAK2	JAK3	TYK2
Tofacitinib*	X	X	X	
Ruxolitinib,† Baricitinib,‡ Momelotinib, CTP-543	X	X		
Oclacitinib,§ Itacitinib, Upadacitinib, Filgotinib, PF04965842, LP0184	X			
ATI-502	X		X	
PF-06700841	X			X
PF-06651600			X	
PF-06826647 BMS-986165				X
Delgocitinib (JTE-052)	X	X	X	X

JAK, Janus kinase; JAKinibs, inhibitors of Janus kinase; FDA, US Food and Drug Administration; TYK, tyrosine kinase.

**FDA approved: rheumatoid arthritis, psoriatic arthritis and ulcerative colitis.*

†FDA approved: adults with polycythemia who have had an inadequate response to or are intolerant of hydroxyurea, adults with intermediate or high-risk myelofibrosis, acute graft-vs.-host disease in adult and pediatric patients 12 years and younger.

‡FDA approved: rheumatoid arthritis.

§FDA approved: atopic dermatitis and pruritus from allergic dermatitis in dogs.

from baseline at Week 4 in EASI score demonstrated a significant improvement and was non-inferior to triamcinolone. Interestingly, significant reductions in itch were noted as early as 1 day after initiation of therapy (64, 65). More recently, pilot studies of topical ATI-502 (JAK1/3) solution (NCT03585296) and PF-06700841 (JAK1/TYK2) cream (NCT03903822) in AD are ongoing. Given the early successes of JAKinibs in AD, ongoing investigation and evaluation is expected to further elucidate the differential effects of JAK selectivity.

ALOPECIA AREATA

Alopecia areata (AA) is an autoimmune disease resulting in partial or complete nonscarring hair loss, with a prevalence of ~1.7 to 2.1% (68). Susceptibility to AA is indiscriminate between the sexes and ethnicities, with initial disease onset often occurring before the third decade of life. Early symptoms are typically characterized by small, well-defined patches of hair loss that may spontaneously resolve with time; however subsequent relapses occur in around a third of cases. Spontaneous remission is rare in patients with alopecia totalis or alopecia universalis. To date, no FDA- or European Medicines Agency–approved treatments exist.

Multiple lines of evidence have demonstrated that AA pathogenesis is autoimmune in nature, with loss of immune privilege and associated T cells infiltration selectively attacking growth at the hair follicle (i.e., anagen phase) (69–72). Healthy hair follicles achieve immune privilege at the anagen phase by downregulation of expression of major histocompatibility complex (MHC) class I and class II molecules (70, 73) and by expression of NK and $CD8^+$ cell inhibitors, such as macrophage migration inhibitory factor (MIF) and transforming growth factors (TGF) β1 and β2, which generate an immunosuppressive microenvironment (74–76). Importantly, hair follicle epithelial stem cells are usually spared during the autoimmune attack, which provides a potential mechanism of hair growth recovery with effective anti-inflammatory treatment (70).

Many different mammalian species, including rodents, are susceptible to AA and this has facilitated preclinical models for the elucidation of cellular and molecular immune pathways (77, 78). The inbred C3H/HeJ strain spontaneously develops alopecia in up to 20% of mice via an IFNγ- and inflammasome-sensitive mechanism (79); however recipient C3H/HeJ animals that receive skin grafts from donor alopecic C3H/HeJ mice develop an accelerated phenotype with nearly 100% disease penetrance (80). Transfer or deletion of effector $CD8^+$ T cells is sufficient to induce or block disease in preclinical models (70, 71, 81), which in consistent with the observation that cytotoxic $CD8^+NKG2D^+$ T cells expressing granzyme B (82) infiltrate around the hair follicles and are major contributors of hair loss (81, 83).

Global transcriptional analyses of mouse and human affected skin identified expression signatures indicative of cytotoxic T-cell infiltration, such as increased production of IFNγ and γ-chain (γc) cytokines, including IL-15 (81, 84). Furthermore, inhibiting IFNγ either by genetic deletion or neutralizing antibody significantly ameliorates AA development and severity (85), supporting the hypothesis that IFNγ drives AA pathogenesis by inducing ectopic expression of MHC molecules and ligands that stimulate NK-cell receptors (NKG2D) in the anagen hair bulb leading to the collapse of the hair follicle immune privilege (70, 86–88). An important cellular source of IFN is plasmacytoid dendritic cells (pDCs), which are normally absent from healthy skin, but migrate into tissues in response to inflammatory stimuli or infection. Infiltrating pDCs have been identified around hair follicles of patients with AA (89) and, upon activation, produce large quantities of type I IFNs (90).

The IFNγ-induced chemokine receptor CXCR3 and its ligands CXCL9 and CXCL10 are upregulated around hair follicles during early AA pathogenesis (**Figure 4**), thereby facilitating lymphocyte recruitment (82, 91). CXCR3 is primarily expressed on Th1 $CD4^+$ T cells, $CD8^+$ T cells, NK, and PDCs during skin inflammation (92), whereas CXCR3 ligands are secreted by many tissue resident cells, including dendritic cells.

Like IFNγ, IL-15 enhances innate and self-reactive memory T-cell immunity, including autoimmune disease pathogenesis (84, 93), and signals via the JAK1/3 pathway with downstream STAT-5 activation (94). Similarly blocking IL-2 or IL-15 receptor beta (IL-15Rβ) ameliorated disease development by inhibiting $CD8^+NKG2D^+$ T-cell accumulation in the skin (81).

The combination of published genome-wide association studies in patients with AA that highlighted JAK signaling (87, 95) and the knowledge that IFNγ primarily signals through JAK1/2 and IL-15 mostly through JAK1/3, provided a compelling rationale for the exploration of small-molecule JAK inhibitors in AA disease (81, 96). Preclinical evaluation of orally administered ruxolitinib and tofacitinib in the skin graft C3H/HeJ mouse model demonstrated disease prevention (81). Marked decreases of CD4, CD8, and MHC class I and II as well as a reduced numbers of $CD8^+/NKG2D^+$ cells were observed in the skin (81). Subsequently, prophylactic and therapeutic baricitinib treatment ameliorated disease and normalized the Alopecia

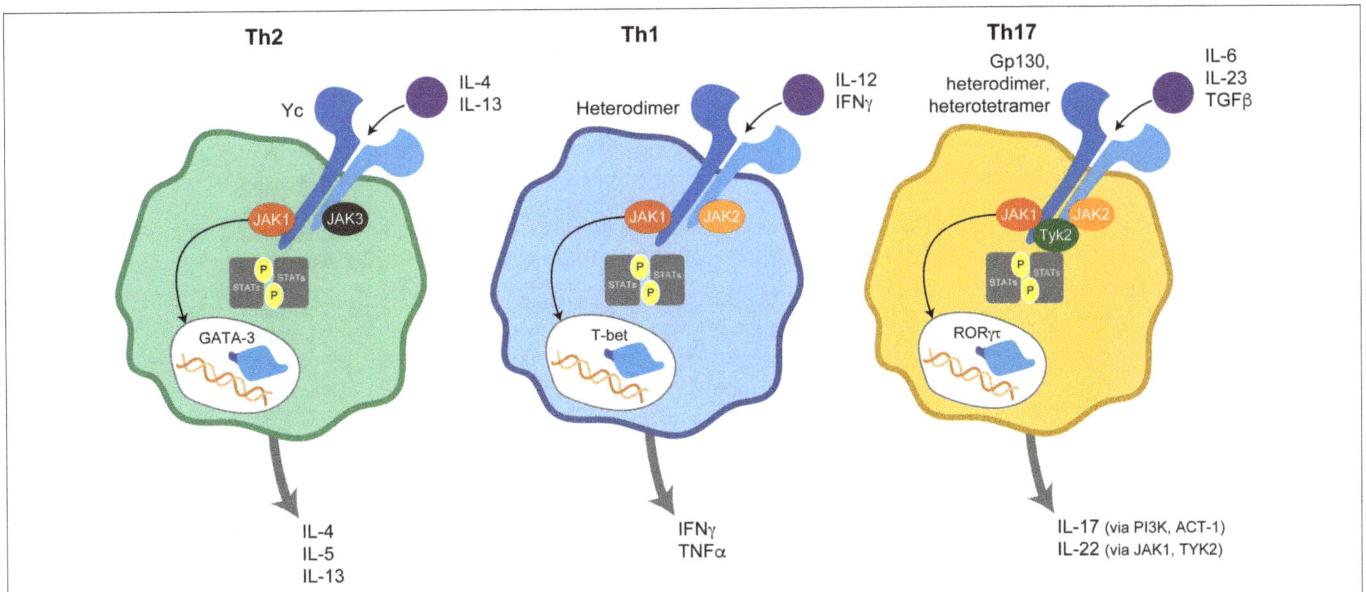

FIGURE 2 | JAK-mediated cytokine signaling in T helper subsets. Ligand binding to its cognate receptor triggers JAK-STAT activation and plays a central role in naive T-cell differentiation into Th1, Th2, and Th17 subsets. ACT, Nuclear factor NF-kappa-B activator 1; GATA, GATA transcription factor 3; IFN, interferon; IL, interleukin; JAK, Janus kinase; PI3K, Phosphoinositide 3-kinases; RORγt, retinoic acid receptor-related orphan receptor γ; STAT, signal transducer and activator of transcription; T-bet, T-box transcription factor TBX21; Th, T helper; TGF, transforming growth factor; TNF, tumor necrosis factor; TYK, tyrosine kinase.

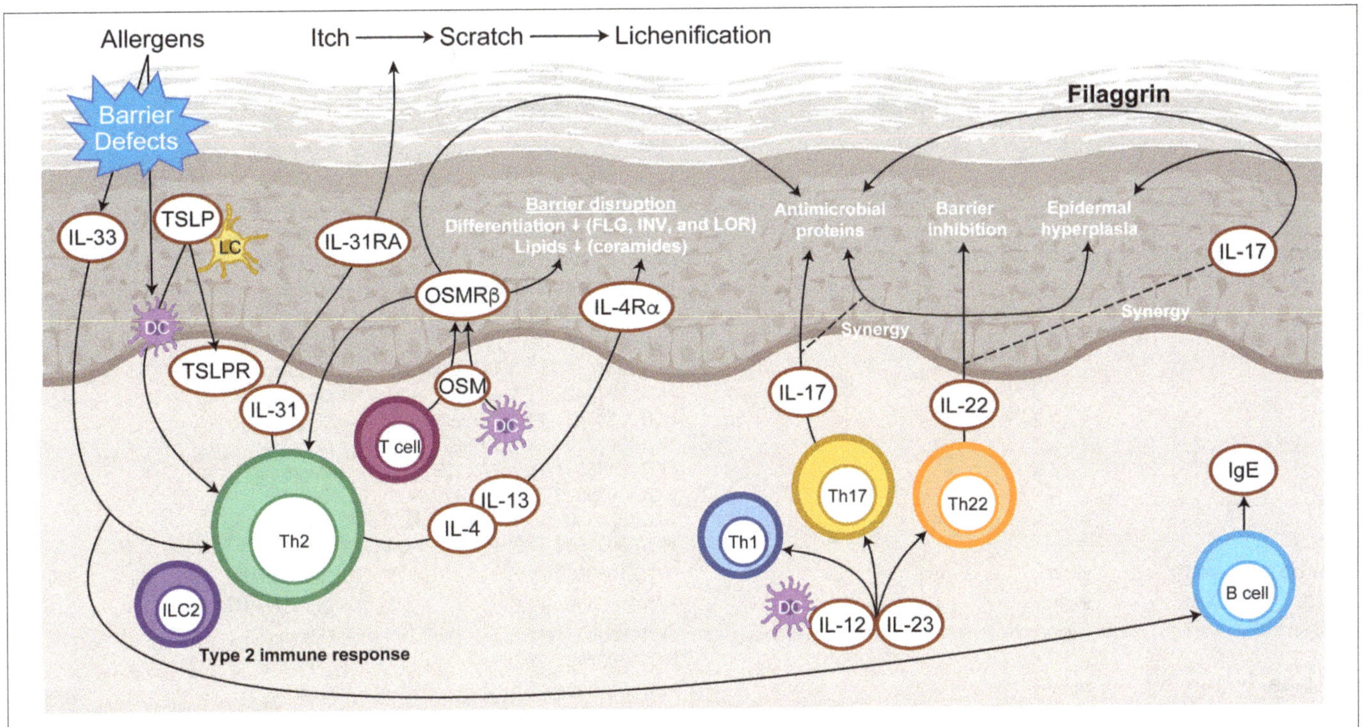

FIGURE 3 | Immunopathogenesis of atopic dermatitis. Allergen entry through the disrupted epidermal barrier stimulates keratinocytes to express cytokines, such as IL-33 and TSLP, which trigger ILC2 and Th2 cell mediated inflammation. Skin-resident dendritic cells take up exogenous and self-antigens released from damaged cells and promote type 2 immunity. CD8+ T cells infiltrate atopic dermatitis skin and activate Th2 cells to further release IL-4 and IL-13, which promotes IgE class switching. Cytokines released from skin infiltrating Th17 and Th22 lymphocytes synergize, leading to further barrier impairment and epidermal hyperplasia. DC, dendritic cell; FLG, Filaggrin; Ig, immunoglobulin; IL, interleukin; ILC2, type 2 innate lymphoid cells; INV, Involucrin; LC, Langerhans cell; LOR, Loricrin; OSM, Oncostatin M; OSMRβ, Oncostatin M receptor β; Th, T helper; TSLP, thymic stromal lymphopoietin.

TABLE 2 | Summary of JAK inhibitor use in the treatment of dermatologic conditions.

Study drug	Target	Company	Dermatology indications	ClinicalTrials.gov identifier	Studystatus	References
ORAL JAK INHIBITORS						
Tofacitinib	JAK 1/2/3	Pfizer	AD	NCT02001181 (Ph2)	Completed	(43)
			Psoriasis	NCT01710046 (Ph2)	Completed	(44)
				NCT01815424 (Ph3)	Completed	(45)
				NCT01309737 (Ph3)	Completed	(46)
				NCT01276639 (Ph3)	Completed	
				NCT01519089 (Ph3)	Completed	(47)
				NCT01241591(Ph3)	Completed	(48)
				NCT01186744 (Ph3)	Completed	(49)
				NCT01163253 (Ph3)	Completed	
			AA, alopecia totalis, alopecia universalis,	NCT02197455 (Ph2)	Completed	(50)
			Dermatomyositis	NCT03002649 (Ph1)	Ongoing	
			Discoid lupus erythematosus,	NCT03159936 (Ph1)	Ongoing	
			cutaneous lupus	NCT03288324 (Ph1/2)	Ongoing	
Abrocitinib (PF04965842)	JAK1	Pfizer	Psoriasis	NCT02201524 (Ph2)	Terminated	(51)
			AD	NCT02780167 (Ph2)	Completed	
				NCT03915496 (Ph2) (JADE MOA)	Ongoing	
				NCT03627767 (Ph2)	Ongoing	
				NCT03349060 (Ph3) (JADE Mono-1)	Completed	
				NCT03575871 (Ph3) (JADE Mono-2)	Completed	
				NCT03422822 (Ph3) (JADE EXTEND)	Ongoing	
				NCT03720470 (Ph3) (JADE Compare)	Ongoing	
				NCT03796676 (Ph3) (JADE TEEN)	Ongoing	
PF-06651600	JAK3	Pfizer	AA	NCT02974868 (Ph2)	Completed	
				NCT03732807 (Ph2/3) (ALLEGRO-2b/3)	Ongoing	
			Vitiligo	NCT03715829 (Ph2)	Ongoing	
PF-06700841	JAK1/ TYK2	Pfizer	Psoriasis	NCT02969018 (Ph2)	Completed	
			AA	NCT02974868 (Ph2)	Completed	
			Vitiligo	NCT03715829 (Ph2)	Ongoing	
PF-06826647	TYK2	Pfizer	Psoriasis	NCT03210961 (Ph1)	Completed	
				NCT03895372 (Ph2)	Ongoing	
Baricitinib	JAK1/2	Eli Lilly/ Incyte	Psoriasis	NCT01490632 (Ph2)	Completed	(52)
			AA	NCT03570749 (Phase 2/3)(BRAVE-AA1)	Ongoing	
				NCT03899259 (Ph3) (BRAVE-AA2)	Ongoing	
			AD	NCT02576938 (Ph2)	Completed	(53)
				NCT03334396 (Ph3) (BREEZE-AD1)	Ongoing	(42)
				NCT03334422 (Ph3) (BREEZE-AD2)	Completed	(42)
				NCT03334435 (Ph3) (BREEZE-AD3)	Ongoing	
				NCT03428100 (Ph3) (BREEZE-AD4)	Ongoing	
				NCT03435081 (Ph3) (BREEZE-AD5)	Ongoing	
				NCT03559270 (Ph3) (BREEZE-AD6)	Ongoing	
				NCT03733301 (Ph3) (BREEZE-AD7)	Ongoing	
				NCT03952559 (Ph3) (BREEZE-AD-PEDS)	Ongoing	
Ruxolitinib	JAK1/2	Incyte	AA	NCT01950780 (Ph2)	Completed	(54)
Itacitinib	JAK1	Incyte	Psoriasis	NCT01634087 (Ph2)	Completed	(55)
INCB054707	JAK1	Incyte	Hidradenitis suppurativa	NCT03569371 (Ph2)	Completed	
				NCT03607487 (Ph2)	Ongoing	
Upadacitinib	JAK1	AbbVie	AD	NCT03646604 (Ph1)	Ongoing	(41)
				NCT02925117 (Ph2)	Completed	
				NCT03569293 (Ph3) (Measure Up 1)	Ongoing	
				NCT03568318 (Ph3) (AD Up)	Ongoing	
				NCT03738397 (Ph3) (Heads Up)	Ongoing	
				NCT03607422 (Ph3)	Ongoing	
				NCT03661138 (Ph3)	Ongoing	
ATI-501	JAK1/3	Aclaris	AA, alopecia totalis, alopecia universalis	NCT03594227 (Ph2)	Completed	

(Continued)

TABLE 2 | Continued

Study drug	Target	Company	Dermatology indications	ClinicalTrials.gov identifier	Studystatus	References
ORAL JAK INHIBITORS						
ASN002	JAK1/2/3 Tyk2 SYK	Asana BioSciences	AD	NCT03139981 (Ph1) NCT03654755 (Ph2) NCT03531957 (Ph2) (RADIANT)	Completed Ongoing Ongoing	(56)
			Chronic hand eczema	NCT03728504 (Ph2)	Ongoing	
Filgotinib	JAK1	Galapagos NV	Cutaneous lupus	NCT03134222 (Ph2)	Ongoing	
GSK2586184	JAK1	GSK	Psoriasis	NCT01782664 (Ph2)	Completed	
BMS-986165	TYK2	BMS	Psoriasis	NCT03004768 (Ph1) NCT02931838 (Ph2) NCT03924427 (Ph3) NCT03624127 (Ph3) (POETYK-PSO-1) NCT03611751 (Ph3) (POETYK-PSO-2)	Completed Completed Ongoing Ongoing Ongoing	(57)
Lestaurtinib	JAK2	Teva/Cephalon	Psoriasis	NCT00236119 (Ph2)	Completed	
Peficitinib	JAK3	Astellas	Psoriasis	NCT01096862 (Ph2)	Completed	(58)
CTP-543	JAK1/2	Concert Pharma-ceuticals	AA	NCT03137381 (Ph2) NCT03898479 (Ph2) NCT03941548 (Ph2) NCT03811912 (Ph2)	Completed Ongoing Ongoing Ongoing	
Study drug	**Target**	**Manufacture**	**Dermatology indications**	**ClinicalTrials.gov identifier**		
TOPICAL JAK INHIBITORS						
Tofacitinib	JAK1/2/3	Pfizer	Psoriasis	NCT01831466 (Ph2) NCT01246583 (Ph2)	Completed Completed	(59) (60)
			AD	NCT02001181 (Ph2)	Completed	(43)
			AA	NCT02812342 (Ph2)	Completed	(61)
PF-06700841	JAK1/ TYK2	Pfizer	Psoriasis	NCT03850483 (Ph2)	Ongoing	
			AD	NCT03903822 (Ph2)	Ongoing	
Ruxolitinib	JAK1/2	Incyte	Psoriasis	NCT00820950 (Ph2) NCT00778700 (Ph2) NCT00617994 (Ph2)	Completed Completed Completed	(62) (63)
			AD	NCT03257644 (Ph2) NCT03011892 (Ph2) NCT03745638 (Ph3) (TRuE-AD1) NCT03745651 (Ph3) (TRuE AD2)	Ongoing Completed Ongoing Ongoing	(64, 65)
			AA	NCT02553330 (Ph2)	Terminated	
			Vitiligo	NCT03099304 (Ph2) NCT02809976 (Ph2)	Ongoing Completed	(66, 67)
ATI-502 (ATI-50002)	JAK1/3	Aclaris	AD	NCT03585296 (Ph2)	Completed	
			AA, alopecia totalis, alopecia universalis	NCT03315689 (Ph2-AU and AT) NCT03551821 (Ph2-eyebrow) NCT03354637 (Ph2) NCT03759340 (Ph2)	Completed Completed Ongoing Ongoing	
			Androgenetic alopecia	NCT03495817 (Ph2)	Ongoing	
			Vitiligo	NCT03468855 (Ph2)	Ongoing	
Delgocitinib (JTE-052)	JAK1/2/3 Tyk Syk	Japan Tobacco Inc.; Leo	AD	NCT03826901 (Ph1) NCT03725722 (Ph2) (mild to severe AD)	Ongoing Ongoing	
			Chronic hand eczema	NCT03683719 (Ph2)	Ongoing	
			AA	NCT02561585 (Ph2) NCT03325296 (Ph2-eyebrow)	Completed Terminated	
			Discoid lupus	NCT03958955 (Ph2)	Ongoing	

AA, alopecia areata; AD, atopic dermatitis; JAK, Janus kinase; TYK, tyrosine kinase.

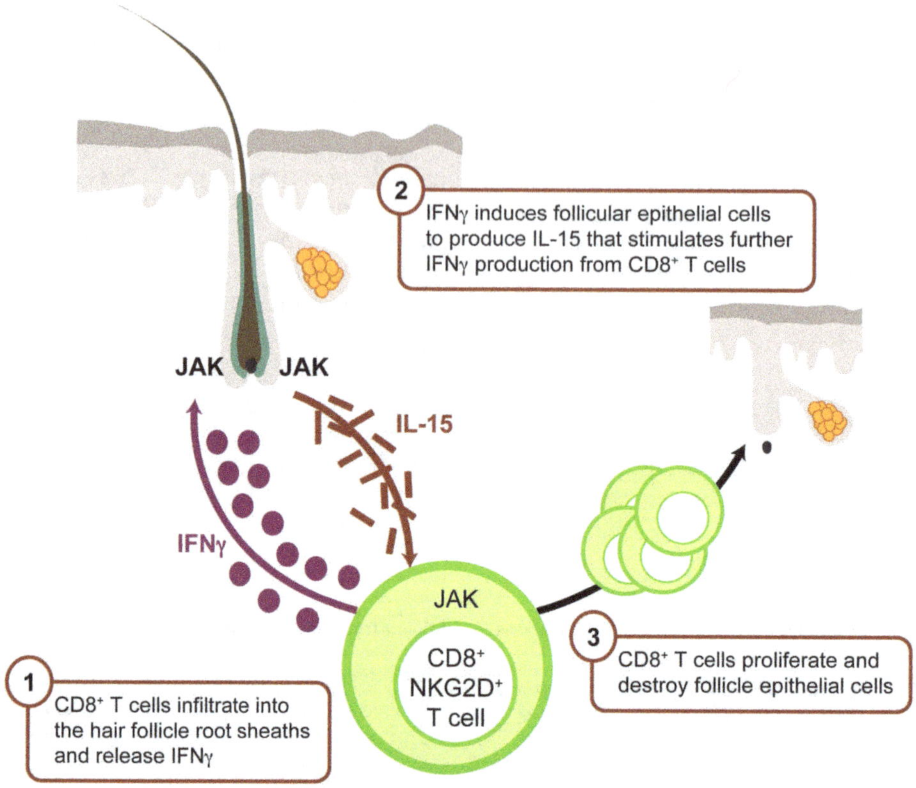

FIGURE 4 | IFNγ-driven inflammation in alopecia areata is JAK mediated. CD8$^+$ T cells infiltrate the dermis, localize to the hair follicle bulb, and release IFNγ. IFNγ binds the IFN receptor on the surface of the follicular epithelial cell, which in turn signals via JAK1 and JAK2 to promote production of IL-15, a mediator of CD8$^+$ T-cell activation. IL-15 binds IL-15 receptor on the CD8$^+$ T cell surface, resulting in signaling via JAK1 and JAK3 to enhance the production of IFNγ and amplify the feedback loop. CD8$^+$ T cells then attack the hair follicle, which causes hair loss. CXCL, chemokine (C-X-C motif) ligand; IFN, interferon; JAK, Janus kinase.

Areata Disease Activity Index (ALADIN) IFNγ gene expression signature (80). Topical administration of JAK inhibitors reversed AA in C3H/HeJ mice (81); however, murine skin is significantly thinner and easier to penetrate, and, therefore the translational validity of these data is still unknown. In addition to its proinflammatory activity, IFNγ-induced JAK/STAT signaling and the recruitment of CD8$^+$ T cells through CXCL9 and CXCL10 can directly interfere with the hair growth cycle via suppressed proliferation and activation of hair stem cells (97) and reduction of angiogenesis (98).

Several case studies have reported improvement of AA in patients who received JAK inhibitors for other autoimmune/autoinflammatory disorders or JAK-STAT gain-of-function mutation diseases (99–103).

Oral tofacitinib has been tested in two open-label studies (NCT02197455 and NCT02312882) and several case reports. In one trial, tofacitinib 5 mg twice daily (BID) was given to patients with severe AA, alopecia totalis, or alopecia universalis. After the 12-week treatment period, nearly two-thirds of patients showed some hair regrowth and 32% of patients achieved a 50% improvement in their Severity of Alopecia Tool (SALT) score (50). The second smaller open-label study in moderate to severe AA demonstrated improved results by increasing the dose of tofacitinib to 10 mg BID (104). Recently, two retrospective studies showed successful treatment of severe AA, alopecia totalis, or alopecia universalis for up to 18 months using tofacitinib, with 58% achieving a 50% improvement 20% achieving a 90% improvement in their SALT score (105–107). Oral ruxolitinib was tested in an open-label study in 12 patients with moderate to severe AA and treatment with 20 mg ruxolitinib BID for 6 months was associated with ≥50% improvement in SALT score for 75% of patients (NCT01950780) (54). Regrowth was seen, in patches as soon as 1 month after study medication was initiated. Following cessation of treatment, shedding was observed, suggesting that pharmacologic JAK inhibition suppresses AA pathogenesis but does deplete autoreactive lymphocytes. Topical formulations of ruxolitinib, tofacitinib, ATI-502 (JAK1/3), and delgocitinib have reported mixed efficacy results in case studies and small proof-of-concept clinical trials (61, 108, 109). At present, there are several clinical trials testing topical JAK inhibitors in patients with different forms of AA, but published results are not yet available (**Table 2**).

PSORIASIS

Psoriasis is a chronic, autoimmune, erythematosquamous dermatosis disorder that affects 2 to 3% of the world population. Skin lesions appear with scaling and redness (110) and are characterized by excessive keratinocyte proliferation (acanthosis), as well as retention of nuclei in the stratum corneum owing to aberrant keratinocyte differentiation (parakeratosis). Multiple inflammatory cell populations are observed within the lesions, including T cells, B cells, neutrophils, and DCs (110). Infiltrating autoreactive T lymphocytes, mainly represented by Th17, Th1, and Th22 cells, release IL-17, IFNγ, IL-22, and TNFα to potentiate disease pathogenesis. All of these cytokines induce keratinocyte-mediated recruitment and activation of additional DCs and lymphocytes, thereby perpetuating the pathogenic cycle (111, 112).

Many of the critical pathogenic mediators of psoriasis are linked to the JAK-STAT signaling pathway. For example, IL-23 engagement with its cognate receptor uses JAK1/2/TYK2 signaling, resulting in downstream STAT3 and STAT4 activation. Within psoriatic skin, dendritic cells and macrophages produce IL-23, which promotes Th17 cell expansion and survival (113). Furthermore, IL-23 together with IL-1β activates γδ T cells to amplify IL-17 production (114). Th17 and γδ T cells found in psoriatic skin are the primary source of IL-22, and this cytokine triggers reduced differentiation, increased proliferation, and acanthosis in psoriatic keratinocytes via STAT3 activation (115). IL-22 binds to its IL-10R2 and IL-22R1 heterodimeric cell surface receptor coupled to JAK1/TYK2 and STAT3 signaling (111, 116). Moreover, gene polymorphisms of *IL23A*, *IL23R*, *STAT3*, *RUNX3*, and *TYK2* have also been identified as susceptibility factors for developing psoriasis (117). More recently, JAK1 expression has been reported to positively correlate with disease duration and Psoriasis Area and Severity Index (PASI) (118) score. Within the inflamed tissue psoriatic lesion microenvironment, other cytokines, such as IL-6 and IL-21, can enhance IL-17 production from Th17 cells in a JAK-STAT–dependent manner (119, 120).

Various rodent models have mechanistically evaluated the importance of JAK-STAT signaling in psoriasis-like lesion formation and disrupted barrier function. Intradermal injection of IL-23 induces a psoriasis-like pathophysiology in mice (121). Oral administration of delgocitinib or topical administration of ruxolitinib significantly inhibited ear swelling (29, 122), and efficacy was associated with reduced IL-22 expression (29). Tofacitinib, modulates both innate and adaptive immunity leading to inhibited pathogenic Th17 cell differentiation via reduced IL-23 expression (123). In human keratinocyte cultures activated with psoriasis-relevant proinflammatory cytokines, tofacitinib suppressed expression of IFNγ-dependent inflammatory genes and normalized keratinocyte responses. Similarly, in the imiquimod-induced psoriasis model that is IL-23/IL-17/IL-22–dependent (121), tofacitinib significantly reduced epidermal thickening and IL-17^{+} or IL-22^{+} lymphocyte infiltration into the dermis (124). Furthermore, a small molecule JAK3 / SYK inhibitor (R348, Rigel Pharmaceuticals), attenuated T-cell–dependent psoriasiform skin lesions in the CD18 mutant PL/J mouse model, including significant reductions in epidermal and dermal lesion scores (125). In T cells, IL-12 induces IFNγ production, IL-23 enhances the differentiation of Th17 cells, and both require TYK2 signaling (126, 127). TYK2 knockout reduced inflammatory response and limited epidermal hyperplasia in the intradermal IL-23 model (128). Furthermore, TYK2-deficient mice were more resistant to several Th1 and Th17 cells autoimmune disorders, including imiquimod-induced psoriasis-like dermatitis (128). The combined JAK1/TYK2 inhibitor, SAR-20347, demonstrated *in vitro* and *in vivo* concentration-dependent reduction of IL-12, IL-22, and IFNγ-mediated inflammation and tissue pathology in the imiquimod-induced psoriasis model (129). Finally, experimentally induced skin trauma in the keratin5.Stat3C transgenic mice (130), which constitutively overexpresses active STAT3 in keratinocytes, develops T-cell– and IL-23–dependent psoriasis-like lesions. Topical administration of a STAT3 inhibitor prevented disease symptoms (130–132). These preclinical findings are consistent with the postulate that the JAK-STAT pathway plays a central role in psoriasis pathogenesis.

Clinically, the efficacy of oral tofacitinib in moderate to severe plaque psoriasis was demonstrated in two phase 3 randomized controlled trials (46). Tofacitinib at 10 mg BID was determined to be non-inferior to etanercept (50 mg subcutaneously twice weekly) (47). Baricitinib was reported to be efficacious in moderate to severe psoriasis in a phase 2 trial (NCT01490632). In this 12-week dose-ranging study, a 75% reduction in PASI was achieved by 43% and 54% of patients treated with baricitinib 8 and 10 mg QD, respectively (52). Itacitinib (JAK1) was evaluated in a phase 2 dose-escalation study in which patients experienced a significant improvement in the Physician Global Assessment (PGA) score at Week 4 with itacitinib 600 mg QD vs. placebo (NCT01634087) (55). Peficitinib (JAK1/3) reported improvements in PASI, PGA, and body surface area at higher dose (50 mg QD) at Day 42 in a phase 2 study (58). In another phase 2 study, 57% of patients treated with GSK2586184 (JAK1) 400 mg QD achieved a 75% reduction in PASI at Week 12 (133).

Topical tofacitinib has been tested in patients with psoriasis, with conflicting results (52, 60, 134). Three psoriasis clinical trials have been completed using topical ruxolitinib cream. In a phase 2 vehicle-controlled study in mild to moderate psoriasis (NCT00778700), ruxolitinib reported PASI reduction, although no clear dose-response was observed. A subsequent trial in 29 patients with psoriasis compared ruxolitinib cream to two active comparators (calcipotriene 0.005% cream and betamethasone dipropionate 0.05% cream; NCT00820950). Both ruxolitinib 1% QD and 1.5% BID achieved clinical efficacy, with 1.5% BID topical ruxolitinib cream being non-inferior to active comparators (62). Finally, a third study conducted in 25 patients with limited psoriasis (covering <20% of the body surface area; NCT00617994) showed that epidermal hyperplasia and dermal inflammation were reduced with ruxolitinib in most patients, along with immunohistochemical markers of inflammation (CD3, CD11c, Ki67, and K16). No significant inhibition of phosphorylated STAT3 in peripheral blood cells was observed, suggesting limited systemic exposure (63). A number of other JAK inhibitors have been studied in psoriasis (**Table 2**).

VITILIGO

Vitiligo is a chronic, autoimmune depigmenting disorder that results from destruction of melanocytes, causing white spots on the affected skin. The global vitiligo prevalence is ~0.5 to 2.0% and varies geographically, with no epidemiologic differences

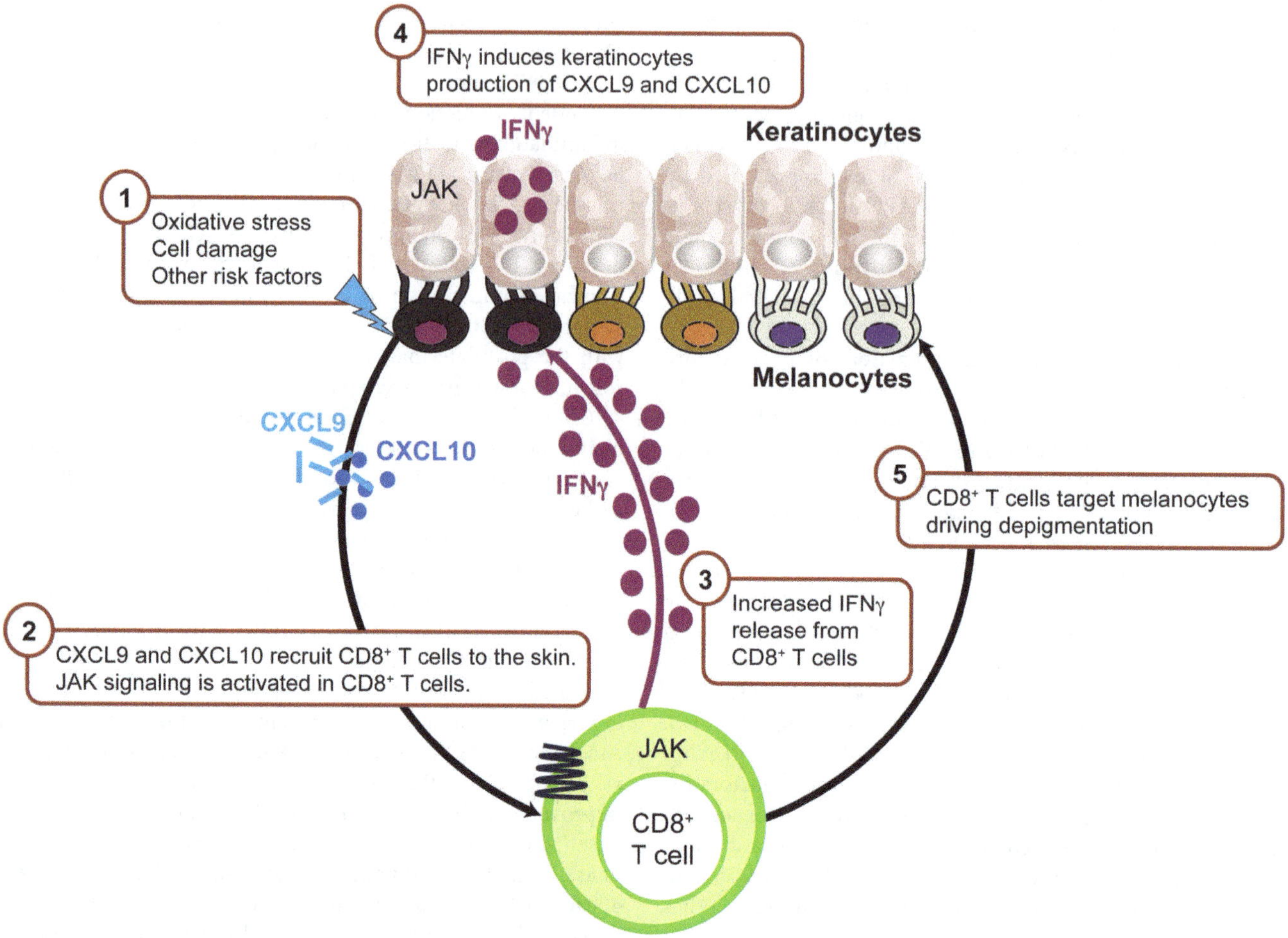

FIGURE 5 | IFNγ-driven inflammation in vitiligo is JAK mediated. Intrinsic and/or extrinsic factors induce the cellular stress response in melanocytes, which then activates innate immunity within the skin to trigger the initial inflammation that leads to autoimmunity. As a result, CXCL9 and CXCL10 are released from keratinocytes leading to recruitment of $CD8^+$ T cells. Activated $CD8^+$T cells produce IFNγ which trigger more CXCL9 and CXCL10 production from keratinocyte through JAK1 and JAK2 signaling and recruit more $CD8^+$ T cells to the inflamed sites. $CD8^+$ T cells then destruct melanocytes and lead to depigmentation. CXCL, chemokine (C-X-C motif) ligand; IFN, interferon; IL, interleukin; JAK, Janus kinase; NKD2D, natural killer group 2D.

between sexes or races (135, 136). Vitiligo can be stigmatized by society, resulting in a significant impact to patient quality of life (137, 138). It is therefore inappropriate to categorize vitiligo as simply a cosmetic problem.

In vitiligo, the frequency of anti-melanocyte $CD8^+$ T cells in the blood and skin correlates with disease severity, and lesional $CD8^+$ T cells *in vitro* induce melanocyte apoptosis in unaffected skin (139, 140). These data support the rationale that cytotoxic T lymphocytes are directly responsible for melanocyte destruction in human vitiligo (**Figure 5**). Expression analysis reveals an IFNγ-specific signature that is associated with infiltrating autoreactive $CD8^+$ T cells (140, 141). Transcriptome analysis on the skin and blood of patients with vitiligo revealed IFNγ-induced chemokines CXCL10 and CXCL9 were increased (142, 143), which is consistent with the observed abundance of autoreactive T cells expressing the cognate CXCR3 receptor (144). Furthermore, serum CXCL10 levels were associated with Vitiligo Area Scoring Index (VASI) of patients with progressive vitiligo, suggesting that the CXCL10/CXCR3 axis mediates T-cell recruitment into the skin of progressive vitiligo.

Consistent with active human vitiligo reports, an adoptive transfer of melanocyte-specific $CD8^+$ mouse model shows epidermal depigmentation but sparing of the hair follicle. Mechanistic studies, including neutralizing antibodies, have demonstrated that depigmentation is IFNγ-dependent via the local accumulation of melanocyte-specific $CD8^+$ T cells within the skin. Adoptive transfer of CXCR3-deficient T cells or inhibition of CXCL10 signaling ameliorated overall disease phenotype, whereas CXCL9 promoted autoreactive T-cell recruitment to the skin but did not significantly contribute to effector function (141, 145). Keratinocytes appear to significantly contribute to the disease process as major chemokine producers via IFN signaling, resulting in augmented autoreactive T-cell homing to the epidermis (146).

Given the apparent critical role for IFNγ in driving vitiligo inflammation and its downstream signaling dependent on the JAK1-JAK2 heterodimer, it is perhaps not surprising that intense and diffuse JAK1 expression is more present within vitiliginous skin compared with healthy tissue. Moreover, high JAK1 expression was associated with short disease duration and a lower percentage of surviving melanocytes (118, 147, 148).

Multiple case reports suggested that orally administered JAK inhibition significantly modulated the vitiligo autoimmune response and facilitated repigmentation (102, 108, 149). Another possible approach to diminish local inflammation and promote repigmentation in vitiligo, but minimize systemic drug exposures, is the use of topical JAK inhibitors. Recently, Rothstein et al. reported a very small open-label trial without placebo control (NCT02809976) in which nine patients completed the 20 week study period. Twice daily ruxolitinib cream demonstrated time-dependent improvement in facial VASI (F-VASI) in the majority of the enrolled vitiligo patients (67). Recently, ruxolitinib cream was tested in a randomized, double-blinded, dose-ranging, vehicle-controlled, phase 2 study in 157 adult patients with vitiligo (NCT03099304). The results show that significantly more patients treated with ruxolitinib cream for 24 weeks achieved a ≥50% percent improvement from baseline in the facial VASI score compared with patients treated with a control vehicle [(66); World Congress of Dermatology; June 2019; Milan, Italy].

CONCLUSIONS

Despite phenotypic differences in the inflammatory mediators responsible for driving disease pathogenesis, these aforementioned dermatoses are characterized by increased inflammatory mediators that signal through the JAK-STAT pathway.

JAK inhibitors are emerging as an exciting class of treatments in the field of dermatology. In murine models of skin inflammation, JAK inhibitors significantly modulated key mechanistic phenotypes that correspond with clinical readouts, such as acanthosis and pruritus. Early phase clinical reports confirmed the positive concept of JAK-STAT antagonism in dermatology, and randomized clinical trials have shown promising results in AD, psoriasis, and vitiligo. Encouraging data were observed in a proportion of AA participants; however, additional studies are needed to fully elucidate the disease pathophysiology and the role for JAK-STAT inhibition.

Larger clinical studies of oral and topical JAK inhibitors in AD, psoriasis, and vitiligo are currently ongoing. These pivotal trials are expected to provide additional insight into the efficacy and safety of JAK inhibitors in dermatology. Safety information for Jakinibs in inflammatory disease indications is mostly based on randomized clinical trials for investigational uses and extension studies. Recent, comprehensive, summaries of the key laboratory changes and clinical adverse events have been reported (150, 151).

Based on the promising results so far and the large number of ongoing clinical trials, it is possible that JAK inhibitors will become an important part of the dermatologist's treatment armamentarium in the future.

AUTHOR CONTRIBUTIONS

All authors listed have made a substantial, direct and intellectual contribution to the work, and approved it for publication.

ACKNOWLEDGMENTS

Editorial and graphical support was provided by Complete Healthcare Communications (North Wales, PA) and was funded by Incyte Corporation.

REFERENCES

1. Villarino AV, Kanno Y, O'shea JJ. Mechanisms and consequences of Jak-STAT signaling in the immune system. *Nat Immunol.* (2017) 18:374–84. doi: 10.1038/ni.3691
2. Rawlings JS, Rosler KM, Harrison DA. The JAK/STAT signaling pathway. *J Cell Sci.* (2004) 117:1281–3. doi: 10.1242/jcs.00963
3. Howell MD, Fitzsimons C, Smith PA. JAK/STAT inhibitors and other small molecule cytokine antagonists for the treatment of allergic disease. *Ann Allergy Asthma Immunol.* (2018) 120:367–75. doi: 10.1016/j.anai.2018.02.012
4. Stark GR, Cheon H, Wang Y. Responses to cytokines and interferons that depend upon JAKs and STATs. *Cold Spring Harb Perspect Biol.* (2018) 10:a028555. doi: 10.1101/cshperspect.a028555
5. Maldonado RA, Soriano MA, Perdomo LC, Sigrist K, Irvine DJ, Decker T, et al. Control of T helper cell differentiation through cytokine receptor inclusion in the immunological synapse. *J Exp Med.* (2009) 206:877–92. doi: 10.1084/jem.20082900
6. Mowen KA, Glimcher LH. Signaling pathways in Th2 development. *Immunol Rev.* (2004) 202:203–22. doi: 10.1111/j.0105-2896.2004.00209.x
7. Chen Z, Laurence A, O'shea JJ. Signal transduction pathways and transcriptional regulation in the control of Th17 differentiation. *Semin Immunol.* (2007) 19:400–8. doi: 10.1016/j.smim.2007.10.015
8. O'shea JJ, Steward-Tharp SM, Laurence A, Watford WT, Wei L, Adamson AS, et al. Signal transduction and Th17 cell differentiation. *Microbes Infect.* (2009) 11:599–611. doi: 10.1016/j.micinf.2009.04.007
9. Wuthrich B, Schmid-Grendelmeier P. The atopic eczema/dermatitis syndrome. Epidemiology, natural course, and immunology of the IgE-associated ("extrinsic") and the nonallergic ("intrinsic"). *AEDS J Investig Allergol Clin Immunol.* (2003) 13:1–5. doi: 10.3109/9780203908877-2
10. Deckers IA, Mclean S, Linssen S, Mommers M, Van Schayck CP, Sheikh A. Investigating international time trends in the incidence and prevalence of atopic eczema 1990-2010: a systematic review of epidemiological studies. *PLoS ONE.* (2012) 7:e39803. doi: 10.1371/journal.pone.0039803
11. Zuberbier T, Orlow SJ, Paller AS, Taieb A, Allen R, Hernanz-Hermosa JM, et al. Patient perspectives on the management of atopic dermatitis. *J Allergy Clin Immunol.* (2006) 118:226–32. doi: 10.1016/j.jaci.2006.02.031
12. Wollenberg A, Oranje A, Deleuran M, Simon D, Szalai Z, Kunz B, et al. ETFAD/EADV Eczema task force 2015 position paper on diagnosis and treatment of atopic dermatitis in adult and paediatric patients. *J Eur Acad Dermatol Venereol.* (2016) 30:729–47. doi: 10.1111/jdv.13599
13. Thyssen JP, Hamann CR, Linneberg A, Dantoft TM, Skov L, Gislason GH,

et al. Atopic dermatitis is associated with anxiety, depression, and suicidal ideation, but not with psychiatric hospitalization or suicide. *Allergy.* (2018) 73:214–20. doi: 10.1111/all.13231

14. Hebert AA, Stingl G, Ho LK, Lynde C, Cappelleri JC, Tallman AM, et al. Patient impact and economic burden of mild-to-moderate atopic dermatitis. *Curr Med Res Opin.* (2018) 34:2177–85. doi: 10.1080/03007995.2018.1498329
15. Weidinger S, Novak N. Atopic dermatitis. *Lancet.* (2016) 387:1109–22. doi: 10.1016/S0140-6736(15)00149-X
16. Neis MM, Peters B, Dreuw A, Wenzel J, Bieber T, Mauch C, et al. Enhanced expression levels of IL-31 correlate with IL-4 and IL-13 in atopic and allergic contact dermatitis. *J Allergy Clin Immunol.* (2006) 118:930–7. doi: 10.1016/j.jaci.2006.07.015
17. Amano W, Nakajima S, Yamamoto Y, Tanimoto A, Matsushita M, Miyachi Y, et al. JAK inhibitor JTE-052 regulates contact hypersensitivity by downmodulating T cell activation and differentiation. *J Dermatol Sci.* (2016) 84:258–65. doi: 10.1016/j.jdermsci.2016.09.007
18. Jin W, Huang W, Chen L, Jin M, Wang Q, Gao Z, et al. Topical application of JAK1/JAK2 inhibitor momelotinib exhibits significant anti-inflammatory responses in DNCB-induced atopic dermatitis model mice. *Int J Mol Sci.* (2018) 19:3973. doi: 10.3390/ijms19123973
19. Fukuyama T, Ehling S, Cook E, Baumer W. Topically administered janus-kinase inhibitors tofacitinib and oclacitinib display impressive antipruritic and anti-inflammatory responses in a model of allergic dermatitis. *J Pharmacol Exp Ther.* (2015) 354:394–405. doi: 10.1124/jpet.115.223784
20. Fujii Y, Sengoku T. Effects of the Janus kinase inhibitor CP-690550 (tofacitinib) in a rat model of oxazolone-induced chronic dermatitis. *Pharmacology.* (2013) 91:207–13. doi: 10.1159/000347184
21. Boniface K, Bernard FX, Garcia M, Gurney AL, Lecron JC, Morel F. IL-22 inhibits epidermal differentiation and induces proinflammatory gene expression and migration of human keratinocytes. *J Immunol.* (2005) 174:3695–702. doi: 10.4049/jimmunol.174.6.3695
22. Lou H, Lu J, Choi EB, Oh MH, Jeong M, Barmettler S, et al. Expression of IL-22 in the Skin Causes Th2-Biased Immunity, Epidermal Barrier Dysfunction, and Pruritus via Stimulating Epithelial Th2 Cytokines and the GRP Pathway. *J Immunol.* (2017) 198:2543–55. doi: 10.4049/jimmunol.1600126
23. Guttman-Yassky E, Brunner PM, Neumann AU, Khattri S, Pavel AB, Malik K, et al. Efficacy and safety of fezakinumab (an IL-22 monoclonal antibody) in adults with moderate-to-severe atopic dermatitis inadequately controlled by conventional treatments: a randomized, double-blind, phase 2a trial. *J Am Acad Dermatol.* (2018) 78:872–81 e876. doi: 10.1016/j.jaad.2018.01.016
24. Lejeune D, Dumoutier L, Constantinescu S, Kruijer W, Schuringa JJ, Renauld JC. Interleukin-22 (IL-22) activates the JAK/STAT, ERK, JNK, and p38 MAP kinase pathways in a rat hepatoma cell line. Pathways that are shared with and distinct from IL-10. *J Biol Chem.* (2002) 277:33676–82. doi: 10.1074/jbc.M204204200
25. Klonowska J, Glen J, Nowicki RJ, Trzeciak M. New cytokines in the pathogenesis of atopic dermatitis-new therapeutic targets. *Int J Mol Sci.* (2018) 19:E3086. doi: 10.3390/ijms19103086
26. Zhang Q, Putheti P, Zhou Q, Liu Q, Gao W. Structures and biological functions of IL-31 and IL-31 receptors. *Cytokine Growth Factor Rev.* (2008) 19:347–56. doi: 10.1016/j.cytogfr.2008.08.003
27. Zhong J, Sharma J, Raju R, Palapetta SM, Prasad TS, Huang TC, et al. TSLP signaling pathway map: a platform for analysis of TSLP-mediated signaling. *Database.* (2014) 2014:bau007. doi: 10.1093/database/bau007
28. Gonzales AJ, Bowman JW, Fici GJ, Zhang M, Mann DW, Mitton-Fry M. Oclacitinib (APOQUEL®) is a novel Janus kinase inhibitor with activity against cytokines involved in allergy. *J Vet Pharmacol Ther.* (2014) 37:317–24. doi: 10.1111/jvp.12101
29. Fridman JS, Scherle PA, Collins R, Burn T, Neilan CL, Hertel D, et al. Preclinical evaluation of local JAK1 and JAK2 inhibition in cutaneous inflammation. *J Invest Dermatol.* (2011) 131:1838–44. doi: 10.1038/jid.2011.140
30. Leyva-Castillo JM, Hener P, Jiang H, Li M. TSLP produced by keratinocytes promotes allergen sensitization through skin and thereby triggers atopic march in mice. *J Invest Dermatol.* (2013) 133:154–63. doi: 10.1038/jid.2012.239
31. Oetjen LK, Mack MR, Feng J, Whelan TM, Niu H, Guo CJ, et al. Sensory neurons co-opt classical immune signaling pathways to mediate chronic itch. *Cell.* (2017) 171:217–28 e213. doi: 10.1016/j.cell.2017.08.006
32. Kim BE, Leung DY, Boguniewicz M, Howell MD. Loricrin and involucrin expression is down-regulated by Th2 cytokines through STAT-6. *Clin Immunol.* (2008) 126:332–7. doi: 10.1016/j.clim.2007.11.006
33. Albanesi C, Fairchild HR, Madonna S, Scarponi C, De Pita O, Leung DY, et al. IL-4 and IL-13 negatively regulate TNF-alpha- and IFN-gamma-induced beta-defensin expression through STAT-6, suppressor of cytokine signaling (SOCS)-1, and SOCS-3. *J Immunol.* (2007) 179:984–92. doi: 10.4049/jimmunol.179.2.984
34. Sehra S, Yao Y, Howell MD, Nguyen ET, Kansas GS, Leung DY, et al. IL-4 regulates skin homeostasis and the predisposition toward allergic skin inflammation. *J Immunol.* (2010) 184:3186–90. doi: 10.4049/jimmunol.0901860
35. Yasuda T, Fukada T, Nishida K, Nakayama M, Matsuda M, Miura I, et al. Hyperactivation of JAK1 tyrosine kinase induces stepwise, progressive pruritic dermatitis. *J Clin Invest.* (2016) 126:2064–76. doi: 10.1172/JCI82887
36. Amano W, Nakajima S, Kunugi H, Numata Y, Kitoh A, Egawa G, et al. The Janus kinase inhibitor JTE-052 improves skin barrier function through suppressing signal transducer and activator of transcription 3 signaling. *J Allergy Clin Immunol.* (2015) 136:667–77 e667. doi: 10.1016/j.jaci.2015.03.051
37. Brauweiler AM, Goleva E, Leung DYM. Th2 cytokines increase Staphylococcus aureus alpha toxin-induced keratinocyte death through the signal transducer and activator of transcription 6 (STAT6). *J Invest Dermatol.* (2014) 134:2114–21. doi: 10.1038/jid.2014.43
38. Koga C, Kabashima K, Shiraishi N, Kobayashi M, Tokura Y. Possible pathogenic role of Th17 cells for atopic dermatitis. *J Invest Dermatol.* (2008) 128:2625–30. doi: 10.1038/jid.2008.111
39. Noda S, Suarez-Farinas M, Ungar B, Kim SJ, De Guzman Strong C, Xu H, et al. The Asian atopic dermatitis phenotype combines features of atopic dermatitis and psoriasis with increased TH17 polarization. *J Allergy Clin Immunol.* (2015) 136:1254–64. doi: 10.1016/j.jaci.2015.08.015
40. Levy LL, Urban J, King BA. Treatment of recalcitrant atopic dermatitis with the oral Janus kinase inhibitor tofacitinib citrate. *J Am Acad Dermatol.* (2015) 73:395–9. doi: 10.1016/j.jaad.2015.06.045
41. Guttman-Yassky E. Primary results from a phase 2b, randomized, placebo-controlled trial of upadacitinib for patients with atopic dermatitis. In: *Presented at: The American Academy of Dermatology (AAD) Annual Meeting, February 16-20.* San Diego, CA (2018).
42. Simpson EL, Lacour E-P, Spelman L, Galimberti R, Eichenfield L, Bissonnette R, et al. Efficacy and safety of baricitinib in moderate to severe atopic dermatitis: results of two phase 3 monotherapy randomized, double-blind, placebo-controlled 16-week trials (BREEZE-AD1 and BREEZA-AD2). In: *Presented at: The 24th World Congress of Dermatology (WCD).* Milan (2019).
43. Bissonnette R, Papp KA, Poulin Y, Gooderham M, Raman M, Mallbris L, et al. Topical tofacitinib for atopic dermatitis: a phase IIa randomized trial. *Br J Dermatol.* (2016) 175:902–11. doi: 10.1111/bjd.14871
44. Krueger J, Clark JD, Suarez-Farinas M, Fuentes-Duculan J, Cueto I, Wang CQ, et al. Tofacitinib attenuates pathologic immune pathways in patients with psoriasis: a randomized phase 2 study. *J Allergy Clin Immunol.* (2016) 137:1079–90. doi: 10.1016/j.jaci.2015.12.1318
45. Zhang J, Tsai TF, Lee MG, Zheng M, Wang G, Jin H, et al. The efficacy and safety of tofacitinib in Asian patients with moderate to severe chronic plaque psoriasis: a Phase 3, randomized, double-blind, placebo-controlled study. *J Dermatol Sci.* (2017) 88:36–45. doi: 10.1016/j.jdermsci.2017.05.004
46. Merola JF, Elewski B, Tatulych S, Lan S, Tallman A, Kaur M. Efficacy of tofacitinib for the treatment of nail psoriasis: two 52-week, randomized, controlled phase 3 studies in patients with moderate-to-severe plaque psoriasis. *J Am Acad Dermatol.* (2017) 77:79–87 e71. doi: 10.1016/j.jaad.2017.01.053
47. Bachelez H, Van De Kerkhof PC, Strohal R, Kubanov A, Valenzuela F, Lee JH, et al. Tofacitinib versus etanercept or placebo in moderate-to-severe chronic plaque psoriasis: a phase 3 randomised non-inferiority trial. *Lancet.* (2015) 386:552–61. doi: 10.1016/S0140-6736(14)62113-9

48. Bissonnette R, Iversen L, Sofen H, Griffiths CE, Foley P, Romiti R, et al. Tofacitinib withdrawal and retreatment in moderate-to-severe chronic plaque psoriasis: a randomized controlled trial. *Br J Dermatol.* (2015) 172:1395–406. doi: 10.1111/bjd.13551
49. Valenzuela F, Korman NJ, Bissonnette R, Bakos N, Tsai TF, Harper MK, et al. Tofacitinib in patients with moderate-to-severe chronic plaque psoriasis: long-term safety and efficacy in an open-label extension study. *Br J Dermatol.* (2018) 179:853–62. doi: 10.1111/bjd.16798
50. Kennedy Crispin M, Ko JM, Craiglow BG, Li S, Shankar G, Urban JR, et al. Safety and efficacy of the JAK inhibitor tofacitinib citrate in patients with alopecia areata. *JCI Insight.* (2016) 1:e89776. doi: 10.1172/jci.insight.89776
51. Schmieder GJ, Draelos ZD, Pariser DM, Banfield C, Cox L, Hodge M, et al. Efficacy and safety of the Janus kinase 1 inhibitor PF-04965842 in patients with moderate-to-severe psoriasis: phase II, randomized, double-blind, placebo-controlled study. *Br J Dermatol.* (2018) 179:54–62. doi: 10.1111/bjd.16004
52. Papp KA, Menter MA, Raman M, Disch D, Schlichting DE, Gaich C, et al. A randomized phase 2b trial of baricitinib, an oral Janus kinase (JAK) 1/JAK2 inhibitor, in patients with moderate-to-severe psoriasis. *Br J Dermatol.* (2016) 174:1266–76. doi: 10.1111/bjd.14403
53. Guttman-Yassky E, Silverberg JI, Nemoto O, Forman SB, Wilke A, Prescilla R, et al. Baricitinib in adult patients with moderate-to-severe atopic dermatitis: a phase 2 parallel, double-blinded, randomized placebo-controlled multiple-dose study. *J Am Acad Dermatol.* (2019) 80:913–21 e919. doi: 10.1016/j.jaad.2018.01.018
54. Mackay-Wiggan J, Jabbari A, Nguyen N, Cerise JE, Clark C, Ulerio G, et al. Oral ruxolitinib induces hair regrowth in patients with moderate-to-severe alopecia areata. *JCI Insight.* (2016) 1:e89790. doi: 10.1172/jci.insight.89790
55. Bissonnette R, Luchi M, Fidelus-Gort R, Jackson S, Zhang H, Flores R, et al. A randomized, double-blind, placebo-controlled, dose-escalation study of the safety and efficacy of INCB039110, an oral janus kinase 1 inhibitor, in patients with stable, chronic plaque psoriasis. *J Dermatolog Treat.* (2016) 27:332–8. doi: 10.3109/09546634.2015.1115819
56. Bissonnette R, Maari C, Forman S, Bhatia N, Lee M, Fowler J, et al. The oral Janus kinase/spleen tyrosine kinase inhibitor ASN002 demonstrates efficacy and improves associated systemic inflammation in patients with moderate-to-severe atopic dermatitis: results from a randomized double-blind placebo-controlled study. *Br J Dermatol.* (2019). doi: 10.1111/bjd.17932. [Epub ahead of print].
57. Papp K, Gordon K, Thaci D, Morita A, Gooderham M, Foley P, et al. Phase 2 trial of selective tyrosine Kinase 2 inhibition in psoriasis. *N Engl J Med.* (2018) 379:1313–21. doi: 10.1056/NEJMoa1806382
58. Papp K, Pariser D, Catlin M, Wierz G, Ball G, Akinlade B, et al. A phase 2a randomized, double-blind, placebo-controlled, sequential dose-escalation study to evaluate the efficacy and safety of ASP015K, a novel Janus kinase inhibitor, in patients with moderate-to-severe psoriasis. *Br J Dermatol.* (2015) 173:767–76. doi: 10.1111/bjd.13745
59. Papp KA, Bissonnette R, Gooderham M, Feldman SR, Iversen L, Soung J, et al. Treatment of plaque psoriasis with an ointment formulation of the Janus kinase inhibitor, tofacitinib: a Phase 2b randomized clinical trial. *BMC Dermatol.* (2016) 16:15. doi: 10.1186/s12895-016-0051-4
60. Ports WC, Khan S, Lan S, Lamba M, Bolduc C, Bissonnette R, et al. A randomized phase 2a efficacy and safety trial of the topical Janus kinase inhibitor tofacitinib in the treatment of chronic plaque psoriasis. *Br J Dermatol.* (2013) 169:137–45. doi: 10.1111/bjd.12266
61. Liu LY, Craiglow BG, King BA. Tofacitinib 2% ointment, a topical Janus kinase inhibitor, for the treatment of alopecia areata: a pilot study of 10 patients. *J Am Acad Dermatol.* (2018) 78:403–4 e401. doi: 10.1016/j.jaad.2017.10.043
62. Punwani N, Scherle P, Flores R, Shi J, Liang J, Yeleswaram S, et al. Preliminary clinical activity of a topical JAK1/2 inhibitor in the treatment of psoriasis. *J Am Acad Dermatol.* (2012) 67:658–64. doi: 10.1016/j.jaad.2011.12.018
63. Punwani N, Burn T, Scherle P, Flores R, Shi J, Collier P, et al. Downmodulation of key inflammatory cell markers with a topical Janus kinase 1/2 inhibitor. *Br J Dermatol.* (2015) 173:989–97. doi: 10.1111/bjd.13994
64. Kim B, Nasir A, Papp K, Parish LC, Kuligowski M, Venturanza M, et al. A phase 2, randomized, dose-ranging, vehicle- and active-controlled study to evaluate the safety and efficacy of topical ruxolitinib in adult patients with atopic dermatitis. In: *Presented at: The 27th European Academy of Dermatology and Venereology (EADV) Congress.* Paris (2018).
65. Raoof T, Kircik L, Kuligowski M, Venturanza M, Sun K, Tan J. 12-Week efficacy and safety data of ruxolitinib cream in adult patients with atopic dermatitis: results from a phase 2 study. In: *Presented at: The 24th World Congress of Dermatology (WCD).* Milan (2019).
66. Rosmarin D, Pandya A, Lebwohl M, Grimes P, Hamzavi I, Gottlieb AB, et al. Efficacy and safety of ruxolitinib cream for the treatment of Vitiligo: results of a 24-week randomized, double-blind, dose-ranging, vehicle-controlled study. In: *Presented at the 24th World Congress of Dermatology.* Milan (2019).
67. Rothstein B, Joshipura D, Saraiya A, Abdat R, Ashkar H, Turkowski Y, et al. Treatment of vitiligo with the topical Janus kinase inhibitor ruxolitinib. *J Am Acad Dermatol.* (2017). 76:1054–60 e1051. doi: 10.1016/j.jaad.2017.02.049
68. Strazzulla LC, Wang EHC, Avila L, Lo Sicco K, Brinster N, Christiano AM, et al. Alopecia areata: Disease characteristics, clinical evaluation, and new perspectives on pathogenesis. *J Am Acad Dermatol.* (2018) 78:1–12. doi: 10.1016/j.jaad.2017.04.1141
69. Paus R, Nickoloff BJ, Ito T. A 'hairy' privilege. *Trends Immunol.* (2005) 26:32–40. doi: 10.1016/j.it.2004.09.014
70. Gilhar A, Etzioni A, Paus R. Alopecia areata. *N Engl J Med.* (2012) 366:1515–25. doi: 10.1056/NEJMra1103442
71. Mcelwee KJ, Gilhar A, Tobin DJ, Ramot Y, Sundberg JP, Nakamura M, et al. What causes alopecia areata? *Exp Dermatol.* (2013) 22:609–26. doi: 10.1111/exd.12209
72. Guo H, Cheng Y, Shapiro J, Mcelwee K. The role of lymphocytes in the development and treatment of alopecia areata. *Expert Rev Clin Immunol.* (2015) 11:1335–51. doi: 10.1586/1744666X.2015.1085306
73. Paus R, Christoph T, Muller-Rover S. Immunology of the hair follicle: a short journey into terra incognita. *J Investig Dermatol Symp Proc.* (1999) 4:226–34. doi: 10.1038/sj.jidsp.5640217
74. Kang H, Wu WY, Lo BK, Yu M, Leung G, Shapiro J, et al. Hair follicles from alopecia areata patients exhibit alterations in immune privilege-associated gene expression in advance of hair loss. *J Invest Dermatol.* (2010) 130:2677–80. doi: 10.1038/jid.2010.180
75. Breitkopf T, Lo BK, Leung G, Wang E, Yu M, Carr N, et al. Somatostatin expression in human hair follicles and its potential role in immune privilege. *J Invest Dermatol.* (2013) 133:1722–30. doi: 10.1038/jid.2013.53
76. Wang X, Marr AK, Breitkopf T, Leung G, Hao J, Wang E, et al. Hair follicle mesenchyme-associated PD-L1 regulates T-cell activation induced apoptosis: a potential mechanism of immune privilege. *J Invest Dermatol.* (2014) 134:736–45. doi: 10.1038/jid.2013.368
77. Mcelwee KJ, Boggess D, King LEJr, Sundberg JP. Experimental induction of alopecia areata-like hair loss in C3H/HeJ mice using full-thickness skin grafts. *J Invest Dermatol.* (1998) 111:797–803. doi: 10.1046/j.1523-1747.1998.00380.x
78. Mcelwee KJ, Boggess D, Olivry T, Oliver RF, Whiting D, Tobin DJ, et al. Comparison of alopecia areata in human and nonhuman mammalian species. *Pathobiology.* (1998) 66:90–107. doi: 10.1159/000028002
79. Shin JM, Choi DK, Sohn KC, Koh JW, Lee YH, Seo YJ, et al. Induction of alopecia areata in C3H/HeJ mice using polyinosinic-polycytidylic acid (poly[I:C]) and interferon-gamma. *Sci Rep.* (2018) 8:12518. doi: 10.1038/s41598-018-30997-3
80. Jabbari A, Dai Z, Xing L, Cerise JE, Ramot Y, Berkun Y, et al. Reversal of alopecia areata following treatment with the JAK1/2 inhibitor baricitinib. *EBioMedicine.* (2015) 2:351–5. doi: 10.1016/j.ebiom.2015.02.015
81. Xing L, Dai Z, Jabbari A, Cerise JE, Higgins CA, Gong W, et al. Alopecia areata is driven by cytotoxic T lymphocytes and is reversed by JAK inhibition. *Nat Med.* (2014) 20:1043–9. doi: 10.1038/nm.3645
82. Ghoreishi M, Martinka M, Dutz JP. Type 1 interferon signature in the scalp lesions of alopecia areata. *Br J Dermatol.* (2010) 163:57–62. doi: 10.1111/j.1365-2133.2010.09775.x
83. De Jong A, Jabbari A, Dai Z, Xing L, Lee D, Li MM, et al. High-throughput T cell receptor sequencing identifies clonally expanded CD8+ T cell populations in alopecia areata. *JCI Insight.* (2018) 3:121949. doi: 10.1172/jci.insight.121949
84. Fuentes-Duculan J, Gulati N, Bonifacio KM, Kunjravia N, Zheng X, Suarez-Farinas M, et al. Biomarkers of alopecia areata disease activity

and response to corticosteroid treatment. *Exp Dermatol.* (2016) 25:282–6. doi: 10.1111/exd.12918

85. Freyschmidt-Paul P, Mcelwee KJ, Hoffmann R, Sundberg JP, Vitacolonna M, Kissling S, et al. Interferon-gamma-deficient mice are resistant to the development of alopecia areata. *Br J Dermatol.* (2006) 155:515–21. doi: 10.1111/j.1365-2133.2006.07377.x
86. Ito T, Ito N, Bettermann A, Tokura Y, Takigawa M, Paus R. Collapse and restoration of MHC class-I-dependent immune privilege: exploiting the human hair follicle as a model. *Am J Pathol.* (2004) 164:623–34. doi: 10.1016/S0002-9440(10)63151-3
87. Petukhova L, Duvic M, Hordinsky M, Norris D, Price V, Shimomura Y, et al. Genome-wide association study in alopecia areata implicates both innate and adaptive immunity. *Nature.* (2010) 466:113–7. doi: 10.1038/nature09114
88. Pratt CH, King LE Jr, Messenger AG, Christiano AM, Sundberg JP. Alopecia areata. *Nat Rev Dis Primers.* (2017) 3:17011. doi: 10.1038/nrdp.2017.11
89. Abou Rahal J, Kurban M, Kibbi AG, Abbas O. Plasmacytoid dendritic cells in alopecia areata: missing link? *J Eur Acad Dermatol Venereol.* (2016) 30:119–23. doi: 10.1111/jdv.12932
90. Charles J, Chaperot L, Salameire D, Di Domizio J, Aspord C, Gressin R, et al. Plasmacytoid dendritic cells and dermatological disorders: focus on their role in autoimmunity and cancer. *Eur J Dermatol.* (2010) 20:16–23. doi: 10.1684/ejd.2010.0816
91. Mcphee CG, Duncan FJ, Silva KA, King LEJr, Hogenesch H, Roopenian DC, et al. Increased expression of Cxcr3 and its ligands, Cxcl9 and Cxcl10, during the development of alopecia areata in the mouse. *J Invest Dermatol.* (2012) 132:1736–8. doi: 10.1038/jid.2012.17
92. Kuo PT, Zeng Z, Salim N, Mattarollo S, Wells JW, Leggatt GR. The role of CXCR3 and its chemokine ligands in skin disease and cancer. *Front Med.* (2018) 5:271. doi: 10.3389/fmed.2018.00271
93. Jabri B, Abadie V. IL-15 functions as a danger signal to regulate tissue-resident T cells and tissue destruction. *Nat Rev Immunol.* (2015) 15:771–83. doi: 10.1038/nri3919
94. Cooley ID, Read KA, Oestreich KJ. Trans-presentation of IL-15 modulates STAT5 activation and Bcl-6 expression in TH1 cells. *Sci Rep.* (2015) 5:15722. doi: 10.1038/srep15722
95. Betz RC, Petukhova L, Ripke S, Huang H, Menelaou A, Redler S, et al. Genome-wide meta-analysis in alopecia areata resolves HLA associations and reveals two new susceptibility loci. *Nat Commun.* (2015) 6:5966. doi: 10.1038/ncomms6966
96. O'shea JJ, Plenge R. JAK and STAT signaling molecules in immunoregulation and immune-mediated disease. *Immunity.* (2012) 36:542–50. doi: 10.1016/j.immuni.2012.03.014
97. Harel S, Higgins CA, Cerise JE, Dai Z, Chen JC, Clynes R, et al. Pharmacologic inhibition of JAK-STAT signaling promotes hair growth. *Sci Adv.* (2015) 1:e1500973. doi: 10.1126/sciadv.1500973
98. Meephansan J, Thummakriengkrai J, Ponnikorn S, Yingmema W, Deenonpoe R, Suchonwanit P. Efficacy of topical tofacitinib in promoting hair growth in non-scarring alopecia: possible mechanism via VEGF induction. *Arch Dermatol Res.* (2017) 309:729–38. doi: 10.1007/s00403-017-1777-5
99. Craiglow BG, King BA. Killing two birds with one stone: oral tofacitinib reverses alopecia universalis in a patient with plaque psoriasis. *J Invest Dermatol.* (2014) 134:2988–90. doi: 10.1038/jid.2014.260
100. Higgins E, Al Shehri T, Mcaleer MA, Conlon N, Feighery C, Lilic D, et al. Use of ruxolitinib to successfully treat chronic mucocutaneous candidiasis caused by gain-of-function signal transducer and activator of transcription 1 (STAT1) mutation. *J Allergy Clin Immunol.* (2015) 135:551–3. doi: 10.1016/j.jaci.2014.12.1867
101. Pieri L, Guglielmelli P, Vannucchi AM. Ruxolitinib-induced reversal of alopecia universalis in a patient with essential thrombocythemia. *Am J Hematol.* (2015) 90:82–3. doi: 10.1002/ajh.23871
102. Harris JE, Rashighi M, Nguyen N, Jabbari A, Ulerio G, Clynes R, et al. Rapid skin repigmentation on oral ruxolitinib in a patient with coexistent vitiligo and alopecia areata (AA). *J Am Acad Dermatol.* (2016) 74:370–1. doi: 10.1016/j.jaad.2015.09.073
103. Boyadzhiev M, Marinov L, Boyadzhiev V, Iotova V, Aksentijevich I, Hambleton S. Disease course and treatment effects of a JAK inhibitor in a patient with CANDLE syndrome. *Pediatr Rheumatol Online J.* (2019) 17:19. doi: 10.1186/s12969-019-0322-9
104. Jabbari A, Sansaricq F, Cerise J, Chen JC, Bitterman A, Ulerio G, et al. An Open-Label Pilot Study to Evaluate the Efficacy of Tofacitinib in Moderate to Severe Patch-Type Alopecia Areata, Totalis, and Universalis. *J Invest Dermatol.* (2018) 138:1539–45. doi: 10.1016/j.jid.2018.01.032
105. Craiglow BG, Liu LY, King BA. Tofacitinib for the treatment of alopecia areata and variants in adolescents. *J Am Acad Dermatol.* (2017) 76:29–32. doi: 10.1016/j.jaad.2016.09.006
106. Liu LY, Craiglow BG, Dai F, King BA. Tofacitinib for the treatment of severe alopecia areata and variants: a study of 90 patients. *J Am Acad Dermatol.* (2017) 76:22–8. doi: 10.1016/j.jaad.2016.09.007
107. Liu LY, Strassner JP, Refat MA, Harris JE, King BA. Repigmentation in vitiligo using the Janus kinase inhibitor tofacitinib may require concomitant light exposure. *J Am Acad Dermatol.* (2017) 77:675–82 e671. doi: 10.1016/j.jaad.2017.05.043
108. Craiglow BG, King BA. Tofacitinib citrate for the treatment of vitiligo: a pathogenesis-directed therapy. *JAMA Dermatol.* (2015) 151:1110–2. doi: 10.1001/jamadermatol.2015.1520
109. Bayart CB, Deniro KL, Brichta L, Craiglow BG, Sidbury R. Topical Janus kinase inhibitors for the treatment of pediatric alopecia areata. *J Am Acad Dermatol.* (2017) 77:167–70. doi: 10.1016/j.jaad.2017.03.024
110. Nestle FO, Kaplan DH, Barker J. Psoriasis. *N Engl J Med.* (2009) 361:496–509. doi: 10.1056/NEJMra0804595
111. Afzali B, Lombardi G, Lechler RI, Lord GM. The role of T helper 17 (Th17) and regulatory T cells (Treg) in human organ transplantation and autoimmune disease. *Clin Exp Immunol.* (2007) 148:32–46. doi: 10.1111/j.1365-2249.2007.03356.x
112. Albanesi C, De Pita O, Girolomoni G. Resident skin cells in psoriasis: a special look at the pathogenetic functions of keratinocytes. *Clin Dermatol.* (2007) 25:581–8. doi: 10.1016/j.clindermatol.2007.08.013
113. Lee E, Trepicchio WL, Oestreicher JL, Pittman D, Wang F, Chamian F, et al. Increased expression of interleukin 23 p19 and p40 in lesional skin of patients with psoriasis vulgaris. *J Exp Med.* (2004) 199:125–30. doi: 10.1084/jem.20030451
114. Sutton CE, Lalor SJ, Sweeney CM, Brereton CF, Lavelle EC, Mills KH. Interleukin-1 and IL-23 induce innate IL-17 production from gammadelta T cells, amplifying Th17 responses and autoimmunity. *Immunity.* (2009) 31:331–41. doi: 10.1016/j.immuni.2009.08.001
115. Zheng Y, Danilenko DM, Valdez P, Kasman I, Eastham-Anderson J, Wu J, et al. Interleukin-22, a T(H)17 cytokine, mediates IL-23-induced dermal inflammation and acanthosis. *Nature.* (2007) 445:648–51. doi: 10.1038/nature05505
116. Boutet MA, Nerviani A, Gallo Afflitto G, Pitzalis C. Role of the IL-23/IL-17 axis in psoriasis and psoriatic arthritis: the clinical importance of its divergence in skin and joints. *Int J Mol Sci.* (2018) 19:E530. doi: 10.3390/ijms19020530
117. Belge K, Bruck J, Ghoreschi K. Advances in treating psoriasis. *F1000Prime Rep.* (2014) 6:4. doi: 10.12703/P6-4
118. Nada HR, El Sharkawy DA, Elmasry MF, Rashed LA, Mamdouh S. Expression of Janus Kinase 1 in vitiligo and psoriasis before and after narrow band UVB: a case-control study. *Arch Dermatol Res.* (2018) 310:39–46. doi: 10.1007/s00403-017-1792-6
119. Wei L, Laurence A, Elias KM, O'shea JJ. IL-21 is produced by Th17 cells and drives IL-17 production in a STAT3-dependent manner. *J Biol Chem.* (2007) 282:34605–10. doi: 10.1074/jbc.M705100200
120. Camporeale A, Poli V. IL-6, IL-17 and STAT3: a holy trinity in auto-immunity? *Front Biosci.* (2012) 17:2306–26. doi: 10.2741/4054
121. Van Der Fits L, Mourits S, Voerman JS, Kant M, Boon L, Laman JD, et al. Imiquimod-induced psoriasis-like skin inflammation in mice is mediated via the IL-23/IL-17 axis. *J Immunol.* (2009) 182:5836–45. doi: 10.4049/jimmunol.0802999
122. Tanimoto A, Shinozaki Y, Yamamoto Y, Katsuda Y, Taniai-Riya E, Toyoda K, et al. A novel JAK inhibitor JTE-052 reduces skin inflammation and ameliorates chronic dermatitis in rodent models: comparison with conventional therapeutic agents. *Exp Dermatol.* (2018) 27:22–9. doi: 10.1111/exd.13370

123. Ghoreschi K, Jesson MI, Li X, Lee JL, Ghosh S, Alsup JW, et al. Modulation of innate and adaptive immune responses by tofacitinib (CP-690,550). *J Immunol.* (2011) 186:4234–43. doi: 10.4049/jimmunol.1003668
124. Morelli M, Scarponi C, Mercurio L, Facchiano F, Pallotta S, Madonna S, et al. Selective immunomodulation of inflammatory pathways in keratinocytes by the Janus Kinase (JAK) inhibitor tofacitinib: implications for the employment of JAK-targeting drugs in psoriasis. *J Immunol Res.* (2018) 2018:7897263. doi: 10.1155/2018/7897263
125. Chang BY, Zhao F, He X, Ren H, Braselmann S, Taylor V, et al. JAK3 inhibition significantly attenuates psoriasiform skin inflammation in CD18 mutant PL/J mice. *J Immunol.* (2009) 183:2183–92. doi: 10.4049/jimmunol.0804063
126. Karaghiosoff M, Neubauer H, Lassnig C, Kovarik P, Schindler H, Pircher H, et al. Partial impairment of cytokine responses in Tyk2-deficient mice. *Immunity.* (2000) 13:549–60. doi: 10.1016/S1074-7613(00)00054-6
127. Shimoda K, Kato K, Aoki K, Matsuda T, Miyamoto A, Shibamori M, et al. Tyk2 plays a restricted role in IFN alpha signaling, although it is required for IL-12-mediated T cell function. *Immunity.* (2000) 13:561–71. doi: 10.1016/S1074-7613(00)00055-8
128. Ishizaki M, Muromoto R, Akimoto T, Sekine Y, Kon S, Diwan M, et al. Tyk2 is a therapeutic target for psoriasis-like skin inflammation. *Int Immunol.* (2014) 26:257–67. doi: 10.1093/intimm/dxt062
129. Works MG, Yin F, Yin CC, Yiu Y, Shew K, Tran TT, et al. Inhibition of TYK2 and JAK1 ameliorates imiquimod-induced psoriasis-like dermatitis by inhibiting IL-22 and the IL-23/IL-17 axis. *J Immunol.* (2014) 193:3278–87. doi: 10.4049/jimmunol.1400205
130. Sano S, Chan KS, Carbajal S, Clifford J, Peavey M, Kiguchi K, et al. Stat3 links activated keratinocytes and immunocytes required for development of psoriasis in a novel transgenic mouse model. *Nat Med.* (2005) 11:43–9. doi: 10.1038/nm1162
131. Miyoshi K, Takaishi M, Nakajima K, Ikeda M, Kanda T, Tarutani M, et al. Stat3 as a therapeutic target for the treatment of psoriasis: a clinical feasibility study with STA-21, a Stat3 inhibitor. *J Invest Dermatol.* (2011) 131:108–17. doi: 10.1038/jid.2010.255
132. Nakajima K, Kanda T, Takaishi M, Shiga T, Miyoshi K, Nakajima H, et al. Distinct roles of IL-23 and IL-17 in the development of psoriasis-like lesions in a mouse model. *J Immunol.* (2011) 186:4481–9. doi: 10.4049/jimmunol.1000148
133. Ludbrook VJ, Hicks KJ, Hanrott KE, Patel JS, Binks MH, Wyres MR, et al. Investigation of selective JAK1 inhibitor GSK2586184 for the treatment of psoriasis in a randomized placebo-controlled phase IIa study. *Br J Dermatol.* (2016) 174:985–95. doi: 10.1111/bjd.14399
134. Ports WC, Feldman SR, Gupta P, Tan H, Johnson TR, Bissonnette R. Randomized pilot clinical trial of tofacitinib solution for plaque psoriasis: challenges of the intra-subject study design. *J Drugs Dermatol.* (2015) 14:777–84.
135. Kruger C, Schallreuter KU. A review of the worldwide prevalence of vitiligo in children/adolescents and adults. *Int J Dermatol.* (2012) 51:1206–12. doi: 10.1111/j.1365-4632.2011.05377.x
136. Boniface K, Seneschal J, Picardo M, Taieb A. Vitiligo: focus on clinical aspects, immunopathogenesis, and therapy. *Clin Rev Allergy Immunol.* (2018) 54:52–67. doi: 10.1007/s12016-017-8622-7
137. Radtke MA, Schafer I, Gajur A, Langenbruch A, Augustin M. Willingness-to-pay and quality of life in patients with vitiligo. *Br J Dermatol.* (2009) 161:134–9. doi: 10.1111/j.1365-2133.2009.09091.x
138. Talsania N, Lamb B, Bewley A. Vitiligo is more than skin deep: a survey of members of the Vitiligo Society. *Clin Exp Dermatol.* (2010) 35:736–9. doi: 10.1111/j.1365-2230.2009.03765.x
139. Ogg GS, Rod Dunbar P, Romero P, Chen JL, Cerundolo V. High frequency of skin-homing melanocyte-specific cytotoxic T lymphocytes in autoimmune vitiligo. *J Exp Med.* (1998) 188:1203–8. doi: 10.1084/jem.188.6.1203
140. Van Den Boorn JG, Konijnenberg D, Dellemijn TA, Van Der Veen JP, Bos JD, Melief CJ, et al. Autoimmune destruction of skin melanocytes by perilesional T cells from vitiligo patients. *J Invest Dermatol.* (2009) 129:2220–32. doi: 10.1038/jid.2009.32
141. Rashighi M, Agarwal P, Richmond JM, Harris TH, Dresser K, Su MW, et al. CXCL10 is critical for the progression and maintenance of depigmentation in a mouse model of vitiligo. *Sci Transl Med.* (2014) 6:223ra223. doi: 10.1126/scitranslmed.3007811
142. Regazzetti C, Joly F, Marty C, Rivier M, Mehul B, Reiniche P, et al. Transcriptional analysis of vitiligo skin reveals the alteration of WNT pathway: a promising target for repigmenting vitiligo patients. *J Invest Dermatol.* (2015) 135:3105–14. doi: 10.1038/jid.2015.335
143. Abdallah M, El-Mofty M, Anbar T, Rasheed H, Esmat S, Al-Tawdy A, et al. CXCL-10 and Interleukin-6 are reliable serum markers for vitiligo activity: a multicenter cross-sectional study. *Pigment Cell Melanoma Res.* (2018) 31:330–6. doi: 10.1111/pcmr.12667
144. Strassner JP, Rashighi M, Ahmed Refat M, Richmond JM, Harris JE. Suction blistering the lesional skin of vitiligo patients reveals useful biomarkers of disease activity. *J Am Acad Dermatol.* (2017) 76:847–55 e845. doi: 10.1016/j.jaad.2016.12.021
145. Richmond JM, Masterjohn E, Chu R, Tedstone J, Youd ME, Harris JE. CXCR3 depleting antibodies prevent and reverse vitiligo in mice. *J Invest Dermatol.* (2017) 137:982–5. doi: 10.1016/j.jid.2016.10.048
146. Richmond JM, Bangari DS, Essien KI, Currimbhoy SD, Groom JR, Pandya AG, et al. Keratinocyte-derived chemokines orchestrate T-cell positioning in the epidermis during vitiligo and may serve as biomarkers of disease. *J Invest Dermatol.* (2017) 137:350–8. doi: 10.1016/j.jid.2016.09.016
147. Abdou AG, Maraee A, Yassien H, Sarhan M. Immunohistochemistry of Janus Kinase 1 (JAK1) Expression in Vitiligo. *J Pathol Transl Med.* (2018) 52:363–8. doi: 10.4132/jptm.2018.09.18
148. Relke N, Gooderham M. The use of janus kinase inhibitors in Vitiligo: a review of the literature. *J Cutan Med Surg.* (2019) 23:298–306. doi: 10.1177/1203475419833609
149. Kim SR, Heaton H, Liu LY, King BA. Rapid repigmentation of vitiligo using tofacitinib plus low-dose, narrowband UV-B phototherapy. *JAMA Dermatol.* (2018) 154:370–1. doi: 10.1001/jamadermatol.2017.5778
150. Choy EH. Clinical significance of Janus Kinase inhibitor selectivity. *Rheumatology.* (2019) 58:953–62. doi: 10.1093/rheumatology/key339
151. Fragoulis GE, Mcinnes IB, Siebert S. JAK-inhibitors. New players in the field of immune-mediated diseases, beyond rheumatoid arthritis. *Rheumatology.* (2019) 58:i43–54. doi: 10.1093/rheumatology/key276

21

Coagulation and Skin Autoimmunity

Massimo Cugno [1,2]*, *Alessandro Borghi* [3], *Simone Garcovich* [4] *and Angelo Valerio Marzano* [1,5]

[1] *Dipartimento di Fisiopatologia Medico-Chirurgica e dei Trapianti, Università degli Studi di Milano, Milan, Italy,* [2] *Medicina Interna, Fondazione IRCCS Ca' Granda Ospedale Maggiore Policlinico, Milan, Italy,* [3] *Sezione di Dermatologia e Malattie Infettive, Dipartimento di Scienze Mediche, Università degli Studi di Ferrara, Ferrara, Italy,* [4] *Istituto di Dermatologia, Università Cattolica del Sacro Cuore, Fondazione Policlinico A. Gemelli IRCCS, Rome, Italy,* [5] *UOC Dermatologia, Fondazione IRCCS Ca' Granda Ospedale Maggiore Policlinico, Milan, Italy*

Correspondence:
Massimo Cugno
massimo.cugno@unimi.it

Several lines of evidence indicate that the immune system, inflammation, and coagulation are simultaneously activated in autoimmune and immune-mediated skin diseases. Pro-inflammatory cytokines such as interleukin-6 and tumor necrosis factor-alpha induce the expression of the main initiator of coagulation, i.e., tissue factor. The proteases of coagulation in turn act on protease-activated receptors inducing the expression of various pro-inflammatory cytokines triggering inflammation. The cross-talk among immune system, inflammation, and coagulation amplifies and maintains the activation of all three pathways. This review focuses on three skin disorders as chronic spontaneous urticaria (CSU), angioedema, and bullous pemphigoid (BP), in which the relationships among the three systems have been investigated or their clinical consequences are relevant. Markers of thrombin generation, fibrinolysis, and inflammation have been reported to be increased in the plasma during flares of CSU and angioedema, as well as in the active phase of BP, with the marker levels reverting to normal during remission. The coagulation activation seems to be important only at local level in CSU and angioedema while both at local and systemic levels in BP which is the only condition associated with an increased thrombotic risk. The prothrombotic state in autoimmune skin diseases raises the question of the indication of anticoagulant treatment, particularly in the presence of other cardiovascular risk factors.

Keywords: coagulation, autoimmunity, urticaria, angioedema, bullous pemphigoid, psoriasis, atopic dermatitis, dermatitis herpetiformis

INTRODUCTION

Immune system, blood coagulation and inflammation strictly interact in providing a defense against a variety of potentially injurious stimuli, such as infections and tissue damages (1). The molecular mechanisms of this interaction have been largely elucidated. Indeed, pro-inflammatory cytokines, like interleukin 1 (IL-1), IL-6, and tumor necrosis factor alpha (TNF-α), induce the expression of tissue factor (TF) the main initiator of blood coagulation whereas downregulate the natural anticoagulants such as antithrombin, protein C, and TF pathway inhibitor (2). On the other hand, the coagulant mediators (FVIIa, FXa, and FIIa) in turn act on protease-activated receptors (PAR) inducing the expression of pro-inflammatory cytokines (3, 4). The relationships between the activation or dysfunction of the immune system and the coagulation system are evident in systemic autoimmune or immune-mediated diseases including lupus erythematosus (5, 6), rheumatoid arthritis (7, 8), and inflammatory bowel diseases (9, 10) which show an increased risk of thrombosis. A few studies suggested the involvement of blood coagulation also in some immune-mediated skin disorders whose aspects will be analyzed in the present review.

Immune-mediated inflammatory skin diseases comprise a group of heterogeneous chronic disorders that share similar immune-mediated pathogenic mechanisms as well as genetic susceptibility. Although their specific etiologies remain often unknown, all are recognized to involve dysregulation of the immune system, including an over-expression of the pro-inflammatory cytokines. In autoimmune and immune-mediated skin disorders, the cross-talk between inflammation and coagulation creates a self-refueling loop which amplifies and sustains the activation of both systems (3). Growing evidence suggests that this has both local and systemic implications.

The aim of the present study is to focus on several skin disorders in which the relationships between immune response, inflammation and blood coagulation have been investigated and/or their clinical consequences are relevant such as chronic spontaneous urticaria, angioedema, and bullous pemphigoid.

CHRONIC SPONTANEOUS URTICARIA

Urticaria is a common skin disease characterized by short-lived swellings, called wheals, which resolve in <24 h. Urticaria can be classified according to duration and etiology as acute or chronic (11). Chronic urticaria is defined as urticaria with or without angioedema lasting more than 6 weeks and can be further classified according to whether it is inducible or not into chronic inducible urticaria or chronic spontaneous urticaria (CSU).

Despite the great research effort of the last 20 years, etiology and pathogenesis of CSU remain largely unclear. However, there is growing evidence that different biologic systems including autoimmunity (12–14), inflammation (15–18), coagulation (19), and auto-allergy (20–23) are involved in the mechanisms leading to mast cell and basophil degranulation and hence to wheal formation (**Figure 1**).

The autoimmune mechanism is based on the presence of circulating histamine-releasing IgG autoantibodies directed against either the high-affinity IgE receptor (FcεRI) on both mast cells and basophils (in most cases) or membrane-bound IgE (in a minority of patients) (12, 13, 24). In a variable proportion (30–60%) of patients with active disease, the intradermal injection of autologous serum (autologous serum skin test, ASST) causes a wheal-and-flare reaction (19). This phenomenon mirrors the activation of mast cells and basophils as well as of the complement cascade by these autoantibodies. Experimental and clinical findings have supported an autoimmune origin in about 30–50% of patients affected with CSU (12, 13). Also other autoantibodies are involved in CSU pathogenesis such as autoantibodies to CD23, the low-affinity IgE receptor (FcεRII), which contribute to eosinophil activation and mast cell degranulation (14, 25). The possible autoimmune nature of CSU is further supported by the association with other autoimmune diseases, notably thyroiditis, and the increased frequency of HLA DRB1*04 (DR4) (26).

Inflammation is involved in the pathophysiology CSU, as demonstrated by the increase in different markers of inflammation, such as matrix metalloproteinase, serum C-reactive protein, IL-6, IL-6 soluble receptor, eosinophil cationic protein (ECP), TNF-α, complement, and others, which are related to CU activity (15–17, 27). On the contrary, adipokines that affect immune responses and exert an anti-inflammatory effect, such as lipocalin 2, have a negative association with CU activity (18).

Coagulation involvement in the pathogenesis of CSU is supported by many lines of evidence (28–33). The original observation that the autologous plasma skin test (APST) may score positive in some ASST-negative patients (29) has given rise to investigation of the coagulation system in CSU patients. In a study that dates back over 10 years, some of us found that CSU patients have elevated plasma levels of prothrombin fragment F1+2, suggesting thrombin generation (29). In subsequent studies, we found that CSU patients show an activation of the tissue factor pathway of coagulation cascade by activated eosinophils (30). Immunohistochemical experiments showed tissue factor expression by eosinophils present in the inflammatory infiltrate of CSU skin lesions (31). These data highlight the relevance of eosinophils in CSU as a source of tissue factor, in accordance with studies showing that eosinophils store tissue factor and transfer it to their cell membrane during activation (34). Eosinophils may be activated directly by autoantibodies directed against the FcεRII CD23 antigen (14) or secondarily to the activation of mast cells by anti-FcεRI and anti-IgE autoantibodies (24). The activation of the tissue factor pathway of coagulation results, in turn, in the generation of thrombin which, in experimental models, has been shown to induce edema through an increase in vascular permeability directly by acting on endothelial cells (35) and indirectly by generating C5a (36, 37), by triggering mast cell degranulation (38–41) and by releasing inflammatory mediators (42, 43). Pro-inflammatory cytokines, such as IL-6 and TNF-α, induce the expression of tissue factor (3, 44), sealing the mutual activation of the two systems, i.e., coagulation and inflammation. The complexes between tissue factor, activated factor VII (FVIIa) and FVa+FXa also activate mast cells via PAR-2, thus amplifying the activation of these cells in CSU (40). On the other hand, mast cell-derived tryptase can induce thrombin generation through a direct activation of prothrombin (45), thus constituting an amplification loop. It must be taken into account also an opposite effect of mast cells on inflammatory response. In fact, recent studies showed that mast cells can also limit thrombin-induced immediate skin inflammatory responses by releasing substances able to reduce the activity of thrombin, for example proteases, like mast cell protease 4 (MCPT4) (46). During severe exacerbations of the disease, CSU patients show marked increase of plasmatic markers of thrombin generation, like prothrombin fragment F1 + 2, FVIIa and thrombin-antithrombin complex (47–49), as well as of fibrinolysis (24, 31, 50). The increase of D-dimer, marker of fibrinolysis, is associated with disease severity (24) and its level resulted higher when compared with that of patients affected with psoriasis (51). Interestingly, a study detected the increase of D-dimer and fibrinogen/fibrin degradation products (FDP), produced by fibrinolysis of either stabilized or non-stabilized fibrin, in patients with CSU, but not in healthy individuals or in patients with inducible type of urticaria (52). Finding that the increase in plasma markers of thrombin generation

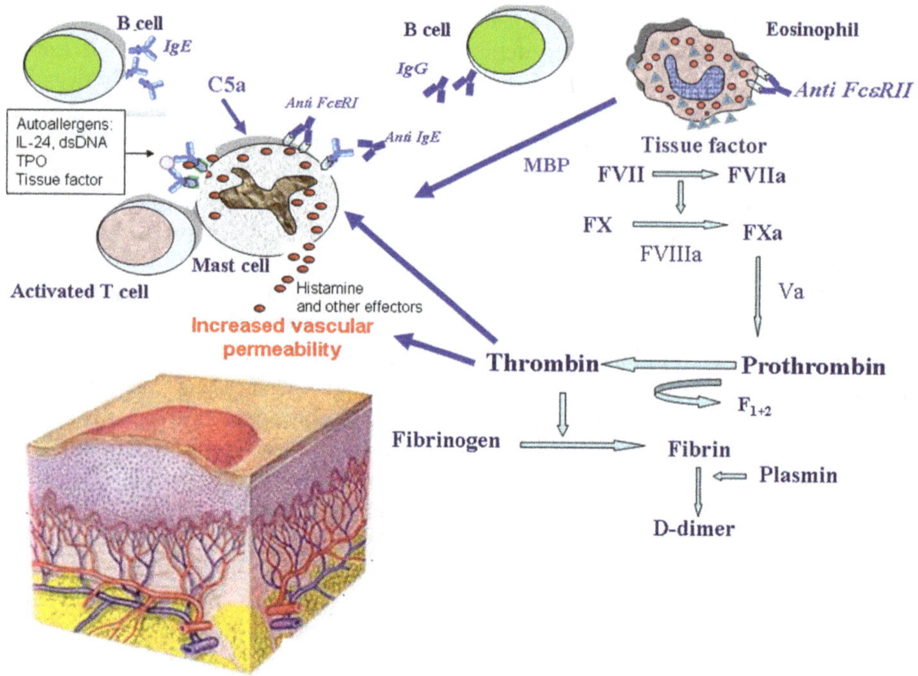

FIGURE 1 | Mechanisms of eosinophil and mast cell activation in chronic spontaneous urticaria. Mast cells release histamine and other effector molecules after stimulation by autoantibodies directed against the high-affinity IgE receptor (FcεRI) and IgE, complement anaphylatoxin C5a, eosinophil-derived major basic protein (MBP), thrombin, and IgE-autoallergen complexes. The most important autoallergens are: interleukin-24 (IL-24), double stranded DNA (dsDNA), thyroperoxidase (TPO), tissue factor. Eosinophils are activated by autoantibodies directed against the low-affinity IgE receptor (FcεRII) and potentially by other factors. Upon their activation, eosinophils release MBP, and express tissue factor which in turn activates the coagulation cascade (factors VII, X, VIII, V, and prothrombin) leading to thrombin generation. Thrombin induces mast cell degranulation as well as increased vascular permeability. Thrombin generation is demonstrated by the presence of fragment F1+2 released from prothrombin after its activation. Finally, fibrin degradation is documented by elevated plasma levels of the fibrin fragment D-dimer during the active phase of the disease.

and fibrinolysis parallels plasma C-reactive protein (CRP) levels further remarks the close link between coagulation activation and inflammation in CSU pathogenesis (53). The interplay between inflammatory and coagulation/fibrinolysis factors in CSU may lead to maintenance and amplification of urticarial inflammation. Both the activation of coagulation and fibrinolysis decrease till complete normalization during remission and biomarker levels return to normal values (31, 49, 54, 55). A limited number of studies investigated the role of platelets in CSU, with no univocal data (56). Platelet activation was found to occur in some skin inflammatory disorders, such as atopic dermatitis and psoriasis (57, 58). Based on these findings, platelets are regarded as a possible link between chronic inflammatory and pro-coagulant states (59). It may be hypothesized that platelet activation may be one of the triggering factors of the coagulation cascade in CSU too, leading to the activation of histamine-releasing effector cells. However, current evidence indicates that the simple determination of platelet indices is not reliable and lacks useful implications in the clinical practice (56).

The activation of the coagulation cascade in CSU pathogenesis may have clinical effects not only in eliciting skin lesions, namely wheal eruption, but also at systemic level. The most important potential clinical consequence of the hypercoagulable state in CSU patients is an increased thrombotic risk (25). In spite of this, patients with CSU are not reported to have an increased risk for thrombotic events. A possible explanation is that the activation of coagulation occurs mostly extravascularly and can be efficiently counteracted by coagulation inhibitors and fibrinolysis. Other potential clinical implications of the recognized involvement of coagulation in the pathogenesis of CSU are the possible therapeutic efficacy of pharmacological agents that interfere with the coagulation pathway. A few reports indicate that heparin, an anticoagulant which potentiates the effect of antithrombin, may be effective in treating CSU (60, 61). An anticoagulant/anti-fibrinolytic therapy, namely nadroparin and tranexamic acid, has been found effective in some patients with refractory CSU and elevated D-dimer levels (62). Moreover, warfarin, an oral anti-vitamin K drug, induced a good response in patients with CU unresponsive to antihistamines in a double-blind, placebo controlled study (63). With reference to further clinical implications of the activation of coagulation and fibrinolysis, elevated D-dimer plasma level has been found to be associated both with a poor response to antihistamines (64) and with a limited response to cyclosporine treatment (65). It is worthy of note that D-dimer plasma levels were observed to parallel the clinical response to omalizumab treatment, dropping in responders and remaining unchanged in non-responders (20, 66). Furthermore, elevated D-dimer plasma levels seem to be a predictive marker of prompt and complete response to the anti-IgE monoclonal antibody (67). It may be assumed that in a subset of CSU patients, the activation of the coagulation cascade has a key role in the pathogenesis of this disorder. In a recent study, the treatment with omalizumab induced a significant decrease in WBC count, platelet count, neutrophil count, ratio of platelet to lymphocyte (PLR), ratio of neutrophil to lymphocyte (NLR) and CRP level and a significant increase in mean platelet volume (MPV) and eosinophil count (68). Taken together, these data suggest that in CSU patients omalizumab may be effective not only antagonizing IgE but also affecting a number of other pathways (69). In particular, it can exert inhibitory effects on inflammation and coagulation cascade, further confirming the strict interaction between immunity, inflammation, and coagulation.

The "autoallergic" mechanism, which has been recently identified, is mediated by specific IgE to different allergens, including double-strained DNA (21), thyroperoxidase (22), IL-24 (23), tissue factor, and thyroglobulin (20). IgE anti-autoallergens seem to cause "autoallergic" mast cell degranulation. In particular, the elevated specific IgE antibodies to tissue factor have been demonstrated to be functionally able to mediate the release of leukotriene C4 by tissue factor-stimulated peripheral basophils (20). Tissue factor, the main initiator of coagulation, is overexpressed in CSU lesional skin (32) where it can activate coagulation and is also accessible to mast cell-bound IgE. Thus, IgE anti-tissue factor could cause "autoallergic" mast cell degranulation, linking the autoallergic and coagulation activation pathways. The presence of autoreactive IgE against several targets in patients with CSU might explain, at least in part, the clinical success of the humanized monoclonal anti-IgE antibody omalizumab.

ANGIOEDEMA

Angioedema refers to a circumscribed, non-itchy edema of the subcutaneous tissues mostly involving lips, face, neck and extremities and/or submucosal tissues affecting oral cavity, larynx and gut (70). It typically lasts from many hours to 3 days before the tissue returns to normal. Angioedema is life-threatening if it occurs in the upper airways and can be very painful if it occurs in the gastrointestinal tract (70). Wheals and angioedema often coexist but may also present alone (71). Most of these conditions are mainly mediated by histamine and other pro-inflammatory mediators released by mast cells and basophils (72). Overall, angioedema can be caused by allergies, inherited or acquired deficiencies of C1-inhibitor protein, or drug reactions. In many cases its pathophysiology remains undetermined (54). Among the vasoactive agents involved in mediating swelling attacks in angioedema, histamine, released by mast cells or basophils, has a prominent role, especially in allergic reactions and in cases of associated urticaria (73). Anti-histamines are effective agents in these forms. However, there are some subtypes of angioedema that do not respond to anti-histamine, such as angioedema due to C1-inhibitor deficiency, angioedema due to ACE inhibitors and a rate of idiopathic angioedema (54). Bradykinin is a recognized mediator of the increased vascular permeability in angioedema. Bradykinin is a vasoactive peptide acting on specific receptors such as B2 receptors that are constitutively present on the endothelium and B1 receptors that are expressed during inflammatory reactions. Bradykinin receptor signaling induces peripheral vasodilatation, enhancement of vascular permeability and subsequent vascular leakage. Bradykinin is the end-product of the contact activation system. This enzymatic cascade circulates in the plasma and consists of factor XII (FXII), plasma prekallikrein (PPK), and high molecular weight kininogen (HK). This system is linked to the intrinsic coagulation system via factor XI (FXI). Animal models showed that production of bradykinin in plasma is ~50% dependent on FXII (74). This suggests the presence of alternative pathways generating bradykinin *in vivo*. The endothelial cell-derived factors *heat shock protein 90* (HSP90) and prolylcarboxypeptidase may be involved in FXII-independent release of bradykinin (75).

Bradykinin was first identified as a mediator for hereditary angioedema (HAE) (76, 77). The genetic form of C1-inhibitor deficiency is due to mutations in one of the two alleles of the C1-inhibitor gene, which leads to either reduced plasma protein levels [hereditary angioedema [HAE] type I] or normal levels but reduced protein function (HAE type II) (78). HAE type III is a rare subtype of HAE that is not connected with C1-inhibitor deficiency but with a dysregulation of the contact (plasma kallikrein-bradykinin) system (79). In a subset of patients with HAE with normal C1-inhibitor, a gain-of-function mutation in FXII has been identified (80). The acquired form of C1-inhibitor deficiency is known as acquired angioedema and is due to C1-inhibitor consumption associated with the presence of anti-C1-inhibitor autoantibodies and/or lymphoproliferative disorders (81). Bradykinin involvement in angioedema pathogenesis is not limited to hereditary forms. Bradykinin is a key mediator in patients with acquired C1-inhibitor deficiency due to underlying auto-immune or lymphoproliferative diseases (82) as well as in those treated with anti-hypertensive drugs that inhibit bradykinin breakdown, such as angiotensin-converting enzyme inhibitors (83). It is also possible that bradykinin may play a supportive role in forms of angioedema that are currently classified as "histaminergic" (84, 85). C1-inhibitor deficiency involves different biological systems that interplay during angioedema attacks. In fact, C1 inhibitor is a serine protease inhibitor (serpin) that blocks the activity of (i) C1r and C1s in the complement system, (ii) factor XII and kallikrein in the contact system, (iii) factor XI and thrombin in the coagulation system, and (iv) tissue plasminogen activator and plasmin in the fibrinolytic system (86). A deficiency in C1 inhibitor results in the hyperactivation of the contact system (87, 88), which leads to the generation of bradykinin. Furthermore, C1-inhibitor deficiencies activate the complement (89) as well as coagulation (90, 91) and fibrinolysis systems (92, 93). Thus, the unregulated activation of coagulation leads to the generation of thrombin, which can potentiate the vasoactive effect of bradykinin both directly (35, 94) and by releasing fibrinopeptides, which enhance the effects of kinins (95). It may be argued that in angioedema due to C1-inhibitor deficiency, thrombin acts synergistically with other vasoactive substances released by the concomitant activation of contact system, complement, or mast cells leading in turn to increased vasopermeability. Plasmin has been assumed to act as a main trigger for contact system activation and bradykinin production in the pathogenesis of most forms of

HAE and specific forms of non-hereditary angioedema (96, 97). Indeed, several clinical observations supported the relevance of plasmin as a natural FXII activator and evidence for plasmin-dependent bradykinin generation as a cause of angioedema during treatment with fibrinolytic agents is accumulating (73). Consistent with this hypothesis, complexes of plasmin with its inhibitor α2-antiplasmin are elevated during attacks of HAE due to C1-inhibitor deficiency, as are the levels of markers of ongoing fibrinolysis, like D-dimer (98). Similarly to CSU, in patients with angioedema there is lack of prothrombotic features (55, 99). Therefore, it may be assumed that in angioedema, factor XII–driven contact system starts inflammatory mechanisms via the bradykinin-producing kallikrein-kinin system, without procoagulant effects (35). Alternatively, it has been proposed that the extreme vascular leakage may move the plasma coagulation factors into the extravascular space, triggering coagulation in the absence of vascular injury or intravascular thrombi (73). Therapy targeting the contact system has been successful in HAE, strongly supporting that angioedema is mediated via bradykinin production (73). Anti-fibrinolytic therapy, mainly tranexamic acid, has been used as prophylactic therapy for HAE attacks for some decades (100).

BULLOUS PEMPHIGOID

Bullous pemphigoid (BP) is an autoimmune blistering disease that mainly affects the elderly and carries a high risk of death (101, 102), mostly due to sepsis and cardiovascular events (103). Either comorbidities or immunosuppressive treatments seem to concur on BP mortality (104). Albeit rare, it is the most common autoimmune blistering disease in Western countries (105). It involves the skin and rarely the mucous membranes and is characterized by the presence of tense blisters usually surrounded by erythematous-edematous, urticaria-like plaques (106, 107). BP has a chronic relapsing evolution, with spontaneous exacerbations and remissions (108). The pathophysiology of BP is linked to the presence of circulating IgG autoantibodies directed against two antigens, BP180 and BP230, which are components of junctional adhesion complexes called hemidesmosomes that promote dermoepidermal cohesion (109, 110) with the contributory role of other pathomechanisms (**Figure 2**). BP180 (type XVII collagen) autoantibodies have been demonstrated to be directly pathogenic by triggering an inflammatory cascade. Inflammatory cells, particularly autoreactive T cells and eosinophils, produce and release a number of cytokines and soluble factors that amplify and maintain tissue damage, which ultimately leads to subepidermal blister formation (111). During acute phase of BP, autoreactive T helper (Th) 1, Th2, and Th17 lymphocytes cooperatively play a role in the development of the disease process (112–114). Although the role of Th17 cells in human BP is not completely defined, recent experimental data showed that IL17A-deficient mice are protected against autoantibody-induced BP, and pharmacological inhibition of IL-17A reduces the induction of BP (115). Moreover, a dysfunction of both T and B regulatory cells, whose immunosurveillance action is critical in preventing autoimmunity, was observed in lesional skin of BP patients (116, 117). The involvement of many cellular players in the BP inflammatory process is supported by elevated serum levels of activation markers, including molecules released by T cells upon their stimulation, molecules involved in B-cell maturation, granule proteins liberated from activated mast cells, neutrophils and eosinophils and adhesion molecules indicative of neutrophil and platelet activation. Complement activation is considered to be critical for blister formation too. Indeed, complement activation by autoantibodies *ex vivo* as measured by the complement-fixation assay in serum was correlated with the clinical disease activity in patients with BP (118). Experimental data in murine models demonstrate that complement-dependent and -independent mechanisms coexist in blister formation. On the basis of knock out mice and pharmacological inhibition studies, the activated 5th component of complement (C5a) appears to be involved, and its receptor 1 (C5aR1) seems to be important during the early phase of the disease while its receptor 2 (C5aR2) seems to be protective. Once the skin inflammation has fully developed, release of reactive oxygen species and proteases from neutrophils and macrophages may become independent of complement (119). Several studies showed that the coagulation cascade is activated in BP and correlates with the severity of the disease (25, 120–123). In particular, coagulation activation markers have been found to be increased at both local level, i.e., in blister fluid, and systemically, i.e., in plasma (123). It has been hypothesized that the activation of blood coagulation is induced by the inflammatory response underlying BP pathogenesis. In this regard, eosinophils are highly represented in the inflammatory infiltrate of the lesional skin and their levels are often increased in peripheral blood (123–125). Elevated concentrations of secretory granules, such as eosinophil cationic protein (ECP) (126, 127) as well as increased levels of IL5, the main cytokine involved in eosinophil biology (128, 129), and IL16, a chemotactic factor for eosinophils (130), in blister fluid and sera of patients with BP confirm the involvement of eosinophils in the pathogenesis of this disease. Eosinophils are recognized to concur in BP elicitation by producing and releasing matrix metalloproteinase (MMP)-9, which plays a key role in degrading BP180 and cleaving the dermal-epidermal junction (131). Release of elastase and gelatinase, namely 92 kDa gelatinase, may further contribute to tissue damage and blister formation (132, 133). Eosinophil degranulation was demonstrated not only in fully developed blisters, but also at the earliest stages of blister development and urticarial lesions of BP (134, 135). Moreover, eosinophils have been postulated as potential intermediates between anti-BP180 IgE autoantibodies, whose pathogenic role in BP has increasingly recognized in recent years, and dermo-epidermal junction separation (136, 137). High-affinity IgE receptors (FcεRI) that are highly expressed on eosinophils in BP patients could enhance the capability of eosinophils to bind IgE and thus influence their subsequent degranulation (138). In recent reports, the monoclonal anti-IgE antibody omalizumab resulted effective in treating patients affected with BP, despite ongoing high levels of anti-skin IgG antibodies (139, 140). This provides further evidence of an independent role for autoreactive IgE-mediated

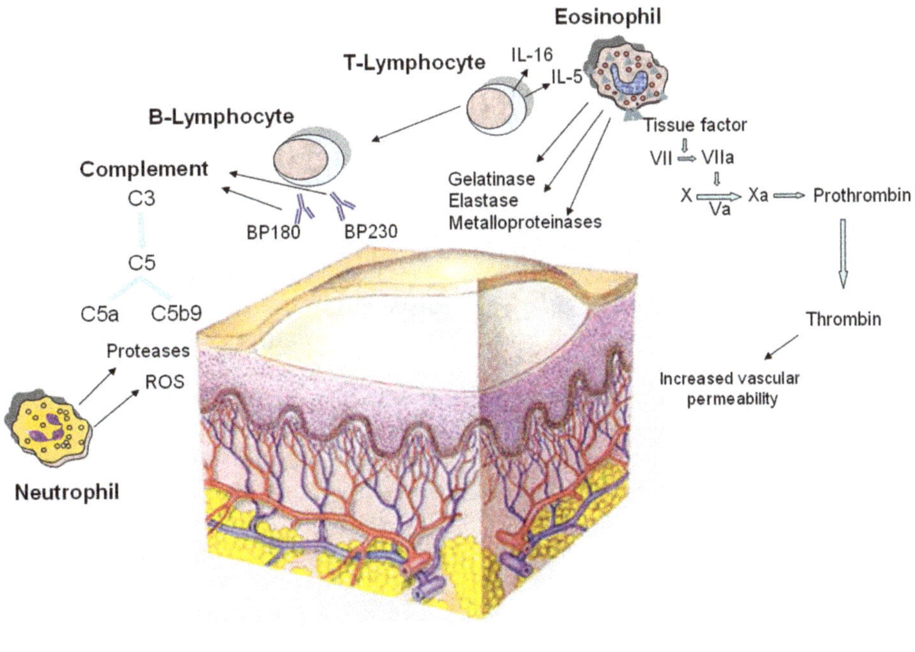

FIGURE 2 | Pathomechanisms of the blister formation in bullous pemphigoid including the involvement of coagulation activation. The dermo-epidermal detachment is due to the interaction of autoantibodies with two hemidesmosomal antigens (BP180 and BP230), followed by complement activation and leukocyte infiltration. Autoreactive T lymphocytes cooperate with B lymphocytes in the autoantibody production; in addition, they release cytokines, most notably IL-5 and IL-16, and other soluble factors responsible for the recruitment and activation of eosinophils. In lesional skin, eosinophils produce and release metalloproteinases, elastase, and gelatinase which contribute to tissue damage. Moreover, eosinophils strongly express tissue factor, which is the main initiator of the coagulation cascade (factors VII, X, VIII, V, and prothrombin) leading to generation of thrombin. This last increases the permeability of blood vessels, amplifying the inflammatory network. Neutrophils contribute in the pathogenesis of bullous pemphigoid by releasing reactive oxygen species (ROS) and proteases. Finally, complement is activated upon binding of the pathogenic autoantibodies to their autoantigens.

inflammation in BP skin lesion development. Eosinophils are also involved in itch induction, mainly due to the release of IL-31 (141, 142). IL31 exerts a chief role in itch, by activating endothelin-1 responsive neurons and by increasing the release of brain natriuretic peptide (BNP), a central mediator of itch (143, 144). With specific reference to the activation of the coagulation cascade in BP, it correlates with eosinophilia other than severity of the disease, thus indicating that eosinophils play a pivotal role in this process (123). Immunohistochemistry showed that eosinophils strongly express TF in lesional skin, as confirmed also by co-localization studies (120, 123). Eosinophils are a major intravascular location for TF storage and exposure. On the other hand, TF facilitates the early transendothelial migration of eosinophils (34). Consistent with these findings, it may be supposed that extrinsic blood coagulation initiated via TF expressed by eosinophils contributes to local inflammation and blister formation (145). In fact, TF plays an important role in the inflammatory process, in addition to its well-documented prothrombotic properties (34). In BP patients, increased skin expression of adhesins and MMPs has been considered an effect of TF action (146). TF is a recognized factor connecting the immune system with coagulation system. Pro-inflammatory cytokines, such as TNF and IL-6, which are increased in BP, induce TF expression (25), as found also in other, very heterogeneous inflammatory conditions (147–149). Activation of the extrinsic coagulation pathway generates thrombin that increases the permeability of blood vessels (150, 151). The presence of thrombin may play a direct role in the pathogenesis of BP by increasing vascular permeability, thus favoring the transendothelial migration of inflammatory cells and their accumulation in the skin. Activated proteases, in turn, act on PARs and induce the expression of various pro-inflammatory cytokines, and this cross-talk between inflammation and coagulation amplifies and maintains the activation of both systems (123). It is noteworthy that BP patients have high levels of coagulation activation markers, such as prothrombin fragment F1+2 (indicating thrombin generation) and D-dimer (indicating fibrin degradation), in plasma samples other than in blister fluid (120, 121, 123). During the disease remission, blood concentration of coagulation activation markers returns to normal (49, 145). Moreover, the concentration of the prothrombin fragment F1+2 correlates with the concentration of immunoglobulins directed against the BP180 antigen (120). All together, these findings clearly indicate that in BP patients there may be an activation of coagulation also at systemic level. A recent study has shown that plasma levels of prothrombotic markers are higher in BP patients when compared with patients affected with CSU (49). In pathological states, especially in inflammatory disorders, the balance between the coagulation and fibrinolysis might be deteriorated (152, 153). It is well known that the inflammatory response inhibits fibrinolysis. The results of a previous study on a group of patients with active BP showed that fibrinolysis is inhibited, due mainly to an increase in the plasma levels of plasminogen activator inhibitor type 1 (PAI-1) activity and antigen (154). The most important clinical consequence of the hypercoagulable state related to both coagulation activation and fibrinolysis inhibition in BP patients is an increased thrombotic risk. It has been consistently reported that the risk of thrombosis is increased in patients with BP (155, 156) and we have found an annual incidence of venous thrombosis of 8% (120), undoubtedly higher than that observed in the general elderly population (157). Langan et al. investigated the main acute medical conditions associated with BP, finding an increased risk for pulmonary embolism (158). A recent multicenter cohort study has shown that the risk of developing venous thromboembolism (VTE) is increased 4-fold in patients with BP as compared with the general population of same age and sex (159). More specifically, the VTE risk increased up to 15 times during the acute phase of the disease, thus indicating a close link between the inflammatory state occurring in active BP and thrombosis. Interestingly, the VTE risk dropped to 1.5 times during clinical remission. This latter finding indicates that a good control of the disease also impacts the occurrence of thrombotic events. This study highlighted in a large cohort of BP patients the close connection between the inflammatory state and risk of VTE. This further emphasizes the tight interplay between inflammation and coagulation cascade. In general, the cardiovascular risk in BP patients may be influenced not only by the inflammatory state but also by the treatment with systemic corticosteroids and immunosuppressive agents (160).

The high thrombotic tendency found in patients with BP, especially during the acute phase of the disease, implies some practical considerations. Firstly, one may wonder whether adding VTE prophylaxis to the immunosuppressive treatments could affect the thrombotic risk of BP patients. Clinical trials on efficacy and safety of antithrombotic drugs administered in the acute phase of the disease could provide some insight into their clinical relevance.

CONCLUSIONS

Coagulation and fibrinolysis activation markers are elevated in many inflammatory conditions, including not only a wide spectrum of systemic diseases of different pathogenesis such as rheumatoid arthritis, inflammatory bowel diseases, and sepsis but also autoimmune or immune-mediated cutaneous disorders. The activation of coagulation in autoimmune skin disorders may have two main consequences: on one hand, a local pathogenic role in inducing the skin lesions and on the other hand a systemic role in increasing the thrombotic risk. Concerning the pathophysiology of the skin lesions, thrombin contributes to increase endothelial vascular permeability, thus amplifying the inflammatory network in CU, angioedema and BP. In the skin microenvironment of CU and BP, eosinophils express tissue factor, which can activate coagulation right there, with the generation of vascular permeability mediators. Concerning the systemic implications of the coagulation involvement, several data indicate an increased thrombotic risk in BP. In contrast, no data are available concerning the incidence of thrombotic complications in patients with CU and angioedema. The retrospective evaluation of a large cohort of patients with BP has shown an increased incidence of venous thrombosis. Although most BP patients are elderly, the incidence of venous thrombosis in this kind of patients appears to be significantly increased as compared to the age-matched population of otherwise healthy subjects. BP is the prototype of autoimmune blistering disorder mediated by autoantibodies but in which an important physiopathological role is played by eosinophils. The intense skin inflammatory infiltrate is in fact characterized by the presence of eosinophils together with autoreactive CD4+ T lymphocytes and a few other inflammatory cells. The increased incidence of thrombosis in autoimmune skin diseases raises the question of the indication of anticoagulant treatment particularly in the presence of other cardiovascular risk factors.

AUTHOR CONTRIBUTIONS

MC, AM, and AB designed and drafted the manuscript. MC, AM, and AB made the literature search. MC, AM, AB, and SG discussed the topics of the manuscript and approved the final version.

REFERENCES

1. Opal SM. Phylogenetic and functional relationships between coagulation and the innate immune response. *Crit Care Med.* (2000) 28:S77–80. doi: 10.1097/00003246-200009001-00017
2. Esmon CT. Crosstalk between inflammation and thrombosis. *Maturitas.* (2008) 61:122–31. doi: 10.1016/j.maturitas.2008.11.008
3. Levi M, van der Poll T. Two-way interactions between inflammation and coagulation. *Trends Cardiovasc Med.* (2005) 15:254–9. doi: 10.1016/j.tcm.2005.07.004
4. Chu AJ. Tissue factor mediates inflammation. *Arch Biochem Biophys.* (2005) 440:123–32. doi: 10.1016/j.abb.2005.06.005
5. Dhar J, Andersen J, Essenmacher L, Ager J, Bentley G, Sokol R. Thrombophilic patterns of coagulation factors in lupus. *Lupus.* (2009) 18:400–6. doi: 10.1177/0961203308097566
6. Kern A, Barabás E, Balog A, Burcsár S, Kiszelák M, Vásárhelyi B. Characterization of the thrombin generation profile in systemic lupus erythematosus. *Physiol Int.* (2017) 104:35–41. doi: 10.1556/2060.104.2017.1.5
7. Ingegnoli F, Fantini F, Favalli EG, Soldi A, Griffini S, Galbiati V, et al. Inflammatory and prothrombotic biomarkers in patients with rheumatoid arthritis: effects of tumor necrosis factor-alpha blockade. *J Autoimmun.* (2008) 31:175–9. doi: 10.1016/j.jaut.2008.07.002
8. Łukasik ZM, Makowski M, Makowska JS. From blood coagulation to innate and adaptive immunity: the role of platelets in the physiology and pathology of autoimmune disorders. *Rheumatol Int.* (2018) 38:959–74. doi: 10.1007/s00296-018-4001-9
9. Borensztajn K, Peppelenbosch MP, Spek CA. Coagulation factor Xa signaling: the link between coagulation and inflammatory bowel disease? *Trends Pharmacol Sci.* (2009) 30:8–16. doi: 10.1016/j.tips.2008.10.007
10. Magro F, Soares JB, Fernandes D. Venous thrombosis and prothrombotic factors in inflammatory bowel disease. *World J Gastroenterol.* (2014) 20:4857–72. doi: 10.3748/wjg.v20.i17.4857
11. Zuberbier T, Aberer W, Asero R, Bindslev-Jensen C, Brzoza Z, Canonica GW, et al. The EAACI/GA^{2}LEN/EDF/WAO Guideline for the definition, classification, diagnosis, and management of urticaria: the 2013 revision and update. *Allergy.* (2014) 69:868–87. doi: 10.1111/all.12313

12. Greaves MW. Pathology and classification of urticaria. *Immunol Allergy Clin North Am.* (2014) 34:1–9. doi: 10.1016/j.iac.2013.07.009
13. Saini SS. Chronic spontaneous urticaria: etiology and pathogenesis. *Immunol Allergy Clin North Am.* (2014) 34:33–52. doi: 10.1016/j.iac.2013.09.012
14. Puccetti A, Bason C, Simeoni S, Millo E, Tinazzi E, Beri R, et al. In chronic idiopathic urticaria autoantibodies against Fc epsilonRII/CD23 induce histamine release via eosinophil activation. *Clin Exp Allergy.* (2005) 35:1599–607. doi: 10.1111/j.1365-2222.2005.02380.x
15. Kasperska-Zajac A, Grzanka A, Damasiewicz-Bodzek A. IL-6 transsignaling in patients with chronic spontaneous urticaria. *PLoS ONE.* (2015) 10:e0145751. doi: 10.1371/journal.pone.0145751
16. Ye YM, Jin HJ, Hwang EK, Nam YH, Kim JH, Shin YS, et al. Co-existence of chronic urticaria and metabolic syndrome: clinical implications. *Acta Derm Venereol.* (2013) 93:156–60. doi: 10.2340/00015555-1443
17. Kolkhir P, Altrichter S, Hawro T, Maurer M. C-reactive protein is linked to disease activity, impact, and response to treatment in patients with chronic spontaneous urticaria. *Allergy.* (2018) 73:940–8. doi: 10.1111/all.13352
18. Trinh HK, Pham DL, Ban GY, Lee HY, Park HS, Ye YM. Altered systemic adipokines in patients with chronic urticaria. *Int Arch Allergy Immunol.* (2016) 171:102–10. doi: 10.1159/000452626
19. Cugno M, Marzano AV, Asero R, Tedeschi A. Activation of blood coagulation in chronic urticaria: pathophysiological and clinical implications. *Intern Emerg Med.* (2010) 5:97–101. doi: 10.1007/s11739-009-0333-5
20. Cugno M, Asero R, Ferrucci S, Lorini M, Carbonelli V, Tedeschi A, et al. Elevated IgE to tissue factor and thyroglobulin are abated by omalizumab in chronic spontaneous urticaria. *Allergy.* (2018) 73:2408–11. doi: 10.1111/all.13587
21. Hatada Y, Kashiwakura J, Hayama K, Fujisawa D, Sasaki-Sakamoto T, Terui T, et al. Significantly high levels of anti-dsDNA immunoglobulin E in sera and the ability of dsDNA to induce the degranulation of basophils from chronic urticaria patients. *Int Arch Allergy Immunol.* (2013) 161:154–8. doi: 10.1159/000350388
22. Altrichter S, Peter HJ, Pisarevskaja D, Metz M, Martus P, Maurer M. IgE mediated autoallergy against thyroid peroxidase–a novel pathomechanism of chronic spontaneous urticaria? *PLoS ONE.* (2011) 6:e14794. doi: 10.1371/journal.pone.0014794
23. Schmetzer O, Lakin E, Topal FA, Preusse P, Freier D, Church MK, et al. IL-24 is a common and specific autoantigen of IgE in patients with chronic spontaneous urticaria. *J Allergy Clin Immunol.* (2018) 142:876–82. doi: 10.1016/j.jaci.2017.10.035
24. Tedeschi A, Kolkhir P, Asero R, Pogorelov D, Olisova O, Kochergin N, et al. Chronic urticaria and coagulation: pathophysiological and clinical aspects. *Allergy.* (2014) 69:683–91. doi: 10.1111/all.12389
25. Cugno M, Tedeschi A, Asero R, Meroni PL, Marzano AV. Skin autoimmunity and blood coagulation. *Autoimmunity.* (2010) 43:189–94. doi: 10.3109/08916930903293086
26. O'Donnell BF, O'Neill CM, Francis DM, Niimi N, Barr RM, Barlow RJ, et al. Human leucocyte antigen class II associations in chronic idiopathic urticaria. *Br J Dermatol.* (1999) 140:853–8. doi: 10.1046/j.1365-2133.1999.02815.x
27. Kessel A, Bishara R, Amital A, Bamberger E, Sabo E, Grushko G, et al. Increased plasma levels of matrix metalloproteinase-9 are associated with the severity of chronic urticaria. *Clin Exp Allergy.* (2005) 35:221–5. doi: 10.1111/j.1365-2222.2005.02168.x
28. Asero R, Tedeschi A, Marzano AV, Cugno M. Chronic urticaria: a focus on pathogenesis. *F1000Res.* (2017) 6:1095. doi: 10.12688/f1000research.11546.1
29. Asero R, Tedeschi A, Riboldi P, Cugno M. Plasma of chronic urticaria patients shows signs of thrombin generation and its intradermal injection causes wheal-and-flare reactions much more frequently than autologous serum. *J Allergy Clin Immunol.* (2006) 117:1113–7. doi: 10.1016/j.jaci.2005.12.1343
30. Asero R, Tedeschi A, Coppola R, Griffini S, Paparella P, Riboldi P, et al. Activation of the tissue pathway of blood coagulation in patients with chronic urticaria. *J Allergy Clin Immunol.* (2007) 119:705–10. doi: 10.1016/j.jaci.2006.08.043
31. Asero R, Tedeschi A, Riboldi P, Griffini S, Bonanni E, Cugno M. Severe chronic urticaria is associated with elevated plasma levels of D-dimer. *Allergy.* (2008) 63:176–80. doi: 10.1111/j.1398-9995.2007.01514.x
32. Cugno M, Marzano AV, Tedeschi A, Fanoni D, Venegoni L, Asero R. Expression of tissue factor by eosinophils in patients with chronic urticaria. *Int Arch Allergy Immunol.* (2009) 148:170–4. doi: 10.1159/000155748
33. Takeda T, Sakurai Y, Takahagi S, Kato J, Yoshida K, Yoshioka A, et al. Increase of coagulation potential in chronic spontaneous urticaria. *Allergy.* (2011) 66:428–33. doi: 10.1111/j.1398-9995.2010.02506.x
34. Moosbauer C, Morgenstern E, Cuvelier SL, Manukyan D, Bidzhekov K, Albrecht S, et al. Eosinophils are a major intravascular location for tissue factor storage and exposure. *Blood.* (2007) 109:995–1002. doi: 10.1182/blood-2006-02-004945
35. Schaeffer RC, Gong F, Bitrick MS, Smith TL. Thrombin and bradykinin initiate discrete endothelial solute permeability mechanisms. *Am J Physiol.* (1993) 264:1798–809. doi: 10.1152/ajpheart.1993.264.6.H1798
36. Asero R, Riboldi P, Tedeschi A, Cugno M, Meroni P. Chronic urticaria: a disease at a crossroad between autoimmunity and coagulation. *Autoimmun Rev.* (2007) 7:71–6. doi: 10.1016/j.autrev.2007.08.002
37. Huber-Lang M, Sarma JV, Zetoune FS, Rittirsch D, Neff TA, McGuire SR, et al. Generation of C5a in the absence of C3: a new complement activation pathway. *Nat Med.* (2006) 12:682–7. doi: 10.1038/nm1419
38. Vliagoftis H. Thrombin induces mast cell adhesion to fibronectin: evidence for the involvement of protease activated receptor-1. *J Immunol.* (2002) 169:4551–8. doi: 10.4049/jimmunol.169.8.4551
39. Razin E, Marx G. Thrombin-induced degranulation of cultured bone marrow derived mast cells. *J Immunol.* (1984) 133:3282–5.
40. Dugina TN, Kiseleva EV, Glusa E, Strukova SM. Activation of mast cells induced by agonists of proteinase-activated receptors under normal conditions and during acute inflammation in rats. *Eur J Pharmacol.* (2003) 471:141–7. doi: 10.1016/S0014-2999(03)01752-7
41. Yanase Y, Takahagi S, Hide M. Chronic spontaneous urticaria and the extrinsic coagulation system. *Allergol Int.* (2018) 67:191–4. doi: 10.1016/j.alit.2017.09.003
42. Cirino G, Cicala C, Bucci MR, Sorrentino L, Maranganore JM, Stone SR. Thrombin functions as an inflammatory mediator through activation of its receptors. *J Exp Med.* (1996) 183:821–7. doi: 10.1084/jem.183.3.821
43. Tedeschi A, Asero R, Lorini M, Marzano AV, Cugno M. Plasma levels of matrix metalloproteinase-9 in chronic urticaria patients correlate with disease severity and C-reactive protein but not with circulating histamine-releasing factors. *Clin Exp Allergy.* (2010) 40:875–81. doi: 10.1111/j.1365-2222.2010.03473.x
44. van der Poll T, de Boer JD, Levi M. The effect of inflammation on coagulation and vice versa. *Curr Opin Infect Dis.* (2011) 24:273–8. doi: 10.1097/QCO.0b013e328344c078
45. Kido H, Fukusen N, Katunuma M, Morita T, Iwanaga S. Tryptase from rat mast cells converts bovine prothrombin to thrombin. *Biochem Biophys Res Commun.* (1985) 132:613–9. doi: 10.1016/0006-291X(85)91177-5
46. Suender CA, Leist M, Åbrink M, Valentin P, Geldmacher A, Steinhoff M, et al. Mast cells are critical for the limitation of thrombin-induced skin inflammation. *Exp Dermatol.* (2018) 27:50–7. doi: 10.1111/exd.13407
47. Wang F, Tang H, Xu JH, Kang KF. Activation of the blood coagulation cascade is involved in patients with chronic urticaria. *J Allergy Clin Immunol.* (2009) 123:972–3. doi: 10.1016/j.jaci.2009.01.039
48. Fujii K, Usuki A, Kan-No Y, Ohgou N. Elevation of circulating thrombin-antithrombin III complex and fibrin degradation products in urticaria. A laboratory finding unrelated to intravascular coagulopathy. *J Dermatol.* (2008) 35:308–10. doi: 10.1111/j.1346-8138.2008.00474.x
49. Cugno M, Tedeschi A, Borghi A, Bucciarelli P, Asero R, Venegoni L, et al. Activation of blood coagulation in two prototypic autoimmune skin diseases: a possible link with thrombotic risk. *PLoS ONE.* (2015) 10:e0129456. doi: 10.1371/journal.pone.0129456
50. Triwongwaranat D, Kulthanan K, Chularojanamontri L, Pinkaew S. Correlation between plasma D-dimer levels and the severity of patients with chronic urticaria. *Asia Pac Allergy.* (2013) 3:100–5. doi: 10.5415/apallergy.2013.3.2.100
51. Criado PR, Antinori LC, Maruta CW, Reis VM. Evaluation of D-dimer serum levels among patients with chronic urticaria, psoriasis and urticarial vasculitis. *An Bras Dermatol.* (2013) 88:355–60. doi: 10.1590/abd1806-4841.20131532

52. Takahagi S, Mihara S, Iwamoto K, Morioke S, Okabe T, Kameyoshi Y, et al. Coagulation/fibrinolysis and inflammation markers are associated with disease activity in patients with chronic urticaria. *Allergy.* (2010) 65:649e56. doi: 10.1111/j.1398-9995.2009.02222.x
53. Grzanka R, Damasiewicz-Bodzek A, Kasperska-Zajac A. Interplay between acute phase response and coagulation/fibrinolysis in chronic spontaneous urticaria. *Allergy Asthma Clin Immunol.* (2018) 18:14. doi: 10.1186/s13223-018-0255-8
54. Khalaf AT, Liu XM, Sheng WX, Tan JQ, Abdalla AN. Efficacy and safety of desloratadine combined with dipyridamole in the treatment of chronic urticaria. *J Eur Acad Dermatol Venereol.* (2008) 22:487–92. doi: 10.1111/j.1468-3083.2007.02511.x
55. Cugno M, Asero R, Tedeschi A, Lazzari R, Marzano AV. Inflammation and coagulation in urticaria and angioedema. *Curr Vasc Pharmacol.* (2012) 10:653–8. doi: 10.2174/157016112801784558
56. Vena GA, Cassano N, Marzano AV, Asero R. The role of platelets in chronic urticaria. *Int Arch Allergy Immunol.* (2016) 169:71–9. doi: 10.1159/000444085
57. Kasperska-Zajac A, Brzoza Z, Rogala B. Platelet function in cutaneous diseases. *Platelets.* (2008) 19:317–21. doi: 10.1080/095371008020 82249
58. Tamagawa-Mineoka R, Katoh N, Kishimoto S. Platelet activation in patients with psoriasis: increased plasma levels of platelet-derived microparticles and soluble P-selectin. *J Am Acad Dermatol.* (2010) 62:621–6. doi: 10.1016/j.jaad.2009.06.053
59. Ghasemzadeh M, Hosseini E. Platelet-leukocyte crosstalk: linking proinflammatory responses to procoagulant state. *Thromb Res.* (2013) 131:191–7. doi: 10.1016/j.thromres.2012.11.028
60. Meyer-De Schmid JJ, Neuman A. Treatment of chronic urticaria with heparin. *Bull Soc Fr Dermatol Syphiligr.* (1952) 59:286–7.
61. Chua SL, Gibbs S. Chronic urticaria responding to subcutaneous heparin sodium. *Br J Dermatol.* (2005) 153:216–7. doi: 10.1111/j.1365-2133.2005.06694.x
62. Asero R, Tedeschi A, Cugno M. Heparin and tranexamic Acid therapy may be effective in treatment-resistant chronic urticaria with elevated d-dimer: a pilot study. *Int Arch Allergy Immunol.* (2010) 152:384–9. doi: 10.1159/000292947
63. Parslew R, Pryce D, Ashworth J, Friedmann PS. Warfarin treatment of chronic idiopathic urticaria and angio-oedema. *Clin Exp Allergy.* (2000) 30:1161–5. doi: 10.1046/j.1365-2222.2000.00857.x
64. Asero R. D-dimer: a biomarker for antihistamine-resistant chronic urticaria. *J Allergy Clin Immunol.* (2013) 132:983–6. doi: 10.1016/j.jaci.2013.04.037
65. Asero R. Plasma D-dimer levels and clinical response to ciclosporin in severe chronic spontaneous urticaria. *J Allergy Clin Immunol.* (2015) 135:1401–3. doi: 10.1016/j.jaci.2014.11.016
66. Cugno M, Genovese G, Ferrucci S, Casazza G, Asero R, Marzano AV. IgE and D-dimer baseline levels are higher in responders than nonresponders to omalizumab in chronic spontaneous urticaria. *Br J Dermatol.* (2018) 179:776–7. doi: 10.1111/bjd.16593
67. Asero R, Marzano AV, Ferrucci S, Cugno M. D-dimer plasma levels parallel the clinical response to omalizumab in patients with severe chronic spontaneous urticaria. *Int Arch Allergy Immunol.* (2017) 172:40–4. doi: 10.1159/000453453
68. Acer E, Kaya Erdogan H, Yüksel Çanak,çi N, Saracoglu ZN. The effect of omalizumab on hematological and inflammatory parameters in patients with chronic spontaneous urticaria. *Cutan Ocul Toxicol.* (2018) 10:1–4. doi: 10.1080/15569527.2018.1495227
69. Kaplan AP, Giménez-Arnau AM, Saini SS. Mechanisms of action that contribute to efficacy of omalizumab in chronic spontaneous urticaria. *Allergy.* (2017) 72:519–33. doi: 10.1111/all.13083
70. Depetri F, Tedeschi A, Cugno M. Angioedema and emergency medicine: from pathophysiology to diagnosis and treatment. *Eur J Intern Med.* (2019) 59:8–13. doi: 10.1016/j.ejim.2018.09.004
71. Antia C, Baquerizo K, Korman A, Bernstein JA, Alikhan A. Urticaria: a comprehensive review: epidemiology, diagnosis, and work-up. *J Am Acad Dermatol.* (2018) 79:599–614. doi: 10.1016/j.jaad.2018.01.020
72. Borriello F, Granata F, Marone G. Basophils and skin disorders. *J Invest Dermatol.* (2014) 134:1202–10. doi: 10.1038/jid.2014.16
73. Hofman Z, de Maat S, Hack CE, Maas C. Bradykinin: inflammatory product of the coagulation system. *Clin Rev Allergy Immunol.* (2016) 51:152–61. doi: 10.1007/s12016-016-8540-0
74. Iwaki T, Castellino FJ. Plasma levels of bradykinin are suppressed in factor XII-deficient mice. *Thromb Haemost.* (2006) 95:1003–10. doi: 10.1160/TH06-03-0128
75. Joseph K, Tholanikunnel BG, Bygum A, Ghebrehiwet B, Kaplan AP. Factor XII-independent activation of the bradykininforming cascade: Implications for the pathogenesis of hereditary angioedema types I and II. *J Allergy Clin Immunol.* (2013) 132:470–5. doi: 10.1016/j.jaci.2013.03.026
76. Nussberger J, Cugno M, Amstutz C, Cicardi M, Pellacani A, Agostoni A. Plasma bradykinin in angio-oedema. *Lancet.* (1998) 351:1693–7. doi: 10.1016/S0140-6736(97)09137-X
77. Nussberger J, Cugno M, Cicardi M, Agostoni A. Local bradykinin generation in hereditary angioedema. *J Allergy Clin Immunol.* (1999) 104:1321–2. doi: 10.1016/S0091-6749(99)70030-8
78. Cugno M, Zanichelli A, Foieni F, Caccia S, Cicardi M. C1-inhibitor deficiency and angioedema: Molecular mechanisms and clinical progress. *Trends Mol Med.* (2009) 15:69–78. doi: 10.1016/j.molmed.2008.12.001
79. Riedl MA. Hereditary angioedema with normal C1-INH (HAE type III). *J Allergy Clin Immunol Pract.* (2013) 1:427–32. doi: 10.1016/j.jaip.2013.06.004
80. Cichon S, Martin L, Hennies HC, Müller F, Van Driessche K, Karpushova A, et al. Increased activity of coagulation factor XII (Hageman factor) causes hereditary angioedema type III. *Am J Hum Genet.* (2006) 79:1098–104. doi: 10.1086/509899
81. Cugno M, Castelli R, Cicardi M. Angioedema due to acquired C1-inhibitor deficiency: a bridging condition between autoimmunity and lymphoproliferation. *Autoimmun Rev.* (2008) 8:156–9. doi: 10.1016/j.autrev.2008.05.003
82. Wu MA, Castelli R. The Janus faces of acquired angioedema: C1-inhibitor deficiency, lymphoproliferation and autoimmunity. *Clin Chem Lab Med.* (2016) 54:207–14. doi: 10.1515/cclm-2015-0195
83. Liau Y, Chua I, Kennedy MA, Maggo S. Pharmacogenetics of angiotensin converting enzyme inhibitor - induced angioedema. *Clin Exp Allergy.* (2019) 49:142–54. doi: 10.1111/cea.13326
84. Nussberger J, Cugno M, Cicardi M. Bradykinin-mediated angioedema. *N Engl J Med.* (2002) 347:621–2. doi: 10.1056/NEJM200208223470820
85. Sala-Cunill A, Björkqvist J, Senter R, Guilarte M, Cardona V, Labrador M, et al. Plasma contact system activation drives anaphylaxis in severe mast cell-mediated allergic reactions. *J Allergy Clin Immunol.* (2014) 135:1031–43. doi: 10.1016/j.jaci.2014.07.057
86. Davis AEIII. C1 inhibitor and hereditary angioneurotic edema. *Annu Rev Immunol.* (1988) 6:595–628. doi: 10.1146/annurev.iy.06.040188.003115
87. Cugno M, Bergamaschini L, Uziel L, Cicardi M, Agostoni A, Jie AF, et al. Haemostasis contact system and fibrinolysis in hereditary angioedema (C1-inhibitor deficiency). *J Clin Chem Clin Biochem.* (1988) 26:423–7. doi: 10.1515/cclm.1988.26.7.423
88. Cugno M, Cicardi M, Coppola R, Agostoni A. Activation of factor XII and cleavage of high molecular weight kininogen during acute attacks in hereditary and acquired C1-inhibitor deficiencies. *Immunopharmacology.* (1996) 33:361–4. doi: 10.1016/0162-3109(96)00086-0
89. Cugno M, Nuijens J, Hack E, Eerenberg A, Frangi D, Agostoni A, et al. Plasma levels of C1-inhibitor complexes and cleaved C1-inhibitor in patients with hereditary angioneurotic edema. *J Clin Invest.* (1990) 85:1215–20. doi: 10.1172/JCI114555
90. Cugno M, Cicardi M, Bottasso B, Coppola R, Paonessa R, Mannucci PM, et al. Activation of the coagulation cascade in C1-inhibitor deficiencies. *Blood.* (1997) 89:3213–8.
91. Cugno M, Zanichelli A, Bellatorre AG, Griffini S, Cicardi M. Plasma biomarkers of acute attacks in patients with angioedema due to C1-inhibitor deficiency. *Allergy.* (2009) 64:254–7. doi: 10.1111/j.1398-9995.2008.01859.x
92. Cugno M, Cicardi M, Agostoni A. Activation of the contact system and fibrinolysis in autoimmune acquired angioedema: a rationale for prophylactic use of tranexamic acid. *J Allergy Clin Immunol.* (1994) 93:870–6. doi: 10.1016/0091-6749(94)90380-8
93. Cugno M, Hack CE, de Boer JP, Eerenberg AJ, Agostoni A, Cicardi M. Generation of plasmin during acute attacks of hereditary angioedema. *J Lab Clin Med.* (1993) 121:38–43.

94. Ehringer WD, Edwards MJ, Miller FN. Mechanisms of a-thrombin, histamine, and bradykinin induced endothelial permeability. *J Cell Physiol.* (1996) 167:562. doi: 10.1002/(SICI)1097-4652(199606)167:3<562::AID-JCP20>3.0.CO;2-4
95. Donaldson VH. Blood coagulation and related plasma enzymes in inflammation. *Ser Haemat.* (1970) 3:39.
96. De Maat S, Hofman ZLM, Maas C. Hereditary angioedema: the plasma contact system out of control. *J Thromb Haemost.* (2018) 16:1674–85. doi: 10.1111/jth.14209
97. Maas C, Renné T. Coagulation factor XII in thrombosis and inflammation. *Blood.* (2018) 131:1903–9. doi: 10.1182/blood-2017-04-569111
98. Varga L, Farkas H. Comprehensive study into the activation of the plasma enzyme systems during attacks of hereditary angioedema due to C1-inhibitor deficiency. *Orphanet J Rare Dis.* (2015) 10:132. doi: 10.1186/s13023-015-0351-5
99. Reshef A, Zanichelli A, Longhurst H, Relan A, Hack CE. Elevated D-dimers in attacks of hereditary angioedema are not associated with increased thrombotic risk. *Allergy.* (2015) 70:506–13. doi: 10.1111/all.12587
100. Mansi M, Zanichelli A, Coerezza A, Suffritti C, Wu MA, Vacchini R, et al. Presentation, diagnosis and treatment of angioedema without wheals: a retrospective analysis of a cohort of 1058 patients. *J Intern Med.* (2015) 277:585–93. doi: 10.1111/joim.12304
101. Kridin K, Shihade W, Bergman R. Mortality in patients with bullous pemphigoid: a retrospective cohort study, systematic review and meta-analysis. *Acta Derm Venereol.* (2018) 99:72–7. doi: 10.2340/00015555-2930
102. Rozenblat M, Halaj A, Rozenblat T, Fisher S, Sah M, Dodiuk-Gad RP, et al. Mortality and risk factors among Israeli bullous pemphigoid patients. *Arch Dermatol Res.* (2019) 311:19–27. doi: 10.1007/s00403-018-1875-z
103. Roujeau JC, Lok C, Bastuji-Garin S, Mhalla S, Enginger V, Bernard P. High risk of death in elderly patients with extensive bullous pemphigoid. *Arch Dermatol.* (1998) 134:465–9. doi: 10.1001/archderm.134.4.465
104. Bernard P, Antonicelli F. Bullous Pemphigoid: A Review of its Diagnosis, Associations and Treatment. *Am J Clin Dermatol.* (2017) 18:513–28. doi: 10.1007/s40257-017-0264-2
105. Kridin K, Ludwig RJ. The growing incidence of bullous pemphigoid: overview and potential explanations. *Front Med.* (2018) 5:220. doi: 10.3389/fmed.2018.00220
106. della Torre R, Combescure C, Cortes B, Marazza G, Beltraminelli H, Naldi L, et al. Clinical presentation and diagnostic delay in bullous pemphigoid: a prospective nationwide cohort. *Br J Dermatol.* (2012) 167:1111–7. doi: 10.1111/j.1365-2133.2012.11108.x
107. Yancey KB, Egan CA. Pemphigoid: clinical, histologic, immunopathologic, and therapeutic considerations. *JAMA.* (2000) 284:350–6. doi: 10.1001/jama.284.3.350
108. Bernard P, Reguiai Z, Tancrède-Bohin E, Cordel N, Plantin P, Pauwels C, et al. Risk factors for relapse in patients with bullous pemphigoid in clinical remission: a multicenter, prospective, cohort study. *Arch Dermatol.* (2009) 145:537–42. doi: 10.1001/archdermatol.2009.53
109. Yancey KB. The pathophysiology of autoimmune blistering diseases. *J Clin Invest.* (2005) 115:825–8. doi: 10.1172/JCI200524855
110. Bagci IS, Horváth ON, Ruzicka T, Sárdy M. Bullous pemphigoid. *Autoimmun Rev.* (2017) 16:445–55. doi: 10.1016/j.autrev.2017.03.010
111. Hertl M, Eming R, Veldman C. T cell control in autoimmune bullous skin disorders. *J Clin Invest.* (2006) 116:1159–66. doi: 10.1172/JCI28547
112. Lo Schiavo A, Ruocco E, Brancaccio G, Caccavale S, Ruocco V, Wolf R. Bullous pemphigoid: etiology, pathogenesis, and inducing factors: facts and controversies. *Clin Dermatol.* (2013) 31:391–9. doi: 10.1016/j.clindermatol.2013.01.006
113. Le Jan S, Plée J, Vallerand D, Dupont A, Delanez E, Durlach A, et al. Innate immune cell-produced IL-17 sustains inflammation in bullous pemphigoid. *J Invest Dermatol.* (2014) 134:2908–17. doi: 10.1038/jid.2014.263
114. Arakawa M, Dainichi T, Ishii N, Hamada T, Karashima T, Nakama T, et al. Lesional Th17 cells and regulatory T cells in bullous pemphigoid. *Exp Dermatol.* (2011) 20:1022–24. doi: 10.1111/j.1600-0625.2011.01378.x
115. Chakievska L, Holtsche MM, Künstner A, Goletz S, Petersen BS, Thaci D, et al. IL-17A is functionally relevant and a potential therapeutic target in bullous pemphigoid. *J Autoimmun.* (2019) 96:104–12. doi: 10.1016/j.jaut.2018.09.003
116. Gambichler T, Tsitlakidon A, Skrygan M, Höxtermann S, Susok L, Hessam S. T regulatory cells and other lymphocyte subsets in patients with bullous pemphigoid. *Clin Exp Dermatol.* (2017) 42:632–7. doi: 10.1111/ced.13135
117. Liu Z, Dang E, Li B, Qiao H, Jin L, Zhang J, et al. Dysfunction of CD19+CD24hiCD27+ B regulatory cells in patients with bullous pemphigoid. *Sci Rep.* (2018) 8:703. doi: 10.1038/s41598-018-19226-z
118. Chiorean RM, Baican A, Mustafa MB, Lischka A, Leucuta DC, Feldrihan V, et al. Complement-activating capacity of autoantibodies correlates with disease activity in bullous pemphigoid patients. *Front Immunol.* (2018) 9:2687. doi: 10.3389/fimmu.2018.02687
119. Karsten CM, Beckmann T, Holtsche MM, Tillmann J, Tofern S, Schulze FS, et al. Tissue destruction in bullous pemphigoid can be complement independent and may be mitigated by C5aR2. *Front Immunol.* (2018) 9:488. doi: 10.3389/fimmu.2018.00488
120. Marzano AV, Tedeschi A, Fanoni D, Bonanni E, Venegoni L, Berti E, et al. Activation of blood coagulation in bullous pemphigoid: role of eosinophils, and local and systemic implications. *Br J Dermatol.* (2009) 160:266–72. doi: 10.1111/j.1365-2133.2008.08880.x
121. Marzano AV, Tedeschi A, Spinelli D, Fanoni D, Crosti C, Cugno M. Coagulation activation in autoimmune bullous diseases. *Clin Exp Immunol.* (2009) 158:31–6. doi: 10.1111/j.1365-2249.2009.03989.x
122. Cugno M, Tedeschi A, Crosti C, Marzano AV. Activation of blood coagulation in autoimmune skin disorders. *Exp Rev Clin Immunol.* (2009) 5:605–13. doi: 10.1586/eci.09.40
123. Marzano AV, Tedeschi A, Berti E, Crosti C, Cugno M. Activation of coagulation in bullous pemphigoid and other eosinophil-related inflammatory skin diseases. *Clin Exp Immunol.* (2011) 165:44–50. doi: 10.1111/j.1365-2249.2011.04391.x
124. de Graauw E, Sitaru C, Horn M, Borradori L, Yousefi S, Simon HU, et al. Evidence for a role of eosinophils in blister formation in bullous pemphigoid. *Allergy.* (2017) 72:1105–13. doi: 10.1111/all.13131
125. Kridin K. Peripheral eosinophilia in bullous pemphigoid: prevalence and influence on the clinical manifestation. *Br J Dermatol.* (2018) 79:1141–7. doi: 10.1111/bjd.16679
126. Giusti D, Gatouillat G, Le Jan S, Plee J, Bernard P, Antonicelli F, et al. Eosinophil Cationic Protein (ECP), a predictive marker of bullous pemphigoid severity and outcome. *Sci Rep.* (2017) 7:4833. doi: 10.1038/s41598-017-04687-5
127. Tedeschi A, Marzano AV, Lorini M, Balice Y, Cugno M. Eosinophil cationic protein levels parallel coagulation activation in the blister fluid of patients with bullous pemphigoid. *J Eur Acad Dermatol Venereol.* (2015) 29:813–7. doi: 10.1111/jdv.12464
128. Wakugawa M, Nakamura K, Hino H, Toyama K, Hattori N, Okochi H, et al. Elevated levels of eotaxin and interleukin-5 in blister fluid of bullous pemphigoid: correlation with tissue eosinophilia. *Br J Dermatol.* (2000) 143:112–6. doi: 10.1046/j.1365-2133.2000.03599.x
129. Engineer L, Bhol K, Kumari S, Razzaque Ahmed A. Bullous pemphigoid: interaction of interleukin 5, anti-basement membrane zone antibodies and eosinophils. A preliminary observation. *Cytokine.* (2001) 13:32–8. doi: 10.1006/cyto.2000.0791
130. Frezzolini A, Cianchini G, Ruffelli M, Cadoni S, Puddu P, De Pità O. Interleukin-16 expression and release in bullous pemphigoid. *Clin Exp Immunol.* (2004) 137:595–600. doi: 10.1111/j.1365-2249.2004.02570.x
131. Amber KT, Valdebran M, Kridin K, Grando SA. The role of eosinophils in bullous pemphigoid: a developing model of eosinophil pathogenicity in mucocutaneous disease. *Front Med.* (2018) 5:201. doi: 10.3389/fmed.2018.00201
132. Shimanovich I, Mihai S, Oostingh GJ, Ilenchuk TT, Bröcker EB, Opdenakker G, et al. Granulocyte-derived elastase and gelatinase B are required for dermal-epidermal separation induced by autoantibodies from patients with epidermolysis bullosa acquisita and bullous pemphigoid. *J Pathol.* (2004) 204:519–27. doi: 10.1002/path.1674
133. Ståhle-Bäckdahl M, Inoue M, Guidice GJ, Parks WC. 92-kD gelatinase is produced by eosinophils at the site of blister formation in bullous pemphigoid and cleaves the extracellular domain of recombinant 180-kD bullous pemphigoid autoantigen. *J Clin Invest.* (1994) 93:2022–30. doi: 10.1172/JCI117196

134. Borrego L, Maynard B, Peterson EA, George T, Iglesias L, Peters MS, et al. Deposition of eosinophil granule proteins precedes blister formation in bullous pemphigoid. Comparison with neutrophil and mast cell granule proteins. *Am J Pathol.* (1996) 148:897–909.
135. Davis MD, Plager DA, George TJ, Weiss EA, Gleich GJ, Leiferman KM. Interactions of eosinophil granule proteins with skin: limits of detection, persistence, and vasopermeabilization. *J Allergy Clin Immunol.* (2003) 112:988–94. doi: 10.1016/j.jaci.2003.08.028
136. Lin L, Hwang BJ, Culton DA, Li N, Burette S, Koller BH, et al. Eosinophils mediate tissue injury in autoimmune skin disease bullous pemphigoid. *J Invest Dermatol.* (2017) 138:1032–43. doi: 10.1016/j.jid.2017.11.031
137. Cozzani E, Gasparini G, Di Zenzo G, Parodi A. Immunoglobulin E and bullous pemphigoid. *Eur J Dermatol.* (2018) 28:440–8. doi: 10.1684/ejd.2018.3366
138. Messingham KN, Holahan HM, Frydman AS, Fullenkamp C, Srikantha R, Fairley JA. Human eosinophils express the high affinity IgE receptor, FcεRI, in bullous pemphigoid. *PLoS ONE.* (2014) 9:e107725. doi: 10.1371/journal.pone.0107725
139. James T, Salman S, Stevenson B, Bundell C, Kelly G, Nolan D, et al. IgE blockade in autoimmunity: omalizumab induced remission of bullous pemphigoid. *Clin Immunol.* (2018) 198:54–6. doi: 10.1016/j.clim.2018.12.015
140. Kremer N, Snast I, Cohen ES, Hodak E, Mimouni D, Lapidoth M, et al. Rituximab and omalizumab for the treatment of bullous pemphigoid: a systematic review of the literature. *Am J Clin Dermatol.* (2018) 2018:6. doi: 10.1007/s40257-018-0401-6
141. Rudrich U, Gehring M, Papakonstantinou E, Rabenhorst A, Engmann J, Kapp A, et al. Eosinophils are a major source of interleukin-31 in bullous pemphigoid. *Acta Derm Venereol.* (2018) 98:766–71. doi: 10.2340/00015555-2951
142. Kunsleben N, Rudrich U, Gehring M, Novak N, Kapp A, Raap U. IL-31 induces chemotaxis, calciummobilization, release of reactive oxygen species, and CCL26 in eosinophils, which are capable to release IL-31. *J Invest Dermatol.* (2015) 135:1908–11. doi: 10.1038/jid.2015.106
143. Bonciani D, Quintarelli L, Del Bianco E, Bianchi B, Caproni M. Serum levels and tissue expression of interleukin-31 in dermatitis herpetiformis and bullous pemphigoid. *J Dermatol Sci.* (2017) 87:210–2. doi: 10.1016/j.jdermsci.2017.04.008
144. Salz M, Haeberle S, Hoffmann J, Enk AH, Hadaschik EN. Elevated IL-31 serum levels in bullous pemphigoid patients correlate with eosinophil numbers and are associated with BP180-IgE. *J Dermatol Sci.* (2017) 87:309–11. doi: 10.1016/j.jdermsci.2017.07.019
145. Zebrowska A, Wagrowska-Danilewicz M, Danilewicz M, Wieczfinska J, Pniewska E, Zebrowski M, et al. Tissue factor in dermatitis herpetiformis and bullous pemphigoid: link between immune and coagulation system in subepidermal autoimmune bullous diseases. *Mediat Inflamm.* (2015) 2015:870428. doi: 10.1155/2015/870428
146. Narbutt J, Waszczykowska E, Lukamowicz J, Sysa-Jedrzejowska A, Kobos J, Zebrowska A. Disturbances of the expression of metalloproteinases and their tissue inhibitors cause destruction of the basement membrane in pemphigoid. *Pol J Pathol.* (2006) 57:71–6.
147. So AK, Varisco PA, Kemkes-Matthes B, Herkenne-Morard C, Chobaz-Péclat V, Gerster JC, et al. Arthritis is linked to local and systemic activation of coagulation and fibrinolysis pathways. *J Thromb Haemost.* (2003) 1:2510–5. doi: 10.1111/j.1538-7836.2003.00462.x
148. Kume K, Yamasaki M, Tashiro M, Yoshikawa I, Otsuki M. Activations of coagulation and fibrinolysis secondary to bowel inflammation in patients with ulcerative colitis. *Intern Med.* (2007) 46:1323–9. doi: 10.2169/internalmedicine.46.0237
149. Liaw PC, Esmon CT, Kahnamoui K, Schmidt S, Kahnamoui S, Ferrell G, et al. Patients with severe sepsis vary markedly in their ability to generate activated protein C. *Blood.* (2004) 104:3958–64. doi: 10.1182/blood-2004-03-1203
150. Garcia JG, Siflinger-Birnboim A, Bizios R, Del Vecchio PJ, Fenton JW II, Malik AB. Thrombin-induced increase in albumin permeability across the endothelium. *J Cell Physiol.* (1986) 128:96–104. doi: 10.1002/jcp.10412 80115
151. DeMichele MA, Moon DG, Fenton JW II, Minnear FL. Thrombin's enzymatic activity increases permeability of endothelial cell monolayers. *J Appl Physiol.* (1990) 69:1599–606. doi: 10.1152/jappl.1990.69.5.1599
152. Saibeni S, Ciscato C, Vecchi M, Boscolo Anzoletti M, Kaczmarek E, Caccia S, et al. Antibodies to tissue-type plasminogen activator (t-PA) in patients with inflammatory bowel disease: high prevalence, interactions with functional domains of t-PA and possible implications in thrombosis. *J Thromb Haemost.* (2006) 4:1510–6. doi: 10.1111/j.1538-7836.2006.01970.x
153. Ingegnoli F, Fantini F, Griffini S, Soldi A, Meroni PL, Cugno M. Anti-tumor necrosis factor alpha therapy normalizes fibrinolysis impairment in patients with active rheumatoid arthritis. *Clin Exp Rheumatol.* (2010) 28:254–7.
154. Marzano AV, Tedeschi A, Polloni I, Crosti C, Cugno M. Prothrombotic state and impaired fibrinolysis in bullous pemphigoid, the most frequent autoimmune blistering disease. *Clin Exp Immunol.* (2013) 171:76–81. doi: 10.1111/j.1365-2249.2012.04674.x
155. Yang YW, Chen YH, Xirasagar S, Lin HC. Increased risk of stroke in patients with bullous pemphigoid: a population-based follow-up study. *Stroke.* (2011) 42:319–23. doi: 10.1161/STROKEAHA.110.596361
156. Joly P, Benichou J, Lok C, Hellot MF, Saiag P, Tancrede-Bohin E, et al. Prediction of survival for patients with bullous pemphigoid: a prospective study. *Arch Dermatol.* (2005) 141:691–8. doi: 10.1001/archderm.141.6.691
157. Rosendaal FR, Van Hylckama Vlieg A, Doggen CJM. Venous thrombosis in the elderly. *J Thromb Haemost.* (2007) 5:310–7. doi: 10.1111/j.1538-7836.2007.02489.x
158. Langan SM, Hubbard R, Fleming K, West J. A population-based study of acute medical conditions associated with bullous pemphigoid. *Br J Dermatol.* (2009) 161:1149–52. doi: 10.1111/j.1365-2133.2009.09350.x
159. Cugno M, Marzano AV, Bucciarelli P, Balice Y, Cianchini G, Quaglino P, et al. Increased risk of venous thromboembolism in patients with bullous pemphigoid. The INVENTEP (INcidence of VENous ThromboEmbolism in bullous Pemphigoid) study. *Thromb Haemost.* (2016) 115:193–9. doi: 10.1160/TH15-04-0309
160. Kibsgaard L, Bay B, Deleuran M, Vestergaard C. A retrospective consecutive case-series study on the effect of systemic treatment, length of admission time, and co-morbidities in 98 bullous pemphigoid patients admitted to a tertiary centre. *Acta Derm Venereol.* (2015) 95:307–11. doi: 10.2340/00015555-1925

Permissions

All chapters in this book were first published Frontiers; hereby published with permission under the Creative Commons Attribution License or equivalent. Every chapter published in this book has been scrutinized by our experts. Their significance has been extensively debated. The topics covered herein carry significant findings which will fuel the growth of the discipline. They may even be implemented as practical applications or may be referred to as a beginning point for another development.

The contributors of this book come from diverse backgrounds, making this book a truly international effort. This book will bring forth new frontiers with its revolutionizing research information and detailed analysis of the nascent developments around the world.

We would like to thank all the contributing authors for lending their expertise to make the book truly unique. They have played a crucial role in the development of this book. Without their invaluable contributions this book wouldn't have been possible. They have made vital efforts to compile up to date information on the varied aspects of this subject to make this book a valuable addition to the collection of many professionals and students.

This book was conceptualized with the vision of imparting up-to-date information and advanced data in this field. To ensure the same, a matchless editorial board was set up. Every individual on the board went through rigorous rounds of assessment to prove their worth. After which they invested a large part of their time researching and compiling the most relevant data for our readers.

The editorial board has been involved in producing this book since its inception. They have spent rigorous hours researching and exploring the diverse topics which have resulted in the successful publishing of this book. They have passed on their knowledge of decades through this book. To expedite this challenging task, the publisher supported the team at every step. A small team of assistant editors was also appointed to further simplify the editing procedure and attain best results for the readers.

Apart from the editorial board, the designing team has also invested a significant amount of their time in understanding the subject and creating the most relevant covers. They scrutinized every image to scout for the most suitable representation of the subject and create an appropriate cover for the book.

The publishing team has been an ardent support to the editorial, designing and production team. Their endless efforts to recruit the best for this project, has resulted in the accomplishment of this book. They are a veteran in the field of academics and their pool of knowledge is as vast as their experience in printing. Their expertise and guidance has proved useful at every step. Their uncompromising quality standards have made this book an exceptional effort. Their encouragement from time to time has been an inspiration for everyone.

The publisher and the editorial board hope that this book will prove to be a valuable piece of knowledge for researchers, students, practitioners and scholars across the globe.

List of Contributors

Nicolo Costantino Brembilla
Department of Pathology and Immunology, Faculty of Medicine, University of Geneva, Geneva, Switzerland

Wolf-Henning Boehncke
Department of Pathology and Immunology, Faculty of Medicine, University of Geneva, Geneva, Switzerland
Divison of Dermatology and Venereology, Geneva University Hospitals, Geneva, Switzerland

Franziska Hübner
Department of Dermatology, University of Lübeck, Lübeck, Germany

Ewan A. Langan
Department of Dermatology, University of Lübeck, Lübeck, Germany
Dermatological Sciences, University of Manchester, Manchester, United Kingdom

Andreas Recke
Department of Dermatology, University of Lübeck, Lübeck, Germany
Lübeck Institute of Dermatological Research, University of Lübeck, Lübeck, Germany

Sandra Saschenbrecker, Ingolf Karl, Lars Komorowski, Christian Probst, Cornelia Dähnrich, Kai Fechner, Winfried Stöcker and Wolfgang Schlumberger
Institute for Experimental Immunology, Euroimmun AG, Lübeck, Germany

Khalaf Kridin
Department of Dermatology, Rambam Health Care Campus, Haifa, Israel

A. Razzaque Ahmed
Department of Dermatology, Center for Blistering Diseases, Tufts University School of Medicine, Boston, MA, United States

Michael P. Schön
Department of Dermatology, Venereology and Allergology, University Medical Center Göttingen, Göttingen, Germany

Ruiling Liu
Center for Antibody Drug, Institute of Biomedicine and Biotechnology, Shenzhen Institutes of Advanced Technology, Chinese Academy of Sciences, Shenzhen, China

University of Chinese Academy of Sciences, Beijing, China

Xiaozhen He and Wenwen Geng
School of Medicine and Life Sciences, University of Jinan, Shandong Academy of Medical Sciences, Jinan, China

Ting Wang
State Key Laboratory Cultivation Base, Shandong Provincial Key Laboratory of Ophthalmology, Shandong Eye Institute, Shandong First Medical University & Shandong Academy of Medical Sciences, Qingdao, China

Qingguo Ruan
Center for Antibody Drug, Institute of Biomedicine and Biotechnology, Shenzhen Institutes of Advanced Technology, Chinese Academy of Sciences, Shenzhen, China
State Key Laboratory Cultivation Base, Shandong Provincial Key Laboratory of Ophthalmology, Shandong Eye Institute, Shandong First Medical University & Shandong Academy of Medical Sciences, Qingdao, China

Jochen H. O. Hoffmann and Alexander H. Enk
Department of Dermatology, University of Heidelberg, Heidelberg, Germany

Sangita Khatri and Kira Astakhova
Department of Chemistry, Technical University of Denmark, Kongens Lyngby, Denmark

Kathryn S. Torok, Emily Mirizio and Christopher Liu
Division of Rheumatology, Department of Pediatrics, Children's Hospital of Pittsburgh, University of Pittsburgh, Pittsburgh, PA, United States

Kata P. Szilveszter, Tamás Németh and Attila Mócsai
Department of Physiology, Semmelweis University School of Medicine, Budapest, Hungary

Stéphane Nesmond, Céline Muller and Sébastien Le Jan
Laboratory of Dermatology, EA7509 IRMAIC, University of Reims-Champagne-Ardenne, Reims, France

Richard Le Naour
Laboratory of Dermatology, EA7509 IRMAIC, University of Reims-Champagne-Ardenne, Reims, France
Department of Biological Sciences, UFR Pharmacy, University of Reims Champagne-Ardenne, Reims, France

Philippe Bernard
Laboratory of Dermatology, EA7509 IRMAIC, University of Reims-Champagne-Ardenne, Reims, France
Department of Dermatology, University Hospital, University of Reims-Champagne-Ardenne, Reims, France

Manuelle Viguier
Department of Dermatology, University Hospital, University of Reims-Champagne-Ardenne, Reims, France

Frank Antonicelli
Laboratory of Dermatology, EA7509 IRMAIC, University of Reims-Champagne-Ardenne, Reims, France
Department of Biological Sciences, Immunology, UFR Odontology, University of Reims-Champagne-Ardenne, Reims, France

Jim Wu
Department of Dermatology and Allergy, Allergie-Centrum-Charité, Berlin Institute of Health, Charité - Universitätsmedizin Berlin, Freie Universität Berlin, Humboldt-Universität zu Berlin, Berlin, Germany

Hanna Bonnekoh, Jörg Scheffel, Marcus Maurer and Karoline Krause
Department of Dermatology and Allergy, Allergie-Centrum-Charité, Berlin Institute of Health, Charité - Universitätsmedizin Berlin, Freie Universität Berlin, Humboldt-Universität zu Berlin, Berlin, Germany
Autoinflammation Reference Center Charité (ARC2), Berlin Institute of Health, Charité - Universitätsmedizin Berlin, Freie Universität Berlin, Humboldt-Universität zu Berlin, Berlin, Germany

Sheila Hoffmann
German Center for Neurodegenerative Diseases, Berlin, Germany

Borros Arneth
Institute of Laboratory Medicine and Pathobiochemistry, Molecular Diagnostics, University Hospital of Giessen and Marburg, Justus Liebig University Giessen, Giessen, Germany

Rebecca L. Krain, Carolyn J. Kushner, Meera Tarazi, Rebecca G. Gaffney, Andrea C. Yeguez, Danielle E. Zamalin and Victoria P. Werth
Corporal Michael J. Crescenz VA Medical Center, Philadelphia, PA, United States
Department of Dermatology, University of Pennsylvania, Philadelphia, PA, United States

Aimee S. Payne
Department of Dermatology, University of Pennsylvania, Philadelphia, PA, United States

David R. Pearson
Corporal Michael J. Crescenz VA Medical Center, Philadelphia, PA, United States
Department of Dermatology, University of Pennsylvania, Philadelphia, PA, United States
Department of Dermatology, University of Minnesota, Minneapolis, MN, United States

Rui Feng
Department of Biostatistics and Epidemiology, University of Pennsylvania, Philadelphia, PA, United States

Tianyu Cao
Department of Dermatology, Tangdu Hospital, Fourth Military Medical University, Xi'an, China

Shuai Shao, Hui Fang, Bing Li and Gang Wang
Department of Dermatology, Xijing Hospital, Fourth Military Medical University, Xi'an, China

Sonali J. Bracken
Department of Internal Medicine, Duke University School of Medicine, Durham, NC, United States

Soman Abraham
Department of Pathology, Duke University Medical Center, Durham, NC, United States
Department of Immunology, Duke University Medical Center, Durham, NC, United States

Amanda S. MacLeod
Department of Immunology, Duke University Medical Center, Durham, NC, United States
Department of Dermatology, Duke University Medical Center, Durham, NC, United States

Julie Plee
Department of Dermatology, University Hospital, University of Reims-Champagne-Ardenne, Reims, France

Anne Durlach
Laboratory Pol Bouin, Hospital Maison Blanche, University Hospital, University of Reims-Champagne-Ardenne, Reims, France

Gareth Edwards and Barbara Horvath
Department of Dermatology, University Medical Center Groningen, Groningen, Netherlands

Gilles F. H. Diercks
Department of Pathology, University Medical Center Groningen, Groningen, Netherlands

Marc A. J. Seelen
Department of Nephrology, University Medical Center Groningen, Groningen, Netherlands

Martijn B. A. van Doorn
Department of Dermatology, Erasmus Medical Center Rotterdam, Rotterdam, Netherlands

Jeffrey Damman
Department of Pathology, Erasmus Medical Center Rotterdam, Rotterdam, Netherlands

Aheen Faisal Mohamad
Aalborg University Hospital, Aalborg, Denmark

Lars Iversen and Rikke Bech
Department of Dermatology, Aarhus University Hospital, Aarhus, Denmark

Natalie E. Stevens, Allison J. Cowin and Zlatko Kopecki
Regenerative Medicine Laboratory, Future Industries Institute, University of South Australia, Adelaide, SA, Australia

Michael D. Howell, Fiona I. Kuo and Paul A. Smith
Incyte Corporation, Wilmington, DE, United States

Massimo Cugno
Dipartimento di Fisiopatologia Medico-Chirurgica e dei Trapianti, Università degli Studi di Milano, Milan, Italy
Medicina Interna, Fondazione IRCCS Ca' Granda Ospedale Maggiore Policlinico, Milan, Italy

Alessandro Borghi
Sezione di Dermatologia e Malattie Infettive, Dipartimento di Scienze Mediche, Università degli Studi di Ferrara, Ferrara, Italy

Simone Garcovich
Istituto di Dermatologia, Università Cattolica del Sacro Cuore, Fondazione Policlinico A. Gemelli IRCCS, Rome, Italy

Angelo Valerio Marzano
Dipartimento di Fisiopatologia Medico-Chirurgica e dei Trapianti, Università degli Studi di Milano, Milan, Italy
UOC Dermatologia, Fondazione IRCCS Ca' Granda Ospedale Maggiore Policlinico, Milan, Italy

Index

www.ingramcontent.com/pod-product-compliance
Lightning Source LLC
LaVergne TN
LVHW082135200926
848484LV00008B/2056